USING NURSING RESEARCH

Editors

Christine A. Tanner

Carol A. Lindeman

Pub. No. 15-2232

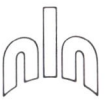

National League for Nursing

Copyright © 1989 by
National League for Nursing.

All right reserved. No part of this book may be reproduced in print, or by photostatic means, or in any other manner, without the express written permission of the publisher.

The views expressed in this book reflect those of the authors and do not necessarily reflect the official views of the National League for Nursing.

ISBN 0-88737-414-X

Manufactured in the United States of America

Contents

Preface	v
Contributors	ix
1 Research in Nursing Practice *Carol A. Lindeman*	1
2 Use of Research in Clinical Judgment *Christine A. Tanner*	19
3 Guidelines for Evaluation of Research for Use in Practice *Christine A. Tanner, Margaret Imle, and Barbara Stewart*	35
4 Basic Concepts, Skills, and Procedures *Charold Baer, Dorothy Bomber, and Audrey Nickodemus*	61
5 Maternity Nursing *Carol Howe, Jennifer Carley-Roe, and Marilyn Parker-Cullen*	97
6 Nursing Care of Children *Sheila Kodadek, Tim Massmann, and Charlyn Wilson*	153
7 Nursing Care of Adults *Charold Baer, Dana Diane Penilton, and Theresa Lerch*	211
8 Nursing Care of the Elderly *Judy Miller, Jelene MacLean, and Gail Perry*	257
9 Mental Health Nursing *Beverly Hoeffer, Laurie Beeson, and Valerie Gowdy*	309
10 Community Health Nursing *Caroline McCoy White, Jean Regier, and Dianne Wheeling*	381

11 Health Promotion and Primary Care Nursing 431
  Pamela Hellings, Grace A. Lin, and Karen S. Davis

12 Nursing Management 473
  Marie S. Berger, Colleen M. Engstrom, and Cynthia Lea Strunk

Preface

This book was inspired by our commitment to research and its potential for improving the quality of patient care. In our work with practicing nurses and students, it has become increasingly clear to us that traditional conceptions of research and research utilization are not likely to result in major improvements in the quality of patient care. Since at least the mid-1970s, nursing leaders have expressed concern about the limited utilization of research in nursing practice. Katefian's (1975) frequently cited study points to the failure on the part of clinicians to take oral temperatures properly even though the procedure yielding the most accurate readings had been well-documented in the literature. More recently, Kirchhoff's (1982) study revealed that nurses have continued to use coronary precautions despite their knowledge of research literature which provided evidence that such practices were unnecessary.

In defense of practicing nurses, Downs (1979) criticized Katefian's conclusions, suggesting that by the time Katefian had conducted her study, electronic thermometers were rapidly replacing the glass thermometers used in the research base. The nurses in Kirchhoff's study may have been making a wise choice in not eliminating coronary precautions on the basis of the research literature. At least one study in the research base was sharply criticized for its methodological and conceptual inadequacies. Moreover, a risk-benefit analysis may well have favored continuance of coronary precautions.

Despite these controversies in nursing, there is substantial evidence that the gap between knowledge production and utilization is on the order of several years. Why does this gap exist? We believe that there are several factors related to the reported failure on the part of nurses to use research: (1) the traditional research paradigm has led to study of problems/issues which are not particularly relevant for practice, but which can be addressed using rigorous methods; (2) the traditional conceptions of research utilization are much too narrow to capture the practice of nurses as they are using new knowledge; and (3) the ways in which nurses are taught research in their undergraduate programs do not necessarily foster the kind of inquiring attitudes that support use of new knowledge, research based and otherwise, in their practice.

The intent of this book is to provide assistance to faculty and students toward resolving some of these issues. In addition, this book differs from other undergraduate research textbooks in several ways. First, it focuses on evaluating research for use in practice. The potential relevance of research to one's practice is central to the evaluation, with issues of scientific credibility being examined secondarily. Second, the book is intended to be used throughout the nursing program, rather than as a text for a single research course. It introduces a framework for evaluating research in early chapters that can be used as students read research throughout their nursing program. Third, the book incorporates recent research on clinical judgment and takes what we believe is a refreshing point of view on how knowledge, including research-based knowledge, might be used during the process of clinical judgment. Finally, it provides opportunities for students to practice the art of critique on carefully selected research reports, drawn from all major areas of clinical nursing practice, then to compare their critiques with those of both faculty experts and other undergraduate students or recently graduated nurses.

The book contains two major sections. The first section includes three introductory chapters that could be used in beginning nursing courses, then re-read at different points throughout the program. Chapter 1 introduces the idea of research in nursing practice, and includes a brief history of the development of nursing research. In Chapter 1, we also present alternative ways to think about research and research utilization. Chapter 2 focuses on the use of knowledge in clinical judgment. We describe knowledge and ways of knowing, as well as the thinking processes of clinical judgment. In Chapter 3, guidelines are presented for the evaluation of research for use in practice.

The second major section of the book was contributed by faculty, undergraduate students, and recently graduated nurses. The chapters are organized around major areas of nursing practice as they might be represented in many undergraduate nursing programs. For each chapter, the senior author (the faculty member) selected three articles from his or her area of practice based on the following criteria:

1. One of the articles should be a classic in the area with continuing relevance for practice, or one which is frequently cited in textbooks.
2. Among the three articles, there should be some sampling of topics within the area of practice. With three articles, we couldn't expect to sample the entire field, but we felt that the utility of the book might be greater if we attempted to have some diversity of content within each area of practice.
3. Among the three articles, there should be some diversity in methods.
4. Each article should be both relevant for practice and of moderate scientific quality, or better.

The first two articles in each chapter are followed by a critique written by the student or new graduate and one written by the faculty member. The final article in each chapter also has critiques prepared by this team, but they are included only in the instructor manual.

The faculty contributors are all part of our dynamic faculty at the Oregon Health Sciences University School of Nursing. They were selected for having a blend of clinical expertise (with most maintaining an active clinical practice) and experience in research. The student contributors were all enrolled in our undergraduate program. They were selected from volunteers for the project on the basis of faculty recommendation, writing ability, and understanding of research. Many of these students have other educational and life experiences that provide a richness and diversity to their views of the research. They were exceptional students. All of the contributors were a joy for us to work with and they made the task of editing unusually easy.

Even with such ease of editing, the book was, in many ways, difficult to write. The difficulty arose primarily from developments in our own thinking and changes in our views of research and its relationship to practice. It was hard to get a fix on our ideas long enough to commit them to paper, then resist the temptation to revise once again, as new thoughts came to us.

We would like to take this opportunity to thank our colleagues and friends, including the contributors to this book, for allowing us to think with them, talk out our ideas, and provide thoughtful criticism.

Christine A. Tanner, PhD, RN, FAAN
Carol A. Lindeman, PhD, RN, FAAN

REFERENCES

Downs, F. S. (1979). Clinical and theoretical research. In F. S. Downs, & J. W. Fleming, (Eds.), *Issues in nursing research*. New York: Appleton-Century-Crofts.

Katefian, S. (1975). Application of selected nursing research findings into nursing practice. *Nursing Research, 24*, 89–93.

Kirchhoff, K. (1982). A diffusion study of coronary precautions. *Nursing Research, 31*, 196–201.

Contributors

This book was developed through the collaborative effort of faculty and undergraduate students at the Oregon Health Sciences University School of Nursing, Portland, Oregon.

Faculty
Charold Baer, PhD, RN, is Professor, Department of Adult Health and Illness Nursing.
Marie S. Berger, PhD, RN, is Associate Professor, Department of Community Health Care Systems.
Pamela Hellings, PhD, RN, is Associate Professor and Chair, Department of Family Nursing.
Beverly Hoeffer, DNSc, RN, is Professor and Chair, Department of Mental Health Nursing.
Carol Howe, DNSc, CNM, RN, is Director of the Midwifery Program and Associate Professor, Department of Family Nursing.
Margaret Imle, PhD, RN, is Associate Professor, Department of Family Nursing and a research facilitator in the Office of Research Development and Utilization.
Sheila Kodadek, PhD, RN, is Associate Professor, Department of Family Nursing.
Carol A. Lindeman, PhD, RN, FAAN is Professor and Dean, School of Nursing.
Judy Miller, MSN, RN, is formerly assistant professor, Department of Adult Health and Illness Nursing, and currently a doctoral student at Oregon Health Sciences University.
Barbara Stewart, PhD, is Professor, Department of Family Nursing, and is a psychometrician and statistician, and currently Director, Office of Research Development and Utilization.
Christine A. Tanner, PhD, RN, FAAN, is formerly Director, Office of Research Development and Utilization, and currently Professor, Department of Adult Health and Illness Nursing.
Caroline McCoy White, DrPH, RN, is Professor, Department of Community Health Care Systems.

Students
The following individuals were students in the School of Nursing at Oregon Health Sciences University. They have since completed the program, and passed their licensure examinations and are now practicing nurses.

Laurie Beeson, BSN, RN
Dorothy Bomber, BSN, RN

Jennifer Carley-Roe, BSN, RN
Karen S. Davis, BSN, RN
Colleen M. Engstrom, BSN, RN
Valerie Gowdy, BSN, RN
Theresa Lerch, BSN, RN
Grace A. Lin, BSN, RN
Jelene MacLean, BSN, RN
Tim Massmann, MA, BSN, RN
Audrey Nickodemus, BSN, RN
Marilyn Parker-Cullen, BSN, RN
Dana Diane Penilton, BSN, RN
Gail Perry, BSN, RN
Jean Regier, BSN, RN
Cynthia Lea Strunk, BSN, RN
Dianne Wheeling, BSN, RN
Charlyn Wilson, BSN, BA, RN

1

Research in Nursing Practice

Carol A. Lindeman, PhD, RN, FAAN

INTRODUCTION

What do motherhood, apple pie, and research all have in common? They are symbols of values held by citizens of the United States. Just as we value the family as an important element in the life of people, we value research as a vehicle for improving the quality of that life. Each year billions of public and private dollars are spent on research. Research is used to evaluate and sell products; the phrase "test after test has shown" is familiar to any television viewer. The daily newspaper carries the results of Gallup polls on such topics as presidential candidates and how Americans feel about the quality of their health care. There is public acceptance of research as the base for action. Researchers that develop technology useful to improving human life are recognized in the history of this country. For example, most readers will be able to match the inventor with the technology in the following quiz.

Inventor	*Invention*
a. Galileo	____ 1. Brassiere
b. Wright Brothers	____ 2. Telescope
c. Koch	____ 3. X-Ray
d. Fleming	____ 4. Airplane
e. Titzling	____ 5. Tuberculosis
f. Von Roentgen	____ 6. Insulin
g. Banting	____ 7. Penicillin

Although health care research was not well funded in the early history of our country, since World War II its funding level has reached into billions of dollars from both public and private sources. Health care research covers a broad range of activities from studies at the molecular level to those dealing with public policy questions. Biomedical science has shown us how to prolong life through the use of complex health technology; and in a relatively short period of time we have come close to conquering some of the age-old killers of humankind. We now look to health research to provide insight into the cure and treatment of disease, to improve the delivery of health care, to enhance health promotion and disease prevention, and to increase our ability to improve the quality of life for underserved groups.

Although the public takes for granted the value of research in producing better cars, televisions, and medications, for example, a first reaction to the thought of nursing research is one of surprise. The lay person usually thinks of nursing in terms of the tasks a nurse can be seen "doing" and not in terms of the knowledge associated with the "doing." Depending on when and how a nurse was educated, he or she may hold the same stereotype of nursing. In fact, nursing research is simply a category of health care research. It serves the same goals as other health care research. However, the phenomena selected for study and the designs used to explore those phenomena reflect the nature and scope of nursing practice. Some noted nurse scientists and their areas of research are shown below:

Nurse Researcher	*Research Contribution*
Hansen	Lactose-free diet: Tube feeding
Jacox and Stewart	Deliberative nursing: Pain reduction
Johnson	Sensation information: Distress reduction
Lindeman	Structured preoperative teaching
Martinsen	Home care for the child with cancer
Norbeck	Social support
Steckel	Mutual goal setting: Attainment
Tanner	Clinical decision making
Verhonick	Decubitus ulcer care and prevention

To better appreciate the current state of the art and science of nursing research, a brief historical perspective is provided.

HISTORICAL PERSPECTIVE

Florence Nightingale, the founder of modern nursing, viewed research as an integral and essential part of nursing practice. She demonstrated this in her own practice and communicated it in her writing. However, in the one hundred years since Nightingale established this model of professional nursing, research has not been a significant part of nursing practice. Almost in contradiction to Nightingale's model of nursing practice, which called for nursing practice to be generated from confirmed facts and epidemiological data, current nursing practice is frequently based on rituals, routines, trial and error, personal preference, imitation, and not on research. In the United States, it is only since the late 1950s that research has once again emerged as a significant component of nursing practice and as a value within the profession.

The history of nursing research in the United States demonstrates an attempt on the part of individual nurse scientists to improve the quality of nursing care and on the part of the profession to use the same process to solve major problems facing the profession.

In describing the use of research to improve the quality of nursing care, a quality assurance framework is used. That framework involves the concepts of *structure*, *process*, and *outcome*. Structure is used to refer to variables in the setting in which care is given and includes appraisal of the facility itself, the equipment and supplies, number and preparation of personnel, and support services and finances. Process variables comprise a second category. Process variables refer to those variables associated with the process of giving care, such as the nursing interventions included in the care of a patient, family involvement in care, and so forth. Outcome, of course, refers to the end result of the interaction of structure and process variables.

During the 1950s, the profession was concerned with the increasing shortage of nursing services in the face of increasing numbers of nurses; a problem that seems to recur. As one response to the feelings of inadequacies of nursing survices, Abdellah and Levine (1958) set up a research design to scientifically test the relationship between the number of nursing personnel employed in hospitals and the feelings of inadequacies of nursing services. Eight thousand seven hundred patients and 9,500 personnel in 57 hospitals with different amounts of professional and total nursing care available served as subjects. On the basis of their statistical analysis, the investigators concluded that in hospitals providing higher professional nursing hours, patients reported fewer unfilled needs. They found no relationship between total nursing hours and the number of unfilled needs reported by patients.

The study by Abdellah and Levine (1958) is a historical landmark in nursing research, and set the stage for nursing research for the next decade and beyond. Their study made it clear that questions of interest to the nursing profession could be pursued through research. In addition, following the pattern of the Abdellah and Levine study, other nurse researchers examined the effects of structural variables on patient outcomes.

Aydelotte and Tener (1960) also studied the impact of increased numbers of nurses on quality patient care. They used an experimental design and made direct observations of the activities of the nursing staff. Their data did not support the conclusion that increasing the number of hours of professional nursing time automatically led to improved patient care. In fact, increasing the number of hours of nursing time available seemed to result in longer coffee breaks and increased socialization among the nursing staff. Although the move to increase the number of hours of professional care available to patients was commendable, it did not ensure quality care.

Following research efforts to link quality of care with numbers of nurses, nurse researchers began to study educational preparation of the nursing staff as the key to quality. Educational preparation is also a structural variable. One study typical of the studies exploring educational preparation was conducted by Georgopolis and Jackson (1970) at the University of Michigan. There, under experimental conditions, the effect of a master's prepared nurse clinician was tested by looking at quality in nursing care plans. The research did not support a measurable, significant effect on nursing care plans from having a master's prepared clinical specialist on the nursing unit. Once again, although the structure variable of educational preparation was viewed as important, it was not the key to quality nursing care.

Nurse researchers have pursued a variety of structure variables and their effect on quality in nursing care. The physical structure of the nursing unit is one such variable (Young, 1980). Round nursing unit designs were contrasted to the more typical long, narrow corridor. The availability of nurse servers and other types of technology including computerized information systems also were studied.

The personality of the nurse is another structure variable on which nurse researchers have focused. This research attempted to specify the right or best personality of the nurse and therby ensure quality of care. Recently, we have seen numerous studies exploring the impact of the method of assignment (team and primary nursing) on quality of care (Young, 1980). Once again from the many studies conducted on this topic, it is clear that the structure variable, by itself, is not the answer to quality nursing care.

While many nurse researchers were studying the effects of structure variables, variables that were easier to isolate and quantify, leaders internal and external to the profession were urging study of nursing practice itself. As early as 1948, Dr. Esther Lucile Brown noted that scientific research and writing by nurses had been negligible. She described a level of professional practice that must be supported by a knowledge base stemming from research. In 1970, the National Commission for the Study of Nursing and Nursing Education noted that nursing had not conducted enough research into its own practices and concluded that a first priority was to increase research into the practice of nursing and the education of nurses.

Over the last two decades, a sizable number of nurse researchers have attempted to study the impact of various nursing interventions (process variable) on patient outcomes. In many instances, results have been dramatic and support the conclusion that scientifically based nursing interventions do lead to measurable benefits for patients. For example, there is the Lindeman and Van Aernam (1971) research study on preoperative teaching. We discuss it at length in the following section as an example of research designed to test the effects of nursing interventions on patient outcomes.

A RESEARCH STUDY

Clinical Concern

The medications and anesthetic administered to a surgical patient have the effect of depressing respiratory and circulatory function. If these body functions are not stimulated in the immediate postoperative period, complications such as pneumonia or emboli (blood clot) could occur. Since the 1940s, nursing care of the surgical patient has included deep breathing, coughing, and bed exercise to prevent complications.

Background

At a registered nurses' staff development program on principles of teaching, a staff member was asked to demonstrate the principles by teaching a skill to the others attending the class. The nurse was to apply the principles to content of her own choice. She selected the postoperative deep breathing, coughing, and bed exercise regime required of most surgical patients. As she proceeded through the demonstration and practice session, many in the class showed surprise over the deep breathing and coughing procedure she described. Immediately class members raised questions asking where she had learned that approach and why she did what she did. Class members began comparing procedures and approaches. It was obvious that personnel were using various procedures. It was also obvious that the quality, quanitity, and timing of the teaching varied from nurse to nurse.

The effects of such variety on patient care is illustrated in an incident reported by one of the surgical head nurses. The nurse approached a patient on this first postoperative day and told him it was time to do his deep breathing and coughing. The patient responded in angry tones, "And which way are *you* going to tell me to do it? Every nurse so far has told me to do it a different way!" Further discussion revealed the patient had been instructed several times by different personnel, including an inhalation therapist, and each required him to perform the procedure in a slightly different manner.

Stimulated by the interest and motivation of the staff, the surgical head nurses met to examine current practice in the area of preoperative teaching. After meeting and reviewing the nursing literature, the head nurses voted to study preoperative teaching of deep breathing, coughing, and bed exercises, commonly called the stir up regime.

Research Question

Broadly stated, the questions of the nursing staff were: (1) what constitutes an effective stir up regime; and (2) does the response a patient gives when asked to deep breathe, cough, and move postoperativley relate to what or how the patient was taught preoperatively?

The nursing problems that led to the studies as identified by nursing personnel were: (1) postoperative respiratory and circulatory complications; (2) patients' frustrations regarding the stir up regime; and (3) nurses' frustrations over an aspect of nursing care that was being practiced in a questionable manner. The immediate goal of the first study was to determine the value of preoperative teaching.

Independent Variable

In research, the term *variable* refers to the characteristic, property, trait, behavior, or attribute of the person or thing observed in a study. To be a variable, the characteristic must vary in the persons or thing under study. In an experimental study, the *independent variable* is the given conditions or behaviors manipulated, modified, or designed by the researcher. In this study, the independent variable was preoperative teaching.

The study was designed to evaluate the effects of two levels of the independent variable: structured and unstructured preoperative teaching. Structured preoperative teaching was defined as the registered nurse imparting knowledge and developing skills in diaphragmatic breathing, coughing, and bed exercises with the presurgical patient, following the lesson plan, and using the audiovisual aides developed for this study. Unstructured preoperative teaching referred to the registered nurse teaching the surgical patient what, how, and when the nurse decided. Perhaps this would have been better labeled "no preoperative teaching" but in deference to those who consider "telling" synonymous with "teaching" or who believe that manual skills can be acquired through strictly mental activity, the term "unstructured" was selected.

Dependent Variable

The *dependent variable* is the condition or behavior thought to result from the manipulation of the independent variable. These variables are observed and measured to determine the effects of the independent variable.

The following measures were selected to determine the value of preoperative teaching: postoperative ventilatory function, number of analgesics administered during the first 72 postoperative hours, and length of hospital stay. Other measures such as chest X-rays had been proposed but were not possible to use because of cost, personnel time, or patient welfare.

Ventilatory function refers to the mechanics of breathing and is measured by tests of vital capacity and expiratory flow rate. The three indices used included:

1. Forced Vital Capacity—the maximal volume of gas that can be expelled from the lungs following a maximal inspiration with expiration as forceful and rapid as possible.
2. Maximum Expiratory Flow Rate—the rate of flow for a specified period of time.
3. Forced Expiratory Volume—the volume of gas exhaled in one given second during the performance of forced vital capacity.

Patient scores were obtained preoperatively and postoperatively.

Preoperative teaching essentially included instruction in the mechanics of breathing and body movement as a means of reducing postoperative complications. The ventilatory function measures were direct measures of the effectiveness of teaching. Length of hospital stay and postoperative analgesics were indirect measures of the effectiveness of reducing postoperative complications.

Design

Design refers to the general plan for setting up and testing a research question. The design specifies the what, who, where, how, and when of the research.

In this study, a pretest/posttest static group design was used. This design was selected to avoid the contamination that most likely would have occurred if the two types of teaching had been conducted concurrently. The design can be diagrammed as follows:

$$S \quad O_1 \quad X_1 \quad O_2 \ldots\ldots\ldots$$
$$S \quad O_3 \quad X_2 \quad O_4$$

"S" stands for static or intact group—in this study the group was all adult surgical patients meeting the identified criteria and admitted to the research site during the specified time. "O" represents observations. "O_1" and "O_3" refer to the preoperative ventilatory function tests. "O_2" and "O_4" refer to the ventilatory function tests, the number of analgesics administered during the first 72 postoperative hours, and the length of hospital stay. "X" represents the independent variable. "X_1" represents unstructured preoperative teaching, the control group. "X_2" represents structured preoperative teaching, the experimental group. The dots represent the passage of time—approximately five months.

Subjects (The Who)

The criteria for subjects were:

1. Fifteen years of age and older.
2. Admitted under nonemergency conditions.
3. Expected to perform the stir up regime postoperatively.
4. Scheduled for a general anesthetic.
5. Able to cooperate for tests of ventilatory function.
6. Not on IPPB therapy preoperatively.

There were 135 subjects in the control group and 126 subjects in the experimental group.

Methodology (The What, How, and When)

The structured teaching plan was based on the following principles for teaching a skill:

1. Analyze the skill from the perspective of a novice before attemping to guide the learner.
2. Demonstrate the skill correctly.
3. Guide the initial practice attempts verbally and, if necessary, physically.
4. Provide for practice—distribute rather than mass the practice.
5. Encourage additional periodic practice.
6. Let the learner know what he or she is doing correctly and what he or she needs to improve.
7. Help the learner learn how to evaluate his or her performance.

To facilitate implementation of the second principle and to ensure consistency in the preoperative teaching, it was decided to develop a sound-on-slide audiovisual program for the demonstration of deep breathing, coughing, and leg and foot exercises.

The sound-on-slide program developed for preoperative teaching consisted of a series of 24 slides and messages. The first slides were introductory including information on why it was important for the patient to do the exercises and what exercises were included in the stir up regime. The remaining slides showed how to do diaphragmatic breathing, effective coughing, and bed exercises including turning and leg and foot exercises. The recorded messages were instructions on how to do the exercises, the slides showed what to do. The program encouraged participation by the observer, included periodic summary slides, and used nontechnical language.

Prior to the start of data collection for structured preoperative teaching, all nursing personnel were instructed in the concept of respiratory control and the approved stir up regime. They practiced diaphragmatic breathing and effective coughing until they could do it correctly and were able to identify whether or not another person was doing it correctly. Personnel further refined their skills over a one-month practice period.

Data Analysis

In experimental studies, the investigator analyzes the data to determine whether the difference between values for the categories of subjects (subjects having structured teaching and subjects having unstructured teaching) could have occurred by chance. Significance is a matter judgement, but is usually set at a level of .05 meaning that five times out of 100 a difference as large or larger could have occurred by chance.

In this study, the t-test for the significance of difference between means for independent samples was applied to the data for each of the three dependent variables. A difference measure was used for the indices of ventilatory function.

Conclusions

The results of the statistical tests applied to the data for three dependent variables support the following conclusions:

1. The ability of subjects to deep breathe and cough postoperatively was significantly improved by the structured preoperative teaching method.
2. The mean length of hospital stay was significantly reduced by the implementation of the structured preoperative teaching method.
3. No differential effect upon postoperative need for analgesia was evident.

Utilization

In nursing research, research utilization refers to the use of the study in clinical settings not involved in the conduct of research.

In the research setting nursing practice changed. The conclusions of the study were supported by the response of the patients themselves. When personnel met to discuss the results of the study, nurse aides, orderlies, staff nurses from the recovery room, and staff head nurses from the units offered illustration after illustration showing the benefits of structured preoperative teaching.

This research and subsequent studies also have been used to change practice in numerous settings across the world. For example, nurses in Canada, China, and Japan have conducted complementary and replication studies. In recent years, investigators have combined data from the various studies to determine the true statistical impact of preoperative teaching and have concluded that it does indeed improve postoperative welfare and lead to shorter hospital stays. Many, if not most, clinical settings now include some type of preoperative teaching of deep breathing, coughing, and bed exercises.

CREATION OF THE NATIONAL CENTER FOR NURSING RESEARCH (NCNR)

The research of investigators such as Lindeman, along with Johnson's (1979) work on reducing painful sensations, Steckel's (1976) work on contracts and compliance, Veronick, Lewis, and Goller's (1972) research on decubitus ulcers, Hansen et al's (1975) work on diarrhea associated with tube feeding, and many other such studies clearly set the stage for further research into the practice of nursing as the key to quality in nursing care. Nursing research that focuses on nursing practice does indeed elevate the practice of nursing and lead to measurable benefits for patients.

The effects of this type of research were so dramatic and offered so much potential that by the 1980s the federal government was willing to increase its commitment to nursing research. The following statement made by congressman Edward R. Madigan (1988) is a succinct expression of this commitment.

> At the beginning of this new year, nursing research has the opportunity to take its place in the mainstream of scientific investigation. The National Center for Nursing Research established within the National Institutes of Health can significantly contribute to basic and clinical research related to the prevention of disease, health promotion, and the care of individuals and families of individuals with chronic illnesses.
>
> When I first offered the amendment to establish a National Institute of Nursing (NIN) in 1983, I recognized that Congress had to take steps to address the changes in the health care delivery system. A more prominent and influential role for nurses in that system was one of the steps I saw as most important. The findings of the Institute of Medicine's study on nursing education policies further convinced me of the need to establish a more visible research activity for nurses. I found that, although a substantial share of the federal health care dollar is expended for care provided by nurses, there is a remarkable absence for funding for research into nursing practice. This has resulted in a critical shortage of nursing leadership in faculties of colleges of nursing and in clinical practice.
>
> The problems in the health care system that I thought required a legislative solution in 1983 were even more evident in 1985. The government's concern for quality health care in the face

of stringent cost-cutting measures; the limitation of acute, hospital-based care in a society that now has chronic—rather than infectious—disease as its most pressing health problem; and the greying of our population, with its corresponding long-term care needs, are just a few of the trends that must be addressed. I believe that nursing research can provide much of the needed data to enhance the provision of high quality effective and efficient health care.

Mission of the National Center for Nursing Research (NCNR)

NCNR was authorized under the Health Research Extension Act of 1985, P.L. 99-158. On April 18, 1986, Secretary Bowen of the Department of Health and Human Services (DHHS) announced its establishment as part of the National Institutes of Health (NIH). The mission of the NCNR is the conduct and support of, and dissemination of information respecting, basic and clinical nursing research, training, and other programs in patient care research. The research programs of the NCNR focus on health promotion and disease prevention, understanding and mitigating the effect of acute and chronic illnesses and disabilities, and the delivery of nursing services. Examples of health promotion research include studies concerning the nutritional requirements of people at various life stages and studies relating the biomedical and behavioral dimensions of human health. Examples of disease prevention research include studies identifying risk factors for particular illnesses and studies of methods that enhance the abilities of people to respond to potential health problems. Examples of research in the area of acute and chronic illness include studies on adaptation and functioning in chronic illness and studies on educational intervention. Examples of research in the area of nursing systems include studies of the outcomes of home care and studies to improve the delivery of nursing care in underserved areas.

If one accepts the premise that nursing practice research is the key to excellence in inpatient care, the next issue is who should conduct such research. Is it primarily the responsibility of nurses in academia or nurses in clinical settings? The following section offers contrasting views regarding responsibility for conducting nursing research.

NURSING RESEARCH: WHOSE RESPONSIBILITY?

Conceptions of Practice

The underlying premise of this book is succinct: if the nurse providing direct care considers theory and research as essential ingredients of nursing practice, quality of care will be higher and the nurse will find work more satisfying and growth promoting. Theory developing, testing, and research are not esoteric activities of a few; rather they are activities that characterize the behaviors of the mass of professional nurses.

To illustrate this point, consider two opposing conceptions of practices. In the first conception, practice is seen as synonymous with *doing*, particularly doing what you have been taught to do. In the second conception, practice is seen as *learning through experience*, and although doing is implicit in this conception it is not the end product. In the first conception, emphasis is on implementation of what is known. In the second conception, emphasis is on what is not known while implementing what is known. In the first conception, the nurse functions as a technology worker; in the second conception, as a knowledge worker.

It is the second conception of nursing practice that is of concern here. Practicing from this conception, the nurse would demonstrate the following behaviors. First, a sense of inquiry would characterize every patient interaction. The nurse would be intellectually alive and constantly alert to the adequacy of the knowledge base for practice. Is the client responding as expected? If so, why? If not, why? Are my preformed ideas congruent with the situation or are there events that I cannot explain?

Second, the nurse is alert to personal or individual ways of knowing. Many excellent clinicians describe "visceral knowing"; they knew it in their "gut" or they felt something "gnawing" at them. Sensations and perceptions are critical to inquiry. Not all ideas generate from reasoning or thinking. The nurse practicing with this in mind will value multiple ways of knowing as part of the knowledge base for practice.

Third, the nurse will think about client interactions, conceptualizing and reconceptualizing those events to isolate the significant phenomena and concepts. For example, both client A and client B have diabetes, and both participated in classes designed to enable safe, effective self-care after discharge from the hospital. Both returned for clinic visits one month after discharge. Client A is doing well; client B is having many problems. Why? Could client B's problems have been indentified earlier? How is client B similar to client A; how is client B dissimilar? How is client B similar to other clients who had difficulty? Considering these events from multiple perspectives until salient concepts can be isolated for further testing is a routine part of practice.

Last, the nurse who views practice as doing coupled with learning through experience will demonstrate well-developed cognitive skills. The nurse will use observation skills to note progress or lack of progress, to identify individual differences within a patient group, and to interpret nonverbal cues. The nurse will draw inferences and generalizations from practice: for example, he or she will be able to reflect on the responses to care from a group of elderly patients and propose how care should be altered when working with the frail elderly. He or she will also be able to apply theory to the care of individuals: for example, knowing that having a clock in a patient's room may help prevent confusion in an elderly patient, the nurse will have relatives bring a clock to the hospital for their elderly patient. Creativity is another cognitive skill evident in this type of nurse. As he or she adapts theory to the individual differences of the patient, he or she will identify alternative ways to implement the nursing care plan.

As this nurse practices at one level of conscious thought, at another level theory is constantly generated or tested and data are collected to accept or reject proposed hypotheses. The nurse practices as a theoretician, as a researcher, and as a scholar. This nurse and this practice also display the highest level of humanism in that all resources of the nurse are brought to bear on the needs of the client as an individual.

Conception of Research

In this book, the research process is viewed as an intellectual adventure beginning with the act of observation and continuing through a range of activities that can be categorized as "description" and "explanation." Until recently, the predominant view of science emphasized validation of existing laws of nature. Today, however, there are multiple views of science and the emphasis is on discovery, validation, and the pragmatic benefits derived from research. In a practice discipline such as nursing, discovering knowledge that can improve practice or the outcomes of practice is vital to the advance of the profession as a whole. We value such knowledge preeminently because it can be used to provide more effective care to patients/clients, families, and society.

Typically, the research process includes a series of steps beginning with a statement of the problem and ending with conclusions and recommendations. This step-by-step approach to research has value in that it takes an abstract concept, "the research process," and focuses on a set of observable behaviors. However, this step-by-step approach to research also has disadvantages in that the *concept* of research may be lost as one focuses on the *concrete steps*. In fact, in nursing there has been a tendency to confuse and possibly even value the concrete steps over the concept. This confusion results in an approach to research that is laden with concerns about "right" or "best" way. Thus, the various steps of the process are valued in and of themselves and not in terms of the goal of generating knowledge.

The fact that the research process is linked with the generation of *scientific* knowledge means that the process must be characterized by efforts to eliminate bias or error. This differs, for example, from the creative process, in which individual bias or expression is assumed. A person likes the work of a certain artist not because the artist has eliminated individual bias but because the art reflects and transforms that bias. On the other hand, nurses value research when individual bias does not alter the results of a study.

In this regard, Cronbach (1973) proposes the concept of disciplined inquiry instead of research, emphasizing the essential ingredients and excitement that characterize research when used under conditions of intellectual freedom.

> Disciplined inquiry has a quality that distinguishes it from other sources of opinion and belief. The disciplined inquiry is conducted and reported in such a way that the argument can be painstakingly examined. The report does not depend for its appeal on the eloquence of the writer or on any surface plausibility.
>
> Whatever the character of a study, if it is disciplined, the investigator has anticipated the traditional questions that are pertinent. He institutes control at each step of information collection and reasoning to avoid the sources of error to which these questions refer. If the errors cannot be eliminated, he takes them into account by discussing the margin for error in his conclusions. Thus, the report of a disciplined inquiry has a texture that displays the raw materials entering the argument and the logical processes by which they were compressed and rearranged to make the conclusion credible.
>
> Disciplined inquiry does not necessarily follow well established, formal procedures. Some of the most excellent inquiry is free-ranging and speculative in its initial stages, trying what might seem to be bizarre combinations of ideas and procedures, or restlessly casting about for ideas.

Encouraged by developments in other disciplines and aware of the difficulties encountered in applying the previous views of the scientific method to the phenomena of nursing, researchers of nursing phenomena began exploring alternate research paradigms and views of science. Initially, these alternate views were cast as dichotomies, such as qualitative verses quantitative data, subjective versus objective, and holism versus reductionism. Today, there is less tendency to view the issues as dichotomous and more tendency for theoretical and scientific pluralism.

Conceptions of Theory

In lay conversation the word *theory* has a connotation that differs from its scientific use. For example, in lay conversation someone may say, "have you heard the latest theory?" implying a speculative or impractical explanation of how things work. In science, however, the word does not express a connotation of values. *Theory* is used to mean a general statement of how and why variables co-vary. A researcher may have tested the stated relationships extensively or minimally. However, the amount of testing is not implicit in the use of the term.

As early as 1969, Ellis claimed that the real theorists in nursing were not ivory tower thinkers, but nurses who worked directly with patients. Edgerton (1973) expanded on this thought by stating that in the process of providing care, the staff nurse must conceptualize and reconceptualize the circumstances as well as available scientific theory. If necessary, the staff nurse would have to create new theory. Practice is not the repeated doing of tasks or technical problem solving; it is the systematic exercise of one's knowledge. It requires imaginative reconstruction of one's knowledge and experience and the ability to isolate significant phenomena.

It should now be clear that an underlying assumption of this book is that the nurse is a knowledge worker and needs to be skilled in the evaluation and application of research-generated knowledge.

Conceptions of Research Utilization

Although most nurses agree that research should be applied in practice, there is still little evidence that it is. We wonder what keeps nurses from using research. Yet nursing is not the only practice discipline that is raising questions about the application of research in practice. Disciplines such as education, psychology, and sociology are raising questions similar to those raised in nursing. Why don't practitioners consciously apply research in practice? Don't they have access to the knowledge? Don't they care? Doesn't the knowledge fit the practice setting?

Figure 1.1 expresses significant characteristics of the traditional view of the relationships between research and practice and, therefore, of research utilization. First, the primary responsibility for developing the knowledge base is ascribed to the scientist. Second, the primary source of knowledge is external to the practitioner–client setting. Third, the practitioner is expected to value and use the scientist-generated knowledge base in practice. Fourth, the practitioner is a conduit for knowledge to be used in the real world. Fifth, the client is not a part of the process of generating or evaluating knowledge. Sixth, research/inquiry is associated with uncovering laws of nature, determining caus-

14 Carol A. Lindeman

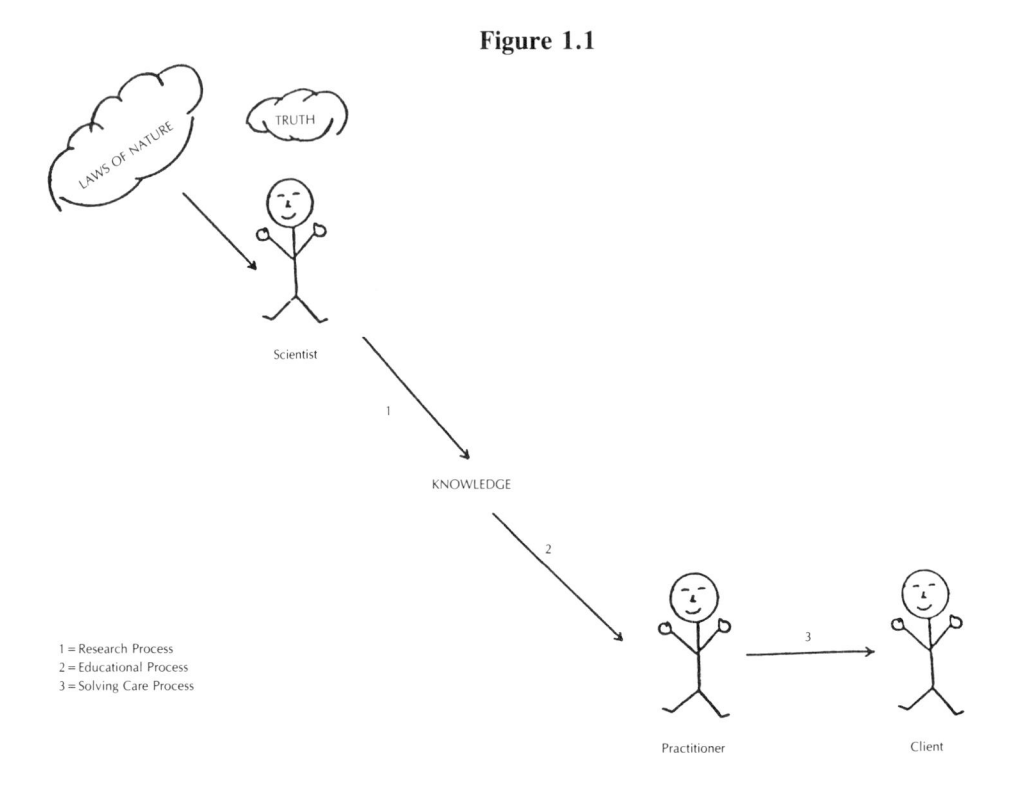

Figure 1.1

[Diagram: Scientist figure receiving from clouds labeled "LAWS OF NATURE" and "TRUTH", arrow labeled 1 pointing to KNOWLEDGE, arrow labeled 2 pointing to Practitioner, arrow labeled 3 from Practitioner to Client]

1 = Research Process
2 = Educational Process
3 = Solving Care Process

ality, and the controlled experiment. Seventh, objective, unbiased observation of *sense* data is essential.

According to Drew (1988), this view of science as epitomized in nursing included these beliefs:

1. *Realism.* Truths about the world are true regardless of what people think, and there is one best way to describe aspects of the world.
2. *The unity of science.* There is just one science about the one real world. The basic sciences (e.g., physics and mathematics) are superior to other sciences (e.g., sociology and psychology). Moreover, all sciences are reducible to the basic sciences.
3. *Mathematics.* Mathematics is the language of nature. There is a sharp distinction between scientific theories and other beliefs (e.g., metaphysics and religion). Scientific theories can be formalized in the language of mathematics and symbolic logic.
4. *Observation–theory distinction.* There is a sharp contrast between reports of observations and statements of theory.
5. *Justification of truth.* Theories are either true or false and can be empirically verified.
6. *Reductionism.* Complex phenomena can be broken down into causal chains or units from which the whole can be understood by reconstituting the parts.

Figure 1.2

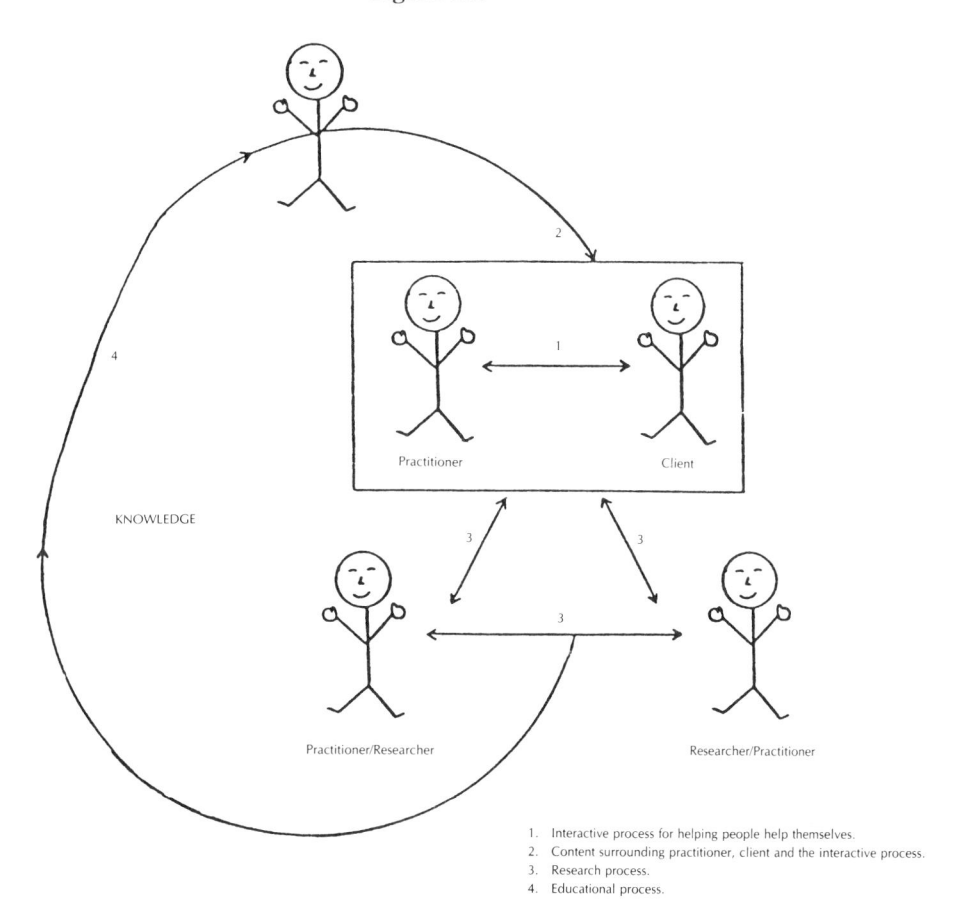

Practitioner ↔ Client

KNOWLEDGE

Practitioner/Researcher   Researcher/Practitioner

1. Interactive process for helping people help themselves.
2. Content surrounding practitioner, client and the interactive process.
3. Research process.
4. Educational process.

7. *Cumulativeness of science.* Science builds on what is already known. Einstein is a generalization from Newton.

An alternate research–practice paradigm consistent with emerging views in philosophy of science would begin with the provider/client component depicted as an interaction and cast within a larger system. Furthermore, the paradigm would have both practitioners and researchers reflecting on practice as a source of knowledge and applying methods of disciplined inquiry to the practice arena. The paradigm would depict an active exchange between client, provider, and researcher regarding knowledge generated through the inquiry of provider and researcher. Figure 1.2 shows one alternative paradigm.

Basic to this paradigm are these assumptions:

1. Thinking and doing are not opposites; thought and conception are means to enhance practice.

2. Knowledge generated from research exists as theory, that is, a set of concepts forming a general framework for guiding practice.
3. Professionals will differ from the public in their abilities to use knowledge to improve the quality of life—not just in possessing knowledge.
4. The art of scientific investigation will be valued once again; approaches will match questions and goals.

The traditional view of the scientific process (refer to Figure 1.1) places the staff nurse in the role of being an instrumental or technical problem solver using research-based knowledge in the form of procedures or protocols. Referring back to the research on structured preoperative teaching, the staff nurse would use this research in practice through the use of procedures regarding preoperative teaching. The preoperative teaching lesson plan and perhaps even the slide-on-sound program would become the standardized procedure for preoperative teaching. This standardized procedure would be used with all patients matching the criteria (elective surgery and general anesthetic). The staff nurse would assume responsibility and accountability for correct implementation of the preoperative teaching plan and for the evaluation of the patient's response to surgery. The underlying assumption is that a research-based procedure is more effective than procedures developed through other methods.

However, in this book, we are promoting an alternate view of research utilization. Here the staff nurse gives more attention to the conceptual components and less attention to the operational components of the preoperative teaching research. The staff nurse, from reflecting on the entire research report and knowledge gained from practice, will note that an important aspect of the preoperative teaching intervention was enabling the patient to be an agent of his or her own care. The patient was less dependent on the nurse and implemented and evaluated activities on his or her own behalf. As the staff nurse applies this knowledge in practice, he or she conceptualizes and reconceptualizes each patient and situation to determine the most effective way to implement these concepts. Depending on his or her assessment, the family may or may not be involved. Depending on the patient's response, the nurse may add additional practice sessions. In the nurse's evaluation of the effectiveness of the teaching, the nurse would focus on the ability of the patient to engage in self-care behaviors in the form of deep breathing, coughing, and bed exercises. Of course, the nurse will also evaluate response to surgery. Over time, the nurse may develop specific routines for implementing these concepts to patients, but such routines will reflect a dynamic use of knowledge in the care of individuals.

CONCLUSION

The profession of nursing is still struggling with questions regarding the relationship of nursing research to nursing practice. Although most practicing nurses would agree that there should be a relationship, there is little agreement on the nature of the relationship. Areas of differing opinion were described in this chapter with regard to conceptions of practice, research, and theory. The authors advocate the view that the professional nurse is a knowledge worker and as such actively applies and evaluates research and theory in practice.

REFERENCES

Abdellah, F., & Levine, E. (1985). *Effects of nursing staffing on satisfactions with nursing care.* Chicago: American Hospital Association, Hospital Monograph Series #4.

Aydelotte, M. K., & Tener, M. E. (1960). An investigation of the relation between nursing activity and patient welfare, Iowa City, IA: State University of Iowa.

Brown, E. L. (1948). *Nursing for the future.* New York: Russell Sage Foundation.

Cronbach, L. J. (1973). Disciplined inquiry. In H. S. Broudy, R. H. Ennis, & L. I. Krimerman, (Eds.), *Philosophy of educational research.* New York: John Wiley & Sons.

Drew, B. J. (1988). Devaluation of biological knowledge. *Image, 20*(1), 25–27.

Edgerton, S. (1973). The technological imagination: A philosopher looks at nursing. *Journal of Thought, 8,* 57-65.

Ellis, R. (1969). The practitioner as theorist. *American Journal of Nursing, 69,* 1434–1438.

Georgopolis, B. S., & Jackson, M. M. (1970). Nursing kardex behavior in an experimental study of patient units with and without clinical nurse specialists. *Nursing Research, 19,* 196–218.

Hanson, R. L., Walkie, B. S., Grant, M., Kubo, W., Bergstrom, N., Padilla, G., & Wong, H. L. (1975, Winter). Patient responses and problems associated with tube feeding. *Washington State Journal of Nursing,* 9–13.

Hinshaw, A. S. (1988). The new national center for nursing research, Patient care research programs. *Applied Nursing Research, 1*(1):2–4.

Johnson, J. E. (1979). Coping with health care events. In *Nursing research: Synopses of selected clinical sites.* Kansas City, MO: American Nurses' Association Commission on Nursing Research.

Lindeman, C., & Van Aernam, B. (1971). Nursing intervention with the pre-surgical patient—The effects of structured and unstructured preoperative teaching. *Nursing Research, 20,* 319–332.

Madigan, E. R. (1988). Nursing research to take its rightful place. *Nursing and Health Care, 7*(1), 3.

National Commission for the study of Nursing and Nursing Education. (1970). *Abstract for action.* New York: McGraw-Hill.

Steckel, S. (1976). Utilization of reinforcement contracts to increase written evidence of the nursing assessment. *Nursing Research, 25,* 58–61.

Veronick, P. J., Lewis, D. W., & Goller, H. O. (1972). Thermography in the study of decubitus ulcers: A pilot study. *Nursing Research, 21,* 233–237.

Young, J., Giovannetti, P., & Lewison, D. (1980). *A comparative study of team and primary nursing care on two surgical inpatient units.* Baltimore, MD: Johns Hopkins University Press.

Young, et al. (1980). *Factors affecting nurse staffing in acute-care hospitals: A review and critique of the literature.* Baltimore, MD: Johns Hopkins University Press.

2

Use of Research in Clinical Judgment

Christine A. Tanner, PhD, RN, FAAN

INTRODUCTION

Clinical judgment is central to nursing practice. In their daily practice, nurses are called upon to make scores of judgments with or on behalf of their patients. Consider the following illustration:

> Mr. Yortz is a 72-year-old man who had a stroke several years ago, leaving the left side of his body paralyzed. He is currently one day postoperative after major abdominal surgery. The nurse knows that it is very important for Mr. Yortz to be as mobile as possible in order to avoid postoperative complications. Mr. Yortz is having quite a bit of pain and, like most postoperative patients, doesn't really want to get up. In this situation, the nurse must make numerous judgments, such as: (1) whether or not to get Mr. Yortz up; (2) given his paralysis, the extent of activity that will be possible, and the ways in which he may be assisted in doing the activity to minimize pain and protect him from injury; (3) the timing of the pain medication with his activity; and (4) the site of and procedure for administration of IM medication.

To the experienced nurse, these judgments seem fairly routine, and unless something unexpected happens, this nurse will care for Mr. Yortz with apparent ease, satisfied with the knowledge he or she has about his needs and with the judgments he or she must make. To the new student, the care of Mr. Yortz may seem overwhelming and every act must be carefully and rationally thought through. These two nurses may have a common knowledge base derived from theory and research: for example, the need for early ambulation postoperatively, the use of principles of physics and body mechanics in patient transfer, and the selection of IM site to minimize discomfort and enhance absorption. But the two nurses probably differ greatly in their experience-based knowledge. And their approach to clinical judgment will probably differ greatly as a result of the differences in their knowledge.

In this chapter, we will examine various approaches to clinical judgment. In addition, we will explore the kinds of knowledge which nurses use for making clinical judgments. Finally, we will examine traditional conceptions of research utilization in light of our understanding about clinical judgment.

CLINICAL JUDGMENT DEFINED

Clinical judgment is defined as the use of knowledge in making one or more of several possible decisions. These decisions are made by the nurse, in interaction with a client, and are directed toward helping the client regain, maintain, or promote health. The decisions that are encompassed in clinical judgment include one or more of the following: (1) the observations to be made in a client situation; (2) the evaluation of the data observed and derivation of meaning; and (3) the nursing actions that should be taken with or on behalf of the client (Kelly, 1966; Tanner, 1987). There are two important aspects to clinical judgment: (1) the thinking processes used by the nurse to reach the judgment; and (2) the knowledge base used by the nurse to make a judgment.

In the literature, several terms are used to describe the processes of clinical judgment. *Clinical decision making* is frequently used to describe the *rational* processes of clinical judgment. Decision making involves collecting and analyzing information, generating alternative approaches, and choosing from alternatives the best way to achieve set goals in patient care. It requires that the nurse break down the situation into elements, weigh each element as to goodness of fit, then arrive at a conclusion. For example, a rational decision-making process in the illustration above might be used to determine the ways to minimize Mr. Yortz's pain postoperatively. One approach to pain reduction which the nurse might consider would be to allow Mr. Yortz to stay in bed. To make the decision about whether this would be a good approach, the nurse must then consider: (1) the likelihood that keeping Mr. Yortz in bed would achieve the goal of minimizing the pain; and (2) the potentially harmful consequences of this approach. In this case, it is unlikely that keeping Mr. Yortz in bed, as the only intervention, would substantially reduce his pain. Also, there are very serious harmful consequences to that decision including increasing the chances of major postoperative complications. Using the rational approach, several other approaches to minimizing pain would be considered and evaluated in terms of achieving the goal and the possibility of harmful consequences.

The *nursing process* is another term frequently used in the literature to describe the processes of clinical judgment. This term describes a systematic, rational process of problem identification and problem solving. Frequently, it is viewed as a step-by-step approach that includes assessment, diagnosis, planning (including goal-setting and prioritizing), intervention, and evaluation. In this view, it is a linear sequence of steps in which each subsequent step flows from the preceding one, so that diagnoses, for example, are derived from assessments, nursing interventions are derived from goals, and so forth (Stevens, 1984; Iyer, Taptich, & Bernocchi-Losi, 1986).

Diagnostic reasoning (Carnevali, Mitchell, Woods, & Tanner, 1984) is a third term more recently introduced to the nursing literature. This is a process in which the nurse attends to presenting signs and symptoms (cues), generates alternative explanations for the cues (diagnostic hypotheses), collects additional data to help rule in or rule out possible explanations, systematically evaluates each explanation in light of the data, and arrives at a diagnosis, or inference, about the client's health status. Again, the process is typically rational and analytic.

As used in this text, the term *clinical judgment* subsumes the processes described by clinical decision making, the nursing process, and diagnostic reasoning as well as including more than these terms imply. Again, the three latter terms refer to a rational, analytic process, in which the nurse breaks the situation down into elements, evaluates systematically each element, and arrives at a conclusion. Futhermore, the processes described by the nursing process and diagnostic reasoning relate to problem situations; that is, the client is either experiencing or is at risk for experiencing some health problem.

Clinical judgment, however, recognizes processes other than the rational/analytic approaches. There are times that experienced nurses identify quite appropriate interventions or recognize the presence of a problem without having gone through a systematic, analytic approach (Pyles & Stern, 1983; Benner & Tanner, 1987). Benner and Tanner have used the term *intuition* as an aspect of clinical judgment to describe "judgment without a rationale." They point out that such judgments are not irrational, meaning crazy or nonsensical, but rather arational. When using intuition, nurses arrive at a decision without being able to describe either the elements of the situation that led to the decision or the process they used to get there.

A second area in which the term *clinical judgment* expands on other frequently used terms is in the focus of that judgment. The focus of both diagnostic reasoning and the nursing process is on actual or potential problems. When there are cues suggesting the possibility of an actual or potential problem, the process of diagnostic reasoning is set into play. The nursing process is a linear sequence of steps used for problem solving or problem prevention. It is our view that clinical judgment includes the aspects of problem identification and problem solving, but is also used in situations where the focus is not on either an actual or potential problem. For example, nurses are routinely involved in teaching new mothers infant care. Establishing the goals for teaching and a suitable approach require much judgment on the part of the nurse. The nurse might think about such teaching in terms of problem prevention, identifying potential problems that infants might experience. The nurse also might view such teaching as a health promotion activity, not directed toward any particular diagnosis or problem, but as an important component of care to help the mother and her infant achieve the highest level of wellness. The thinking that actually goes into this teaching may be very different than that described by the nursing process or the diagnostic reasoning process (Henderson, 1982; Shamansky & Yanni, 1983; McHugh, 1986).

Up to this point, we have indicated that clinical judgment includes at least two interrelated sets of processes: analytic and intuitive. Let us explore each of these in more detail.

PROCESSES OF CLINICAL JUDGMENT

In the last 20 years, over 20 studies have been conducted to examine the thinking processes used by nurses as they make clinical judgments (Tanner, 1987). Our understanding about these processes is far from complete. However, examples are taken from this research to serve several purposes: (1) to illustrate how nurses may approach situations in which they must make a judgment; (2) to provide fodder for our thinking about how research might be used in clinical judgment; and (3) to help stimulate you to reflect on your own processes of judgment.

Analytic Processes

Several nurse researchers have conducted research aimed at describing the rational/analytic processes involved in aspects of clinical judgment. Hammond, Kelly, Schneider, and Vancini (1966) studied nurses' use of information in drawing inferences about postoperative patients. Corcoran (1986a; 1986b) and Grier (1976) examined the processes nurses use in planning care. In the early 1980s, our research group (Westfall, Tanner, Putzier, & Padrick, 1986; Tanner, Padrick, Westfall, & Putzier, 1987; Padrick, Tanner, Putzier, & Westfall, 1987) became interested in the processes which nurses use in moving from assessment data to diagnosis. We had noticed that students could usually complete an accurate assessment, but had some difficulty in interpreting assessment data to formulate diagnoses. We asked these questions: (1) What thinking processes are used by both nurses and nursing students in the development of diagnoses? (2) What are differences in thinking processes between nurses and nursing students?

To reveal the thinking processes, we used a procedure that combined videotaped patient simulations as a stimulus for students and nurses to think aloud as they analyzed the situation. A brief videotape portraying a patient experiencing some signs or symptoms of a problem was first shown to the subjects. The subjects were then instructed to ask the examiner questions, much as they would in practice, until they obtained enough information to determine a diagnosis or take nursing action. During the question asking, they were also instructed to think aloud, expressing themselves however they wished. This was then tape recorded and transcribed for analysis.

Figure 2.1 is an excerpt and analysis from one subject's think-aloud interview. The subject is responding to this situation:

> Mr. Seymour is a 72-year-old man who was admitted to the hospital for a work-up of severe abdominal pain. (The simulation was developed back in the days patients were admitted to the hospital for noninvasive diagnostic work). He is an insulin dependent diabetic who has a history of alcoholism. Two days ago, he spiked a fever and his chest film showed evidence of pneumonia.
>
> The videotape portrays an elderly man, supine in bed, yelling out 'Elsie, bring the cows back to the barn' and other statements that don't make much sense in the context. The nurse tries to arouse Mr. Seymour, telling him that he is in the hospital, but Mr. Seymour continues being restless and yelling out to 'Elsie.' The tape also shows that Mr. Seymour has an IV running; on the bedside are a pair of thick glasses and hearing aids.

In this study, we derived a framework modeled on previous studies of physicians and medical students (Elstein, Shulman, & Sprafka, 1978). The model is comprised of four basic components: (1) problem sensing—paying attention to initially available cues and recognizing that they indicate some problem or problems; (2) activating diagnostic hypotheses, or tentative explanations for the

Figure 2.1
Excerpt and Analysis from Diagnostic Reasoning Study

In the left column is an excerpt from a senior nursing student's thinking aloud: (I = interviewer; S = subject). In the right column are notes indicating the kind of thinking process that's being used.

I: Tell me what you're thinking now after seeing the videotape.

S: Not much! Actually a lot. This guy's really confused. Who was Elsie anyway? — Cue
Well, I guess that doesn't matter, right now. He's diabetic and I'd be worried — Cue
that he might be having an insulin reaction. He also reminded me of those guys — Hypothesis, Experience
over at the VA, you know, in DTs, so I'd want to look into that. But first I'd put on — Hypothesis, Action
his glasses and hearing aid. Is his vision pretty bad? — Question—unclear purpose

I: Tell me what you're thinking?

S: All right. I was just thinking that he might be having sensory deprivation or — Hypothesis
something. You know, when people are deaf or blind, then are put in the — Statement of knowledge
hospital or any kind of strange environment, they can get real crazy. This is
worse with older people. So, how's his vision? — Question—hypothesis-driven

I: He needs his glasses to see. He said on admission that he's practically blind without them. He had cataracts removed several years ago.

S: And he's obviously hard of hearing. Well, let's see. Has he had any visitors? — Inference from cue
You know, meaningful kind of stimulation? — Question—hypothesis-driven

I: His son was in earlier in the day.

S: Well, let's move along. This could still be a problem, but I'm worrying about — Hypothesis
his blood sugar, and probably I should've gone after that first. Has he had
blood sugars done? — Question—hypothesis-driven

---

cues; (3) collecting additional information, directed toward ruling in and ruling out the hypotheses; and (4) evaluating the hypotheses.

We found, as illustrated in the excerpt above, that both junior and senior level baccalaureate students and practicing nurses activate hypotheses very early in the encounter. The model described how both nurses and nursing students approach diagnostic reasoning. Other approaches to information gathering than those described by Elstein, Shulman, and Sprafka (1978) were found. As suggested by the Elstein model, both nurses and nursing students collected data that were clearly directed toward one or more of their hypotheses. They also collected data apparently for the purpose of further describing the cues presented—for example, aggravating factors, alleviating factors, associated manifestations, etc.—which were not related to any particular hypotheses. Numerous other, yet less frequently used strategies, were also described (Tanner, 1987).

In the illustration in Figure 2.1, the student had sufficient knowledge to know where to focus her attention—she knew what cues were salient in the situation. She paid attention to the cue that the patient was confused. (Not all students did—some focused on the cause of the abdominal pain, completely ignoring the patient's confusion.) She also had sufficient knowledge to activate some diagnostic hypotheses based on tentative explanations for cues, and to determine what additional data she needed in order to reach a diagnosis. She used her experience at the VA to activate the hypothesis of delirium tremens. She also had knowledge of how older people, particularly those with sensory impairments, might become confused with a change in environment. In this excerpt, the student asked some questions which were hypothesis driven—that is, they were used to help her rule in or rule out the possible explanations that she was considering. There was one question for which the purpose was not clear. In the entire transcript, this student considered eight different hypotheses, and eventually decided that the patient simply needed his glasses and hearing aid put back on, although she indicated that she could not rule out the possibility of the confusion being caused by some of the medications that the patient was on.

This example illustrates the use of an analytic approach in arriving at a diagnosis, or inference, about the state of the patient. Analytic approaches to determining appropriate interventions also have been described by Corcoran (1986a, 1986b).

Intuitive Processes

The approach our team used to study diagnostic reasoning caused us concern, however. We were worried that the use of simulation and the procedure of the subject asking for one bit of information at a time actually promoted analytic methods, when, in fact, other approaches to clinical judgment might be used by nurses in practice. So we turned to Patricia Benner for assistance in using naturalistic and interpretive approaches to the study of clinical judgment. We conducted a study on the role of intuition in clinical judgment that relied on intensive interviews with nurses about actual caregiving episodes, and observations of them in their practice (Benner & Tanner, 1987). We based our study, in part, on the work of Dreyfus and Dreyfus (1986), and we described six aspects of intuition that seemed to figure prominantly in the clinical judgment of expert nurses. Two of these aspects will be described briefly to enhance your sense of how intuition appears.

Pattern Recognition. Pattern recognition is the perceptual ability that enables human beings to recognize configurations and relationships without analytically specifying the components of the patterns. Face recognition provides an immediate example of this ability. In daily life, people do not analyze an individual's facial features, yet they are able to recognize people they have met by referring to a memory of the overall facial "pattern." Similarly, patients present patterns that expert nurses learn to attend to. In contrast to this view of pattern recognition, however, analytical models of clinical judgment treat pattern recognition either as a feature detection system, in which a list of features held in memory is matched against the features presented by the patient, or as a template matching scheme.

Pattern recognition ability in a clinical situation is illustrated in the following excerpt of an interview (Benner & Tanner, 1987):

> This patient had a lot of cerebral edema, so they put him on fluid restriction. Somehow I knew that he was going to have a rough time, and I knew that he was at high risk for a pulmonary embolus. I accidentally overheard his wife say 'My husband is not feeling well. He's just getting very anxious. Can someone help me get him back to bed?'

Even though I wasn't taking care of him that night, I wanted to investigate. I had a suspicion that there was something wrong with him. He was sort of pale and anxious. He had all the classic signs of a pulmonary embolus. He was still conscious. We called the doctor, and then he coded. (p. 24)

For this nurse, an essential part of the pattern was the patient's history, which she knew. She also had expectations that this patient was at high risk for a pulmonary embolus. Her wariness sensitized her for instant pattern recognition. In this case, it might have been possible for the nurse to list individual cues—in fact, she did say that the patient was pale and anxious. To a novice, however, these cues alone, even with the history, would not set up the *pattern* of pulmonary embolus. The ability to recognize patterns comes only after many hours of direct observation, seeing similar patterns, and learning their meaning from experience.

Sense of Salience. Sense of salience, or the perception of things as being more or less important, is a second aspect of intuition. The expert nurse, who has a sense of salience, will not consider all observations as pertinent. Some will stand out as more or less important. Skilled observations of the patient over a long period of time allow the nurse to understand what is salient for *this* situation. A routine assessment checklist will not as likely be effective in situations that require highly individualized observations, such as the subtle changes occuring in head-injured patients.

Several other aspects of intuition have been described, and there are undoubtedly many others which will surface in our ongoing research. It is clear, even in these early stages of research on clinical judgment, that neither analytic nor intuitive processes can be effective in the absence of knowledge relevant for the situation. We turn now to a discussion of the knowledge base for clinical judgment, then we will return to the use of this knowledge, including research-based knowledge, in clinical judgment.

KNOWLEDGE USED FOR CLINICAL JUDGMENT

The last decade has seen an enormous increase in the number of writings on the relationship between theory and practice, with most writers taking the position that scientifically based theory is essential for quality nursing practice. While theory can be a useful guide for practice, it is clearly not the only way of knowing that guides nurses in their day-to-day decision making. This assertion is based on consideration of the large number of decisions that nurses must make on a daily basis; many of these decisions have no research or explicit theoretic base. Yet these same decisions result in care that seems to work well for their patients.

Benner (1983, 1984) has introduced to nursing the notion that there are two broad categories of knowledge that guide nursing action: theoretical and practical. Theoretical knowledge, or "knowing that," is the category of knowledge that usually comes to mind when we think about knowledge. It is formalized in terms of general, abstract rules and principles. It is typically taught in the classroom and conveyed in textbooks. In effect, theoretical knowledge provides guideposts for clinical judgement, but it often requires adaptation in a particular situation.

A simple example of theoretical knowledge, or "knowing that," is the basic procedure for administering an injection. A nurse can describe the steps for administration in clear language, and in a sufficiently abstract way that can be applied in many situations. But there will be other situations in which the general procedure will not work; for example, a patient who cannot assume any position other than a supine position. In that case, the theoretical knowledge may not be enough to decide on the best way to approach administering the injection. The nurse might be able to figure out the best approach based on reasoning from other abstract principles, or he or she may base the approach on experience.

Theoretical knowledge is derived from several sources. A major source for theoretical knowledge used in nursing practice is that derived from research in other sciences. For example, in coronary care units there is the common practice to avoid rectal stimulation through such procedures as taking rectal temperatures or giving enemas. The reasoning went something like this: A patient with an injured myocardium is more likely to experience arrythmias. Rectal stimulation may in turn stimulate the vagus nerve, causing slowing of the heart and allowing ectopic foci to arise, resulting in arrhythmias. Another example of this derived source of theoretical knowledge is in the area of patient education. Many of the principles for patient teaching are drawn from studies of learning in healthy college students as well as laboratory studies of learning using animal models.

A second source for theoretical knowledge is research within the discipline of nursing. This research may be directed toward *description* of phenomena that are of concern to nurses, such as the phenomenon of sensory deprivation, or it may be directed toward *prescription* of specific nursing action. In some instances, the research may be used to test the application of principles derived from basic or other sciences to nursing practice. For example, nurses have tested the effects of rectal temperature taking on patients who have had a heart attack in order to determine if the precautions derived from basic sciences are really necessary.

A third source for theoretical knowledge is theory derived from reflection on practice. For example, there is Elizabeth Kubler-Ross's (1969) well-known theory of the grief process, derived from her extensive work as a psychiatrist with dying patients. Another illustration of this source for theoretical knowledge was provided in Chapter 1. In this case, the nurse combined her review of the research on patient education and reflections on her own practice to recognize a more important concept that might be used—that of enabling the patient to be an agent of his own care. Her theoretical knowledge base will be expanded as she attempts to use this concept in her practice, reflecting on the practice, refining the concept, and trying it in different ways.

In contrast to theoretical knowledge is practical knowledge, or "knowing how." In nursing, as well as in other professions, there is a growing understanding of the role of practical knowledge in making astute clinical judgments. Practical knowledge is a "knowing how" derived from experience; it is a knowing-in-action, as Schon (1983) describes it:

> When we go about the spontaneous, intuitive performance of the actions of everyday life, we show ourselves to be knowledgeable in a special way. Often we cannot say what it is that we know. When we try to describe it we find ourselves at a loss, or we produce descriptions that are obviously incomplete. Our knowing is ordinarily tacit, implicit in our patterns of action

and in our feel for the stuff with which we are dealing. It seems right the way that our knowing is in our action.

Similarly, the workaday life of the professional depends on tacit knowing-in-action. Every competent practitioner can recognize phenomena—families of symptoms associated with a particular disease, peculiarities of a certain kind of building site, irregularities of materials in structures—for which he cannot give a reasonably accurate or complete description. In his day-to-day practice he makes innumerable judgments of quality for which he cannot state adequate criteria, and he displays skills for which he cannot state the rules and procedures. Even when he makes conscious use of research-based theories and techniques, he is dependent on tacit recognitions, judgments and skillful performances. (pp. 49–50)

Clinical expertise or practical knowledge is essential for skilled clinical judgment. In the instance of assessing patients for complications, for example, the nurse may use guidelines that are derived from research literature or from theory to begin the assessment. However, the experienced nurse has probably developed a much more extensive knowledge base for this assessment; this nurse is able to recognize subtle cues, patterns, and relationships long before a beginning nurse may be aware of changes. This ability is the result of clinical expertise derived from many hours of direct observation and care of patients (Benner, 1984).

Characteristics of practical knowledge include the following: (1) it is seldom formalized in language, in part, because there is no language to describe some of the qualitative aspects of this knowledge, in part, because it is tacit—that is, unrecognized by the clinician using it; (2) it may be in the form of past, concrete whole situations—experiences that the clinician has had with similar and dissimilar patients; (3) it falls into two general categories: knowledge of the particular patient that serves as a rich background of understanding and knowledge across patients with similar characteristics; and (4) it is solicited in the context of a particular situation and is dependent on that context for meaning. By observing nurses' actions in a particular situation, their practical knowledge becomes more apparent.

Theoretical and practical knowledge are highly interrelated, but, in some ways, distinct kinds of knowledge. Practical knowledge is developed through experience in which the nurse tests and refines propositions, hypotheses, and expectations. According to Benner (1984), experience is not the mere passage of time, but rather results when "preconceived notions and expectations are challenged, refined or disconfirmed by the actual situation" (p. 3). Hence theoretical knowledge guides acquisition of practical knowledge. However, as Kuhn (1970) and Polanyi (1958) have pointed out, humans acquire many skills without theoretical knowledge. Moreover, it is not always possible to give theoretical accounts for common activities, such as riding a bicycle. In short, some practical knowledge will escape formalization in language or in ways that can be tested scientifically.

Clearly both theoretical and practical knowledge are necessary for clinical judgment. For an experienced nurse encountering a familiar situation, the needed knowledge is readily solicited. The beginning nurse, however, must: (1) learn how to recognize a situation in which a particular aspect of theoretical knowledge applies; and (2) begin to develop a practical knowledge that allows refinement, extension, and possible adjustment of the appropriate theoretical base. But even the beginning nurse is not without useful practical knowledge. For example, students who are skilled in interpersonal relationships have learned to recognize certain facial expressions and body language as carrying a certain meaning within their culture. They have learned to respond to these expressions through their life experience and perhaps without the benefit of theory on therapeutic communication.

USE OF KNOWLEDGE IN CLINICAL JUDGMENT

We have discussed two major approaches to clinical judgment: the analytic and the intuitive. The use of either of these approaches in clinical judgment relies on the availability of knowledge, both theoretical and practical. The relationships between the process of clinical judgment and the knowledge available to the clinician in the context of a particular patient situation is depicted in Figure 2.2. What the nurse notices in the particular situation, and what has immediate relevance, will depend in large measure on the knowledge available to the nurse. Applicable theoretical or practical knowledge will be solicited by the situation.

The processes of clinical judgment used in a particular situation are dependent, in part, on the nurse's experience with similar/dissimilar situations, and the extent to which the presenting situation matches preconceived notions and expectations. Generally, the less experienced clinician will rely more heavily on analytic approaches, while the more experienced clinician will rely on intuitive approaches (Benner, 1984). Intuition requires practical knowledge, while analytic approaches can be used predominantly with theoretical knowledge. (Benner, 1984; Benner & Tanner, 1987).

While we have discussed the two approaches to clinical judgment and the two kinds of knowledge as if they were distinct entities, in the practice of the experienced clinician a hybrid performance is likely to appear. In any particular situation, there are likely to be instances when both intuitive and analytic judgments appear. The source of knowledge for the judgment also is likely to be a blend of theoretical with practical knowledge, some of which the nurse will be able to make explicit and some that will remain tacit.

**Figure 2.2
Model of Clinical Judgment**

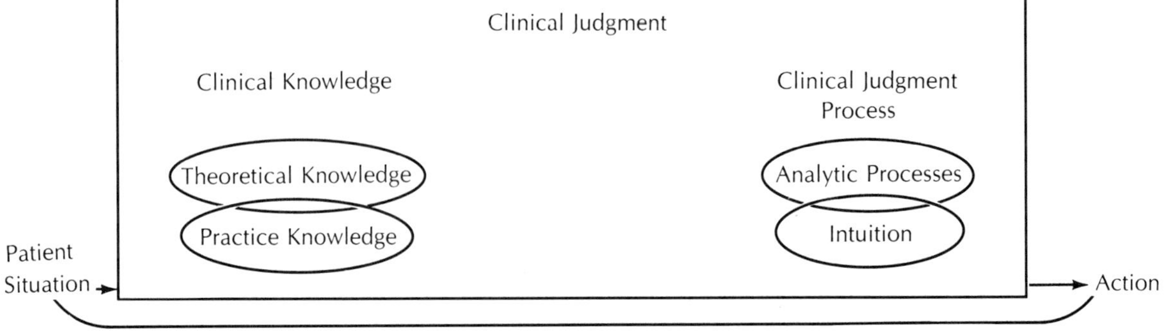

In Figure 2.2, judgment on the part of the nurse leads to some action. Actions include nursing interventions, such as teaching or coaching the patient, or keeping a watchful eye on the patient, and continuing to monitor those aspects that are salient in the situation. The judgment, the action, and the consequences for the patient have the potential of contributing to both the practical and theoretical knowledge of the clinician. The clinician might remember the situation as a paradigm case, a form of practical knowledge, in which the nurse's sets, expectations or hypotheses were so altered by the experience that he or she remembers it clearly as a whole, concrete illustration. If the clinician reflects on the situation, abstracting from it concepts that seem to apply, then the experience of judging, of deciding upon a particular action, will also contribute to his or her theoretical knowledge.

Within this view of clinical judgment, the clinician may use knowledge gained from research in a variety of ways. The most obvious, of course, is research that contributes to the clinician's theoretical knowledge base. In general, researchers express a basic assumption in regard to the "use" of theoretical knowledge. In practice, research was "used" when it was implemented as part of a program or directly led to some decision, that is, that some specific action could be attributable to use of research findings. When it was clear that a clinician had analyzed a particular situation, drawing on findings from research to guide or support the analysis, then one might say that the clinician had used the research findings. However, this "instrumental" utilization is only one kind of use, and is rather unusual.

Another use for research might be its contribution to the clinician's way of thinking about an issue or particular situation. Reading a research report might lead the clinician to reflect on his or her practice, recognizing instances from practice that may be similar or dissimilar to what the research reports. Additionally, the clinician might not put the research to any particular documentable use but rather allow it to serve as a more general form of "enlightenment" (Weiss, 1980). The way in which nurses approach future situations might be different because of extension and refinement of their clinical knowledge, but the change would not be traceable to a particular study. Caplan and Rich (1975) use the term "conceptual utilization" to describe this use of research.

The notion of instrumental research utilization is based on traditional views of science and the nature of scientifically derived knowledge. The most central assumption to this traditional view is that of unity of science—that is, that the human sciences are the same as the natural sciences. This, in turn, assumes that humans behave with law-like regularity (as do molecules in a chamber), and that covering laws can be discovered exposing causal chains—that is, that one event leads predictably to another event. Several other assumptions underlying the traditional view of science were described in Chapter 1.

Unfortunately, this mechanistic view does not seem to hold up in the practice of nursing. Part of the difficulty is that humans are fundamentally different from objects of study in the natural sciences. As Taylor (1985), a contemporary philosopher, points out:

> There are matters of significance for human beings which are peculiarly human, and have no analogue with animals. These are just the ones I mentioned earlier, matters of pride, shame, moral goodness, evil, dignity, the sense of worth, the various forms of human love, and so

on. If we look at goals like survival and reproduction, we can perhaps convince ourselves that the difference between man and animals lies in a strategic superiority of the former: we can pursue the same ends much more effectively than our dumb cousins. But when we consider these human emotions, we can see that the ends which make up a human life are *sui generis*. And then even the ends of survival and reproduction will appear in a new light. What it is to maintain and hand on a human form of life, that is, a given culture, is also a peculiarly human affair. (p. 102)

This is not to say that research conducted within the traditional approach to science cannot be used as a basis for clinical judgment in nursing practice. Such research in both nursing and other health sciences has led to significant advances in the theoretical knowledge base for nursing practice. But an understanding of personhood, as Taylor (1985) has described, suggests that science is not likely to lead us to the *certainty* that we would like to have about aspects of our practice. And it cannot give us prescriptions that will work in every situation.

Again, Chapter 1 presented an example of instrumental utilization of research that indicated that patients did better postoperatively if they received structured preoperative teaching (Lindeman & VanAernam, 1971). For the nurse who wishes to use this research instrumentally, he or she would conclude that there was evidence of a direct causal chain: preoperative teaching (as operationalized in the study) led to better pulmonary function that, in turn, led to shorter length of hospital stay. The nurse would use this research in practice through specific procedures regarding preoperative teaching. The teaching lesson plan, perhaps including the slide and tape program, would become his or her standardized procedure for preoperative teaching. However, this notion of a causal chain, using the concrete operationalization of the causative agent, is much too simplistic in light of our understanding of the complexities of emotions, meanings, and intentions integral to humans.

There are instances, however, where nurses can apply research instrumentally, to some extent, rather than conceptually. One example is research that focuses on aspects of nursing practice in which the unique characteristics of humanness (e.g., emotions, meanings, intentions) are not critical to the specific nursing care. For example, determining the best procedure for endotracheal suctioning has prompted extensive research. Suctioning is necessary to remove accumulated secretions in patients have who endotracheal tubes in place since the natural mechanism (coughing) is not effective. But suctioning also is traumatic to the trachea and can cause hypoxemia. Numerous studies have been conducted to determine aspects of the procedure (e.g., length of time the catheter is in place, administering 100% oxygen before suctioning) that minimize complications. A nurse could use this research to follow the procedure that has been documented to cause the least hypoxemia and tracheal trauma.

Even within this instrumental application, there are limits to the precision of a prescription that will work in every situation. For example, research has been contradictory about the best way to deliver 100% oxygen prior to endotracheal suctioning in order to prevent or minimize hypoxemia (Barnes & Kirchhoff, 1986). Some patients seem to do better if the oxygen is delivered by a hand ventilator, others with a mechanical ventilator. In this case, after numerous studies, we may have reached the limits of what can be prescribed to work in every situation.

Table 1.1
Illustrative Subset of Data from Study on Preoxygenation Methods

Patient number	Hand ventilator postsuctioning pO2	Mechanical ventilator postsuctioning pO2
1	84	70
2	52	70
3	90	64
4	88	68
5	71	78

Even if the results among studies had not been contradictory, there are difficulties in translating research on *populations* to the care of the *individual* patient. When two or more procedures are tested, the results are usually reported in terms of differences between the average scores of the comparison groups. In the above illustration, clinicians might have preoxygenated patients with the hand ventilator, then later preoxygenated them with the mechanical ventilator. The researcher might then have compared the patient's average blood oxygen level prior to and after suctioning under the two preoxygenation conditions. Table 1.1 shows a fictitious set of data that might be used for such a comparison. The total sample for this study was 25 patients; these data are for five of that sample.

In the total sample, the mean for condition 1 was 82.4 and the mean for condition 2 was 58. There were statistically significant differences between the two conditions, with condition 1 being superior. However, two individual patients shown in the subset of data apparently fared better under condition 2 than condition 1. This might have been a chance occurrence. The point is that research is reported in such a way that we know only that patients *on the average, with other things being equal*, will do better under condition 1 than condition 2. The clinician can use this research as a guide, but must be on the alert for those situations in which the patient does not respond in the same manner, or is in some other way different from the average patient in the study.

Utilization of research in clinical practice always requires the clinician to exercise judgment, and to take the stance of disciplined inquiry advocated in Chapter 1. The care that the nurse provides will reflect a dynamic use of knowledge, subject to modification in individual care situations, and open to revision as experience over time suggests.

The clinical knowledge of the inquiring nurse is thus informed by research, theory, and practice experiences. This knowledge forms the basis for several aspects of clinical judgment:

1. Knowledge, both theoretical and practical, often determines what stands out as important in a particular patient situation. In the illustration of the expert nurse's use of pattern recognition, her knowledge allowed her to see that the patient was at risk for pulmonary embolus and to instantly recognize the pattern of cues when the patient deteriorated. Research-based knowledge can contribute to the nurse's overall knowledge base for assessing risks. For example, research on pressure sore formation conducted over the last two decades has provided clear indications as to which patients are at high risk for pressure sores and,

therefore, may require more aggressive preventive measures. This research contributes to the nurse's knowledge base and allows the nurse to recognize that particular patients may be at risk. Features such as nutritional status, condition of the skin, and age of the person will stand out as important to the knowledgeable nurse when he or she is caring for an immobilized patient, but may recede in the background when caring for a young active person.

2. Knowledge helps the nurse selectively observe. In the section on the analytic processes of clinical judgment, we described the processes of hypothesis activation and hypothesis directed data gathering. Research directed toward describing phenomena of concern to nurses helps provide information about what cues are highly associated with particular problems. This allows the nurse, using this knowledge base, to select data relevant to determining the problem(s) the patient may be experiencing. For example, research on sensory deprivation has provided rich descriptions of its symptomatology, providing guidance to nurses who suspect that a patient may be experiencing the consequences of sensory deprivation.

3. Knowledge may also guide action. Research-based knowledge may contribute to the nurse's repertoire of possible interventions that are likely to produce desired outcomes or reduce the probability of complications.

CONCLUSION

Our understanding of clinical judgment and the use of knowledge in clinical judgment is far from complete. We know that judgment can be guided by theoretical knowledge, but practical knowledge of the situation is also needed. We do not advocate the instrumental application of research in practice, meaning strict adherence in applying the research protocol to the actual situation. Rather, we believe that the use of research in practice requires skilled judgment and an inquiring attitude.

A prerequisite to research utilization is the critical evaluation of the research itself. Traditional models of research utilization require that the knowledge discovered or verified in the research be reasonably certain—that is, that the research meet fairly stringent criteria of scientific merit and that enough study and samples exist to accept results as true. We also believe that evaluation of the research along these lines is important, but that scientific merit and replication are only two of many criteria one should use in determining if some or all aspects of the research ought to be incorporated into one's knowledge base for practice. Clearly not all published research is ready for use in practice. Some of it was never intended to be directly carried into practice; some of it was not of high enough quality to trust the results. Additionally, in some, the proposed nursing actions are of such great risk to the patient, or cost to the institution, that we would rather have a great deal of confidence in the findings before even attempting to use the action, even in a single situation. On the other hand, many research reports have redeeming characteristics, even if the specific action(s) evaluated by the study is not sufficiently supported to use in practice.

In order for you to determine which aspects of research may be considered "redeemed" and ready for use, and which are so worrisome that you would not want to use the ideas in practice, the remainder of this book is devoted to helping you read and evaluate research reports.

REFERENCES

Barnes, C. A., & Kirchhoff, K. T. (1986). Minimizing hypoxemia due to endotracheal suctioning: A review of the literature. *Heart and Lung: The Journal of Critical Care, 15,* 164–178.

Benner, P. (1984). *From novice to expert: Power and excellence in nursing practice.* Palo Alto, CA: Addison-Wesley.

Benner, P. (1983). Uncovering the knowledge embedded in clinical practice. *Image: The Journal of Nursing Scholarship, 15*(2), 36–41.

Benner, P., & Wrubel, J. (1982). Skilled clinical knowledge: The value of perceptual awareness. *Nurse Educator, 7*(3), 11–17.

Benner, P., & Tanner, C. (1987). Clinical judgment: How expert nurses use intuition. *American Journal of Nursing, 87,* 23–31.

Caplan, N., & Rich, R. F. (1975). *The use of social science knowledge in policy decisions at the national level.* Ann Arbor: Institute for Social Research, University of Michigan.

Carnevali, D., Mitchell, P., Woods, N., & Tanner, C. (1984). *Diagnostic reasoning in nursing.* Philadelphia: Lippincott.

Corcoran, S. (1986a). Task complexity and nursing expertise as factors in decision making. *Nursing Research, 35,* 107–112.

Corcoran, S. (1986b). Planning by expert and novice nurses in cases of varying complexity. *Research in Nursing and Health, 9,* 155–162.

Dreyfus, H. L. (1979). *What computers can't do: The limits of artificial intelligence.* New York: Harper and Row.

Dreyfus, H. L., & Dreyfus, S. E. (1986). *Mind over machine.* New York: The Free Press.

Elstein, A., Shulman, L., & Sprafka, S. (1978). *Medical problem solving.* Cambridge, MA: MIT Press.

Grier, M. (1976). Decision making about patient care. *Nursing Research, 25*(2), 105–110.

Hammond, K. R., Kelly, K. J., Schneider, R. J., & Vancini, M. (1966). Clinical inference in nursing: Information units used. *Nursing Research, 15,* 236–243.

Henderson, V. (1982). Nursing process—Is the title right? *Journal of Advanced Nursing, 7,* 103–109.

Iyer, P., Taptich, B., & Bernocchi-Losey, D. (1986). *Nursing process and nursing diagnosis.* Philadelphia: W.B. Saunders.

Kelly, K. J. (1966). Clinical inference in nursing: I. A nurses' viewpoint. *Nursing Research, 15,* 23–26.

Kubler-Ross, E. (1969). *On death and dying.* New York: MacMillan.

Kuhn, T. S. (1970). *The structure of scientific revolutions.* Chicago: University of Chicago Press.

Lindeman. C., & Van Aernam, B. (1971). Nursing intervention with the pre-surgical patient: The effects of structured and unstructured preoperative teaching. *Nursing Research, 20,* 319–332.

McHugh, M. (1986). Nursing process: Musings on the method. *Holistic Nursing Practice, 1*(1), 21–28.

Newell, A., & Simon, H. (1972). *Human problem solving.* Englewood Cliffs, NJ: Prentice Hall.

Padrick, K. P., Tanner, C. A., Putzier, D. J., & Westfall, U. E. (1987). Hypothesis evaluation: A component of diagnostic reasoning in nursing. In A. McLane (Ed.), *Classification of Nursing Diagnoses: Proceedings of the Seventh National Conference.* St. Louis: C. V. Mosby.

Polanyi, M. (1958). *Personal knowledge*. London: Routledge & Kegan Paul.

Pyles, S. H., & Stern, P. N. (1983). Discovery of nursing gestalt in critical care nursing: The importance of the grey gorilla syndrome. *Image: The Journal of Nursing Scholarship, 15*(2), 51–57.

Schon, D. A. (1983). *The reflective practitioner*. New York: Basic Books.

Shamansky, S., & Yanni, C. (1983). In opposition to nursing diagnosis: A minority opinion. *Image: The Journal of Nursing Scholarship, 15*(2), 47–50.

Stevens, B. (1984). *Nursing theory, analysis, application, evaluation*. Boston: Little, Brown.

Tanner, C. A. (1987). Teaching clinical judgment. In J. J. Fitzpatrick & R. L. Tauton (Eds.) *Annual review of nursing research*, (pp. 153–173). New York: Wiley & Sons.

Tanner, C. A., Padrick, K. P., Westfall, U. E., & Putzier, D. J. (1987). Diagnostic reasoning strategies of nurses and nursing students. *Nursing Research, 36*(6), 358–363.

Taylor, C. (1985). *Human agency and language: Philosophical papers*. Cambridge, England: Cambridge University Press.

Weiss, C. (1980). Knowledge creep and decision accretion. *Knowledge: Creation, Diffusion, Utilization, 1,* 381–386.

Westfall, U. E., Tanner, C. A., Putzier, D. J., & Padrick, K. P. (1986). Clinical inference in nursing: A preliminary analysis of cognitive strategies. *Research in Nursing and Health, 9,* 269–277.

3

Guidelines for Evaluation of Research for Use in Practice*

Christine A. Tanner, PhD, RN, FAAN
Margaret Imle, PhD, RN
Barbara Stewart, PhD

INTRODUCTION

At first, reading a research article may seem like traveling in a foreign country where you are trying to understand a new language. For this journey, there are several strategies that our students have found useful. First, learning research jargon to feel conversational with that language is quite helpful; keep a research text handy for looking up unfamiliar terms. Second, our students have learned that reading research cannot be done in the same way as reading a novel; rather it is necessary to attend to nearly every sentence. Many articles need to be reread, sometimes several times, before the pieces fall in place. This also is true for more experienced reviewers. Third, students have told us that they often have to describe in their own words what the researcher did before they even attempt to evaluate the strengths and limitations of the article. Finally, it is helpful to approach an article with confidence that you *can* understand it. By rereading an article or asking a colleague who has expertise in the clinical content or research methods described in the article, you can clarify aspects that at first appear unintelligible. At the same time, do not automatically decide that an article that sounds

---
*This chapter is based, in part, on Tanner, C. A. (1987). Evaluating research for use in practice: Guidelines for the clinician. *Heart and Lung: The Journal of Critical Care*, 16, 424–430.

esoteric contains the most significant research. From our experience, we can assure you the clearest writing comes from nursing's most literate and thorough researchers.

Most research articles will be composed of four basic sections. The first section usually states the problem under study, reviews past literature regarding that problem, defines a conceptual framework that identifies the logical connections among the variables related to the problem, and states hypotheses or research questions that the researcher hopes to address using the results of the study. The second section describes the method employed by the researcher in doing the study. This section includes information about the selection of subjects, the intervention if the study is experimental, the measures used, and the procedures employed to implement the intervention or collect the data. The third section describes results from the analysis of the data. The fourth section contains the researcher's interpretation of these results.

The research critique guidelines described in this chapter will lead you through all four sections of the research article. The guidelines emphasize (1) the potential utility of the research in clinical nursing practice, (2) the critical components of scientific merit, and (3) other factors that ought to influence the decision to use the research in practice.

The guidelines are derived from our approaches to reading research articles critically and to deciding if and how we want to use the research in our practice. We begin by skimming the entire research article. Then we reread it more carefully with particular attention to the first and second sections; that is, those sections that describe the questions under study and the methods used to investigate them. Through careful reading of these two sections, it is possible to make a preliminary judgment that an article is or is not of relevance to one's clinical practice.

Once we judge a particular study to have relevance to our practice, we proceed with a careful review of the remainder of the article. As a result, a complex critique of the article can arise that examines both scientific merit and other factors in the decision to use the research in practice. However, at the end of each part, there is an opportunity to judge the potential utility and scientific merit of the study before investing more effort in its full evaluation.

EVALUATING A STUDY FOR CLINICAL RELEVANCE

A useful preliminary step in evaluating a study is to classify the study by its primary purpose and type of data. This is important because different kinds of questions addressed in the critique apply, depending on the classification of the study. The initial parts of the article, including the research questions and methods section, provide the information needed to classify the study by purpose and type of data. The 2 × 2 table shown in Figure 3.1 summarizes the four types of studies found in nursing research literature. An example for each one will be used to illustrate the differences.

As you read nursing research, the most common type of study you will encounter is that which seeks to describe some nursing phenomenon by way of quantitative data (Brown, Tanner, & Padrick, 1984). These *descriptive, quantitative* studies tend to summarize what the subjects in the study are like on the measures obtained. In addition, they frequently seek to determine whether the scores of subjects on one measure are related in some way to their scores on another measure. The term *quantitative data* usually refers to numerical scores that are obtained from measuring the subjects with some instrument.

Figure 3.1
Classification of Studies in Nursing Literature

		Primary Type of Data	
		Quantitative	Qualitative
Primary Purpose	To describe a phenomenon of interest to nursing	Descriptive/ Quantitative	Descriptive/ Qualitative
	To test the effects of an intervention of interest to nursing	Experimental/ Quantitative	Experimental/ Qualitative

Davidhizar, Austin, and McBride (1986) provide an example of a descriptive, quantitative study in Chapter 9 of this book. In this study, attitudes of schizophrenic patients toward taking their medication were described, using a "fixed-response" quantitative measure. On this attitude measure of 26 questions, the range of possible scores was −52 to 130. In addition, a measure of the patients' insights into their illness was developed and administered; the range of possible scores on the insight instrument was 10 to 50, with 10 showing the least insight, and 50 showing the most insight. In the research report, the patients' scores on these instruments were reported, as well as the extent to which there was a relationship between the two scores; for example, a positive relationship indicated that the more insight a patient had about his or her illness, the better his or her attitude about taking medications.

A second type of study you will encounter is *experimental*, which usually employs *quantitative* data to answer its research questions. In its simplest form, the researcher uses some "treatment" or nursing intervention with one group of subjects, usually referred to as the experimental group. The researcher wants to determine if the intervention has an "effect" on some measured characteristic of the experimental group. In order to determine if the intervention has had an effect, the researcher compares the mean score of this experimental group on the measured characteristic with the mean score of a control group which has not received the intervention. If the experimental and control groups differ enough on the measured characteristic in the direction the researcher has hypothesized, then the researcher concludes that his or her intervention "had an effect" on the characteristic.

Brown and Hurlock (1975) present an example of this kind of study in Chapter 5 of this book. In this study, three different methods of preparing the breast to reduce breastfeeding trauma were examined. The women were assigned to one of three treatment groups to determine, more specifically, if any of the three methods was superior in preventing nipple sensitivity and trauma. In addition, the women did the breast preparation on only one breast, so that one breast served as the control.

In research reports about experimental studies, the intervention is often referred to by the special term, *independent variable*. In an experimental study, the independent variable is the variable that the researcher manipulates; in this case, whether a subject received the intervention (i.e., was in the experimental group) or did not receive the intervention (i.e., was in the control group). In the Brown and Hurlock (1975) study, the independent variable was type of nipple preparation. On the other hand, the *dependent variable* in an experimental study is the characteristic of the subjects that the researcher thinks his or her intervention will influence. Sometimes the dependent variable is called the "outcome" or "criterion" variable. In this study, there were two main dependent variables: the objective and subjective indications of nipple pain after breastfeeding was initiated.

A third type of study you will encounter is one that has *description* as its main purpose and uses *qualitative data* as a basis for describing the phenomenon of interest. The term *qualitative data* refers to data which are in the form of words rather than numbers. Raw qualitative data may be in the form of field notes or tape recordings of events. These raw data are subjected to some processing before they are analyzed, however: field notes are converted to "write-ups" which are intelligible to anyone, not just the note taker. Audiotapes are transcribed; actions on videotapes are described. All of these methods of data collection use words, rather than numbers, as the medium, and analysis continues to depend on use of words.

Olshansky (1987) presents an example of a qualitative descriptive study in Chapter 5 of this book. This study was conducted to explore the meaning of infertility to couples experiencing it. The couples were interviewed about how infertility had affected their lives, how it had affected their relationships with significant others, and how they had dealt with their feelings engendered by infertility. Responses to these interviews were tape recorded and transcribed. According to Olshansky, "The researcher constructed codes, or words, that captured the meanings of the transcripts, a process referred to as open coding. Eventually several codes were grouped into categories that subsumed these codes" (p. 56). Through the process of coding, identifying categories and eventually relationships among categories, a beginning theory describing the process of dealing with infertility was developed.

A fourth type of study you will encounter, and which is found least often in nursing literature, we have termed *experimental/qualitative*. In this type of study, the investigator seeks to determine the effectiveness of some nursing intervention and uses qualitative data as the dependent or outcome variable. Tudor (1952) presents an example of such a case study involving only one or a few subjects in Chapter 9 of this book. In her article, Tudor described the process of mutual withdrawal among patients and staff on a psychiatric ward. The investigator intervened with two patients and observed the effects on both the patients' way of relating and the staff's response to them. The effects were described using words rather than a numerical score.

Once the purpose of the study and the type of data used are identified, then one may begin critical review of the study contents. Of prime interest at this point is *relevance for clinical practice*. The questions on the research critique examine several possible uses of research: (1) to solve a particular problem encountered by nurses in their practice; (2) as an aid to clinical judgment; (3) as a potentially generalizable theory which has been generated or tested through research; and (4) using instruments employed in a study which appear to have utility for making decisions in practice (see Figure 3.2).

Using Research to Solve Problems

The most obvious way that research may be used in practice is for solving a particular problem encountered by nurses. For example, nurses may recognize that the incidence of phlebitis seems

Figure 3.2
Evaluation for Clinical Relevance

Type of Study:

1. Is the purpose of the study primarily (a) to describe a phenomenon of concern to nursing or (b) to test the effects of one or more independent variables, such as a nursing intervention?
2. Is the kind of data collected primarily quantitative or qualitative?

Potential Use in Practice Through Direct Application:

1. What was the clinical problem that was studied? Does this study have the potential to help solve a problem which you currently face in your practice?
2. Does the study have the potential to help you with any of the following types of decisions:
   - Deciding on appropriate observations to make in order to infer both patient problems and strengths.
   - Identifying the extent to which patients may be at risk for certain problems or complications.
   - Deciding on the intervention most likely to produce desired outcomes and/or reduce the probability of complications.
3. Is a theory or proposition which might serve to guide practice generated, developed or tested by the study? What kinds of clinical nursing decisions might be guided by this theory?
4. How did the investigator measure the dependent variables or outcomes? Do you see the potential for using any of these measures in your practice?

Other Uses for Research: Enlightenment

Please describe any other aspect of the research report which you particularly appreciate or find enlightening. What applications of the research do you see that the investigator did not see? What are applications other than the categories described above?

Pause for Reflection:

If the answer to any of the above questions is positive, then the study deserves further consideration. It has potential for use in practice. If you answered no to *all* of the questions, then the study is probably not relevant to your practice and there is no need to evaluate it further (unless you are reviewing the study for other reasons).

---

to be high on their unit and review the research literature for possible causes of phlebitis; they may discover that recent research suggests that IV dressings should be changed more frequently than has been the practice on the unit. Other examples of research directed toward specific problems in practice include: (1) prevention of diarrhea in tube-fed patients (Walike, et al., 1975); (2) prevention of wandering in elderly, cognitively impaired nursing home residents; (3) reducing attrition from exercise programs (Jordan-Marsh, 1985); and (4) verifying amount and frequency of urinary incontinence in elderly ambulatory care patients (Robb, 1985).

Using Research as an Aid to Clinical Judgment

As described in Chapter 2, clinical judgment requires a series of decisions including: (1) the selection of cues that are important to observe in particular situations; (2) the identification of risk factors which may predispose an individual to health problems or complications of treatment; and

(3) the selection of an intervention which will result in a desired outcome with a minimum of risk to the patient. Descriptive research, whether qualitative or quantitative, may help in the first two of these decisions. For example, descriptive research about the experience of infertility may provide guidance to the nurse in assessing his or her clients (Olshansky, 1987). Descriptive research in the signs and symptoms of sensory deprivation assists the nurse in evaluating patients for the presence or absence of this condition. The descriptive study about the relationship between insight and attitude toward medication taking may help the nurse identify patients who are at risk for noncompliance in medication taking (Davidhizur, Austin, & McBride, 1986).

The third kind of decision, selecting an appropriate intervention, may be supported by either descriptive or experimental research. The research may be directed toward investigating which intervention will cause the least negative consequences. For example, numerous studies on tracheobronchial suctioning have examined ways in which hypoxemia and tracheal trauma may be minimized (Barnes & Kirchhoff, 1986). Studies on oxygen uptake and cardiovascular responses during bathing are directed toward identifying the best method of bathing to minimize complications in patients with myocardial infarction (Winslow, Lane, & Gaffney, 1985). Other studies are directed toward investigating the effectiveness of selected interventions in creating desired outcomes. For example, Lamontagne, Mason, and Hepworth (1985) investigated the effects of relaxation on school-age children in order to evaluate its potential benefits in helping children learn to cope with stress.

Use of Research-Based Theory to Guide Practice

Another way that research may be used in practice is through either the generation or testing of a theory. Theory is an abstraction which serves to make scientific findings meaningful and generalizable.

A theory may describe a phenomenon of interest, such as Ohlshanky's (1987) beginning theory of the experience of infertility. Or a theory may help explain relationships among several phenomena, such as the description of the relationship among social support, stress, and health offered by Norbeck and Tilden (1983). A theory also may prescribe nursing action, such as the theory of mutual goal setting discussed by Alexy (1985). In each of these cases, a theory goes beyond the specific aspects of the study—the sample, the particular instruments—to be more generally applicable.

Research may be used either to generate a new theory or test an existing one. Sometimes there is no previous research about a nursing phenomenon or further development of a theory is needed. Perhaps a clinical practice problem is not yet described in the research literature and many aspects of it are not sufficiently understood to develop appropriate means to intervene. Research questions to study these situations are exploratory in nature, and include: (1) what are the experiences of patients in a complex intensive care environment? or (2) how do new parents cope with sleep deprivation in the immediate postpartum period? Studies would be designed to identify and define categories of patient experiences in the ICU or to describe and categorize ways in which parents cope with sleep deprivation. Theories derived from such studies may be useful in helping nurses identify factors they should consider in caring for ICU patients or in working with new parents who are struggling with a wakeful infant. Typically, studies designed to generate theory rely on qualitative data, primarily because what is sought is precisely what qualitative data are intended to reveal: description of the phenomenon in terms of new concepts and relationships among concepts.

Studies designed to test theory may use a variety of approaches. A theory may suggest that there is a relationship between two or more concepts. For example, current conceptions of social support suggest that there is a strong relationship between stress and episodes of illness which can be mitigated by a responsive support network. Research, using quantitative measures of stress, health status, and social support could be designed to test these relationships in a descriptive study.

There are some theories used by nurses which support the application of particular nursing interventions. In a classic series of studies conducted by Johnson (Johnson, 1972, 1973; Johnson & Rice, 1974; Johnson, Kirchhoff, & Endress, 1975; Johnson, Morrissey, & Levinthal, 1973), the effectiveness of theoretically derived interventions in reducing the distress associated with medical procedures was tested. The theory underlying the intervention proposes that a discrepancy between expectations about sensations and the actual experience of sensations during a threatening event results in distress. The intervention is aimed at reducing the discrepancy between expectations and actual experience. It involves providing information to patients about what they can expect to experience during medical procedures. The intervention has been tested in both laboratory and clinical studies with adult patients undergoing endoscopy and children undergoing orthopedic cast removal. (The latter study is reprinted in Chapter 6 of this text.) Although the populations have differed, and the precise way in which the intervention was developed has varied from study to study, there has been substantial support of the generalizability of the theory to other populations undergoing medical procedures.

Use of an Instrument in Practice

Instruments which are used for particular studies or have been developed and tested through research may be useful to nurses in their day-to-day practice. The Braden scale is an example of an instrument developed specifically for use in practice (Bergstrom, Braden, Laguzza, & Holman, 1987). The Braden scale was developed to assist nurses in the early identification of patients who may be at risk for developing pressure sores. Even when other aspects of the study may not be particularly useful, a nurse may find the instrument relevant for his or her practice.

EVALUATING A STUDY FOR SCIENTIFIC MERIT

Once the research report has passed critical review for clinical relevance, then the evaluation of its scientific merit becomes salient. Three aspects of this evaluation are included in the guidelines: (1) the extent to which the conceptualization or justification for the study makes sense and thereby provides a sound basis for the remainder of the report (internal consistency); (2) the degree to which there has been sufficient methodological rigor for the reader to believe the results and conclusions;

Figure 3.3
Evaluation of the Conceptualization and Internal Consistency

1. Overall, does the report hang together? Does the investigator end up studying what you thought he or she would study when reading the introductory paragraphs? Does the language of the report make sense to you?
2. Does the underlying conceptualization make sense, specifically:
   - Is there justification for the study?
   - Do the study questions relate to the justification?
   - Is there an overall fit among the conceptualization of the nursing practice questions, the concepts used as a basis for the research, and the operational definitions of the concepts as variables in the study?
3. Do the investigators do the study in a way that allows them to answer the questions they posed? Are the answers/conclusions consistent with the type of research questions and the methods of the study? In other words, are the beginning, middle, and end of the research report clearly related to each other? Specifically:
   - Are the independent and dependent variables logically related?
   - Are the subjects consistent with the population of interest?
   - Are the instruments likely to measure the phenomenon of interest?
   - Are the data collection procedures such that they won't interfere with usual practice and therefore bias the results?

Pause for Reflection:

If there are major conceptual problems (i.e., the underlying justification doesn't make sense), or if there is not internal consistency in the report (i.e., the methods don't fit with the conceptualization or the research questions aren't really addressed), then you have several possible options: (1) to continue with more detailed evaluation of the study, hoping that additional reading will clarify the confusing aspects of the report; (2) to seek consultation from a person with some expertise in research methods who may be able to clarify some of your questions; and (3) to evaluate the report no further, because it is sufficiently confusing that its usefulness in practice is jeopardized.

---

and (3) the representativeness of the sample and setting, and evidence of replication of the study allowing for some confidence in the generalizability of the results.

Conceptualization and Internal Consistency

The questions in this part of the critique (see Figure 3.3) examine several basic aspects of the report which are important to the potential usefulness of the study in practice. First, assuming that the reader has a basic understanding of research language and a good grasp of the practice phenomenon which the study addresses, it seems appropriate that the report should make sense to him or her and should flow logically from beginning to end.

The justification for a study may be derived from the research literature, from theory, or from concerns in practice. Basically the justification is an explanation of why the study is important for nursing. For example, the investigators may identify either gaps in the research literature or inconsistencies in results which this study is designed to resolve. Or the justification for the study may lie in a description of a theoretical proposition which has not been adequately tested. In other situations, because the phenomenon under investigation may not have had prior study, an exploratory, qualitative, and descriptive approach is justified. The investigators may simply describe observations or clinical hunches from their practice which they wish to test empirically. The investigators may think that the replication of a previous study in a different setting would contribute to the generalizability of the previous study's findings. These are all illustrations of an appropriate justification for a study. *What should be clear in the study justification and conceptualization is why these particular research questions make sense to study now, given prior research, available theoretical perspectives, and clinical observation.*

The internal consistency of the study refers to the extent to which the justification for the study, its conceptualization, and the specific research questions frame the remainder of the study report. We would expect that the variables studied would be clearly linked to the study's conceptualization. The way in which the variables are operationalized as interventions or as measures should make sense in light of the justification for the study. For example, an investigator may wish to study the extent to which selected factors in the intensive care environment cause stress in patients. The identification of environmental variables may flow from the investigator's clinical observations or from a theoretical framework which describes an inclusive categorization of potentially stressful environmental factors. The measure(s) of the dependent variable of stress in patients should be based on a logical argument for a relationship between those measures and measures of the potentially stressful environmental factors. The results and conclusions should specifically address the research questions.

At this point in the research critique, the reader should pause and reflect on the study's merit so far. If there appear to be major conceptual problems (e.g., the justification simply does not make sense) or if there is not internal consistency in the report (the methods do not fit with the conceptualization or the research questions are not really addressed), then you have several possible options. You may decide that the study is of sufficient importance to your practice that you are willing to overlook weak justification or some conceptual inconsistencies, at least for the time being. You may find that if you continue with more detailed evaluation of the study, the additional reading will clarify some confusing aspects of the report. You may wish to seek consultation from a person with more expertise in research methods who may be able to clarify some questions. Or you may choose to evaluate the report no further, because it is simply too confusing.

Believability of Results

In this part of the critique, the methods, results, discussion, and conclusion sections of the report should be reread with more attention to details. Here questions regarding the report concern matters of *screening*. Their purpose is to alert you to major methodological issues which might cause you to question the validity of the results and, therefore, their applicability to practice. Screening questions are organized by the categorization of research in terms of primary purpose and type of data: (1) for all studies regardless of the purpose of the study and kind of data (see Figure 3.4); (2) for both descriptive studies and those testing the effects of some independent variable using quantitative data (see Figure 3.5); and (3) for descriptive studies using qualitative data (see Figure 3.6). No specific criteria are offered for experimental/qualitative studies. Their evaluation relies on guidelines provided for other categories of research.

Critique Questions Relevant to all Studies: Method

Sample. As you read the sections of a research report that describe the subjects and their selection, there are several important factors to consider. First, textbooks on research emphasize the importance of drawing a *random sample* from the population of interest. Because it is rarely feasible to study an entire population of interest (e.g., all persons having their first child in 1988 or all persons currently caring for an older relative or friend), we rely on findings from a randomly selected sample to make generalizations about the larger population. The most important reason for using random sampling is that many of the statistical procedures we use to analyze data rely on random selection of subjects from the population of interest in order for statements of statistical significance to be accurate.

Despite the desirability of using random samples, researchers in nursing, as well as those in related fields, are rarely able to select a sample randomly from the population of interest. Often, for reasons related to the constraints imposed by doing research in practice settings, these researchers rely on convenience samples for their studies. This lack of random sampling does not mean that the research findings from such studies are useless. If, as you read research reports about studies that have used convenience samples, you find that the researcher has provided an adequate description of the sample in terms of such characteristics as age, gender, ethnicity, educational level, income, and living situation, you can make some assessment of the strengths and limitations of the sample. A good research report will also include a statement of limitations of the generalizability of the findings if a convenience sample has been used. It also is worthwhile to note that, although most nursing research uses clients, patients, or nurses—people—as subjects, some studies use other types

**Figure 3.4
Believability of Results: Questions Relevant to all Studies**

1. *Methods:*
   - What subjects were studied and how were they selected? If a convenience sample was used, did the investigator take into consideration sample characteristics which might influence the results of the study? Are the subjects involved in some way in the phenomenon of interest?
   - Does the investigator discuss potential biases and intervening variables and ways in which these were accounted for?
   - Does the investigator discuss reliability of the measures? Is reliability satisfactory? Does the investigator report on procedures for achieving consistency between two or more data collectors?
   - Does the investigator discuss validity of the measures? Are you confident of the instrument validity? Does the investigator describe how the interview guide, if used, was developed?
2. *Conclusions:*
   - Does the investigator stay within the boundaries indicated by the subjects, types of interventions attempted and the measures used?

of subjects, for example, community health care agencies. In such cases, the kinds of characteristics that might be considered relevant to the study are agency size, whether it is public or private, and organizational complexity.

One important feature of the sample that you should look for concerns what proportion of those persons or agencies asked to participate did agree to participate. You should feel more confident about the results of a study where 80 to 90 percent of those invited to participate did so compared to a study where only 33 or 50 percent of those invited did agree to participate. Because many nursing studies involve subjects who are vulnerable, and because nurse researchers have an ethical obligation to give any subject the right to refuse to participate, participation rates are sometimes low. In such instances, you should look for an explanation of the reasons for the low participation rate and for some qualification of the results in light of the reasons for nonparticipation. Cotanch and Strum (1987) present an example of a succinct description of participation rate in Chapter 7 of this book. They state:

> Sixty-eight patients who were considered were eligible for the study. Six patients refused to participate and two patients began the study but withdrew immediately after the initial intervention training session (both withdrawals were in the placebo group). The results are based on 60 patients. (p. 35)

In studies where mailed questionnaires are used for data collection, the researcher should report the percentage of those returned with usable responses.

A common question that is often asked about the study sample is, "How big is big enough?" There is no single rule about the optimum sample size. Some kinds of research questions and designs require samples that number in the hundreds or even thousands, while others need only a few or in some cases one subject. Some general guidelines may assist you in your critique. Studies using qualitative data usually use fewer subjects than studies using quantitative data. It is not uncommon to see studies using qualitative data obtained on 15 or 20 subjects or fewer.

Unless researchers have gathered extensive quantitative data on just one or a handful of subjects (e.g., they observed one subject during 40 observation sessions), most quantitative studies will probably involve at least 25 or 30 subjects. As a general rule, you will probably see somewhat smaller sample sizes in experimental studies than in descriptive correlations studies. Unless the availability of subjects is very limited or the type of data being collected is very costly in terms of time or apparatus, most experimental studies will have a least 10 or 20 subjects per group, and often will have 30 to 50 subjects per group, especially if there is only one control and one experimental group. Many quantitative/descriptive studies use multivariate statistics to analyze their data and consequently use at least moderately large samples of 75 to 100 subjects or more. The more variables that the researchers want to analyze using multivariate statistics, the more subjects they will need. Sometimes the number of subjects needed is several hundred or more in situations where there are many variables.

Other aspects of the research being equal, we feel more confident about research findings when the sample size is reasonably large so that the range of possible responses from subjects has probably been obtained from the study sample. If 10 in every 100 patients had a negative reaction to a particular nursing intervention, then having 20 patients in an experimental group may be too few to detect such a problem. On the other hand, a sample size can also be too large in that a researcher obtains statistically significant results simply because, with very large samples, even very small differences between groups or very small relationships among variables will be detected as significant. We will discuss the issue of statistical versus practical significance later. For now, we will say that sometimes researchers use an unnecessarily large sample. In the early stages of research, it is frequently advisable to put energy into small but well-designed exploratory projects. If the results of those look promising, then studies with larger samples are in order.

Potential Biases. Sometimes researchers draw conclusions about the relationships between two variables or the difference between groups on some characteristic and fail to take into account other factors that may be affecting the relationship or difference they have found. Sometimes researchers include these other factors in the way they conceptualize the phenomenon but do not or cannot include the factors in the actual design of the study. Sometimes it is only after the data have been collected and analyzed that the researchers realize that some other variables should have been taken into account. In reading a research article, you may find such issues presented in the discussion of findings.

Many of the aticles reprinted in this book include discussion of possible biases. Wolfer and Visintainer (1975) present an excellent example of this kind of discussion in Chapter 6. The section of their article entitled "Limitations and Suggestions for Further Study" illustrates a candid and thorough consideration of alternative explanations for study results.

Reliability of Measures. *Reliability* refers to the accuracy and stability of the instrument. When we attempt to measure some phenomenon quantitatively, there is often some degree of error; that is, we aren't perfectly precise in the extent to which a score reflects the amount of the attribute we are attempting to measure. For example, if an individual is weighed daily and a wide variation in weight is obtained, then there is considerable measurement error (assuming that the individual is not actually gaining and losing a lot of weight). When there is a large amount of measurement error, the instrument is unreliable.

We cannot determine the amount of measurement error directly, but we can estimate it indirectly. Two ways which are frequently reported in the literature are internal consistency reliability (using the statistic referred to as Cronbach's alpha or the Kuder Richardson formula) and test–retest reliability (using a correlation coefficient). Internal consistency reliability estimates the extent to which all items on a test measure the same thing—essentially, how cohesive the test is. This method works well for most kinds of written tools with a number of items to be answered by the subjects; with computerized data analysis it is a relatively easy estimate to obtain. However, it may not be appropriate for all measures.

Test–retest reliability requires that the instrument be administered twice to the same sample, with some reasonable time interval—usually two weeks—between the two administrations; however, the interval should be determined by several factors including consideration of how much might be learned or remembered in the first administration. The scores from the first administration are correlated with scores from the second administration to determine how stable the measure is.

Both internal consistency reliability and test–retest reliability are reported in terms of a reliability coefficient which is expected to be positive and to have a possible range of 0.00 to 1.00. Usually, the reliability coefficient will fall between .40 and .90. The general rule of thumb states that a reliability coefficient above .70 is considered adequate, but some consider it preferable to have it above .80 or even .90 for special uses of the measure (Nunnally, 1978).

Reliability of the measure is very important to the believability of the results. First, minimizing the amount of measurement error is necessary in order to find a relationship between two or more variables or to determine the effectiveness of a treatment. Suppose, for example, that we wanted to evaluate the effectiveness of a weight loss program. If one of the outcome measures was weight loss, and the scales were unreliable (i.e., there was a great deal of variation from day to day in weight, even though the actual weight was unchanged), then it would be unlikely that we would see any effects of the weight loss program. Another reason that some estimate of reliability is important is the idea that reliability is a necessary (although not sufficient) condition for validity. Validity refers to the extent to which the instrument measures what it is supposed to measure. If there is a great deal of measurement error (i.e., the instrument is unreliable), then it cannot measure the phenomenon it is supposed to measure. (This does not mean that reliability must be established *before* there is any assessment of validity. Some forms of validity must be established prior to testing for reliability.)

Despite the importance of reliability to a study, many published research reports do not include any indication of the reliability of the measures. Strickland and Waltz (1986) examined 99 articles published in 1984 and found that 58.4 percent did not include information on the reliability of instruments.

In the critique guidelines, two questions address the reliability of instruments: (1) is an estimate of reliability reported? and (2) is the reported reliability adequate? If the answer to these two questions is no, you might well ask if the study should be dismissed as totally unbelievable. However, as in nearly everything concerning reliability, the answer to this questions is "it depends." Sometimes instruments are so well known or widely used that the investigators assume that the reader will know that the instrument has been repeatedly evaluated for its reliability. Sometimes the instrument is such that one could expect a minimum of measurement error, although we still would prefer to see reliability reported in these cases. Sometimes, in the procedures section of the report, the investigators have described ways in which the instruments were calibrated and checked frequently, but they may not have estimated reliability per se. For example, a scale may have been calibrated against a standard and checked periodically so that one is assured that it is weighing accurately. If the reliability is not reported and none of these other conditions exist, then the believability of the results—particularly findings which are contrary to what is predicted or which are not statistically significant—should be seriously questioned.

Validity of Measures. As indicated above, the term *validity* refers to the extent to which the instrument measures what it is supposed to measure. For example, a paper-and-pencil instrument on anxiety is frequently used to measure the level of anxiety of hospitalized patients. There are two components to this instrument—the trait, presumably a stable characteristic of the person, and the state, the amount of anxiety created by current events. While a measure of trait anxiety would not be a valid measure of the anxiety caused by hospitalization, a measure of state anxiety might be.

Validity of a measure is never proven. Rather one gathers evidence for its validity. In this regard, the term *content* validity refers to the extent to which: (1) the instrument has content (or items) on the instrument representative of the attribute or phenomenon being measured; and (2) the extent to which the attribute is "covered" by the items. Usually, content validity is a concern during the development of the instrument and relies on the use of a panel of experts who assist the investigator in making sure that the items are representative of the attribute being measured. Other kinds of validity are estimated after the instrument has been developed and are referred to by such names as criterion-related validity, predicitive validity, construct validity, divergent validity, and so on. These all refer to various ways that investigators may evaluate the extent to which an instrument is measuring what it is intended to measure.

Like reliability, validity is very important to the believability of study results. And, as with reliability, the validity of measures is not consistently reported in the research literature. Strickland and Waltz (1986) found that 58 percent of the studies in their sample contained no reference to the validity of the measures used in the study. The questions in the guidelines thus ask you to consider: (1) if validity is reported or discussed; and (2) your confidence in the validity of the instruments. The extent to which failure to report validity jeopardizes the believability of the study is a matter of judgment, just as it is with reliability.

Critique Questions for Studies Using Quantitative Measures: Method
(Descriptive and Experimental)

Studies using quantitative measures may be descriptive or experimental. Descriptive studies may be designed to either describe the sample on one or more attributes or to determine the extent to which one or more attributes correlate with other attributes. Most studies will do both, that is, describe the sample and examine the data for relationships among the attributes. In descriptive studies, the investigator does not manipulate any variables, but rather collects data to see if relationships exist. In contrast, experimental studies are frequently directed toward testing the effectiveness of interventions; the investigator will manipulate one or more variables. Although many books on research imply that experimental studies are superior to descriptive studies, this is not the case. The choice of the type of study depends on the kind of question the investigator wishes to answer.

Experimental Studies: Treatment Groups. The term *experimental study*, when used strictly, means the random assignment of subjects to an experimental group and one or more control groups. The experimental group receives the experimental treatment (the nursing intervention) while the control group receives an alternative treatment, sometimes termed a placebo, or no treatment.

Random assignment to treatment groups involves first identifying a sample from the population of interest, giving a separate number to each subject, and then using a random numbers table to assign subjects to the various treatment conditions. This "randomization" procedure ensures that systematic biases have not been built into how subjects are assigned to experimental and control groups.

If the experimental and control groups differ on the dependent variable before the study even starts or if they differ on other variables that might influence the effectiveness of the treatment, then the independent variable will not actually be "independent" of these other variables but instead

Figure 3.5
Believability of Results: Questions for Quantitative Descriptive and Experimental Studies

1. *Methods:*
   - If an intervention was tested with different treatment groups, were the subjects randomly assigned to these groups? If yes, did that result in other methodological or clinical problems? If not, did the investigator control for possible initial differences between the groups? Does the control group receive a treatment reflecting the current standard of practice? Is there a reasonable comparison?

2. *Results:*
   - Are the results thoroughly reported?
   - Are the statistics used appropriate for the type of data collected and the kind of research questions asked?

3. *Conclusions:*
   - If there were statistically significant findings (e.g., a positive correlation between two variables; a difference between two treatment groups), what explanation does the investigator offer? Based on your knowledge and experience, what other explanation might there be for these results (e.g., did a large sample size contribute to statistically significant findings?) In the real world, would a difference of that magnitude be important?
   - Does the investigator use statistics to replace professional judgment? Or alternately, does the investigator use professional judgment to refute the statistical findings?
   - If the findings were not as expected, or not statistically significant, does the investigator provide a reasonable explanation? Could any of the following be possible explanations for these results: small sample size, invalid or insensitive measures, a very heterogeneous sample, not a strong enough intervention.

---

will be "confounded" with these other variables. If a researcher cannot randomly assign subjects to a treatment group, then the design is referred to as a quasiexperimental rather than a true experimental design. Such quasiexperimental designs are often the only option available for nursing research. Cook and Campbell (1979) discuss the strengths and limitations of such designs.

An example of the kind of problem that might arise if a researcher could not use random assignment will illustrate the importance of randomization. Brailey's (1986) study (in Chapter 10 of this book) had two primary purposes: "to examine the effects of group and individual teaching by nurses in the workplace on 140 female office employees' health knowledge, beliefs, and practices regarding breast self-examination and to identify factors associated with frequency of practice" (p. 223).* The independent variable was teaching approach, with three different kinds: group, individual, and no teaching. It evidently was not possible to randomly assign subjects to the kind of teaching approach. Hence, the groups might be different from one another in ways other than the teaching approach. Random assignment is a way to help the groups be as similar as possible on all relevant variables except the independent variable.

---

*Note that these two purposes imply both experimental and descriptive approaches. It is quite common to include both purposes in one study. The first purpose implies a comparison between two or more groups—comparing two levels of an independent variable—and is therefore "experimental." The second purpose is to examine for relationships between variables—specifically to identify factors related to the frequency of self-breast examination. The purpose is descriptive in nature.

To deal with this potential problem, Brailey (1986) did what was appropriate: she measured the subject on numerous variables to determine pre-intervention differences between groups. It turned out that there were initial differences among the groups on several potentially important variables: perceived benefits of breast self-examination, confidence in skill of technique, and frequency of breast self-examination. The control group scored highest on these measures. The net effect of these pre-intervention differences in this study might have been to mute any effect of the teaching intervention. We assume that through randomization we evenly distribute the subjects between the groups on variables which may be important to the study.

Sometimes, despite random assignment, experimental and control groups differ on important demographic or personal characteristics. Researchers often present evidence to demonstrate how well the randomization worked. If the groups did, in fact, differ on some of these characteristics, statistical techniques, such as analysis of covariance, may have been employed to control in part for the differences between the groups. Brailey (1986), in the example above, did not use these statistical procedures.

Results. In evaluating the thoroughness of results of quantitative studies, there are several components that you should look for. First, you should look to see what statistics are presented. Table 3.1 lists frequently used statistics and their general purpose.

Regardless of whether their studies are descriptive or experimental in nature, researchers frequently use such statistics as the mean and the standard deviation to describe characteristics of their samples. In *almost all studies* using quantitative data, you should expect to see some statistical evidence regarding the average subject, such as the mean or median, and the range or spread of scores. You should also look for some mention of how missing responses were handled and how much missing data existed. You can sometimes determine this by looking at the sample size mentioned earlier in the article and comparing it to the sample size reported in the results section or tables.

In *descriptive* studies which examine relationships between two or more variables, one of several statistics might be used depending on the nature of the data. Pearson's correlation coefficient (Pearson's r) is used when the data are continuous; chi square (χ^2) is used when the data are

Table 3.1
Purposes of Commonly Used Statistics

Statistic	Purpose
Mean or Median	To represent what the typical or average subject is like.
Range of scores	To indicate how spread out the scores are.
Pearson correlation; Kendall's tau; Spearman's rho	To reflect the degree of relationship between two variables.
Chi square	To reflect a relationship between two variables for categorical data.
T-test	To test if there is a difference between the mean scores of two groups.
Analysis of variance	An extension of the *t*-test to test if there are significant differences among mean scores of 3 or more groups or with two or more independent variables.

categorical. In *experimental* or *quasiexperimental* studies, when the investigator wishes to compare two groups on continuous data, the *t*-test might be used. If there are more than two groups or more than one independent variable, analysis of variance might be used.

All statistics require that certain assumptions be met. For example, using analysis of variance usually assumes that the group sizes are equal (although there are some conditions when group sizes are unequal). When you consult with a statistician or nurse researcher about the appropriateness of your statistical procedures, your consultation is based partly on the extent to which these assumptions have been met. Good basic courses in statistics also will prepare you to evaluate a study on this basis.

Hellmann and Grimm (1984) present an example of the use of multiple kinds of statistics (in Chapter 4 of this book). In this study, "The Influence of Talking on Diastolic Blood Pressure Readings," the investigators reported the mean diastolic blood pressure as 87.10 in the "no talking" condition, as 88.96 in the "talking during cuff inflation" condition, and as 95.35 in the "talking during entire procedure" condition. These three means convey useful descriptive information for practicing nurses. Hellmann and Grimm also used the inferential statistical procedure of analysis of variance to determine if the differences among these means are larger than would have been expected by chance alone. Based on this analysis, they found that "reading conditions have a significant effect on diastolic blood pressure, $F(2.94) = 74.07, p < .0001$ ... the mean diastolic blood pressure increases as the amount of talking during a particular treatment condition increases" (p. 255). Then they employed Dunn's procedure to show that the mean diastolic blood pressure readings under both talking conditions were significantly higher ($p < .01$) than that when no talking was allowed.

In the last sentence of the previous paragraph, the $p < .01$ refers to the statistical significance of the findings as well as the probability of making what statistician's call a Type I error. What this "$p < .01$" means is that *if* the mean diastolic blood pressure in the "no talking" condition was really *equal* to the mean diastolic blood pressure in the "talking during entire procedure" (i.e., talking does not really have any effect at all on blood pressure), then obtaining a difference in mean blood pressure scores as large as the one obtained in this study would occur in less than 1 out of 100 studies conducted using the same method as Hellmann and Grimm's. In other words, if talking really has no effect at all on blood pressure, finding any difference between the mean blood pressure in the "no talking" and "talking" conditions would occur only because of chance, or what statisticians would call sampling error. Furthermore, finding a difference as large as that reported in the Hellmann and Grimm (1984) study by chance alone is highly improbable; it would occur less than once in every 100 similarly conducted studies. Because it is so improbable that such a large difference would occur by chance alone, the researcher concludes that the large difference is a real difference caused by a patient's talking during the blood pressure reading procedure.

Although the use of statistical hypothesis testing is more complicated than the above description, most researchers usually require that the statistical significance of a specific result be .05 or smaller before they consider that result significant. Most of the significance tests in nursing research involve a comparison of the central tendency (e.g., means) of two or more groups to see if they are different from one another or a test of whether a relationship (e.g., a correlation) between two variables is large enough to conclude the two variables are associated in some way.

Conclusion. As you read a researcher's conclusions based on the results of his or her study, you might want to review some of the conceptual and methodological issues we have presented in this chapter and see whether you think the researcher should have commented on such issues in explaining or qualifying his or her findings. In general, we think that a researcher should not suggest that there is a difference between two groups or that a relationship exists between two variables unless the statistical evidence supporting such findings is significant. In other words, a researcher should not discuss statistically nonsignificant findings as if they were significant. On the other hand, the presence of a statistically significant finding does not necessarily mean that the finding has clinical importance.

The question of whether or not a statistically significant finding is clinically significant is important to address when considering the use of the research in practice. When a finding is statistically significant, it is quite unlikely that the finding is due to chance. For example, in the Brown and Hurlock (1975) study on breast preparation for breast feeding, three methods were studied for their effectiveness in reducing nipple pain and trauma. The investigators determined that nipple rolling was significantly effective in preventing nipple trauma. This statement of statistical significance means only that if the study were repeated 100 times, drawing from the same population of mothers, 95 times out of 100 nipple rolling would be found to be effective. Another way of saying this is that there are 5 chances out of 100 that the finding of nipple rolling effectiveness is due to chance alone. Yet another way of saying this is that we can be 95 percent confident that nipple rolling is effective in reducing nipple trauma. There are several ways that investigators, in the design of their study, can improve their chances of finding statistically significant differences if such differences truly exist. One way is to increase the sample size. With a very large sample size, not much difference between group means is required to have statistically significant findings.

Clearly, statistical significance is not the same as clinical significance. Brown and Hurlock (1975) indicate that their finding is not clinically significant. Although they do not provide reason for this judgment, it is probably related to the small magnitude of difference between the two groups. For example, suppose that nipple trauma were rated on a scale of 1 to 5, with 1 being practically no apparent trauma and 5 being redness and cracking. (Since insufficient information is provided, we don't actually know how nipple trauma was measured in this study.) Let us suppose that the average nipple trauma for the experimental group is 3.2 and the control group is 3.8. If the sample size is large enough, this difference might be statistically significant, but there would be little practical difference in the mothers' perceptions of their nipple trauma. Hence, this would be considered a clinically insignificant result.

A study by Keller and Bzdek (1986) provides a positive illustration of clinical significance. In their study, they examined the effectiveness of therapeutic touch on tension headache pain. They describe therapeutic touch as a "modern derivative of the laying on of hands that involves touching with the intent to help or heal" (p. 101). They randomly divided 60 volunteer subjects with tension headaches into treatment and placebo groups. They used a standardized pain questionnaire to measure headache pain levels before each intervention, immediately afterward, and four hours later. They reported that the experimental group had a 77 percent decrease in pain scores from pretest levels while the control group experienced a 49 percent reduction. More striking was the report that the experimental group experienced a 66 percent reduction in pain intensity while the control group experienced only a 24 percent reduction. These differences are both statistically and clinically significant.

The judgment of clinical significance comes from at least two considerations: (1) an understanding of the measures used and how sensitive they may be to the phenomenon under study; and (2) what an individual patient's experience might be with the magnitude of change or difference in the measure employed. The former should be information which is at least partially provided in the research report. The latter may be based largely on your own clinical experience and observations.

Regardless of whether the findings are statistically significant or not, the researcher should discuss their theoretical and clinical importance. The researcher also should discuss any limitations of the study or other variables that might have influenced the findings by making them appear more or less significant than they actually are. If the findings were not as expected or not statistically significant, the researcher should provide a reasonable explanation. Such an explanation should include consideration of the issues discussed in this chapter and describe the adequacy of the sample, psychometric quality of the measures, and strength of the intervention.

Critique Questions for Descriptive Qualitative Studies: Method

Sample. One of the first methodological features to be examined in a qualitative study is "who were the subjects?" The subjects should be representative of the phenomenon of interest. Note that this is a different concern than in quantitative studies in which the ideal is to select a sample who are representative of a population of people. Subjects who represent the phenomenon of interest make it possible for the researcher to learn about the experiences of these subjects with that phenomenon. Subjects in qualitative research are frequently referred to as informants since they provide such direct access to the phenomenon.

For qualitative research to result in complete descriptions of a nursing phenomenon, the subjects must be accessed carefully, making sure to tap all possible experiences with and viewpoints about the phenomenon. Such a sample is termed *theoretical* (Glaser & Strauss, 1967). When all views have been tapped, the researcher finds that data from additional subjects yields no new information, only a confirmation of what previous subjects have said. When this happens, the concept, or category of interest, is termed *saturated*.

Suppose, for example, that an investigator is conducting a study to answer the research question "How do new postpartum parents cope with sleep deprivation?" The sample of subjects would not be appropriate if it included pregnant women, or hospital labor-and-delivery nurses, as subjects. Neither has an ongoing experience with the phenomenon of interest, even thought they might have heard someone else's account of the experiences. Appropriate subjects might initially be new parents of both sexes, who have a variety of home situations which are likely to influence the amount of sleep they are able to get (e.g., the presence of another adult in the home to help with night feedings). The range of home situations would be important to sample since new information about coping with sleep deprivation might be obtained from famlies with differing situations.

Data Collection. Data collection devices in qualitative research are frequently observations or

Figure 3.6
Believability of Results: Questions for Descriptive Qualitative Studies

1. *Methods:*
   - Is the sampling adequate to tap all viewpoints on the nursing phenomenon and to saturate the concept(s)?
   - Does the investigator report his or her data gathering and analysis process in some detail, describing changes in data collection and reasons for such changes?

2. *Results:*
   - Are the observations that support each concept internally consistent? Do the observations in one category seem more similar to each other or to observations put in other categories?
   - Are the categories representative of the group of observations? What else might the observations suggest in addition to, or different from, the categories as they are named or defined?
   - Are there concepts which did not emerge but which you would have expected from your clinical experience? Would the sample used in the study have yielded these concepts or were different types of subjects needed?
   - Are relationships between and among concepts as described by the investigator supported by the data? Do these relationships make sense to you? Are there other possible related concepts?
   - Does the investigator describe changes in the coding categories as data analysis proceeds?

Pause for Reflection:

The set of questions addressing methodology identify potentially critical issues. If any of these aspects is not adequately addressed in the research report, it *may* be grounds for the reader to decide on nonutilization—depending on the risk involved in using the results and depending on the availability of other studies which corroborate the results of this study.

If the methodological issues are adequately addressed, the reader then evaluates if the results described and conclusions drawn are appropriate. There frequently will be other explanations/conclusions than those that the investigator provides; negative review on this aspect is not sufficient by itself to decide on nonutilization. However, if results can be clearly attributed to factors other than those raised in the original research question, additional caution in using the study is warranted.

---

interviews, often unstructured interviews. If an interview guide is used, the researcher should report how the guide was developed and what types of responses are expected from using it. If more than one person collects data, whether an interview guide or an observational tool is used, the study should report the way in which the researcher ascertained that each person collected the data in a consistent way. This is similar to the reliability issue for instruments. In qualitative research, the data collectors themselves are the data collection instruments. When two or more researchers work together on a study, they should report how they determined if they observed or interviewed in a consistent way, particularly if there was no interview guide or observational tool.

Results.   Analysis of qualitative data is quite different from analysis of quantitative data. In the latter, the data are used, in part, to determine the extent to which predicted relationships exist. In an experimental study, it is predicted that the experimental group will do better (e.g., show more of a trait) than the control gorup; data are gathered and statistical tests are used to determine if there is a difference between the two groups. In the analysis of qualitative data, the purpose often is to generate a theory rather than to test it. According to Phillips (1986), the process of inductive reasoning is used, that is, ''supporting logical relationships by using specific observations to formulate general theoretical statements'' (p. 124). Thus the qualitative researcher classifies specific observations together according to rules that guide the clustering of these observations into categories. Then a category or concept label is derived from the meaning of the observations within the category. As observations are clustered a more general or abstract label, like an umbrella, is developed to subsume or cover all previous categories (Spradley, 1979; Phillips, 1986).

Unlike quantitative studies, qualitative exploratory and descriptive studies use an interactive process to draw conclusions, even early in the study. The interaction is between the data, the researcher's analytic thinking, and the subjects who may be asked to provide more information and to confirm findings. Qualitative methods require that data analysis be concurrent with data collections. The data analysis involves drawing tentative conclusions about categories. These tentative conclusions will be continually modified and refined as new data are collected and analyzed. The emergent conclusions guide the collection of subsequent data. Thus, it is not uncommon for the researcher to modify interview questions during the course of the study, if only to focus them with greater clarity on the concepts as they emerge from the data. Olshansky (1987) illustrates this in Chapter 5 of this book.

Throughout the data analysis process, the researcher reads, codes, and organizes data, then recodes and reorganizes to reflect higher levels of conceptual analysis. The actual data and concepts grounded in actual data guide the researcher toward final conclusions. As the researcher analyzes the data, he or she selectively samples pertinent literature to help substantiate conceptualizations. The researcher also will selectively sample additional subjects to test findings, and refine the resultant analysis to validate or refute initial, tentative conclusions. From these interactive processes of data collection and analysis, concepts are generated and refined.

Because of the interactive process between researcher and data, and between data collection and data analysis, the researcher should leave an "audit trail" behind him or her in the report (Lincoln & Guba, 1985). Such an audit trail provides the reader, or another researcher, the benefit of insight into the researcher's thought processes during analysis and resultant alterations in data gathering. When the reader knows the process steps taken by the researcher, the ideas considered, and the decision points, he or she can assess conclusions for believability by placing him or herself in the place of the researcher.

The questions included in the critique guidelines relate to: (1) the internal consistency of the concepts derived during the analysis; (2) the representativeness of the categories in terms of the observations identified; (3) the extent to which the concepts that have emerged are what you would expect from your clinical experience; (4) the relationships among concepts and the extent to which the data support these relationships; and (5) the adequacy of the description of the data analysis process, specifically the major modifications in coding categories that occurred during the data collection and analysis processes.

Key to evaluating the findings and conclusions of a qualitative study are your own clinical observations of the phenomenon under study. You should examine the researcher's empirically grounded concepts and supporting data to determine if they represent your own experience with the phenomenon. In addition, you will want to examine the extent to which the data are similar to your observations of the phenomenon, considering similarities and differences between your clients and the informants for the study.

Summary. The set of questions addressing believability of results, for all studies and for studies classified by type, does not include all aspects that an experienced reviewer looks for in doing a critique. However, they touch on major areas we have found to contribute to our confidence in research findings and our willingness to implement research results in practice. If any of these aspects is not adequately addressed in the research report, it *may* be grounds for you to decide on nonutilization—depending on the risk involved in using the results and on the availability of other studies that corroborate the results of this study. Frequently, there will be at least one or two method areas which could have benefitted from further elaboration or clarity. However, before rejecting a study on methodological grounds alone, particularly one that otherwise holds promise for usefulness in your practice, we recommend continuing the evaluation of the study for its generalizability and for evaluation of potential risks and costs.

Generalizability of Results

To determine if the results of the study are applicable in your setting and with your patients, consider these several factors. The first set of questions addresses the extent to which the sample and setting are similar to your patients and setting. Questions about sampling procedures used and, therefore, the presumed representativeness of the sample are salient here. If the researcher uses random selection from the target population of both persons and settings, then you might assume that your setting and patients are sufficiently similar to the sample included in the study. However, true random selection is rarely possible in clinical research. Therefore, you must rely on the researcher's description of the sample to ensure that persons similar to those you wish to generalize the results to were included in the sample; similarly you must evaluate the representativeness of settings. You must ascertain if those who implemented the procedures in the study were like those who might implement the procedures in your setting. It may be that special training will be required for you to use the interventions in your practice.

Often the study sample and setting will differ from the sample and setting that you wish to generalize. In this case, replication of the study takes on great importance. If replication has occurred, if other researchers have tested and supported the theory in a variety of studies, and if these other researchers have evaluated the measure with several different samples, then the reader can have greater confidence in the results—and in achieving some degree of success in using the research in decision making with specific patients. However, with nursing research still in its infancy (or perhaps early childhood), replication is more the exception than the rule. We do not believe, however, that use of research in practice should be limited only to those studies that have been replicated. Instead, we encourage you to consider the possibility of replication in your own practice and to evaluate the costs, risks, and benefits of using and of not using the research.

Other Factors to Consider in Utilization

In this part of the guidelines, we suggest questions which can be addressed either from the standpoint of the individual nurse making a judgment as to whether to use the research in the care of a particular patient or from the standpoint of the nurse instituting a major change in practice

Figure 3.7
Evaluation of Generalizability of the Results

1. Are there similarities between the methods and procedures of the study and those typically employed in current practice? Specifically:
   - Is the sample and setting similar or dissimilar to the sample and setting which you wish to generalize (target population)?
   - Were the individuals doing the testing typical of practicing nurses? Were they specially trained?
   - In an experimental study, were the individuals implementing the intervention typical or were they specially selected or trained?
2. Are you aware of other studies that address the same problem, test the same intervention, evaluate the same measure or test the same theory (replication)? Were the results similar to the results obtained in the present study?

Pause for Reflection:

In the ideal situation, there will be considerable similarity between the study sample, procedures, and the target population, *and* the study will have been replicated. The nurse can have confidence in the study findings and have more confidence in using the study in his or her practice. More frequently, one or both of the above criteria are not met. If, however, the study has met other criteria, and it is possible to do systematic evaluation of the use of the study in practice, then utilization is recommended. Failure to meet the criteria of generalizability, alone, is not sufficient justification for a non-utilization decision.

---

throughout the institution. If the intended scope is the latter, then you will need to anticipate a major effort in planning, with involvement of multiple groups. The questions in this section are designed to balance your judgment about utility and merit of the research with practical considerations. The consideration of these questions allows for the decision to use some research which may not meet all the criteria for scientific merit, but which holds some promise of leading to beneficial outcomes.

Figure 3.8
Other Factors to Consider in Utilization

1. What is the feasibility of doing systematic evaluation of the research-based practice?
2. What are the benefits and risks using the research in practice? Do the benefits outweigh the risks? Consider:
   - What is the risk of changing practice based on the research?
   - What is the risk of maintaining current practice—that is, not trying the practice suggested by the research?
   - What are the benefits of changing practice?
3. What is the cost of changing practice based on this research? Do the potential benefits outweigh the costs?

Pause for Reflection and Final Judgment:

If the benefits outweigh the costs, there are virtually no risks, and it is feasible to systematically evaluate the outcomes, even with a single patient, it is appropriate, then, to proceed using the research in clinical practice. This is true, even if not all the criteria for scientific merit have been met. If costs are high or there is some risk involved, and some aspect of scientific merit is questionable, then additional research should be conducted before practice is changed based on the research.

The first question, that of the feasibility of doing a systematic evaluation of the research-based practice, is critical regardless of the strengths of the research report and the degree of generalizability evident. As Barlow, Hayes, and Nelson (1984) have pointed out, the individual clinician's decision to use research for an individual patient rests on the judgments that: (1) the patient to which he or she wishes to apply the new practice is like the average patient in the study who benefitted from the practice; and (2) that a clinically significant improvement will result from the research-based practice when only statistically significant results have been reported. It would greatly advance the science of nursing if nurses in practice, who attempt to use research-based practices, would document the effectiveness (or ineffectiveness) of the practice with individual patients. Such documentation is the result of planning for systematic evaluation.

The remaining questions probe risk and cost/benefit issues. Both the risk of changing practice based on the research and the risk of not changing practice should be explored. You may make a judgment that the latter risk is greater and, therefore, decide to implement the practice even though other criteria have not been completely met. You may find that, although benefits in patient outcomes might accrue from a change in practice, such benefits are not of sufficient magnitude to warrant the added cost. You must consider each of these practical aspects before deciding whether to implement an institution-wide change in practice or not.

CONCLUSION

Research in nursing has the potential to contribute substantially to quality of patient care. But this potential can only be realized if the research base is critically evaluated and used appropriately as a basis for practice. At best, research will always only be a guide for practice. The astute clinician will combine his or her practical wisdom derived from experience, with an understanding of the individual patient's situation, and with knowledge derived from research to make a clinical judgment thought to be of benefit to the patient.

REFERENCES

Alexy, B. (1985). Goal setting and health risk reduction. *Nursing Research, 34,* 283–288.

Barlow, D. H., Hayes, S. C., & Nelson, R. O. (1984). *The scientist practitioner: Research and accountability in clinical and educational settings.* New York: Pergamon Press.

Barnes, C. A., & Kirchhoff, T.K. (1986). Minimizing hypoxemia due to endotracheal suctioning: A review of the literature. *Heart and Lung: The Journal of Critical Care, 15,* 164–178.

Bergstrom, N., Braden, B. J., Laguzza, A., & Holman, V. (1987). The Braden Scale for predicting pressure sore risk. *Nursing Research, 36,* 205–210.

Brailey, L. J. (1986). Effects of health teaching in the workplace on women's knowledge, beliefs and practices regarding breast self-examination. *Research in Nursing and Health, 9,* 223–231.

Brown, J. S., Tanner, C. A., & Padrick, K. P. (1984). Nursing's search for knowledge. *Nursing Research, 33,* 26–32.

Brown, M. S., & Hurlock, J. T. (1975). Preparation of the breast for breastfeeding. *Nursing Research, 24,* 448–551.

Cook, T. D., & Campbell, D. T. (1979). *Quasi-Experimentation: Design and analysis issues for field settings.* Chicago: Rand McNalley.

Cotanch, P. H., & Strum, S. (1987). Progressive muscle relaxation as antiemetic therapy for cancer patients. *Oncology Nursing Forum, 14*(1), 33–37.

Davidhizar, R. E., Austin, J. K., & McBride, A. B. (1986). Attitudes of patients with schizophrenia toward taking medication, *Research in Nursing and Health, 9,* 139–146.

Glaser, B. G., & Strauss, A. L. (1967). *The Discovery of grounded theory: Strategies for qualitative research.* Chicago: Aldine Publishing Company.

Hellmann, R., & Grimm, S. A. (1984). The influence of talking on diastolic pressure readings. *Research in Nursing and Health, 7,* 253–256.

Johnson, J. E. (1972). Effects of structuring patients' expectations on their reactions to threatening events. *Nursing Research, 21,* 499–504.

Johnson, J. E. (1973). Effects of accurate expectations about sensations on the sensory and distress components of pain. *Journal of Personality and Social Psychology, 27,* 261–275.

Johnson, J. E., Morrissey, J. F., & Leventhal, H. (1973). Psychological preparation for endoscopic examination. *Gastrointestinal Endoscopy, 19,* 180–182.

Johnson, J. E., & Rice, V. H. (1974). Sensory and distress components of pain: Implications for the study of clinical pain. *Nursing Research, 23,* 203–209.

Johnson, J. E., Kirchhoff, K. T., & Endress, M. P. (1975). Altering children's distress behavior during orthopedic cast removal. *Nursing Research, 24,* 404–410.

Jordan-Marsh, M. (1985). Development of a tool for diagnosing changes in concern about exercise: A means for enhancing compliance. *Nursing Research, 34,* 103–107.

Keller, E., & Bdzek, V. M. (1986). Effects of therapeutic touch on tension headache pain. *Nursing Research, 35,* 101–105.

Lamontagne, L. L., Mason, K. R., & Hepworth, J. T. (1985). Effects of relaxation on anxiety in children: Implications of coping with stress. *Nursing Research, 34,* 289–292.

Lincoln, Y. S., & Guba, E. G. (1985). *Naturalistic inquiry.* Beverly Hills: Sage Publications.

Norbeck, J. S., & Tilden, V. P. (1983). Life stress, social support, and emotional disequilibrium in complications of pregnancy: A prospective, multivariate study. *Journal of Health and Social Behavior, 24,* 30–46.

Nunnally, J. C. (1978). *Psychometric theory* (2nd ed.). New York: McGraw-Hill.

Olshansky, E. F. (1987). Identity of self as infertile: An example of theory-generating research. *Advances in Nursing Science, 9*(2), 54–63.

Phillips, L. R. F. (1986). *A clinician's guide to the critique and utilization of nursing research.* New York: Appleton-Century-Crofts.

Robb, S. S. (1985). Urinary incontinence verification in elderly men. *Nursing Research, 34,* 278–282.

Spradley, J. (1979). *The ethnographic interview.* New York: Holt, Rinehart, & Winston.

Strickland, O. L., & Waltz, C. F. (1986). Measurement of research variables in nursing. In P. Chinn (Ed.), *Nursing research methodology: Issues and implementation*. Rockville, MD: Aspen, pp. 79-90.

Tanner, C. A. (1987). Evaluating research for use in practice: Guidelines for the clinician. *Heart and Lung: The Journal of Critical Care, 16*, 424–430.

Tudor, G. E. (1952). A sociopsychiatric nursing approach to intervention in a problem of mutual withdrawal on a mental hospital ward. *Psychiatry: Journal for the Study of Interpersonal Processes, 15*(2). Reprinted in *Perspectives in Psychiatric Care*, 1970, 8(1), 11–35.

Walike, B. C., Padilla, G., Bergstrom, N., Hanson, R. L., Kubo, W., Grant, M., & Wong, H. L. (1975). Patient problems related to tube feeding. In M. V. Batey (Ed.), *Communicating nursing research: Critical issues in access to data*. Boulder, CO: Western Interstate Commission for Higher Education in Nursing.

Winslow, E. H., Lane, L. D., & Gaffney, F. A. (1985). Oxygen uptake and cardiovascular responses in control adults and acute myocardial infarction patients during bathing. *Nursing Research, 34*, 164–169.

Wolfer, J. A., & Visintainer, M. A. (1975). Pediatric surgical patients' and parents' stress responses and adjustment. *Nursing Research, 24*, 244–255.

4

Basic Concepts, Skills, and Procedures

Charold Baer, PhD, RN
Dorothy Bomber, BSN, RN
Audrey Nickodemus, BSN, RN

INTRODUCTION BY: CHAROLD L. BAER, PhD, RN

There are numerous skills and procedures inherent in the practice of nursing. Concomitant with those skills and procedures are clinical decisions that guide their performance in the practice setting often involving modifications in the technique for performing a specific skill or procedure, or factors that interfere with the correct performance of a procedure. Unfortunately, few of the multitude of skills and procedures involved in patient care have a research base to guide their implementation or modification in practice. Instead, nurses usually use tradition and intuition to guide the clinical decision making related to skills and procedures. Nurses also continue to ask the difficult questions surrounding the performance of skills and procedures. They want to know why a specific procedure should be done in a certain way, or at a certain time. They want to know how certain patient characteristics, activities, or responses will affect the performance of skills and procedures.

Fortunately, such questions have had a practical effect. Today more nurses are conducting research related to basic skills and procedures than ever before. In addition, while many of the initial studies were descriptive, more recently, nurses have focused their research efforts on correlational or experimental designs. The studies selected for inclusion in this chapter demonstrate the progress occurring in this area of clinical practice research.

Keen's study was included for two major reasons: (1) it used an experimental design to evaluate the effectiveness of two types of intramuscular injection techniques in reducing site discomfort and lesion formation, and (2) the phenomenon of interest is of concern to almost every clinician. The results, accompanied by other supporting studies, could significantly impact nursing practice and patient care. In addition, the investigators' efforts to quantify such a subjective response as pain, as well as the objective response of lesion formation, are worthy of consideration. Potential utilization of the results for clinicians is included in a section entitled "Clinical Implications." The inclusion of this section demonstrates an awareness of the need to involve clinicians in the change process if research is to have significant impact on nursing practice.

The article by Hellmann and Grimm was included because it addresses a patient variable that may interfere with the accuracy of the results obtained from the implementation of a basic procedure: the effect of patient talking on diastolic blood pressure measurements. This study is an example of research involving variables that could impact the clinical decision making surrounding the performance of a skill or procedure. Such studies may increase the clinician's awareness of the many other variables that are present in patient care that might interfere with the accuracy of results obtained from performing routine skills or procedures. In addition, the methodology and definition of the variables are worthy of note.

The Samples, Van Cott, Long, King, and Kersenbrock study was selected for inclusion because it addresses an assessment parameter that is frequently measured and used in clinical decision making by practicing clinicians. In addition, it demonstrates what appears to be a mismatch between one of the questions being asked and the study design. Furthermore, it indirectly validates that clinical decision making, professional autonomy, and overall assessment parameters are more useful in patient care, than is a single assessment parameter, whether it is performed routinely or in concert with circadian rhythm changes.

These three studies are reflective of the maturational process that continues as the data base accumulates for answering the practitioner's questions related to basic skills and procedures.

Comparison of Intramuscular Injection Techniques to Reduce Site Discomfort and Lesions

Mary Frances Keen, DNSc, RN
Associate Professor
School of Nursing
University of Miami
Coral Gables, FL

The Z-track intramuscular injection technique was compared with the standard injection technique for incidence and severity of discomfort and lesions at the injection site. Fifty subjects received injections of meperidine hydrochloride alone or in combination with promethazine hydrochloride every 3 to 4 hours for a total of two to eight injections. Subjects served as their own controls by receiving both techniques. They were evaluated for the presence and severity of discomfort on a 4-point Likert scale. Injection site lesions were determined by visualization and palpation. The Z-track technique significantly decreased incidence of selected descriptors of discomfort and lesions at selected time intervals, severity of discomfort at selected time intervals, and severity of lesions at all time intervals postinjection.

Intramuscular injections are a common therapeutic technique performed by nurses. However, adverse effects of frequent injections may include pain (Joubert, de Menezes, & Fernandez, 1972; Travell, 1955) and the formation of cutaneous, subcutaneous, and intramuscular lesions (Aberfield, Bienenstock, Shapiro, Namba, & Grob, 1968; DeHaan, Schellenberg, & Sobota, 1974; Hanson, 1966). The purpose of this study was to compare the effects of Z-track intramuscular injection and standard intramuscular injection techniques on the incidence and severity of discomfort and lesions in subjects receiving frequent injections. Although the Z-track technique has periodically been recommended for all intramuscular injections, the technique has primarily been reserved for use with iron dextran preparations which are known to be particularly irritating and permanently staining to the subcutaneous tissues.

REVIEW OF THE LITERATURE

Although reports of adverse effects secondary to injection therapy in selected patients are common in the literature, the actual frequency of such occurrences is insufficiently documented. Roberts (1975) conducted a systematic study to determine the frequency of discomfort and skin reactions in a hospitalized population receiving injections as part of a prescribed medical regimen. Prolonged discomfort was defined as any pain, burning, numbness, or other uncomfortable sensation experienced by the subject longer than 15 minutes after an intramuscular injection; prolonged discomfort was noted in 20 of the 60 subjects (33%).

Roberts (1975) defined injection site lesions as any palpable or observable aberration (e.g., ecchymosis, erythema, papules, or nodules) at the injection site. Fifty-three subjects (88%) had at least one visible injection site lesion; nine of the lesions were judged to be unacceptable injection reactions (e.g., one or more nodules). Subjects with acceptable injection reactions received a mean number of 16.3 injections; those with unacceptable reactions received a mean number of 25.7 injections. Roberts' study suggests that the population at highest risk are patients receiving repeated injections over a period of days or weeks.

One suggested cause for the development of lesions and subsequent postinjection discomfort has been the deposition of the injected solution into the subcutaneous tissue rather than the intended musculature. Erroneous deposition of the injected solution may be due to a variety of factors, e.g., needles of insufficient length. The leakage of solution into the subcutaneous tissue after withdrawal of the needle due to the use of a straight injection pathway is another suggested factor. Shaffer (1929), using roentgenograms of intramuscular injections of heavy metals, e.g., bismuth, demonstrated that a straight injection pathway, such as that created by a standard intramuscular injection, permits flowback of injected solution along the injection path. Shaffer also demonstrated on roentgenogram that a broken injection pathway produced by the Z-track injection method would prevent this flowback of injected solution.

HYPOTHESES

I. The incidence and degree of severity of subject discomfort will be less following administration of the Z-track intramuscular injection technique than following administration of the standard intramuscular injection technique.

II. The incidence and degree of severity of injection site lesions will be less following administration of the Z-track intramuscular injection technique than following administration of the standard intramuscular injection technique.

METHOD

Sample

A sample of 50 subjects was chosen, based on review of the literature and consultation with a statistician. Thirty-seven subjects were male, 13 were female; 30 subjects were black, 20 were white. Ages ranged from 21 to 57 years (M age = 35.5 years ± 5.3 years). The largest part of the sample were diagnosed as acute and/or chronic pancreatitis (34%) or sickle cell anemia (28%); these two diagnoses were prevalent because the study required that subjects be receiving prescribed doses of intramuscular meperidine hydrochloride at regular intervals. All subjects were within 20% limits of normal weight for height (Metropolitan Life Insurance Company, 1959) and gave informed consent.

The convenience sample was composed of available subjects who met the study requirements and who had no interfering illnesses, such as generalized or localized edema or coagulation abnormalities, or preexisting injection site aberrations, such as skin rash, neurosensory loss, or unilateral changes.

Subjects were inpatients on selected medical and surgical units of a university medical center hospital. They received a minimum of two intramuscular injections of meperidine hydrochloride alone or in combination with promethazine hydrochloride every 3 to 4 hours as part of a prescribed medical regimen. Individual subjects received the same medication or combination of medications at each injection.

Measurement: Discomfort was interpreted as subjects' experience of burning, stinging, aching, being sore, or hurting when touched or moving the leg. Intensity of the sensation was rated on a 4-point Likert scale (0-3) by descriptors of none, mild, moderate, or severe. The discomfort questionnaire was administered by the nurse researcher verbally after each injection (one treatment interval postinjection) and by the research assistant each evening the subject was enrolled in the study.

Site lesions at the time of injection were interpreted as the development of resistance to needle penetration, resistance to injection of the solution, or seepage of the injected solution from the injection site following withdrawal of the needle.

Postinjection site lesions were interpreted as a finding of (a) pigmentation changes observed by comparison with the surrounding skin color (the site was measured for color using a paint chip color scale and for size using a clear metric ruler); (b) skin sloughing measured by observation for local peeling or flaking of skin; (c) swelling as determined by palpation and measurement with a clear metric ruler; and (d) induration as determined by palpation and measurement with a clear metric ruler.

If an area of discoloration, swelling, or induration was irregularly shaped, the size was recorded by using a clear piece of cellophane and a black felt-tip marking pen to duplicate the area. At the conclusion of the study, areas of discoloration, induration, or swelling were reproduced on 3 × 5 cards and sorted by three nurses to determine a scale of severity for point assignment. Observations of injection site lesions were recorded by the researcher at the time of injection, at the time of each subsequent injection (two treatment intervals postinjection), and by the research assistant each evening the subject was enrolled in the study.

Pilot Study: Interrater reliability was established during a pilot study using eight subjects. The subjects were examined by the nurse researcher using the measures of site lesions, given an injection, and then interviewed using the measures of discomfort. One-half hour later, the subjects were reexamined and interviewed by the research assistant. Scores were compared using the Pearson product moment correlation test. Interrater reliability for measures of discomfort was $\tau = .88$; interrater reliability for measures of site lesions was $\tau = .70$.

Procedure

Subjects were assigned to a treatment group upon entry into the study by use of a table of random numbers. Treatment Group A received the Z-track technique in the left ventrogluteal site and the standard technique in the right ventrogluteal site; Treatment Group B received the standard technique in the left ventrogluteal site and the Z-track technique in the right ventrogluteal site. By receiving both injection techniques, subjects served as their own controls, given the assumption that the right and left ventrogluteal sites were not significantly different, a criterion for entry into the study. Information as to the specific injection method being used in each site was withheld from the research assistant, the subjects, and the staff nurses caring for the subjects.

The right and left ventrogluteal sites were used exclusively during the course of the study and had not been used for at least one month prior to entry into the study. Subjects began the study with the first injection in the left ventrogluteal site, and the method of injection (standard or Z-track) remained constant for the site. The ventrogluteal site was chosen because of the absence of major nerves and blood vessels, the visibility of the site, and the infrequency with which the site is used by others.

All injections were given by the nurse researcher with a 1½-inch, 22-gauge, disposable needle with a 3cc disposable syringe. The meperidine hydrochloride was withdrawn from a single dose vial using one needle. If the subject was to also receive promethazine hydrochloride, the medication was drawn into the syringe following the meperidine hydrochloride. Then ¼cc of air was drawn into the syringe, and the needle was changed to another 1½-inch, 22-gauge needle. The total volume of medication received in each injection varied from 0.75 to 3cc ($M = 1.65 \pm 0.65$cc). The most frequently occurring volume was 1cc (30%). During the study, volumes received in the right and left ventrogluteal sites remained equal but not necessarily constant. For example, at injections 1 and 2, a subject might have received 1cc in each site, but at injections 3 and 4, the subject could have received 2cc in each site.

Subjects were placed in a side-lying position with the upper leg flexed in a 20° angle (Kruszewski, Lang, & Johnson, 1979), and the ventrogluteal area was adequately exposed. The area was examined by visualization and palpation for the presence of tenderness or lesions that would prohibit further use of the site. Subjects' report of pain or extreme discomfort precluded use of the site.

The ventrogluteal site was localized using the procedure described by von Hochstetter (1956). Four injection points within the designated site were used by the investigator for purposes of site rotation. A maximum of four injections per ventrogluteal site was given due to the limited size of the area.

The skin was cleansed with two 70% isopropyl alcohol swabs using a circular motion, starting at the center and moving outward, for a period of 15 seconds for each swab (Story, 1952). The alcohol was then allowed to dry. Needle puncture was made rapidly to a depth of 1½ inches at a near 90° angle to the skin with the needle directed slightly upward toward the crest of the ilium (von Hochstetter, 1956). The needle was aspirated for five seconds (Stokes, Beerman, & Ingraham, 1944); if clear of blood, the fluid was injected with a slow, steady pressure over a period of 10 seconds/cc (Zelman, 1961). The needle was withdrawn rapidly and light finger massage was applied with a dry 2 × 2 gauze square for 15 seconds (Zelman, 1961). The Z-track technique differed from the standard technique only in the use of lateral displacement of the cutaneous tissues prior to site cleansing and needle insertion. The lateral tension was released immediately after withdrawal of the needle.

Immediately following the injection, the subject was questioned about feelings of discomfort at the present injection site as well as the prior injection site. Each evening the subject was in the study the research assistant examined the left and right sites by visualization and palpation and questioned the subject about discomfort in both sites.

Data Analysis: Data were tabulated to determine incidence of discomfort and site lesions at four time intervals: immediately postinjection, one treatment interval postinjection (discomfort only), two treatment intervals postinjection (lesions only), and in the evening of each day. Frequencies of discomfort and lesions of specific descriptors were examined using chi square. Discomfort and lesions scores were examined using a t test for related measures.

RESULTS

During the course of the study 240 injections were given. The total number of injections administered to each subject varied from two to eight; the most frequent numbers were four (40%) and six (44%). Each subject received an equal number of injections in the left and right ventrogluteal sites. The treatment interval between injections varied from 2.5 to 5 hours (M time interval = 3.5 ± 1 hour). The interval between injections for each subject remained constant at the time interval ordered by the physician and requested by the subject (± .5 hours). Seventeen subjects (34%) received only meperidine hydrochloride, and 33 subjects (66%) received the combination of meperidine hydrochloride and promethazine hydrochloride.

Incidence of Discomfort: Immediately postinjection, 45 of the 50 subjects (90%) reported the presence of some form of discomfort with the standard technique, and 43 subjects (86%) reported some form of discomfort with the Z-track technique. When complaints of discomfort immediately postinjection for the total number of injections given (N = 240) were examined, the presence of discomfort was noted for 95 of the 120 standard injections (79%) and 92 of the 120 Z-track injections (77%). At one treatment interval postinjection, 33 of the 50 subjects (66%) reported discomfort in the standard site, but 10 of the 50 subjects (20%) who had received the Z-track technique reported discomfort. When the total number of discomfort questionnaires administered at one-treatment interval (N = 190) was examined, discomfort was noted in 50 of the 95 standard injections (53%) and in 28 of the 95 Z-track injections (29%).

On the evening of the first study day, 19 of the 29 subjects (66%) who had received a standard injection as their last injection reported discomfort. Of the 21 subjects who had received the Z-track as their last injection, 14 (67%) reported discomfort; of these 21 subjects, 12 (57%) reported discomfort in the standard injection site (they had received a standard injection prior to the Z-track). Of the 29 subjects who had received a Z-track injection prior to the standard injection, 12 (41%) reported discomfort in the Z-track injection site.

When the frequencies of the specific descriptors of discomfort were examined using the chi-square test, the following complaints were found to be statistically significant: (a) The Z-track injection method caused a significantly greater number of hurt-when-touched responses (at the injection site) immediately postinjection, $x^2 = 4.47$, $p < .05$. (b) The standard injection method caused a significantly greater number of aches, $\chi^2 = 7.00$, $p < .05$, and hurts-when-touched responses, $\chi^2 = 6.19$, $p < .05$, at one-treatment interval postinjection. (c) The standard injection method caused a significantly greater number of aches, $\chi^2 = 5.39$, $p < .05$, and hurts, $\chi^2 = 1.50$, $p < .05$, during the first evening at the previous injection site.

Severity of Discomfort: Using a t test for related measures, combined discomfort scores for all time intervals, discomfort scores recorded immediately postinjection, and discomfort scores at one-treatment interval postinjection demonstrated no significant difference between the standard and Z-track injection techniques. However, discomfort scores in the evening of the subjects' first day in the study showed significance, supporting hypothesis I at $p < .02$, $t = 2.58$, $n = 50$.

Incidence of Lesions: At the time of injection, 35 incidences of resistance to needle penetration and to injection of solution, or seepage of solution from the injection site, were noted in a total of 120 standard injections (30%). Of the 120 Z-track injections, 13 incidences of resistance or seepage were recorded (11%).

At two-treatment intervals, when the site for reinjection was examined, the presence of a lesion was reported in 30 of the 72 observations (42%) at the site of a standard injection compared to 5 in 72 observations (7%) at the site of a Z-track injection. If the incidence of lesions is determined by number of subjects rather than by number of site observations, 22 of the 50 subjects (44%) had some type of lesion at the standard site; with use of the Z-track, only 12 of the 50 subjects (25%) had a lesion.

In the first evening of the study, lesions were reported in 20 of the 50 subjects (40%) at the standard injection site, compared with 8 of the 50 subjects (16%) at the Z-track site.

When frequencies of the specific indicators of injection site lesions were examined using chi square, the following indicators were found to be statistically significant: (a) The standard injection method was associated with significantly greater resistance to the injection of solution at the time of injection, $\chi^2 = 13.78$, $p < .05$. (b) The standard injection method caused a significantly greater number of pigmentation changes at two-treatment intervals post injection, $\chi^2 = 16.99$, $p < .05$. (c) The standard injection method caused a significantly greater number of pigmentation changes, $\chi^2 = 11.58$, $p < .05$, and swellings, $\chi^2 = 6.66$, $p < .05$, in the evening of the first day.

Severity of Lesions: Using a t test for related measures, the combined lesion scores for all observations demonstrated significance at the $p < .001$ level ($N = 50$) in support of the Z-track method, $t = 6.70$. Objective scores recorded at the time of injection, $t = 5.30$, and at two-treatment intervals postinjection, $t = 4.74$, also showed significance supporting hypothesis II at the $p < .001$ level. Objective scores recorded in the evening of the subject's first day on the study supported the hypothesis at the $p < .01$ level, ($t = 2.90$).

T tests for related measures performed on the specific indicators of injection site lesions demonstrated that the significant indicators were pigmentation changes at two-treatment intervals postinjection, $t = 2.48$, $p < .02$, pigmentation changes in the evening of the first day, $t = 3.86$, $p < .001$, and swelling in the first evening, $t = $

3.05, $p < .001$. Pearson product moment correlations were demonstrated at $p < .001$ between: (a) pigmentation changes at two-treatment intervals postinjection and in the first evening, $\tau = .40$; (b) pigmentation changes and swelling in the first evening, $\tau = .38$; (c) swelling and induration at two-treatment intervals, $\tau = .28$; (d) pigmentation changes at two-treatment intervals and swelling in the first evening, $\tau = .22$.

DISCUSSION

The mixed results in relation to the incidence of discomfort are interesting. Immediately postinjection the Z-track method increased the incidence of discomfort, but at one-treatment interval postinjection the discomfort was decreased. The same was true the evening of the first day for the site used previously but not for the site used most recently. These findings support a theory that the Z-track technique would not cause a decrease in the initial discomfort of injection; instead, the Z-track may affect discomfort secondary to leakage and deposition of the injected solution into the subcutaneous tissue.

This theory is further supported by findings related to the severity of discomfort. Subjective scores immediately postinjection and at one-treatment interval did not demonstrate a significant difference; however, subjective scores recorded in the evening of the first day did demonstrate that the Z-track method caused significantly less severe discomfort than did the standard method. A time interval may be necessary before injection lesions develop. Development of significant pigmentation changes and swelling at the standard site the first evening would support this explanation; expressions of discomfort thus would be assumed to coincide with lesion development.

Another possible explanation for the mixed results may be that the earlier complaints of discomfort were gathered by the nurse researcher, the same person who gave the injections. Complaints of discomfort in the evening were gathered by the research assistant. The research assistant may have been more objective in the manner of asking questions on the questionnaire, or the subjects may have been influenced by awareness of the testing situation and hesitant to report discomfort to the person giving the needed injection.

Although the potential for investigator bias may have been a major drawback of the study design, the pilot study determining interrater reliability on the measures of discomfort and lesions did not support this notion. If the observations of the research assistant only had been reported in this study, the hypotheses would continue to be supported by the severity of discomfort, $p < .02$, and lesions, $p < .01$, as well as the frequency of specific descriptors of complaints of aching and hurting, pigmentation changes, and swelling, $p < .05$.

Strengths of the design that helped minimize the effects of investigator bias were: (a) Subjects served as their own controls by receiving both injection techniques. (b) All injections were given by the nurse researcher in accordance with strict injection procedures. (c) The research assistant and the subjects were aware of the two techniques being investigated but knew nothing of the treatment method being used in each ventrogluteal site.

Clinical Implications: The results of this study illustrate that nurses can decrease the incidence and severity of injection site lesions and possible subsequent discomfort by using the Z-track injection method. Although this method has previously been reserved primarily for use with iron dextran preparations, the literature and theoretical framework suggest that the technique would be appropriate for all injections. This study points out that the method could be particularly helpful for patients who receive frequent injections over extended periods of time.

REFERENCES

Aberfield, D. C., Bienenstock, H., Shapiro, M. S., Namba, I., & Grob, D. (1968). Diffuse myopathy related to meperidine addiction in a mother and child. *Archives of Neurology, 19,* 384–388.

DeHaan, R. M., Schellenberg, M. A., & Sobota, J. T. (1974). Assessing local reactions and serum enzyme changes from intramuscular injections: A preliminary evaluation. *Journal of Clinical Pharmacology, 14,* 183–191.

Hanson, D.J. (1966). Acute and chronic lesions from intramuscular injections. *Hospital Formularly Management, 1*(9), 31–34.

Joubert, L., De Menezes, J. P., & Fernandez, C. A. (1972). Measurement of variations in pain associated with intramuscular injections. *Journal of International Medical Research, 1*, 61–64.

Kruszewski, A. Z., Lang, S. H., & Johnson, J. E. (1979). Effects of positioning on discomfort. *Nursing Research, 28* (2), 103–105.

Metropolitan Life Insurance Company (1959, November-December). New weight standards for men and women. *Statistical Bulletin, 40*, 1–4.

Roberts, R. A., (1975). *Frequency of discomfort and skin reactions from intramuscular injections*. Master's thesis. Case Western Reserve University, Cleveland, OH.

Shaffer, L. W. (1929). The fate of intragluteal injections. *Archives of Dermatology and Syphilogy, 19*, 347–364.

Stokes, J. H., Beerman, H., & Ingraham, R., Jr. (1944). *Modern clinical syphilogy* (3rd ed.). Philadelphia: W. B. Saunders, pp. 302–309.

Story, P. (1952). Testing of skin disinfectants. *British Medical Journal, 2*, 1128.

Travell, J. (1955). Factors affecting pain of injection. *Journal of the American Medical Association, 158*, 368–371.

von Hochstetter, A. V. (1956). Problems and technique of intragluteal injection. Part II. Influence of injection technique on the development of syringe injection injuries. *Schweizerische Medizinische Wochenschrift, 86*, 69–76.

Zelman, S. (1961). Notes on techniques of intramuscular injections. The avoidance of needless pain and morbidity. *American Journal of the Medical Sciences, 241*, 563–574.

This article is printed with permission of *Nursing Research*.
Copyright 1986 American Journal of Nursing Company.

Original article:
Keen, M. F. (1986). Comparison of intramuscular injection techniques to reduce site discomfort and lesions. *Nursing Research, 35*(4), 207–210.

CRITIQUE BY: DOROTHY BOMBER, BSN, RN

Part I: Clinical Relevance

The administration of medications is a major responsibility of clinical nurses. Because this includes giving injections, it would be beneficial to nurses to discover the least painful and injurious techniques to use in administering injections. Keen proposes that the Z-track technique, which "has primarily been reserved for use with preparations which are known to be particularly irritating and permanently staining to the subcutaneous tissues," might be the best method for giving all intramuscular injections.

It is not uncommon to see patients with bruises or localized swelling or redness at the site of an IM injection, or to hear them complain about painful "shots," sometimes even hours after the injection was administered. It would certainly be of benefit to these patients and their nurses to utilize a technique that minimizes the occurrence of such incidents.

In her literature review, Keen reports that the "population at highest risk for adverse effects secondary to injection therapy are patients receiving repeated injections over a period of days or weeks." Therefore, it follows that these are the patients who would benefit most from routine use of the Z-track technique, if it is in fact less injurious. Keen proposes, however, that all patients receiving IM injections could be best treated with routine use of the Z-track technique.

If a nurse accepted Keen's theory and chose to use this technique for all IM injections, it is within the scope of practice to do so without the permission of a physician or other health care professional. Both techniques are supposedly demonstrated to nurses during their education and the Z-track method is not reserved just for irritating solutions because it is otherwise damaging or dangerous. If this study remains sound after further evaluation and a nurse is convinced of the possible benefits of routinely using the Z-track method to give injections instead of the standard technique, and a review of the literature does not reveal possible adverse side effects of this technique, it is within the scope of a nurse's professional judgement to utilize the Z-track technique.

In short, the article appears to offer clinical relevance and potential utility for all nurse clinicians who administer IM injections.

Part II: Conceptualization and Internal Consistency

In the introductory portions of the study, Keen stated that her purpose was to investigate whether the Z-track technique would produce fewer adverse effects than the standard intramuscular injection technique. She then presented two hypotheses which logically followed this inquiry: that the Z-track technique would decrease "the incidence and degree of (1) subject discomfort and (2) injection site lesions" when compared with those following standard IM injections. Her study variables were clearly related to the independent variable, type of injection technique, and directly influenced the dependent variable, subject discomforts and lesions. In addition, the study design fit her purpose. Her sample consisted of patients who received multiple injections and thus were most at risk for experiencing adverse effects. These patients received both types of injections allowing for comparison and some degree of control. Following the treatment, the researchers interviewed the patients to obtain subjective discomfort information, measured the lesions with rulers, and evaluated the skin color with paint chips for objective data regarding the severity of resultant lesions.

Ultimately, the conclusions Keen drew from the data were consistent with the questions originally posed and with the data obtained. She related, with clear logic, the original research question/hypotheses, study methods, and conclusions. In addition, she wrote her study with satisfactory concision. It definitely warrants further evaluation.

Part III: Believability of Results

Keen's study purported to compare the adverse effects of two alternate IM injection techniques. To collect data on these effects, she used both qualitative and quantitative measures. Discomfort was evaluated using patient interviews and a Likert-type scale. In response to a verbal questionnaire, the patients indicated the quality of their pain (burning or aching), and the intensity of their sensations. Site lesions were measured quantitatively. The researchers measured any areas of discoloration, swelling, or induration with rulers and recorded irregularly shaped lesions on cellophane for more accurate estimations of size.

As previously mentioned, the sample consisted of patients receiving multiple injections. Keen admits that the sample is one of convenience with patients from "selected medical and surgical units at a university medical center hospital." She excluded patients who had "interfering illnesses or preexisting injection site aberrations." By limiting her sample, she apparently wanted to obtain clearer results, with the results being due to the intervention, not due to preexisting conditions. For even greater clarity in her analysis, Keen limited her subjects to those receiving injections of either "meperidine hydrochloride alone or in combination with promethazine hydrochloride every three to four hours." This controlled for differences caused by medications rather than technique. Keen's sample also excluded pediatric and geriatric patients. Subjects' ages ranged from 21 to 57 years. Thus, Keen chose to control possible intervening variables by excluding as many as possible from the study.

The sample size was quite small with 50 subjects, who served as their own controls, randomly assigned to treatment groups. Each patient received injections with the Z-track technique in one ventrogluteal site and the standard technique in the other. Keen states that the patients were not told which injection technique was used in each site, but it is difficult to believe that this information could be withheld from them. If they knew how the two techniques differed, they would probably be able to discern if the nurse laterally displaced the cutaneous tissue (Z-track) or not. This could have introduced bias into their subjective responses.

Keen conducted a pilot study with eight patients to establish interrater reliability between the nurse researcher and research assistant. Measures of discomfort and of site lesions "were compared using the Pearson product moment correlation test," with scores of $r = .88$ and $r = .70$. Since I am not familiar with this statistical test, I cannot determine if these scores are significant. Consultation with a nurse researcher would be helpful in determining the appropriateness of the applicability of the test, as well as its meaningfulness.

Unfortunately, Keen did not discuss the validity of her measures. While her measures for site lesions seemed valid, assuming that the size of a lesion reflects its severity, this is not necessarily the case. Nonetheless, researchers in previous studies did utilize this method which lends some validity to the measures. In addition, Keen did not offer specific information regarding the questionnaire she used to collect discomfort data. She mentioned it was administered verbally both by the nurse researcher and the research assistant and that it included a description of the type of sensation and a Likert scale of intensity. However, she did not mention how it was developed, by whom, and whether or not it had been used before—a significant omission.

On the other hand, Keen presented a thorough report of the results of her study. She summarized the raw data, converting the number of patients with a given complaint or lesion to percentages of the whole sample. Then she analyzed the frequencies of discomfort and the specific lesions (using chi square) and the scores for discomfort and lesions (using a t-test), and presented the statistically significant data. Again, consultation with a nurse researcher would be necessary to gain assurance of the appropriateness of these statistical measures for the type of data provided, but the data are clearly appropriate to the research questions Keen originally posed.

In the discussion section of her article, Keen further analyzed the results of her study. She admitted some "mixed results in relation to the incidence of discomfort." It seemed that Z-track injections were initially more painful than standard injections, though by evening this fact was reversed.

In explanation she referred to a theory presented in the literature review. "One suggested cause for postinjection discomfort has been the deposition of the injected solution into the subcutaneous tissue rather than the intended musculature." She proposed that her findings supported this theory stating that "the Z-track technique would not cause a decrease in the initial discomfort of injection; instead, the Z-track may affect discomfort secondary to leakage and deposition of the injected solution into the subcutaneous tissue." Clearly, this is one possible explanation. However, it also is possible that the subjects could tell which injections were given with the Z-track technique, because of the position of the nurse's hand holding the skin taut and the resulting displacement of skin, and unconsciously decided these were less painful.

In relation to the incidence of lesions, the study results seemed to support Keen's theory: the Z-track technique is superior to the standard technique in reducing lesions. These findings seem less vulnerable to bias introduced by the subjects, or the research assistant, who did not know which technique was used in which site. However, they still could have been biased by the nurse researcher. Since she gave the injections, she knew which techniques were used in each site and could have biased her descriptions of the lesions either consciously or unconsciously. Keen admitted that "the potential for investigator bias may have been a major drawback of the study design," but stated that the interrater reliability determined through the pilot study "did not support this notion."

There are several weaknesses in this study. The sample is small, one of convenience, and quite limited. The measures used have questionable validity. Furthermore, there are some potential biases and, subsequently, other potential conclusions. However, the study does offer support, however limited, for Keen's theory. Replication of this study, with a larger sample and possibly different measures, would add credibility to Keen's claim.

Part IV: Generalizability of Results

The generalizability of Keen's study is severely compromised by the limits she placed on her sample: an adult, medical-surgical population receiving meperidine hydrochloride alone or in combination with promethazine hydrochloride. This obviously differs greatly from most clinical settings.

On the other hand, if nursing administration did choose to implement the practice promoted by Keen, it would be a relatively easy and feasible action. The technique itself, the Z-track method, is already well known. If it was to replace the standard technique, several demonstrations or a workshop would be sufficient for nurses to brush up on their technique and begin to implement it.

Part V: Other Factors to Consider in Utilization

Notwithstanding the weaknesses in Keen's study and its need for replication, utilization, at least on a trial basis, may be justified. This becomes apparent when looking at utilization from a cost-benefit perspective. As previously stated, the technique seems to be easily implemented and the cost to the hospital would be minimal. More importantly, the Z-track technique is apparently not any more harmful than the standard technique—patients are not put at risk by changing techniques, but stand only to gain from it. Therefore, the possible benefits outweigh the costs and implementation on a trial basis could be recommended.

Original article:
Keen, M. F. (1986). Comparison of intramuscular injection techniques to reduce site discomfort and lesions. *Nursing Research, 35*(4), 207–210.

CRITIQUE BY: CHAROLD BAER, PhD, RN

Part I: Clinical Relevance

The clinical problem studied by Keen involved determining which intramuscular injection technique resulted in the fewest incidents and least severe occurrences of site discomfort and lesions. These phenomena are of interest to clinicians because nurses: (1) often spend a significant amount of their time with patients in administering medications via intramuscular injection; (2) engage in clinical decision making surrounding the administration of intramuscular injections; (3) assess the patients' physiologic responses to intramuscular injections in order to alter or reaffirm the plan of care; and

(4) care about the patients' subjective responses to intramuscular injections. Thus, the results of this study could add to the body of knowledge available to guide nursing practice related to this aspect of patient care. It could assist in delineating patient assessment parameters, risk factors, and an appropriate injection technique to decrease complications.

Keen's research focused on a specific technique used in implementing an interdependent nursing intervention: administering intramuscular injections. This intervention is interdependent for two reasons: (1) the prescribing of medications surpasses the scope of practice for the general clinician; and (2) the medication must be prescribed before it can be administered. The selection of a specific administration technique, however, is an independent nursing decision that is consistent with the general scope of practice. In terms of this study, validating that the Z-track method results in reduced site discomfort and lesions might encourage nurses to reassess the technique they currently use, replicate the study, and institute the use of the Z-track method for all intramuscular injections.

Again, the independent variable consisted of the type of intramuscular injection administered while dependent variables included site discomfort and lesions. The investigator operationally defined site discomfort as the "subjects' experience of burning, stinging, aching, being sore, or hurting when touched or moving the leg." She measured this variable using a verbally administered questionnaire that categorized the intensity of the patients' sensations according to a 4-point Likert scale comprised of the following descriptions: none, mild, moderate, or severe. The second dependent variable, site lesions, has two operational definitions, one applicable at the time of injection and one for postinjection evaluations. At the time of the injection, site lesions were defined and measured according to "the development of resistance to needle penetration, resistance to injection of the solution, or seepage of the injected solution from the injection site following withdrawal of the needle." After the injection, site lesions were defined according to degree of pigmentation changes measured by a paint chip color scale and a clear metric ruler; skin sloughing measured by the presence of locally peeling or flaking skin; degree of swelling measured by palpation and a clear metric ruler; and induration measured by palpation and a clear metric ruler. Irregularly shaped lesions were traced on clear cellophane with a felt pen for further analysis at the conclusion of the study. Any and all of these measures could easily be used by a clinician in the patient care setting. In fact, most of them are currently being used as general data collection procedures with patients at the nurse's discretion. Such measures can provide valuable data when used to assess any type of lesion, not just those resulting from intramuscular injections.

In general, this study is clinically relevant and could contribute to the body of knowledge necessary to guide nursing practice. From this perspective, it merits continuing evaluation.

Part II: Conceptualization and Internal Consistency

Keen's study is clearly articulated, logically sequenced, and internally consistent. She relates justification to the frequency of use of intramuscular injections as a nursing intervention and the potential for patient complications to occur. She acknowledges that "the actual frequency of patient complications resulting from intramuscular injections is insufficiently documented," but suggests that the literature review supports the fact that those patients who receive repeated injections for prolonged periods are at high risk for developing such complications. She derives the research question logically from the justification and literature review to reflect conceptual clarity. She relates the independent variable, defined as the type of intramuscular injection technique, to the dependent variables: complications of site discomfort and lesions. The operational definitions of the dependent variables are conceptually consistent, with site discomfort designated as a subjective expression and lesions as objective measurements.

Keen designed this study appropriately to answer the clinical question. Because her sample included patients receiving repeated intramuscular injections, it was consistent with the target population of interest. The measurement instruments seemed valid for assessing the dependent variables. However, it is possible that the data collection procedures could have introduced some bias into the study because the individual who administered the injections also participated in the measurements of the dependent variables.

In general, the study is logically conceptualized and consistent. Even with the possible threat of bias, it is still potentially useful for clinical practice.

Part III: Believability of Results

This study purported to compare the effects of two types of intramuscular injections, Z-track and standard, on the incidence and severity of site discomfort and lesions in subjects receiving frequent injections. The data collected consisted of quantitative subjective and objective measurements.

Keen selected a convenience sample of 50 subjects for her study. The criteria for inclusion in the study appeared to involve: (1) inpatient status on selected medical and surgical units of a university medical center hospital; (2) reception of a minimum of two intramuscular injections of meperidine hydrochloride alone, or in combination with promethazine hydrochloride, every three to four hours; (3) a weight for height ratio that was within 20 percent of the normal limits as defined by life insurance standards; (4) the absence of interfering illnesses, such as preexisting injection site skin problems; and (5) right and left ventrogluteal sites that were not significantly different. The sample consisted of 37 males and 13 females, of whom 30 were black and 20 white. The age range was from 21 to 57 years, with a mean of 35.5 years. The predominant medical diagnoses for the subjects were acute or chronic pancreatitis (34 percent) and sickle cell anemia (28 percent). However, the composition of the sample poses interesting questions regarding its ability to be truly representative of the target population.

Keen randomly assigned subjects to treatment groups; subjects served as their own controls, which negated the differences between the two treatment groups. However, because both treatment groups received both types of injections, one type in the left ventrogluteal site and the other in the right, comparison of the effects of the two types of injections was enhanced.

As previously suggested, the study design expresses a potential for investigator bias—the individual who gave the injections also recorded the first data sets. Keen states that the following design strengths helped to minimize the effects of investigator bias: "(a) subjects served as their own controls by receiving both injection techniques; (b) all injections were given by the nurse researcher in accordance with strict injection procedures; and (c) the research assistant and subjects were aware of the two techniques being investigated but knew nothing of the treatment method being used in each ventrolguteal site." Yet, to this reviewer, these factors are not convincing enough as controls to negate the effects of investigator bias because all could result in compounding the effect. For example, patients can usually identify when skin is laterally displaced rather than uniformly tautened. There were, however, two facts cited that indicated that investigator bias may have been minimized: (1) interrater reliabilities of $r = .88$ and $.70$; and (2) that if only the research assistants' observations were used, the hypotheses would still be supported at $p = < .02$ and $< .01$.

The investigator does not discuss the reliability and validity data for the measures used to assess the dependent variables, nor does she document their developmental process. The measures appear to have content validity, and, therefore, are appropriate for the study. The lack of reliability information, however, is distressing.

Keen analyzed data using chi square and a t-test for related measures. While the t-test for related measures seems appropriate for analyzing the discomfort and lesions scores, chi square does not seem equally appropriate for analyzing frequency data. While using chi square to analyze frequency data is appropriate for nominal levels of measurement, using it to analyze data from a sample in which subjects served as their own controls violates an underlying assumption of independent samples. Consequently, it would seem more appropriate to use another nonparametric statistical test—for example, the McNemar test—which is designed for use with nominal level measurements for two sample cases in which the samples are related or dependent. In fact, it also might be more appropriate to substitute the correlated t-test for the t-test for repeated measures, based on the relatedness of the sample.

Keen reported and discussed her results thoroughly, thereby enhancing their logical relation to the study question. She explained statistically significant results by using data from previous research studies and normal physiologic parameters. She discussed unexpected results, such as the increased discomfort that accompanied the Z-tract method immediately postinjection but which had dissipated by the next measurement interval, in terms of previous studies and potential areas of faulty design in this study. In general, she strived to interpret the results based on their clinical applicability and utility for nurses.

Unfortunately, the use of statistical measures designed for independent samples, rather than related or dependent samples, decreases the credibility of the study. Certainly, additional studies supporting these results, in addition to reanalysis of the data, would enhance credibility. Prior to recommending widespread implementation of the technique, such reanalysis would be important to obtain.

Part IV: Generalizability of Results

There are distinct similarities between the methods and procedures employed in this study and those currently used in nursing practice. For example, the individual administering the injections was a professional nurse with clinical experience. He or she administered injections using the protocol currently being taught and implemented in clinical settings. In addition, the research assistant who participated in obtaining the measurements of the dependent variable was a master's prepared nurse. The fact that data collection was completed by nurses suggests that nurses in the clinical setting could easily obtain the same data by using the same measurements.

The setting is representative of current practice. However, the sample composition limits the generalizability of results. Because there were 37 males and 13 females (30 blacks and 20 whites), and an age range of 21 to 57 years, the convenience sample was not representative of the target population. In general, one would expect gender, race, and age to be represented in different quantities in the population at large. In addition, acute and chronic pancreatitis (34 percent) and sickle cell anemia (28 percent) are probably not as prevalent in the population as they were in the sample. Also, meperidine hydrochloride is not necessarily the intramuscular pain medication of choice for most patients. Certainly, all of these sample and study characteristics may be applicable to specific geographic patient populations, but they do not seem to be representative of the entire patient population that might experience the phenomena of concern addressed by this study.

While this study has limited generalizability and has not been replicated, it is still possible that the results, if implemented, could be beneficial for patients in the clinical setting. In this case, the clinician would need to decide if the possibility of a patient experiencing less pain during the evening following an injection, and fewer lesions overall, are sufficient reasons to change current practice. The clinician also would need to consider potential negative consequences of implementing the Z-track method for all patients.

Part V: Other Factors to Consider in Utilization

Changing standard practice to include the Z-track method for administering intramuscular injections to all patients involves few risks. The technique is currently used for administering certain types of medications, and would require no additional time, equipment, or education to include all intramuscular injections. Also, every nurse learns both techniques during the formal nursing education process and is prepared to implement either technique in the clinical setting. Thus, it would seem that the benefits of implementing the study results outweigh potential risks, particularly when one considers the alternative. If the standard technique continues to be used, nurses can expect patients who receive frequent injections to continue to experience more site discomfort and lesions.

Implementation of the study results also would provide an opportunity for continuing evaluation of the effects of the Z-track technique. Indeed, it would be feasible to conduct ongoing, systematic evaluation using either the measures defined in this study, or others determined as defined by clinicians. Feasibility is enhanced by the nature of the measures: they are compatible with the usual patient assessment techniques employed by clinicians.

The cost of implementing the change in practice would be minimal, primarily because it is already being implemented on a reduced scale. Expansion of the use of the Z-track technique would not involve additional personnel time or education, more equipment, or sanction by another professional group. Essentially, it would only entail a commitment by clinicians to use this technique for administering all intramuscular injections. Based on these factors, it is appropriate to recommend that clinicians implement this research-based practice.

The Influence of Talking on Diastolic Blood Pressure Readings

Rosemary Hellmann
Doctoral Student
Department of Epidemiology
State University of New York
Buffalo, NY

Dr. Susan A. Grimm
Manchester, NH

Recent research disclosed a number of variables which may distort blood pressure readings, but little attention has been paid to talking as such a variable. To investigate the effect of talking on diastolic blood pressure, 48 subjects with one previous diastolic blood pressure reading of 90 mm Hg or more and not taking antihypertensives, were recruited from an outpatient hypertension clinic. Three diastolic blood pressure readings under each of three sequentially counter-balanced treatment conditions were obtained: no talking, reading neutral material for part of the procedure, and reading neutral material continuously. Blood pressure increased significantly (p < .01) under both talking conditions. Implications for nursing education, practice, and future research are discussed.

Within the last decade, hypertension has come to the forefront as a life-threatening disease. Mass public screening for hypertension was instituted in 1972 as part of the National High Blood Pressure Education Program of the Department of Health, Education, and Welfare (Moyer, 1973). Since then it has been widely recommended that blood pressures be monitored whenever possible and considered a routine procedure in physician and dentist offices, clinics, etc. (Kochar, 1976). However, it is important that blood-pressure readings be accurate since the consequences of inaccurate readings are potentially serious.

Improper equipment and techniques were cited as causes for error in blood pressure measurements. Kirkendall (1974) listed improper position of the patient or arm, improper position and/or size of cuff, inaccuracy of the manometer, improper speed of the cuff inflation and deflation, lack of rest for the patient's limb between readings, and lack of multiple readings as factors producing inaccurate blood pressure readings. Skidmore and Marshall (1976) also reported improper cuff wrapping (e.g., too loose or too tight) as a cause of inaccuracy. Guidelines for taking blood pressures on thighs, infants, or children were described by Kaplan (1973), who also delineated methods of increasing the volume of the Korotkoff sounds when they are not audible.

Maxwell (1977) identified other variables, i.e., the time of day, fear, physical discomfort, apprehension, a full bladder, the physical setting, body position, or appearance, position, and attitude of the person recording the measurement, as factors influencing blood pressure readings. Kirkendall (1974) recommended that patients avoid eating, smoking, or exposure to cold for at least 30 minutes prior to having their blood pressure measured to avoid measurement error. Medications that effect the blood pressure also must be considered (Kaplan, 1973).

A variable which has not received much attention is the effect on blood pressure of talking during the measurement procedure. While working in a hypertension screening unit, the senior researcher observed a differential effect on blood pressure when the patient talked during the measurement procedure. A pilot study, investigating the effect of talking on diastolic blood pressure showed that blood pressure was higher ($p < .05$) when normotensive subjects ($N = 20$) talked during the measurement procedure than when they did not (Hellmann & Carlo, 1980). The impact of conversation on blood pressure was measured by Lynch, Thomas, Long, Malinow, Chickandonz, and Katcher (1980). They suggested that the emotional content and/or context of the communication at the time of measurement, and the personality of the participant effected the blood pressure. The significant increase in blood pressure during verbal communication also may have a physiological basis. The act of word formation and articulation, independent of the content of verbalization, could raise the blood pressure readings.

A valid measurement of blood pressure is of particular importance in making clinical judgments about people with hypertension. This study was done to investigate one variable thought to elevate blood pressure readings, verbalization during measurements.

METHOD

Subjects

Forty-six male and two female outpatients ($N = 48$) ranging in age from 27 to 69 years were recruited from the hypertension clinic of a large Veterans Administration Medical Center. (Subjects were chosen from the approximately 65 to 75 patients who had appointments for blood pressure rechecks on Tuesday or Thursday mornings from October through January. A number of those scheduled, 10 to 20 patients, did not keep their rescreening appointment (possibly due to holidays).

Patients with at least one previous blood pressure reading of 90 mm Hg or greater, who were not currently taking antihypertensive medication, and could read simple words in English, were asked to participate in the study. Eight subjects had taken antihypertensive medication previously. Medication history was obtained from chart review or from participants who could name their medication(s). Five persons refused to participate in the study because of time constraints.

Measures

Blood Pressure Readings. Systolic and diastolic blood pressures were obtained with a standard sphygmomanometer. The criteria of the American Heart Association for measuring blood pressure (Kirkendall, Feinleib, Fries, & Mark, 1980) were followed throughout: right arm at level of heart, mercury manometer, auscultatory method, patient seated, cuff size appropriate, cuff inflation to 180 mm Hg, cuff deflation 2 to 3 mm Hg/sec, and record 1st and 5th Korotkoff sounds.

Reading Task. The card which subjects read was designed to maximize simplicity and minimize affective response(s). It was developed by Hellmann and Carlo (1980) using the level of words found in the newspaper. Colleagues were asked about the simplicity and the potential of an emotional response when reading the card. Further evaluation of the content validity or the reliability of the card was not conducted. The card which was read by the subjects contained the following statements:

> One and one equals two. Two and two equals four. Four and four equals eight. If eight and eight equals sixteen then sixteen and sixteen equals thirty-two. Only if thirty-two and thirty-two equals sixty-four can we be sure of the number.

Procedure

All subjects who had rescreening appointments were asked to participate in the study. They were given information concerning the study procedures and risks. Subjects were randomly assigned, by means of a random number table, to a particular sequence of the three treatment conditions. The order of the conditions was varied to control any order effects.

Following an initial rest period of 5 minutes, three blood pressure readings were obtained at 2-minute intervals, under each of three conditions, for a total of nine blood pressure readings on each subject.

Condition 1: Subjects were instructed not to talk before, during, or after the blood pressure measurement.

Condition 2: Subjects were instructed to read aloud the words on the card while the blood pressure cuff was inflated. Once the cuff was inflated, they were told to stop reading and the blood pressure was measured.

Condition 3: Subjects were asked to read aloud the words on the card while the blood pressure measurement was taken. They were told to repeat the reading until they were instructed to stop.

Subjects did not practice reading the card before the measures were made, however, the subjects were told that the material to-be-read was simple to read. No one had difficulty reading the card aloud. After completing the procedure, subjects were debriefed, and given an opportunity to ask questions.

Data were analyzed using a one-way ANOVA for repeated measures. Such a within-subjects design was chosen because it allowed each subject to serve as his/her own control, and because within-subject variation was the criterion of interest rather than group comparisons. The mean of the three diastolic blood pressure readings obtained under each treatment condition was calculated since the mean of three readings is the best measure of blood pressure status (Souchek, Stamler, Dyer, Paul, & Lepper, 1979, p. 197).

RESULTS

The reading conditions have a significant effect on diastolic blood pressure, $F(2.94) = 74.07$, $p < .0001$. As shown in Table 1, the mean diastolic blood pressure increases as the amount of talking during a particular treatment condition increases.

Confidence intervals (see Table 2) for the treatment conditions were calculated using Dunn's procedure (Keppel, 1973, pp. 147–149). The mean readings under both talking conditions are significantly higher ($p < .01$) than those when no talking was allowed. No effect is noted from the order of treatment conditions.

Subjects (16%) who have normal readings (diastolic < 90 mm Hg) under the no talking condition became mildly hypertensive (diastolic 90

Table 1
Diastolic Blood Pressure (mm Hg) Under Each Treatment Condition

Condition	M	SD
No talking	87.10	9.17
Talking during cuff inflation	88.96	8.98
Talking during entire procedure	95.35	10.09

Note. Means were based on three readings for each of the 48 subjects under each of the three conditions.

Table 2
Confidence Intervals of Diastolic Blood Pressure Readings for No Talking Compared With Talking

		.99 Confidence Interval	
Condition	Mean Difference	Lower Limit	Upper Limit
Talking during cuff inflation vs. No talking	1.86*	.40	3.32
Talking during whole procedure vs. No talking	8.25*	6.79	9.71

Note. Means were based on three readings for each of the 48 subjects under each of the three conditions.
*$p < .01$.

to 104 mm Hg) under the condition of continuous talking. An additional 16% of subjects whose no talking readings are in the mildly hypertensive range became moderately hypertensive (diastolic 105 to 115 mm Hg) under the continuous talking condition.

DISCUSSION

While the mean diastolic blood pressure readings for the subjects increased significantly under two talking conditions, only the no talking mean compared with the continuous talking mean is clinically significant. Similar results of an increase in blood pressure when the subject either reads a text or talks were reported by Lynch et al. (1980). This finding has a number of clinical implications. For instance, allowing talking while blood pressure is measured may give a misleading picture of an individual's blood pressure. If such a reading falls into the hypertensive range, it may result in an unwarranted or incorrect diagnosis of hypertension. Once made, such a diagnosis is difficult to retract and is likely to remain with an individual. Such an incorrect diagnosis may lead to initiation or increase of antihypertensive medication which has risks and potentially adverse consequences.

The implications these findings have for nursing are clear: Both nurse clinicians and educators should be aware that blood pressure readings may be artificially high if taken while an individual is talking. Nurses should be educated in the proper technique for measuring blood pressure which, in addition to several precautions noted earlier (cold exposure, smoking, etc.), should include the discouragement of patients' talking. Since any individual blood pressure reading is potentially atypical (for a particular person), the mean of several readings is a more reliable baseline for making clinical judgments (Souchek et al., 1979, Gordon, Sorlie, & Kannel, 1976). This finding was thought to have even greater clinical significance for labile hypertensives, individuals whose blood pressure readings fluctuate. In view of the multiplicity of circumstances surrounding the measurement of blood pressure which could lead to error in readings, clinicians should be cautious before labeling an individual as normotensive or hypertensive, and placing an individual on antihypertensive medication with its potentially adverse side-effects.

We recommend that future research on blood pressure measurement include a replication of the present study with a larger, more representative sample of the general population. Since the population of veterans studied is not representative of the population at large, one might question the extent to which our findings will generalize to other populations. A valuable addition to any future replication would be the use of automated equipment to control for any experimenter effects. While our study attempted to minimize the emotional content of subjects' verbalizations, further research relating emotional content of speech and blood pressure also is desirable to evaluate if this would further influence the magnitude of blood pressure changes.

REFERENCES

Gordon, T., Sorlie, P., & Kannel, W. (1976). Problems in the assessment of blood pressures: The Framingham study. *International Journal of Epidemiology, 5*, 327–333.

Hellmann, R., & Carlo, S. (1980). The effects of talking on diastolic blood pressure. *American Journal of Nursing, 12*, 2190.

Kaplan, N. M. (1973). *Clinical hypertension*. New York: Medcom Press.

Keppel, G. (1973). *Design and analysis: A researcher's handbook*. New Jersey: Prentice Hall.

Kirkendall, W. M. (1974). How to get a reliable blood pressure. *Dialogues in Hypertension, 1*, 8–12.

Kirkendall, W. M., Feinleib, M., Fries, E. D., & Mark, A. L. (1980). Recommendations for human blood pressure determination by sphygmomanometers. *Circulation, 62*, 1145A–1155A.

Kochar, M. S. (1976). Hypertension screen. *Journal of the American Medical Association, 236*, 2551.

Lynch, J. J., Thomas, S. A., Long, J. M., Malinow, K. L., Chickandonz, G., & Katcher, A. H. (1980). Human speech and blood pressure. *Journal of Nervous and Mental Disease, 168,* 526–534.

Maxwell, M. H. (1977). A functional approach to screening. In *The hypertensive handbook.* West Point: Merch, Sharp & Dohme.

Moyer, J. H. (1973, May). Nation's attention focused on hypertension. *Pennsylvania Medicine, 76,* 34-35.

Skidmore, E., & Marshall, A. (1976, March 11). Towards a more accurate measurement of blood pressure. *Nursing Times, 72,* 376–378.

Souchek, J., Stamler, J., Dyer, A. R., Paul, O., & Lepper, M. H. (1979). The value of two or three versus a single reading of blood pressure at first visit. *Journal of Chronic Diseases, 32,* 197–210.

This article is printed with permission of *Research in Nursing and Health.*
Copyright © 1984 John Wiley & Sons.

Original article:
Hellmann, R., & Grimm, S. A. (1984). The influence of talking on diastolic blood pressure readings. *Research in Nursing and Health*, 7(4), 253–256.

CRITIQUE BY: AUDREY NICKODEMUS, BSN, RN

Part I: Clinical Relevance

Hellmann and Grimm studied a variable that decreases the accuracy of diastolic blood pressure readings in clients. Certainly students and new graduates are concerned with the variances identified in both procedure and patient status that affect blood pressure measurement. Since the measurement of blood pressures is a widely accepted nursing function, research that identifies potential inaccuracies is of concern to all nurses. Indeed, blood pressure readings have a high potential to be incorrectly performed. In this regard, Hellmann and Grimm cite factors contributing to incorrect readings in their literature review. Specifically, their study focuses on the potential of verbalization to skew diastolic readings.

However, because it may be difficult to separate verbalization as a source of error from the content and emotions of an individual's conversation, the study has only limited clinical application. The investigators cite the work of Lynch, Thomas, Long, Malinow, Chickandonz, and Katcher (1980) in demonstrating the need for research to separate an inaccurate diastolic blood pressure reading due to verbalization (the dependent variable) from variations due to conversation and emotional content. Although the nurse clinician may be aware that talking and other patient activities may increase an individual's blood pressure reading, it is logical and scientifically critical to investigate these components separately. The clinician's awareness of the impact of specific activities that raise blood pressure is helpful in identifying the degree of risk for a particular patient.

Hellmann and Grimm have proposed that accurate blood pressure readings are critical to the clinical management of patients. In fact, they base the original research question regarding verbalization as an error factor on clinical observations of one of the researchers. Hellmann and Grimm also cite instances where the treatment of hypertensive patients was initiated when unnecessary, or delayed when needed, based on inaccurate blood pressure readings. The nurse clinician can readily identify the impact of accuracy in taking blood pressures. However, because this study uses readings on hypertensive patients exclusively, general clinical relevance becomes problematic.

In their study, Hellmann and Grimm tested a specific intervention: the reading of mean diastolic blood pressures primarily in male hypertensive outpatient clients ($n = 48$) under three sets of conditions. These randomly sequenced conditions included: (1) no verbalization; (2) verbalization through part of the procedure; and (3) verbalization throughout the entire blood pressure reading. Individuals served as their own controls using verbalization as the independent variable, with the accuracy of the blood pressure measurements being increased by three serial measurements for each condition. To enhance study control, the subjects read a predetermined set of words chosen by the investigators for simplicity and lack of emotional content. While measuring blood pressures is a traditional nursing practice, in this study it is altered by the placement of controls by the researchers, a factor that must be taken into account when considering results.

Therefore, though this study measures an artificial phenomenon (controlled verbalization), the study indicates to the clinician that hypertensive clients who talk during blood pressure readings may be at high risk for inaccurate measurements of diastolic pressure. Obtaining accurate blood pressure readings is an important function in determining diagnoses. This study, then, though inconclusive in its specific results, is important for its review of the correct procedure for blood pressure readings, its attention to the need for accuracy in technique, and its stressing the many factors that can play a part in producing inaccurate readings. As a reslt, all clinicians concerned with accurate blood pressure readings would find in this research some relevance to their practice.

Part II: Conceptualization and Internal Consistency

The investigators justify their concept by the clinical relevance of accurate blood pressure measurements. In addition, they clearly define their basis for the study of talking as a physiological process separate from the content of an individual's conversation.

However, the merit of the study is decreased by the small sample size and the choice of primarily male subjects from a hypertension treatment clinic, thereby limiting the generalizability of specific conclusions. In addition, because of an artificially created situation (controlled verbalization), the study limits generalizability even further; although such limitations seem necessary for internal consistency and control of extraneous variables.

The investigators define the limits of hypertension as being a diastolic measurement of greater than 90 mm Hg and also define verbalization, as well as the controls that they are placing on those definitions. Yet, while the conclusions drawn are overextended (due to the above mentioned limitations), they are stimulating. They present to the nurse clinician a challenge to increase the accuracy of blood pressure readings in practice.

The scientific merit of this study is focused on its potential for replication and the evaluation of a clinical technique involved in a widely used (and seemingly simplistic) nursing procedure.

Part III: Believability of Results

This study focuses on testing the logical connection between increases in diastolic blood pressure readings and the act of talking among subjects, although the readings are subject to many other variables. The data collected are quantitative and subjected to statistical analysis.

In the convenience sample used, all but two of the subjects are male: the setting involved was a Veteran's Administration outpatient clinic. Hellmann and Grimm recognize but do not discuss the potential bias of this overrepresentation of male subjects. In addition, while they chose subjects from among all rescreening patients, they failed to supply criteria concerning clinic guidelines for rescreening. The investigators also provide no rationale for the exclusion of subjects receiving antihypertensive medication, nor do they provide data on other medications these subjects may be taking, nor other interventions (such as dietary) that they may be using to control hypertension.

In the introduction and literature review, the investigators highlight their concern regarding the correct identification of hypertensive patients. Additional medical reports currently available in consumer publications have raised the issue of patients being labeled as hypertensive with only one increased diastolic blood pressure reading. A variable to be considered in this group of subjects is how accurately screened they were on their initial visit. Did this clinic use multiple diastolic measurements in the initial screening? Were the subjects' baseline blood pressure measurements measured with the same accuracy and attention to the American Heart Association guidelines as the study readings? With such concerns in mind, the reader should question the significance of 16 percent of the subjects having normal blood pressures (a diastolic less than 90 mm Hg) on initial measurement.

All of the variables related to the inaccuracies of blood pressure measurement must be considered as possible extraneous variables in this study. For example, the variables cited from Maxwell (1977) in the literature review list a number of variables that are not addressed by the investigators: "time of day, fear, physical discomfort, apprehension, a full bladder, the physical setting, body position, or appearance, position, and attitude of the person recording the measurement."

In addition, the hypertensive subjects may be emotionally invested in the study due to their "hypertensive" label and their reaction to being tested. Also, the researchers do not provide an explanation of their "debriefing" procedure, nor do they mention a standardized format for the explanation of the research to their subjects.

Further weaknesses in the study include the card used containing the standardized words read by the subject, which was not tested for validity or reliability. While Hellmann and Grimm acknowledge this weakness, they also imply content validity from positive responses from colleagues. However, there is no testing of this assumption. Using numbers and mathematics may be devoid of emotional content, but do any of the subjects have the potential to react due to "math anxiety"? The reader also cannot be assured that the act of reading aloud in front of the researchers is not more anxiety provoking than normal conversation for certain individuals.

The data collection procedure is limited by lack of information about the number of clinicians involved in data collection, or information about interrater reliability. Hellmann and Grimm have carefully detailed the procedure to be followed through the use of the American Heart Association guidelines, but provide no information about the accuracy of following that procedure among individuals measuring diastolic blood pressure. Equipment reliability is not documented according to the manufacturer's reliability or by any clinical testing of accuracy between the number of cuffs used, or differences between sphygmomanometers involved in the collection of data.

The investigators were careful to randomly sequence the testing conditions, with each subject acting as his or her own control. Serial data collection occurred only once for a series of three readings for each subject and the mean was subject to distortion by any number of variables occurring at the time (such as discomfort, time of day, or room temperature).

The statistical analysis of the data, a one-way ANOVA, is appropriate for testing the difference between means of three or more sets of conditions. The one-way ANOVA is specifically applicable to the subjects' comparison design chosen by the investigators. The mathematical interpretation of the data adds to the believability of the results. While Hellmann and Grimm allude to a difference between statistical and clinical significance in their analysis of blood pressure results, they do not define that difference with greater specificity.

Hellmann and Grimm conclude their study by identifying a general "need to increase awareness," consistent with their small, limited sample and lack of control over extraneous variables. They also stress the "multiplicity of circumstances" which may lead to blood pressure errors. The number of potential variables that could result in blood pressure measurement errors generates a number of alternate conclusions to this study, as well. Each extraneous variable previously identified could skew the statistical significance of the results. Such potential variables limit the conclusiveness of the study.

The conclusions focus on the need for attention to procedure, education, and replication. Replication with additional control of variables is imperative. However, while Hellmann and Grimm recognize that it would be difficult to make further conclusions without replication, they do view their work as being statistically significant.

Part IV: Generalizability of Results

For the clinician, this study assumes importance by way of its description of the correct procedure for measuring blood pressure (according to the American Heart Association) and the listing of the many variables noted to create inaccuracies in blood pressure readings. It would be safe to estimate that few clinicians implement the American Heart Association standards for blood pressure measurement in any particular setting. Therefore, clinicians may be forced to scrutinize their own procedure against those standards and identified variances.

Unfortunately, the small, hypertensive, male sample from a clinic and the artificial intervention that was tested in the study does not contribute to immediate usefulness for the clinician. However, it does contribute to a body of knowledge that clinicians can draw from in evaluating their practice and increasing their awareness of the intricacies of a commonly performed nursing procedure. Any additional attention by the clinician to perfecting technique in measuring blood pressure should be considered as a gain.

Part V: Other Factors to Consider in Utilization

Hypertension screening has become a nationally recognized health need, and continuing research-based practice to correctly identify hypertensive patients is critical to patient management. However, in a review of the sources the investigators utilized in their literature search, the reader can identify only two nursing sources; the balance of these studies are medical. It would seem that nurses, who obtain many blood pressure readings, should be in the forefront of research to identify correct procedures and variances in accuracy.

The question of need for accuracy in hypertensive screenings is without dispute. However, the changes in practice this would require and the attention given to variance in the hospital setting may prove more controversial. It would be of great benefit to all patients to have more accurate blood pressure measurements obtained in all situations, of course. Yet, because critically ill patients may be increasingly monitored by technology rather than hands-on nursing procedure, other considerations not dealt with in this study arise. In addition, for varying institutions to implement changes in blood pressure technique, questions concerning cost effectiveness will arise, especially if the procedure will consume more time than is now usual. Also important to consider is this possibility: as this decade's nursing shortage looms on the horizon, the measuring of blood pressures may be increasingly delegated to auxiliary personnel.

The attention to accuracy in the treatment of hypertensive patients is well worth continuing research. The investigators made valid references to the cost of unneeded or missed treatment. However, the use of serial measurements and the control of a large number of identified variances may be more difficult to manipulate in a hospital setting, where the variance in blood pressure may be slight and have no application to a client's treatment plan or overall care. Application of this study will be to a specialized population and setting. Attention to the ramifications of the variances inherent in blood pressure readings should be stressed at all educational levels, with an attempt to expand the American Heart Association guidelines to assimilate the newest well-documented variances in readings.

Original article:
Hellmann, R., & Grimm, S. A. (1984). The influence of talking on diastolic blood pressure readings. *Research in Nursing and Health*, 7(4), 253–256.

CRITIQUE BY: CHAROLD BAER, PhD, RN

Part I: Clinical Relevance

This research focused on a specific clinical problem: the effect of talking on diastolic blood pressure. This problem could hold clinical significance because of the amount of time that nurses expend with patients in obtaining blood pressure measurements, the need for those measurements to be as precise as possible, and the increasing incidence of misdiagnosis and treatment of patients experiencing transient elevations in blood pressure. In order to decrease incidences of transient elevations in measurement, study results also suggest an additional, research-based criterion that the nurse would assess prior to obtaining a blood pressure measurement. The inclusion of such a criterion could assist the nurse in obtaining more accurate blood pressure measurements, and would constitute a clinically significant contribution to patient care.

In this investigation, the phenomenon of concern is the effect of an extraneous variable—talking—on a patient's blood pressure measurement. A comparison of the effects of no talking, talking during part of the procedure, and talking during the entire procedure could result in clinically applicable data. Based on the results, a nurse could elect to alter the procedure for obtaining blood pressure measurements by including a directive to the patient to refrain from talking during the procedure. In addition, the nurse could consider valid only those measurements that were obtained while the patient was silent. Instituting these alterations in the performance of a basic procedure is within an individual nurse's scope of practice and requires no consultation with, or permission from, other individuals within the health care hierarchy.

The independent variable in this study was the amount of talking the patient engaged in during the blood pressure measurement. The dependent variable was the patient's diastolic blood pressure reading as measured using a standard mercury sphygmomanometer in accordance with the American Heart Association guidelines. Measuring patients' blood pressures is a frequent activity for nurses and one at which they become highly skilled. Although nurses may use varying types of equipment, and may modify the American Heart Association guidelines based on a patient's status, nurses do adhere to the basic principles inherent in the guidelines for obtaining an accurate measurement. Thus, from a technical aspect, the measurements they obtain should be accurate. However, the results of this study could suggest that nurses control the variable of talking in order to increase the accuracy of the measurements they obtain. The results also might suggest that nurses control the amount of reading that a patient does during the blood pressure measurement process. This application of the results is deduced from the methodology presented: subjects were to read words from a card rather than engage in normal conversation. Perhaps it is not just the physiologic formation and expression of words that induces variation in diastolic blood pressure; perhaps the reading, comprehension, and interpretation of those words also induces a similar variation.

Part II: Conceptualization and Internal Consistency

Hellmann and Grimm have clearly articulated and logically sequenced their study. They seem to have dealt with the intended variables, if reading words aloud from a card is equivalent to talking. While both activities include similar pyschologic, physiologic, and interpretive behaviors, that does not necessarily mean that they are identical, however. Perhaps it requires more "stress" on physiologic processing to converse than it does to read words aloud from a card, or vice versa. If such is the case, then using one as an operational definition of the other would be inappropriate.

The investigators have drawn justification for the study from the following: (1) the current national concern about hypertension as a chronic, life-threatening disease; (2) an awareness of the consequences of the misdiagnosis and treatment of patients due to inaccurate measurements; (3) previous research indicating the numerous types of variables that can influence a patient's blood pressure; (4) previous research concerning the impact of conversation on a patient's blood pressure; and (5) the importance of an accurate blood pressure measurement as a component of a nurse's clinical decision making. In addition, the investigators have logically related the clinical question to their justification for the study. Again, the conceptualization of the study is consistent with the current knowledge base, if talking and reading aloud are considered equivalent behaviors.

The investigators have appropriately designed their study to answer the clinical question they posed. They logically relate independent and dependent variables and enhance their validity by referring to previous research. In addition, the convenience sample selected for this study is consistent with some, but not all, segments of the population of interest. The sample, recruited from a hypertension clinic at a large Veterans Administration Medical Center, was comprised of 46 males and 2 females, ranging in age from 27 to 69 years.

Data collection procedures, which are consistent with normal standards of practice, including the two-minute intervals between the three serial blood pressure measurements, should not bias study results. In general, the conceptualization and internal consistency of the study are appropriate, with one possible exception—the operational definition of talking.

Part III: Believability of Results

This study purported to test the effect of an influencing variable—amount of talking—on a patient's diastolic blood pressure reading. The data collected are numerically quantified blood pressure measurements. The subjects served as their own controls and were randomly assigned to a particular sequence of the three treatment conditions, which included no talking, talking only during cuff inflation, and talking during the entire procedure.

The investigators selected a convenience sample from those patients who elected to return to a hypertension clinic at a large Veterans Administration Medical Center for blood pressure rescreening. To determine subject inclusion, they used three criteria: (1) at least one previous diastolic blood pressure reading of 90 mm Hg or greater; (2) not currently taking antihypertension medications; and (3) an ability to read simple words in English. However, the first criterion seems inappropriate. The investigators include a series of three blood pressure measurements in the study to ensure validity, but are willing to accept only one for subject inclusion. The use of this double standard could lead to the inclusion of subjects who were not actually hypertensive.

The investigators do not discuss potential biases, intervening variables, reliability of measures, number of data collectors, or interrater reliability, if more than one data collector was involved. Perhaps they felt that reliability data were superfluous in connection with a frequently performed and accepted procedure, such as blood pressure measurement. If so, it would have been helpful if they had stated their views on this subject. However, they did, if tangentially, discuss the validity of the measures.

In this respect, they elected to use the mean of a series of three blood pressure measurements in order to increase the validity of the outcome measure. They also had colleagues assess the simplicity and emotive evoking potential of the card used to standardize the subjects' verbalizations during the study. They state that no further content validity or reliability studies were conducted concerning the card. Unfortunately, they fail to address their rationale for not conducting such studies, or the potential effects on the study of not having those data.

In addition, the investigators did not adequately discuss the standardized card representing the operational definition of the independent variable. They mention who developed the card's content and that it includes words common to newspapers, but they fail to discuss the inclusion of numerical content. Perhaps subjects would consider such content anxiety provoking, particularly if they disliked numbers or math. Also, while the card's content is straight forward, it is made convoluted by the addition of "if" and "only if" statements.

The statistical analysis employed, a one-way ANOVA for repeated measures, is appropriate for a study involving dependent or related samples and an interval or ratio-level measurement for the dependent variable. Also, the selection of a within subjects design was appropriate because the subjects served as their own controls.

Conclusions drawn from the results of this study are appropriate in terms of the clinical question posed, subjects tested, and design employed. However, the investigators do not adequately discuss, or attempt to explain, the results of the study. While they make two statements regarding the results and a previous study that supports the findings of this study, they devote the remainder of their discussion to implications for clinical practice and suggestions for replication studies. It does appear that there is a significant change in a patient's diastolic blood pressure reading when the patient progresses from a silent state to one in which verbalizations occur. Whether or not that change is due to talking, reading aloud, physiologic variations, or psychologic interpretations remains unclear based on this study. Regardless of the cause, a change of 10 points is significant enough to warrant that additional attention be given to controlling intervening variables while the measurement is being obtained.

In general, while the results appear believable, they are not without question. The ambiguities surrounding the operational definition of the independent variable and its true relationship to the variable of "talking" could lead one to draw alternate conclusions about the study.

Part IV: Generalizability of Results

Sample selection poses the major threat to external validity or generalizability of this study. Certainly the Hawthorn effect and novelty also may be threats, but they do not appear to be as significant as the selection problem. In this sample, the subjects are not representative of the entire target population. The sample is overrepresentative of the male gender and may be underrepresentative of hypertensive patients based on the inclusion criteria of at least one previous diastolic blood pressure reading of 90 mm Hg or greater and not currently taking antihypertensive medications.

The setting for the study also may not be representative of the typical settings that the target population might select for health care. Government-organized hypertension clinics may be different than private or public clinics. However, one would anticipate that the procedure for measuring a patient's blood pressure would be implemented identically, regardless of the type of clinic. Nevertheless, the generalizability of the study still would be limited by the type of setting selected.

The individuals involved in the data collection were not identified. If one assumes that the investigators were the data collectors, then it can be further assumed, since both investigators are nurses, that the data collection procedures could be implemented by typical staff nurses. In addition, because most nurses routinely obtain blood pressure measurements according to principles inherent in the American Heart Association guidelines, it can be inferred that the study measurements and those obtained in clinical practice result from the implementation of a standard assessment procedure.

Previous studies that have investigated the effects of talking on diastolic blood pressure seem to have had problems similar to this study. Primarily, the problem seems to revolve around the operational definition of talking and how the physiologic, psychologic, and interpretive components are controlled in the study. Despite or perhaps because of this problem the results of those studies do corroborate the results of this investigation.

In general, even though the results of this study have limited generalizability, there is sufficient clinical relevance and significance to suggest utilization of the results. However, the limitations of the study decrease its credibility and circumscribe the clinician's confidence in implementing the results.

Part V: Other Factors to Consider in Utilization

The results of this study could easily be implemented and systematically evaluated in clinical practice. Implementation would only require the nurse to request that the patient refrain from talking or reading during the blood pressure measurement. Evaluation could consist of chart audits, because blood pressure measurements are recorded at least once a day for every patient in a clinical setting. If preferred, more elaborate evaluation plans also could be instituted.

Only minimal risks are involved in changing practice by implementing the results of this study. If the request to the patient to refrain from talking or reading during the blood pressure measurement is made in a caring manner and accompanied by an explanation, it is unlikely that the patient will be offended. However, it is possible that some patients might view this request as an infringement on their personal rights and thus respond in an emotional manner. Such an emotional response might then have a more pronounced effect on their diastolic blood pressure reading than talking would.

If nurses do not change practice by implementing these results, they risk obtaining falsely inflated diastolic readings by allowing patients to talk during the procedure. On the other hand, if nurses change practice as prescribed by the study results, they would benefit by an increase in accuracy in blood pressure measurements.

Costs for implementing the results of this study would be virtually negligible. Any additional cost would be expended in terms of the increased nursing time required to make the request of the patient and to explain why it was being made. It is unlikely that the time spent in actually measuring the blood pressure would be altered. Therefore, it seems that the benefits to patient care in implementing study results would outweigh any costs accrued, and that implementation could be recommended.

Circadian Rhythms: Basis for Screening for Fever

Julie F. Samples, MSN, ARNP
Instructor
College of Nursing
University of South Florida
Tampa, FL

Mary Lou Van Cott, MS, RN
Instructor
College of Nursing
University of South Florida
Tampa, FL

Charlene Long, MS, RN
Assistant Professor
College of Nursing
University of South Florida Tampa, FL

Imogene M. King, EdD, RN
Professor and Director of Nursing Research
College of Nursing
University of South Florida
Tampa, FL

Angela Kersenbrock, MS, RN
Instructor
College of Nursing
University of South Florida
Tampa, FL

Elevation in body temperature is one of the most frequently used indicators of the presence of a physical illness or potential threat to health. An individual's temperature is often used as the basis for decisions about diagnosis, treatment, and discharge from the hospital. Routine temperature measurements are taken in most hospitals early in the morning and before 5 P.M. Temperatures are measured in the evening only in individuals who exhibit elevations during the routine times. The rationale for this routine of temperature measurement is often based on tradition or convenience rather than on research findings.

Research in biological rhythms has identified endogenous and exogenous factors that influence human behavior in health and illness. One common expression of an endogenous rhythm in human beings is the circadian thermal rhythm called body temperature (Aschoff, 1960; Lobban, 1960). Body temperature rhythm is one of the most stable rhythms in humans. Based on circadian rhythm, studies of temperature measurement have identified 5 P.M. to 7 P.M. as the peak of the daily cycle, the time when the temperature is likely to be elevated (Selle, 1952).

The purpose of this study was to determine: (a) if the peak of the circadian thermal rhythm is the optimal time to screen adult hospitalization patients for fever, and (b) the necessary frequency for measurement of oral body temperature.

REVIEW OF THE LITERATURE

For more than a century researchers have reported that core body temperature exhibits a circadian rhythm. Wunderlich and Sequin (1871) reported that the time of the lowest body temperature was 7 A.M. to 9 A.M.; the highest temperature, from 4 P.M. to 6 P.M. Studies over the past 30 years have shown that body temperature rhythm is stable and does not differ significantly in normal healthy people (Aschoff, 1960; Minors & Waterhouse, 1981; Stephens & Halberg, 1965).

In an early study in nursing, Schmidt (1958) measured temperatures of medical-surgical patients at 6 A.M. and 2 P.M. for 21 days. Of 1,876 observations recorded, over 90% were within normal limits. Findings resulted in a change in routine temperature measurement at the hospital studied from twice a day to once a day at 2 P.M. Sims (1965) examined temperature measurement records of 130 medical-surgical patients and recommended that one temperature measurement at 7 P.M., in relatively stable patients, effectively screened for fever. In a study of frequency and time of routine temperature measurement in one hospital (DeRisi, 1968), oral body temperature of 100 adult male medical-surgical patients was measured five times a day (6 A.M., 10 A.M., 2 P.M., 6 P.M., 10 P.M.) for 3 days. In relating circadian thermal rhythm studies to routine body temperature measurement, DeRisi found that routine times did not coincide with the peak of the thermal rhythm and recommended measuring body temperature at the peak of the circadian rhythm to effectively screen for fever.

In a retrospective survey of oral body temperature measurements of 717 adult medical-surgical patients at 4 P.M., 8 A.M., and 4 P.M., Bell (1969) found that 2.23% of patients had elevated temperatures at 7 A.M. that had not been elevated the previous day. The 2.23% reflected 16 patients who either were critically ill or were admitted with fever of undetermined origin. A recommendation was made that temperatures should be taken once a day between the hours of 4 P.M. and 8 P.M. Angerami (1980) studied 225 patients to determine the optimal time for temperature measurement to detect hyperthermia. Axillary temperatures were measured with an electronic thermometer eight times (7 A.M., 9 A.M., 11 A.M., 1 P.M., 3 P.M, 5 P.M., 7 P.M., 9 P.M.) for one day. The most sensitive hour to detect hyperthermia was found to be 7 P.M.

Measurement of oral body temperature has been shown to be a more accurate indicator of body core temperature than rectal or axillary measurement (Blainey, 1974; Cranston, 1966). Erickson (1980) noted that the validity of oral temperature measurement depends on the placement of the thermometer. In a study of three sublingual areas, oral temperatures were significantly higher in the right and left posterior sublingual pockets compared to the area located beneath the tongue at the front of the mouth where the frenulum attaches to the mouth floor, when measured with predictive electronic thermometers.

The inaccuracy of mercury thermometers has been reported in several studies (Beck & St. Cyr, 1974; Palmer, 1949; Purintun & Bishop, 1969). Knapp (1966) reported electronic thermometers to be more accurate then mercury in glass thermometers when tested in a standard water bath. Beck and St. Cyr (1974) also reported the electronic thermometer to be superior to mercury during in vitro experiments but inaccurate in a clinical setting due to inadequate and inconsistent placement of the thermometer probe.

Effects of variables such as the ingestion of ice water, oxygen therapy, and mouth breathing on the accuracy of measurement of body temperatures have been evaluated. Forster, Adler, and Davis (1970) and Woodman, Parry, and Simms (1967) studied the effect of ice water ingestion on oral temperatures. Both studies reported a lowered body temperature; however, measurement showed a return to the preingestion temperature within 15 minutes. Lim-Levy (1982) studied 100 healthy adults and found that oxygen inhalation using a nasal cannula did not effect oral body temperature taken with an electronic thermometer. A similar finding was reported by Yorkman (1982) when patients used cooled and heated aerosol masks. Dressler, Smejkal, and Ruffolo (1983) found a greater difference in body temperature between the oral and rectal sites in patients using oxygen masks. This finding may have been related to temperature sensitivity of the acutely ill compared to healthy adults. Cooper and Abrams (1981) studied mouth breathers and found that body temperature was not significantly affected by mouth breathing.

This study used predictive knowledge from research in circadian rhythms such as body temperature in the natural environment of hospitals to determine if the routine procedure of taking body temperatures was essential to effective patient care. The theoretical framework for the study is based on predictive knowledge from circadian rhythm studies and nursing studies. If existing knowledge about biological rhythms and body temperature is used in taking routine temperatures of hospitalized adults, two outcomes are possible: (1) a more accurate measure of body temperature will be recorded and (2) the dollar savings in manpower hours could have an impact on cost containment programs in hospitals.

METHOD

The proposal for this study was approved by the institutional review board of the medical center. Directors of nursing of participating hospitals granted permission for data collection. Subjects were selected from medical-surgical units in three community hospitals. Male and female adult subjects over 18 years of age, hospitalized for medical, diagnostic, or surgical treatments, were selected the evening prior to the initial 6 A.M. temperature. Individuals with the following conditions ere excluded: disorders of the central nervous system, oral pathology, oral paralysis, oral surgery, less than 24 hours postoperative, or receiving total parental nutrition.

The nursing Kardex® was initially reviewed to select patients. Patient medical records and medication Kardexes® were also reviewed to further screen selected subjects. When possible, the list of subjects was reviewed with the head nurse to see if there were contraindications to participation in the study. Members of the research team then instructed each subject on the purpose and plan of the study and verbal consent for participation was obtained. This type of consent was approved by the institutional review board because temperature taking is a routine hospital procedure. Patients were told they could withdraw from the study at any time during the three days of data collection. The sample selected for analysis for one 24-hour period consisted of 49 men who ranged in age from 18 to 91 years and 58 women whose age ranged from 19 to 87.

Oral body temperature of each subject was measured and recorded during six time intervals throughout the day: 6 P.M., 10 P.M., 6 A.M., 10 A.M., 2 P.M., and 6 P.M. The same procedure was used by all data collectors. The thermometer probe was placed in the left or right posterior sublingual pocket of the oral cavity. The probe remained in place until the electronic thermometer signaled by sound that the body temperature had been measured. The measurement was recorded on a data collection form designed for this study. Prior to each of the six measurement time periods, the electronic thermometers were tested for accuracy, using the method recommended by the manufacturer.

RESULTS

Data analysis of measurements for one 24-hour period, 6 P.M. one day to 6 P.M. the next day, revealed no first fevers at 6 A.M. or 10 A.M. Of 107 subjects, 38 (36%) had febrile readings during the 24-hour cycle. Of these 38 subjects, 23 (60%) were first febrile at the first 6 P.M. measurement; 9 (24%) were first febrile at 10 P.M.; 3 (8%) were first febrile at 2 P.M.; and 3 (8%) were first febrile at the second 6 P.M. measurement. Results indicated that the optimal time to measure body temperature to screen for fever is 6 P.M. and the frequency is once a day.

Of the 38 subjects who had febrile readings, 8 were not febrile at either of the 6 P.M. measurements. Six of these 8 had an elevation only at that one time interval and not at any other time period. A seventh had an elevation at 10 P.M., and again at 6 A.M. but was afebrile at the other readings. The eighth subject had an evaluation at 10 P.M., 10 A.M., and 2 P.M.

Two additional subjects were afebrile at the first 6 P.M. measurement, but they were febrile 4 hours later at 10 P.M. and throughout the study. These two subjects' temperature elevations would not have been detected until the 6 P.M. measurement on the following day (20 hours) if temperature measurements were taken only routinely at 6 P.M. each day. However, temperature is only one variable observed by nurses in assessing progress or changes in health status.

DISCUSSION

From the sample of 107 subjects analyzed for one 24-hour period, 38 subjects had febrile temperatures. Thirty of the 38 subjects who had febrile readings were detected by measuring temperatures at 6 P.M., the peak of the circadian thermal rhythm. If temperatures had been taken only at this time, 8 (7%) subjects who had febrile readings at other times would have been undetected. If in this group of 107 subjects, body temperatures had been measured at 6 P.M. only, 2 subjects would have had febrile readings from 10 P.M. that would have been undetected for 20 hours. A change in body temperature may represent a significant change in patient status but temperature change frequently has accompanying symptoms that nurses assess routinely.

The findings of this study indicate that one daily routine temperature recording at the peak of the circadian thermal rhythm (5 P.M. to 7 P.M.) is adequate to screen for fever in adult hospitalized patients. Body temperature may be measured more than once daily, based on professional nursing judgment about the status of patients.

Recommendations

Nurses should replicate the design of this study by measuring patients' body temperature for a 24-hour period from 6 P.M. to 6 P.M. in their institutions. If their findings support the hypothesis, results should be used by nursing service committees to change policy for routine measurement of body temperature. Reduction of routine temperature measurement procedures in health care agencies has implications for cost containment.

The findings of this study may have significance for rehabilitation and nursing home facilities in which nurses could replicate the study with implications for change in routine nursing care. Nurses in areas in which patients have neurological dysfunction that might affect body temperature should implement a similar study to determine if circadian thermal rhythm is present and the relationship of this rhythm to routine measurement of the body temperature. Nurse educators may incorporate in their teaching a concept of circadian rhythms related to body temperature so that as students develop skill in measuring temperature, they are able to gain some theoretical knowledge as a basis for measurement.

REFERENCES

Angerami, E. L. S. (1980). Epidemiological study of a body temperature in patients in a teaching hospital. *International Journal of Nursing Studies, 17*(2), 91–99.

Aschoff, J. (1960). Circadian rhythms in man. *Science, 148,* 1427–1432.

Beck, W. C., & St. Cyr, B. (1974). Oral thermometry. *The Guthrie Bulletin, 43,* 170–185.

Bell, S. (1969). Early morning temperatures? *American Journal of Nursing, 69*(4), 764–766.

Blainey, C. G. (1974). Site selection in taking body temperature. *American Journal of Nursing, 74*(10), 1859–1861.

Cooper, K. H., & Abrams, R. (1981). Attributes of the oral cavity as a site for basal body temperature measurements. *Journal of Obstetric, Gynecologic and Neonatal Nursing, 13*(2), 125–129.

Cranston, W. I. (1966). Temperature regulation. *British Medical Journal, 2,* 69–75.

DeRisi, L. (1968). Body temperature measurements in relation to circadian rhythmicity in hospitalized male patients. In *American nurses association clinical sessions* (pp. 251–258). New York: Appleton-Century-Crofts.

Dressler, D., Smejkal, C. & Ruffolo, M. (1983). A comparison of oral and rectal temperature measurements on receiving oxygen by mask. *Nursing Research, 32*(6), 373–375.

Erickson, R. (1980). Oral temperature differences in relation to thermometer and technique. *Nursing Research, 29*(3), 157–164.

Forster, B., Adler, D., & Davis, M. (1970). Duration of effects of drinking iced water on oral temperature. *Nursing Research, 19*(2), 169–170.

Knapp, H. (1966). Accuracy of glass clinical thermometers compared to electronic thermometers. *American Journal of Surgery, 112,* 139–141.

Lim-Levy, F. (1982). The effect of oxygen inhalation on oral temperature. *Nursing Research, 31*(3), 150–152.

Lobban, M. (1960). The entrainment of circadian rhythms in man. *Cold Spring Harbor Symposia on Quantitative Biology, 25,* 325.

Minors, D. S., & Waterhouse, J. M. (1981). *Circadian rhythms and the human.* Bristol: John Wright & Sons, Stonebridge Ltd. Press.

Palmer, D. H. (1949). A check on acceptability of clinical thermometers. *Hospitals, 23*(5), 87–88.

Purintun, L. R., & Bishop, B. E. (1969). How accurate are clinical thermometers? *American Journal of Nursing, 69*(1), 99–100.

Schmidt, M. A. (1958). Are all TPRs necessary? *American Journal of Nursing, 58,* 559.

Selle, W. A. (1952). *Body temperature: Its changes with environment, disease and therapy.* Springfield, IL: Charles C. Thomas, Publisher.

Sims, R. S. (1965). Temperature recording in a teaching hospital. *The Lancet, 2*(9), 535–536.

Stephens, G. J., & Halberg, F. (1965). Human time estimation. *Nursing Research, 14*(4), 310–317.

Woodman, E., Parry, & Simms, L. (1967). Sources of unreliability in oral temperatures. *Nursing Research, 16,* 276–279.

Wunderlich, C. A., & Sequin, E. (1871). *Medical thermometry and human temperature.* New York: William Wood & Company, pp. 26–27.

Yorkman, C. A. (1982). Cool and heated aerosol and the measurement of oral temperature. *Nursing Research, 31*(6), 354–357.

This article is printed with permission of *Nursing Research.* Copyright 1985 American Journal of Nursing Company.

5

Maternity Nursing

Carol Howe, DNSc, RN, CNM
Jennifer Carley-Roe, BSN, RN
Marilyn Parker-Cullen, BSN, RN

INTRODUCTION BY: CAROL HOWE, DNSc, RN, CNM

The scope of maternity nursing has expanded significantly in recent years. Far beyond caring for laboring and postpartum mothers, nurses today address the broad spectrum of high-tech/high-risk childbearing as well as the return to a less interventive "natural" birth experience. Moreover, "women's health" issues, largely ignored by nursing curricula in the past, keep seeping into the sphere of the maternity nurse.

New science and new technology have made the experience of maternity possible for women who previously could not conceive to bear children. Preterm babies previously considered nonviable are now survivors. Their mothers require long-term nursing support to cope with their high-risk pregnancies and the loss of a normal birth and newborn. Women also are demanding more control over their birth experiences and nursing strategies are changing to support these demands.

Some women remain childless either by choice or by chance. Those who choose not to have children still have reproductive health care needs, such as family planning or menstrual disorders, as well as the need to maximize their health potential through diet, exercises, and stress reduction. Those for whom childlessness is a bitter twist of fate need the additional assistance of coming to terms with their infertility.

Nurses interact with women in a variety of settings and roles. Inpatient nursing roles may encompass labor and delivery or postpartum nursing as well as surgical nursing on units where infertility evaluation or gynecological surgery is conducted. Outpatient settings may include clinics or offices whether as staff nurses or as nurse-midwives and women's health care nurse practitioners.

Regardless of role or setting, nursing research can improve the quality of care delivered. Nonetheless, frequently in maternity nursing, care has emanated from tradition rather than science. One of the articles selected for critique in this chapter is a good example. Brown and Hurlock studied the effect of selected nursing interventions in breast feeding. An excellent experimental study published over a decade ago, this research failed to demonstrate any beneficial effect for those nursing interventions that are still standard of care today. Had nurses heeded the evidence and moved onward to the development of new, more efficacious interventions, successful long-term breast feeding might be the norm rather than the exception that it is today.

The studies selected for critique in this chapter reflect the broad scope of maternity nursing today as well as the varied methodological approaches which characterize nursing research in this specialty. Brown and Hurlock's study, mentioned earlier, is a classic experiment designed to test the effectiveness of nursing interventions with breastfeeding mothers. Norbeck and Tilden's study is a multifactorial, correlational design to explore the relationship of social support to obstetrical outcome. Olshansky's study uses grounded theory methodology to explore the feelings of infertile couples. Each provides knowledge to guide the nursing care of women and their families.

The scope of materinty nursing is expanding almost exponentially. Traditional roles are becoming more demanding and new roles are emerging as technology expands and as women's health care needs change. Only research well developed and consistently utilized will allow nursing to keep pace with the health care needs of clients.

Preparation of the Breast for Breastfeeding

Marie Scott Brown, PhD
Assistant Professor
School of Nursing
University of Colorado
Denver, CO

Joan T. Hurlock, MS
Assistant Professor
University of Northern Colorado
Greeley, CO

To evaluate effectiveness of three commonly suggested methods of preparing the breasts for breastfeeding—nipple rolling, application of cream, and expression of colostrum—57 women volunteered to prepare one breast and not the other. One-third of the group used one each of the three methods. After delivery, the women completed data sheets on the subjective tenderness of both breasts, and an investigator visited them to evaluate objective measures of nipple irritation. When the treated and untreated breasts were compared, no significant differences in either objective or subjective measures of nipple sensitivity or trauma were found in any of the three groups. These findings imply that these traditional methods of preparing the breasts for breastfeeding are ineffective.

Most of the literature (Adebonojo, 1972; Applebaum, 1970; Barnes et al., 1953; Baum, 1971; Beal, 1969) and most clinicians who work with young infants advocate breastfeeding as a superior method of feeding. But problems with breastfeeding are common as witnessed by the fact that only 25 percent of the women in this country nurse their child for even one week and only 10-15 percent continue for two months (Fomon, 1974, p.8). Reasons for this infrequency need to be explored and ameliorated. In particular, why do half the women who begin breastfeeding stop before two months? Many reasons have been given; motivation (Applebaum, 1970), nipple pain (Newton, 1952), breast engorgement (Newton and Newton, 1951), and inverted nipples (Wennen, 1969) have been implicated. Preventive measures to eliminate or lessen these problems seem important.

According to preventive measures with which this research was concerned, the breasts are prepared for breastfeeding prenatally in order to prevent postnatal nipple pain and trauma. Although many methods of doing this have been suggested, basically the methods fall into three categories: 1) nipple friction such as brisk rubbing with a washcloth or ripple rolling, the purpose of which is to "toughen" the epithelium of the nipple so that it is more impervious to the trauma of sucking; 2) applications of various types of creams (lanolin, Masse®, A and D®, Mammol®, and similar substances) to "lubricate" and soften the nipple, making it more supple and hence less susceptible to damage; 3) the prenatal expression of colostrum. Although variations of these methods are generally advocated in the literature, little research has been done to substantiate their usefulness.

REVIEW OF THE LITERATURE

As stated, the literature recommends one of the three types of prenatal preparation of the breasts for breastfeeding. Although some sources question the validity of such preparation (Gunther, 1945), most assume its usefulness (Applebaum, 1970). The fact that pain and damaged nipples are important factors in the course of lactation has been investigated to some extent. In 1950, Newton and Newton found that more than 80 percent of breastfeeding mothers experienced such pain. The following year they found that such pain often caused sucking time to be limited with a resulting decrease in stimulation and consequent fall in the amount of milk secreted (Newton and Newton, 1951). They also showed that such pain frequently inhibits the letdown reflex, resulting in poor milk flow and less effective sucking (Newton and Newton, 1948).

Research concerning preventive measures appears to be scarce. Newton (1952) studied various types of care given to the nipples. The methods of care were given during the first five days following birth, although some of the same methods frequently advocated for prenatal care were studied. Women studied included one group who washed their nipples with a soap solution before feeding, one who treated them with 70 percent alcohol, one who used A and D Ointment®, one who used A and D Concentrate®, one who used lanolin, and one who used plain water. The results of the study showed that the groups which used soap, alcohol, and the A and D Concentrate® suffered more problems than the control group which used water. The other groups were not significantly different from the control group. The study, though suggestive regarding prenatal preparation, was concerned only with postnatal care, and its results should not be directly applied to prenatal preparation of the breasts.

Two studies dealt directly with the antenatal preventive measures designed to decrease nipple pain and damage postnatally. The first (Gans, 1958) focused on three groups—one untreated, one which applied a .5 percent stilbestrol cream in hydrous ointment form, and one which used a "releasil 7" water-repellent silicone barrier type of cream available in Great Britain. The treatments were begun four months before the expected date of confinement. Neither of the treatments significantly decreased problems with nipple pain or damage. The "control" group, unfortunately, was instructed to dry their nipples with a towel so that they actually used one method suggested in the literature for hardening nipples. The results are difficult to evaluate since no group was studied which in fact did nothing to the breast.

Ingelman-Sundberg (1958) compared the amount of milk present on the twelfth day of lactation and the amount of objective nipple damage present during the first five days between a control group who did not prepare their nipples prenatally and a group who massaged their nipples and expressed colostrum from their breasts beginning with the fifth month of pregnancy. Little detail is available concerning how these preparations were carried out. No differences were found between the two groups.

STATEMENT OF THE PROBLEM

The purpose of this study was to evaluate three specific types of prenatal breast preparations (representing the three categories described in the literature as effective) in reducing objective and subjective signs and symptoms of nipple problems that may lead to ineffective nursing.

Hypotheses

Four major and two minor null hypotheses were investigated.

Major Hypotheses. Four major hypotheses were stated:

I. Nipples prepared prenatally by the technique of nipple rolling for a period of three to six weeks will not differ on measures of objective or subjective damage or pain from those nipples not prepared in any way.

II. Nipples prepared prenatally by the application of Masse® cream for a period of three to six weeks will not differ significantly on measures of objective or subjective damage or pain from nipples receiving no preparation.

III. Breasts prepared prenatally by expression of colostrum for a period of three to six weeks will not differ significantly on measures of objective or subjective damage or pain from breasts receiving no such preparation.

IV. The three methods of preparation (i.e., nipple rolling, application of Masse ® cream, and expression of colostrum) will not differ significantly from each other in their effectiveness in reducing the incidence of objective or subjective nipple trauma or pain.

Minor Hypotheses. The minor hypotheses were not directly related to the major problem, but were seen as important clinical problems that easily fall in the realm of this research:

V. Light-haired (i.e., redheaded and blonde), fair-skinned women are not more subject to objective or subjective nipple damage and pain, than are dark (brown or black-haired), dark-skinned individuals.

VI. Weight gain (as an indication of amount of milk ingested) will not be significantly greater in infants who suck from breasts prenatally prepared by the expression of colostrum. (This would indicate that the amount of milk flow has not been increased by this method of preparation.)

Method

The Population. Fifty-seven women were chosen, some from a metropolitan area and some from a rural area of Colorado. Of lower or middle-income brackets, they were obtained through prenatal classes or private physicians' practices. There was a racial mix between Anglo- and Chicano-Americans. No mother was accepted into the study if she had previously breastfed an infant, and any mother-baby pair who had enough difficulties postpartum to be kept in the hospital longer than the average stay was discarded from the sample. Important variables such as hair color, skin color, and other physical characteristics were recorded. A matched sample was automatically obtained on all these variables.

Prenatal Preparation. Three weeks before the expected date of confinement subjects were sought who were willing to participate in the experiment. Each woman was assigned randomly to one of the three groups (nipple rolling, application of cream, and expression of colostrum). She was then taught this method of preparation by the nurse investigators and instructed to perform it twice daily on one breast only. The other breast was to receive no preparation. Subjects were asked postnatally if they had indeed maintained this schedule, and those who did not were discarded from the sample. The breast to be prepared was chosen randomly by a coin toss and was recorded, but the woman was asked not to reveal this information to the nurse who would inspect her breasts postnatally. This would avoid bias in the nurse's evaluation of the objective evidence of nipple damage. There was, of course, no way to avoid the bias that the woman herself might display toward (or perhaps away from) the breast she knew she had prepared.

Postnatal Evaluation. Two main dependent variables were measured postnatally, the objective and subjective indications of nipple pain. The objective measures were taken by the investigators and a small number of research assistants (primarily nurses with experience in maternal-child nursing and nursing students who had finished their maternal-child student experience.) All were thoroughly trained and checked by the investigators before making the evaluations on their own. The breasts were examined by the nurse investigators each day in the hospital and every other day after returning home for a period of ten days. Form A (see Figure 1) was completed, including information on the amount of filling of the breast, amount of redness within and outside the areola (measured in millimeters), number and size of fissures, and amount of protrusion. The size of the areola was also measured and the apparent intensity of sucking action of the infant was estimated (each hospital visit included an observation of a feeding period). A column for problems or comments was included for anything the nurse noted, particularly for any asymmetrical condition. The infant was also weighed at each visit.

The subjective measurement of nipple prob-

Figure 1
Objective Nipple Rating by Nurse Observer

Name _____
Number _____
Hair color _____
Skin color (fair, medium, dark, other) _____

	Date					Day 10	
		Day 1					
		Right	Left			Right	Left
Condition of breast a) soft							
b) filling							
c) firm							
d) engorged							
Redness within areola (mm)							
Redness from border of areola out (in mm)							
Number and size of fissures (in mm)							
Size of areola							
Nipple check a) protruding							
b) flat							
c) inverted							
Sucking intensity a) strong							
b) good							
c) fair							
d) poor							
Baby's weight							
Comments							

lems was obtained by asking the mother to fill out a questionnaire (Figure 2) immediately after each feeding. This questionnaire ascertained the time of feeding, number of minutes the infant nursed on each breast, and which breast was used first. The mother was then asked to rate nipple sensitivity on a scale of one to four for each side (from comfortable to painful) and to comment specifically on the use of supplements, pain medication, nipple shields, ointment, or other measures. The comments column was usually generously filled out. Information on the number of

Figure 2
Excerpt from the Subjective Rating of Nipple Tenderness by Patient
(Example of Two Days' Ratings)

Name _____
Number _____
Date and time of delivery _____

KEY: C = completely comfortable
 T = some tenderness
 VT = very tender
 P = painful

FEEDING OF THE DAY	(1st)	(2nd)	(3rd)	(4th)	(5th)	(6th)	(7th)
Day of delivery	R L	R L	R L	R L	R L	R L	R L
a) just prior to feeding							
b) beginning feeding							
c) during feeding							
d) right after feeding							
e) between feedings							
f) minutes per breast							
g) first breast used							
h) time of feeding							
i) comments[1]							
First day after delivery							
a) just prior to feeding							
b) beginning feeding							
c) during feeding							
d) right after feeding							
e) between feedings							
f) minutes per breast							
g) first breast used							
h) time of feeding							
i) comments[1]							

[1] Comments: Please put down any comments you think would be helpful. For instance, we would like to know if you used ointments, creams, heat, pain medications, or a nipple shield at each feeding. Other comments would also be appreciated.

feedings per day and their frequency was computed from the information the mothers filled out on time of day.

Variables Considered Confounding. The method of preparing one breast and not the other on an individual woman was believed by the investigators to offer a distinct advantage in the control of variables. It meant the vast majority of possibly influential variables (e.g., nutritional status of mother, health conditions, socioeconomic status, race) were held constant since they were true, of course, for both breasts. In effect, a matched sample design was obtained. A few local conditions, such as protrusion, could not be controlled in this way, but these differences were carefully recorded and examined. Other variables such as the handedness, faithfulness of preparation, number of days of preparation, which breast was used to begin each feeding, the number of minutes the infant sucked at each breast, and the length of time since the last feeding were all recorded and analyzed.

Data Analysis. All variables were compared between groups. Faithfulness of preparation, hair color, and skin color were compared by use of chi square; the rest were compared by use of an F test. The first four null hypotheses were tested by the t test. Level of significance was set at .05.

Results

The three groups did not differ from each other on any of the measures except the average length of time between feedings. In this variable, the groups which prepared their breasts by nipple rolling appeared to have a longer average length of time between feedings. The reason for this is not known.

Hypotheses. Null hypotheses II and III could not be rejected ($p > .05$). In testing null hypothesis I the t test was significant. While this difference may be statistically significant, it probably is not clinically significant. In testing null hypothesis IV, no significant difference was found among the three groups on either objective or subjective measures of nipple trauma or pain.

Null hypothesis V could not be rejected by means of the F test ($p > .05$); and null hypothesis VI was tested by chi square and accepted ($p > .05$).

DISCUSSION

Although health professionals and lay organizations concerned with breastfeeding still tell mothers that various methods of preparing their breasts prenatally will enhance their chances of success of avoiding pain and nipple trauma, these

Table 1
Subjective Difference between Treated and Untreated Breasts of Three Groups of 19 Subjects Each as Measured by t Test

Subject	I Nipple Rolling	II Masse Cream	III Expression of Colostrum
1	-.525	.026	-.006
2	.172	.739	0.000
3	-.577	-.095	-.257
4	.200	-.040	-.070
5	.040	.006	.107
6	-.143	-.600	.362
7	.043	.007	-.263
8	.010	.008	.010
9	.000	.000	-.080
10	-.522	-.100	-.010
11	.007	.000	.048
12	-.122	.000	.300
13	-.040	.060	.182
14	.000	-.180	-.378
15	-.100	.000	-.075
16	.050	.040	-.040
17	-.575	.080	-.080
18	.031	-.450	-.100
19	-.060	.000	-.020
S*	.248	-.453	-.454
I	.061	.247	.173
X̄*	-.111	.061	.030
τ	1.95*	-.025	.018

*$p > .05$
*S represents the estimate of standard deviation for different scores in each column; V, the corresponding variant (= S'); X̄, the corresponding areas; t, the value for the one-sample t test.

statements were not verified by this study. This finding appeared to be in accordance with the other two studies cited in the literature. Of interest also was the fact that the frequently heard clinical impression that light-haired, fair-skinned women have more difficulty with nipple damage was not substantiated by this study. Again, this finding was consistent with Gans' (1958) study. The idea that expression of colostrum prenatally will increase milk flow was not supported, as in this study infants fed by this method did not gain more weight than infants fed from breasts not so prepared.

Implications for Nursing. Two contributions to nursing resulted from this study—one methodological, one clinical. The method of asking subjects to prepare only one breast was a highly effective way of controlling for possibly confounding variables. The method is applicable to other types of clinical research in which local topical physiologic responses are measured.

Also of significance was the finding that the traditional methods of preparing breasts for breastfeeding appeared to be ineffective in relieving nipple soreness. For nursing to grow in its scientific acceptability and body of knowledge, the basis of clinical teaching should be thoroughly researched. Some nurses believe the value of these three methods of preparation is to help a woman become familiar with her breasts before her child is born so that her anxiety in handling them during the nursing process is reduced. If this familiarization process is the importance of such preparation, the rationale should be clearly stated. A nurse should not state that these methods will reduce nipple pain or trauma, since there is no evidence to support this statement. Indeed, this research would indicate that such an assumption is untrue.

REFERENCES

Adebonojo, F. O. (1972). Artificial vs. breast feeding. *Clinical Pediatrics, 11,* 25–29.

Applebaum, R. M. (1970). The physician and a common sense approach to breast feeding. *Southern Medical Journal, 63,* 793–799.

Barnes, G. R., Jr. (1953). Management of breast feeding. *Journal of the American Medical Association, 151,* 192–199.

Baum, J. D. (1971). Nutritional value of human milk. *Obstetrics and Gynecology, 37,* 126–129.

Beal, V. A. (1969). Breast- and formula-feeding of infants. *Journal of the American Dietary Association, 55,* 31–37.

Fomon, S. J. (1974). *Infant nutrition* (2nd ed.). Philadelphia: W. B. Saunders.

Gans, B. (1958). Breast and nipple pain in early stages of lactation. *British Medical Journal, 5100,* 830–832.

Gunther, M. (1945). Sore nipples causes and prevention. *Lancet,* 590–593.

Ingelman-Sundberg, A. (1958). The value of antenatal massage of nipples and expression of colostrum. *Journal of Obstetrics and Gynecology of the British Commons, 65,* 448–449.

Newton, M., & Newton, N. R. (1948). The let down reflex in human lactation. *Journal of Pediatrics, 33,* 698–704.

Newton, M., & Newton, N.R. (1948). Breast abscess: A result of lactation failure. *Surgery, Gynecology, and Obstetrics, 91,* 651–655.

Newton, M., & Newton, N.R. (1951). Postpartum engorgement of the breast. *American Journal of Obstetrics and Gynecology, 61,* 664–667. 667.

Newton, N. (1952). Nipple pain and nipple damage. *Journal of Pediatrics, 41,* 411–423.

Wennen, C. A. (1969). Breast feeding by mothers with flat nipples. *Journal of Tropical Pediatrics, 15,* 163–166.

This article is printed with permission of *Nursing Research.* Copyright 1975 American Journal of Nursing Company.

Original article:
Brown, M. S., & Hurlock, J. T. (1975). Preparation of the breast for breastfeeding. *Nursing Research, 24*(6), 448–451.

CRITIQUE BY: MARILYN PARKER-CULLEN, BSN, RN

Part 1: Clinical Relevance

The clinical problem under study concerns what antepartal methods, if any, help to decrease nipple pain and trauma associated with breastfeeding. Brown and Hurlock relate this problem to the more encompassing concern of poor breastfeeding statistics in the United States. According to Brown and Hurlock, a principal reason that women stop breastfeeding soon after delivery is nipple pain. Therefore, they feel that measures used to prevent such pain are worthy of study.

Although I am not currently working with an obstetrical population, I do recall concerns of expectant mothers during my experience in maternity nursing. Usually, questions about various methods of "nipple toughening" arose. Some women mentioned the use of sandpaper and nipple stretching. These methods usually evoked an agonized look from me and sounded more injurious and traumatic to the nipples than the most aggressive baby with teeth. I was left with suggesting the less rigorous "nipple rolling" yet knew nothing about actual benefit. Other professionals in the clinic could not offer enlightening information on the topic as well. Therefore, research on this topic appears to have use in the clinical setting.

Specifically, Brown and Hurlock's research has the potential of providing a nurse with additional clinical information. This, in turn, facilitates decision making regarding the use of interventions; or, in this case, ruling out interventions due to their inability to produce results.

While Brown and Hurlock did not generate a new hypothesis by their research, they did test four primary and two minor hypotheses. While these latter hypotheses are not related directly to the primary problem under question, they are strong enough for future research and potential application to practice.

In terms of specific nursing interventions, the investigators tested three: nipple rolling, cream application, and colostrum expression. These interventions recommended by the lay as well as professional medical population, are undertaken by some women prior to delivery to "toughen" up their nipples for breastfeeding.

Brown and Hurlock sought to determine if there was a relationship between nipple preparation and decreased nipple pain and trauma during breastfeeding.

The dependent variable, or status of the nipple after breastfeeding, was measured both subjectively and objectively. Investigators, research assistants, and nursing students measured nipple trauma on the basis of color and skin condition (as evidenced by lesions) over a period of 10 days immediately postpartum. Other objective data included infant weight gain and sucking intensity. Subjective data included the mothers descriptions of nipple sensitivity throughout the feeding process.

Of the measures mentioned above, the most useful for clinical practice is that of assessing growth, or more accurately, weight gain. In a well-baby clinic, a care provider assesses infant weight. Any variation from the norm warrants investigation. The care provider looks at the child's feeding habits so as to reveal a possible problem within the breastfeeding mother. As used in this research, subjective and objective examination might reveal nipple pain or trauma. These measures are all within the realm of nursing and can be undertaken without prior approval or permission of other health care professionals.

In conclusion, this study appears of potential use to those working within maternal–child nursing.

Part II: Conceptualization and Internal Consistency

Brown and Hurlock wrote their report with clarity and succinctness. It held my attention and did not require an advanced course in statistics to understand. They did not sway from the topic and followed through with intentions indicated in the first few paragraphs.

The underlying concept addressed is a basic one. Essentially, if pregnant women "prepared" their breasts for breastfeeding, would this lead to decreased nipple pain and trauma, and, therefore, to an increased chance of successful nursing? The concept, successful breastfeeding, is supported by the literature review which yielded research stating that one of the reasons for poor breastfeeding statistics in America is due to nipple pain and trauma in the nursing mother. Also, it is this literature that provides justification for the study.

The underlying concept relates coherently to the questions under study; they are logically operationalized as variables in the research. The independent variable, antepartal nipple preparation, was comprised of the three possible treatments mentioned previously.

The investigators decided on a research design which would most likely support their hypotheses. However, it was a traditional design that I have not often seen in nursing research. Scientifically testing interventions is not common, I assume, because nursing is somewhat new as a science and still largely involved with theory generation.

Brown and Hurlock chose a representation of the population under study (pregnant women) and divided them so as to test each intervention. Three weeks prior to their delivery date the subjects were taught one method of nipple preparation and instructed to perform it twice daily. The investigators did not assess the usefulness of these interventions until after delivery.

The instruments used to assess interventions were both subjective and objective. The latter instruments included the physical assessment and measurement of the nursing mother's breasts; the former instrument included a scale rating nipple sensation by the mother. In general, the instruments appear sound in measuring nipple pain and trauma and are commonly used by nurses in maternal–child practice.

Part III: Believability of Results

This study purported to test actual nursing interventions. Application of these interventions leads the investigator to data of a quantitative nature. These data allowed Brown and Hurlock to form concrete appraisals of the relationships between the independent and dependent variables.

Subjects were selected from rural and metropolitan areas in the state of Colorado. Brown and Hurlock specify that the women were Anglo and Chicano, of a lower to middle income bracket, and came from private physicians or prenatal classes. It is not clear as to how the investigators made subject choices but it appears to be nonprobable in nature. Since Brown and Hurlock wanted some representativeness of the population, quota sampling would account for the racial mix as well as income variation. However, although nipple pain may be related to skin color, the sample did not include all racial groups, hence limiting generalizability of the findings.

Brown and Hurlock address three potential biases regarding subjects: women who have previously breast fed; women whose postpartum stay in the hospital exceeded the average; and varying physical characteristics. The first two variables were dealt with by omission from the study. The latter variable was attended to by recording hair and skin color. This informaton was used later in the data analysis and applied to one of the minor hypothesis not directly related to the research problem.

However, Brown and Hurlock are weak in discussing the reliability and validity of the measures. For example, they did not address the reliability or consistency of results obtained postnatally. Was there interrater reliability? In essence, were the investigators, research assistants, and nursing students all objectively measuring and assessing breasts with uniform results. Brown and Hurlock state only that they were "trained and checked by investigators before making evaluations on their own." However, it is difficult for researchers to accurately and consistently assess such nebulous physical characteristics as breast states of engorgement, texture, and color.

Since the objective instrument may not be reliable, its validity must be questioned. Examples of validity problems include the instrument's attention to redness, and sucking intensity. These items do not necessarily measure the degree of nipple trauma or pain. In addition, nipple redness might be undetectable in a dark skinned woman or excessive in a woman with less pigment. Sucking intensity also is subject to criticism because a child, though sucking poorly, may have latched only on to the nipple, which could be more painful than the child having latched on to the areola with a vigorous suck.

Which breast the infant first starts to feed on is another concern of significance. Although this concern is incorporated into the instrument, my experience with new mothers proves that infants tend to spend more time and suck with more vigor at the breast first offered. I would have liked to see this variable controlled for by intentionally alternating the breast first offered at each feeding.

The subjective questionnaire completed by mothers after each feeding appears straight forward. The scale assessing pain is useful in that it assigns a measurable value to a sensation. In general, the investigators stayed within the confines of the proposed problem in the use of subjects, measurement, and instrumentation.

The investigators tested the three interventions or independent variables on randomly assigned groups. From a total sample of 57, 19 women were chosen for each test group. Brown and Hurlock mention no methodological or clinical problems arising from this randomization other than some minor physical variations in women which could not be controlled for. In general, control was uniquely achieved within the study by virtue of the fact that women have two breasts. One breast received the treatment and the other nothing. As Brown and Hurlock point out, this controlled for such variables as "nutritional status of mother, health conditions, socioeconomic status, and race."

The overall results of this study were presented concisely. Given my limited understanding of statistics, I trust that Brown and Hurlock provided accurate information regarding outcome. I am unable to say if the statistical testing they used is appropriate for the data collection, however. To do so, I would have to consult with a more qualified source before making any statements regarding the use of chi square and t-test in this study.

All hypotheses tested exceeded the upper limit of what is probable ($p > .05$). In relation to the primary hypothesis, Brown and Hurlock state that "no significant difference was found among the three groups on either objective or subjective measures of nipple trauma or pain." The outcome data seems quite realistic given the variables and indicative of the "real" world, although sample sizes were quite small. However, with a larger sample population, significant differences might then appear.

The conclusions drawn by the investigators do not reach beyond the boundaries of the study. Results appear to be directly related to the primary research question, thus warranting use of the information in practice.

Part IV: Generalizability of Results

Generalizability of this research is dependent upon numerous factors. An initial factor that supports utilization of this research is that procedures and methods used in the study are common and familiar to the maternal–child setting.

Another factor, the sample, although small and missing representatives from higher income levels, is similar enough to patients where I have practiced to allow generalizability. The primary investigators enhanced generalizability by obtaining subjects from both metropolitan and rural settings.

Brown and Hurlock state that investigators were trained to assess the postpartum mothers. It is conceivable that those teaching the interventions and doing the postnatal evaluations are typical of nursing professionals in antepartal and postpartal settings, thus another positive factor supporting generalizability.

Personally, I am not aware of other studies which addressed the same nursing issues presented in Brown and Hurlock's research. However, in reading their literature review, I see that studies have been done rendering similar data, providing more credence to the application and clinical use of their results.

Brown and Hurlock did their research in 1975. Because of the span of years between then and now, I would be hesitant to incorporate their results in practice until I looked at more recent research. Ideally, I would like to find research in the same problem with a larger sample that substantiates Brown and Hurlock's findings.

Part V: Other Factors to Consider in Utilization

Incorporating Brown and Hurlock's research into practice has little risk in that the study findings support doing away with interventions rather than implementing them. Time and energy would have to be expended in educating practitioners and patients on the possible futility of antepartal nipple preparation. However, this could be done with little cost via a short inservice or newsletter to fellow care providers.

On the other hand, it is that "little risk" that remains problematic. A potential and perhaps unrecognized risk may exist in dissuading women from preparing their nipples for breastfeeding. For example, there could be women who have benefited from the intervention physically or mentally. In this regard, Brown and Hurlock's sample is not of sufficient size for me to grant total conviction to their results. While the research is encouraging and with strong scientific merit, it is not entirely without risk.

Original article:
Brown, M. S., Hurlock, J. T. (1975). Preparation of the breast for breastfeeding. *Nursing Research, 24*(6), 448–451.

CRITIQUE BY: CAROL HOWE, DNSc, RN, CNM

This study was selected for critique because it exemplifies a classic approach to nursing research. In addition to being a well controlled, tightly designed experimental study, its results are as applicable today as they were when first published 12 years ago. The investigators identified a particular clinical problem: breastfeeding failure caused by painful nipples or the inability of the infant to "latch on" as a result of inverted nipples. They then selected for examination a number of commonly recommended therapies which had not been adequately tested.

Part I: Clinical Relevance

The clinical problem remains today. Documentation exists that breastfeeding offers many advantages over bottle feeding to both mother and infant. Breastfeeding has regained much of the popularity it lost during the 1950s, 1960s, and 1970s. The rate of initiation of breastfeeding has increased from a low of 20–25 percent in the 1970s to 80 percent in the early 1980s (Steinmetz, 1985). From the perspective of infant health, nursing throughout the first year of life is recommended. However, studies indicate that as many as 20–40 percent discontinue breastfeeding by the sixth week, and only 5–20 percent of mothers continue to nurse by six months.

Nurses interact with breastfeeding mothers in a variety of settings, including childbirth education, primary health care roles, inpatient labor and postpartum settings, and physician's offices. Infant feeding has resided within the independent domain of nursing for many years. The only exceptions are when the mother is advised not to nurse as a result of illness or complications that make breastfeeding contraindicated. However, physicians are rarely versed on the "how to" of breastfeeding, and assistance for the mother in this area comes from nurses.

In this study, the investigators tested three breast preparation interventions that nurses have commonly recommended to mothers who plan to breastfeed: nipple rolling, expression of colostrum, and the use of Masse' Cream. It is interesting to note that in spite of a number of good studies (including this one) that have shown little or no effect from these interventions, they are still commonly recommended. Each of these interventions is reputed to prevent nipple trauma, either by "toughening" the nipple, soothing the nipple, or helping it to evert to allow the infant to latch on more easily. Nipple trauma was measured both subjectively (by a perception of pain score) and objectively by investigator inspection (for redness, fissures, and eversion of the nipple). Expression of colostrum is also reputed to increase milk supply. Therefore, infant weight gain was measured as a proxy variable for the amount of milk produced.

The clinical problem remains relevant to nursing practice in a variety of settings. The tested interventions are also still in evidence, making the results of this study worthy of reconsideration.

Part II: Conceptualization and Internal Consistency

In general, this study is well designed to test the variables of interest. As an intervention study, it is logically experimental with tight controls. Each woman served as her own control, preparing one breast and not the other. The investigator remained blind to which breast had received the intervention. Women were randomly assigned to groups, each group using a different method of nipple preparation. The variables were clearly defined and measures were used that intuitively were valid, and, equally as important, usable by nurses in any setting. Nipple preparations were carried out in the home setting by the subjects themselves, mimicking the "real life" situation in which nurses would apply the interventions.

Part III: Believability of Results

As noted, this study was quantitative and experimental, and designed to evaluate the effectiveness of three commonly used nursing interventions to prepare nipples for nursing and thus decrease nipple trauma in the postpartum period.

The investigators selected their subjects from physicians' offices and prenatal clinics in both rural and urban settings. Both whites and Chicanos from lower and middle income families were included. Fifty-seven women who had not nursed an infant before were recruited and assigned randomly to one of the three interventions. Three weeks before their estimated date of birth, they were asked to begin twice daily preparation of one breast. Which breast was prepared was determined by coin flip. Postnatally, each mother kept a record of each feeding, including length of feeding, which breast was used first at each feeding, and a subjective measure of pain perception. Each mother was visited daily in the hospital, and every other day at home for the first 10 days after birth. The breasts were inspected for nipple redness, fissures, and eversion. In addition, the infant was weighed.

Four major and two minor hypotheses were tested. The first three hypothesized that each of the three treatments would make no significant difference in subjective or objective measures of nipple trauma. The fourth stated that no one of the three treatments would be more effective than any other. The minor hypotheses related to the testing of two common clinical impressions: (1) that fair haired women experienced more nipple trauma; and (2) that expression of colostrum would increase milk supply.

Objective measures of nipple trauma included inspection of the breast by an investigator blind to which nipple had been prepared. Subjective measures included the subjects' perception of pain. Infant weight served as a proxy measure of the amount of milk produced. Additional potential interacting variables also were recorded, including mothers' report of number of days of preparation, length of feedings, and the faithfulness of preparation.

Within each treatment group only nipple rolling was found to be significantly effective in preventing nipple trauma. Brown and Hurlock comment, however, that the difference is probably only statistically rather than clinically significant. Further, no significant difference in pain or trauma was noted between intervention groups. In addition, fair haired women were not found to experience more nipple trauma and mothers who expressed colostrum did not make more milk (as measured by infant weight gain).

The mechanism of sample selection is not clear, but appears to be a convenience selection of essentially normal new mothers. There is no reason to believe that this group of women is inherently different from other nursing mothers to whom the results of the study might be applied. Use of the contralateral breast as control and random assignment to groups enhances the tightness of the design and decreases the potential impact of interacting or intervening variables. Brown and Hurlock note, however, that the mother's subjective belief regarding the efficacy of the method may serve as a source of bias in reports of pain.

Reliability was addressed by ensuring that all investigators and research assistants were "thoroughly trained and checked" before evaluation of nipple trauma. The procedure for training was not described.

The objective measures of nipple trauma have face validity. They were, in fact, the measures used by clinicians to idenify the clinical problem. Use of infant weight as a measure of breast milk supply is a bit more troublesome. Other variables such as supplementation could easily influence early infant weight gain. Difficulties in "latching on" could retard weight gain even in the presence of adequate milk. Finally, there may not be sufficient variation weight gain in the first 10 days of infant life to create a significant difference either statistically or clinically.

Analysis of the first four hypotheses was done by t-test. A matched pair t-test for measurement of differences between prepared and unprepared breasts within treatment groups would be appropriate. However, the use of the t-test to analyze differences among the three treatment groups is not as clear. The use of multiple t-test to compare more than two groups results in a greater chance of finding a difference. A mean difference score obtained for each group would allow use of one-way analysis of variance. It is not clear from the report, however, how individual or group trauma scores were calculated. Nominal data, such as hair and skin color and faithfulness of preparation, were appropriately tested by chi square.

Interpretation of the statistical findings was the most difficult aspect of this critique. In addition to the questions raised in the preceding paragraph, two other issues seem relevant. Why was nipple rolling statistically significant, but viewed as not clinically effective? In this case, the investigators have overridden their own results, but without adequate explanation as to why in their professional judgement the treatment was not effective. It is important, however, that investigators not lose sight of the issue to clinical significance. Depending upon the type of analysis, the size of the sample and so forth, minor differences in scores may obtain statistical significance but have little clinical relevance. Perhaps in this study, major differences were in the objective signs of trauma, but there was little difference in patient perception of pain. In that case, the clinical significance would be markedly diminished even in the face of a statistical difference in scores. The data, however, are not reported in a manner that would allow the reader to understand the rationale for the investigators' judgement. Although the objective measures of nipple trauma were conceptually sound and clearly defined, it is not clear how a nipple trauma score was obtained. Therefore, it is difficult to make judgements regarding the appropriateness of statistical analysis.

Alternate explanations for the findings are not explored in sufficient detail. The sample size seemed large enough to show differences given the type of analysis performed and the number of variables tested. The measures, as noted earlier, seem valid. However, the most logical explanation for the result is that the interventions that nursing commonly recommends to prevent nipple trauma are simply not effective.

Part IV: Generalizability of Results

The results of this study should be generalizable to most nursing mothers. The interventions tested are used commonly and were performed in the same manner that would characterize clinical practice settings. There is no obvious difference between this sample and other samples of normal nursing mothers. The investigators are perhaps not typical of many practicing nurses by virtue of their advanced preparation and academic focus. However, they have designed a study that is clinically relevant to nurses practicing at any level and in many settings.

Part V: Other Factors to Consider in Utilization

This study could be easily replicated in a variety of settings. It involves a population easily accessible to nurses and clearly within the purview of nursing. The design is clear and the measurement is not difficult. The major difficulties encountered would be obtaining time or personnel for the 10-day follow up. This is especially true as a result of the movement toward early discharge from the hospital in recent years. It would be difficult to replicate the daily inspection that was accomplished in the hospital in this study

Adopting the results of this study into practice, however, involves certain atypical difficulties. One usually is concerned with the introduction of new knowledge, new skills, or new procedures into practice. However, adopting the results of this study requires analysis of cost/benefit, the introduction of change, and frequently, teaching or training of staff. In this instance, the difficulty is in convincing nurses to drop a conventional teaching which has not been shown to be effective. In addition to the difficulty of convincing nurses that what they have been taught is not correct, the loss of these suggestions for nipple preparation leaves little for nurses to offer patients for preparation for breastfeeding. Furthermore, and without documentation, the major tests in nursing continue to list these techniques of preparation as dogma (Varney, 1986; Neeson & May, 1986). It is difficult to institute change in the face of long accepted practice. The benefits of accepting the results of this research seem to lie in the potential to stimulate nurses to search for other more effective methods of preventing nipple trauma rather than continuing to rely upon ritual.

REFERENCES

Neeson, J., & May, K. (1986). *Comprehensive maternity nursing.* New York: Lippincott.

Steinmetz, K. (1985). *Informational correlates of successful breastfeeding: A replication.* Unpublished master's thesis, Oregon Health Sciences University: Portland, OR.

Varney, H. (1986). *Nurse-midwifery.* Boston: Blackwell Scientific Publishers.

Life Stress, Social Support, and Emotional Disequilibrium in Complications of Pregnancy: A Prospective, Multivariate Study

Jane S. Norbeck
University of California
San Francisco, CA

Virginia Peterson Tilden
Oregon Health Sciences University
Portland, OR

This study used a multivariate approach to determine the effects of selected psychosocial variables on pregnancy complications in a naturally-occurring population of medically-normal women from various racial, marital, and socioeconomic groups. Pregnant women between 12 and 20 weeks' gestation (N = 117) were tested with standardized instruments that measured life stress; social support; and the emotion-state variables of anxiety, depression, and self-esteem. Life stress during pregnancy was measured in the last prenatal month. Outcome was determined by postpartum chart review. Life stress and social support (emotional) were significantly related to emotional disequilibrium. Significant main effects were found for life stress (prior year) on overall and gestation complications and for emotional disequilibrium on infant-condition complications. A significant interaction of life stress (during pregnancy) and social support (tangible) was found for all three types of complications, but not for overall pregnancy complications.

Complications of pregnancy have been associated with life stress, psychosocial assets (including social support, anxiety, and other psychological variables (Gorsuch and Key, 1974; Nuckolls et al., 1972; McDonald, 1968). However, among the studies conducted over the past two decades, findings have often been inconsistent or contradictory. Direct comparison of studies is difficult because constructs have been selected and defined differently from study to study; measurement has occurred at various temporal points of the pregnancy; and samples have differed in parity, race, marital status, and socioeconomic level.

Table 1 outlines studies that have demonstrated significant relationships between psychological variables and complications of pregnancy. Although these are prospective studies, limitations in design give rise to rival hypotheses to explain the findings.

The first rival hypothesis is the presence of a third variable that explains the apparent relationship between a predictor and an outcome variable. With one exception, these studies did not control for preexisting medical risk factors, either through sampling criteria or statistical analysis. A significant relationship between a psychological variable and complications may be spurious because the medical condition might be the direct cause of both the elevated score on the psychological test and the occurrence of complications. For example, a diabetic woman is medically at risk for complications of pregnancy. Knowledge of this

Table 1
Outline of Prospective Studies on Psychological Variables and Pregnancy Complications[a]

Author and Date	Sample Size	Preexisting Medical Risk	Parity	Demographic Characteristics	Significant Variables[b]	Time Measured	Comments
Davids, DeVault, & Talmadge, 1961	48	Not Controlled	Mixed	Age 14–40 (Other characteristics not reported)	Anxiety (MAS) "Alienation" Personality Traits (TAT)	7th Month Gestation	Complication list did not include gestation period
Davids & DeVault, 1962	50	Not Controlled	Mixed	Not Reported	Anxiety (MAS, TAT, Sentence Completion)	Third Trimester	Complication list did not include gestation period
McDonald & Christakos, 1963	86	Not Controlled	Mixed	Age 16–37, Mean Education 9.1 Yrs., Very Low SES, 99% Married, White	Anxiety (MAS) Depressive or Neurotic Personality (MMPI), Low Self-Esteem & Ego Strength	6th Month Gestation	
McDonald & Parham, 1964	160	Not Controlled	Primiparas	Age 14–32, Mean Education 11.2 Yrs., Low-Middle SES, White, Unmarried	Anxiety (MAS) Neuroticism (MMPI) Unmarried	7th Month Gestation	
Nuckolls, Cassel, & Kaplan, 1972	170	Subjects Excluded for a Few Preexisting Factors	Primiparas	38.8% Adolescent, Middle to Lower SES, White, Married (Military Dependents)	"Psychosocial Assets" (Social Support, Ego Strength, Attitudes toward Pregnancy)	Prior to 24th Week Gestation	Significant findings are from a subsample of 26 subjects
Gorsuch & Key, 1974	111	Not Controlled	Mixed	Age 17–41, 61% White, 39% Black, 54% Married	Life Events, Anxiety (STAI)	32nd Week Varied 2–32 Weeks Gestation	Significant Life Events time period was not measured prospectively
Crandon, 1979a, 1979b	146	Not Controlled	Not Reported	Age 15–35 (Other characteristics not reported)	Life Events During Preg. Anxiety (IPAT)	Measured Post-Deliv. Third Trimester	

[a] Unless otherwise noted, the complication list included complications of gestation, labor and delivery, and infant condition.
[b] Abbreviated instruments are: MAS (Manifest Anxiety Scale), TAT (Thematic Apperception Test), MMPI (Minnesota Multiphasic Personality Inventory), STAI (State-Trait Anxiety Inventory), IPAT (Institute for Personality and Ability Testing—anxiety battery).

increased risk may lead to higher anxiety, but anxiety itself may not have a causal relationship to the outcome.

A second rival hypothesis concerns lack of control for age. Pregnant adolescents are known to be at higher risk for complications than adult women under age 40, yet very young subjects were included in each sample. Although age was not significantly related to complications in studies that reported this analysis, univariate tests may not tap the actual influence of age on complications. In the case of advanced age, for example, age is considered a medical risk factor at a younger age for primiparas than for multiparas.

Without the joint analysis of age and parity, the findings of these studies are subject to contamination from sampling.

Finally, some of these studies may not be truly prospective because the predictor variables were measured so late in the pregnancy that complications such as preeclampsia may have been experienced prior to the measurement of the predictor variables. In one study (Gorsuch and Key, 1974), life events occurring during the pregnancy were measured after delivery. In these cases, it is reasonable to speculate that the complicated patient might report a greater number of stressful events (or other phenomena) in an attempt to explain the negative outcome that she had experienced.

In light of these rival hypotheses, it is of interest that two recent studies (Jones, 1978; Beck et al., 1980), which did control preexisting medical risk factors and used multivariate approaches to study the effects of age, parity, socioeconomic level, and/or race, did not find significant relationships between complications and anxiety, personality, or maternal attitudes. Furthermore, Jones found an opposite effect for life stress: *low* levels of life change were significantly associated with complications.

Nuckolls et al. (1972) did partially control for preexisting medical risk factors. This is the only study that examined the influence of social support on complications of pregnancy; however, social support was imbedded in a construct, psychosocial assets, that included measures of ego strength and attitudes toward the pregnancy. Neither psychosocial assets nor life stresses were significantly related to complications; however, when analyzed together, psychosocial assets were found to have a buffering effect on life stress. In a subsample of 26 subjects who reported high life-stress both during the pregnancy and for the two years preceding the pregnancy, those with low psychosocial assets had a complication rate of 91 percent, compared to 33 percent for subjects with high psychosocial assets. No significant effects were found when life stress was high at only one of the two time periods.

The findings from the Nuckolls et al. (1972) study have been influential in the development of research on social support. Direct confirmation of the stress-buffering effects of social support, in which social support was not confounded with other constructs, was reported by Wilcox (1981) in a study of psychological symptoms. Whether social support, distinct from psychosocial assets, is significantly related to complications of pregnancy is not known.

A final note on previous studies concerns generalizability of the findings. Nuckolls et al. (1972) studied wives of enlisted men; these women may have very different life-stress and social-support patterns from women who live in the context of their naturally-occurring social networks. Many of the other samples were restricted to specific social class levels, racial groups, or marital status groups. The statistical control possible through multivariate techniques allows the study of a naturally-occurring population and the examination of demographic variables in conjunction with predictor variables as they might jointly influence outcomes.

THEORETICAL MODEL

The studies outlined in Table 1 have not evolved from or contributed to a comprehensive theoretical model to explain how various psychological and social factors might work together to influence pregnancy outcomes. In other health and mental health areas, research has been reported in which empirical clarification for theoretical models has been developed (Langlie, 1977; LaRocco et al, 1980; Lin et al., 1979; Pearlin et al., 1981).

The theoretical model of stress developed by Sarason (1979) was used to guide the design and analysis of this study. In this model, psychological stress involves "appraisals of (1) situations or tasks confronting the individual and (2) the individual's ability to deal successfully with them" (p. 3). Five elements are described in this process (see Figure 1): The *situation* (an event or task with demands, constraints, and opportunities) involves a *call to action* that leads the individual to *appraise the situation*. Stress follows a call for action when the individual perceives personal capabilities as fall-

Figure 1
Elements from Sarason's Theoretical Model of Stress with Operationalized Interpretation in Parenthesis

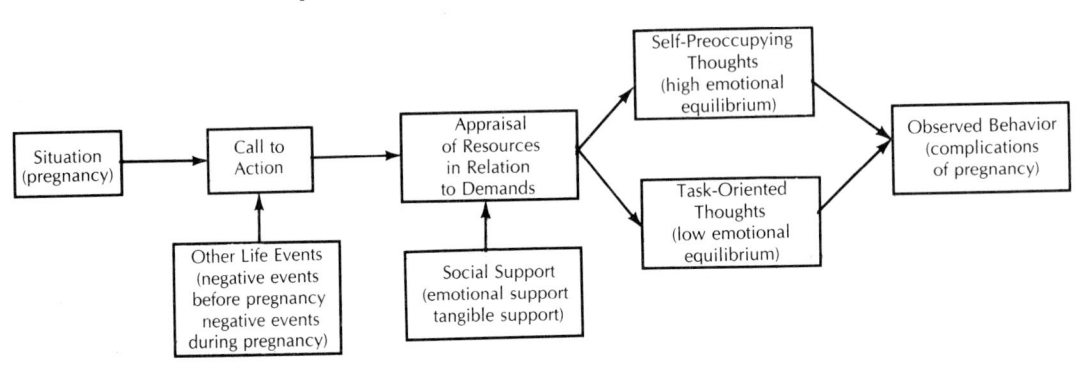

ing short of the needed personal resources. Depending on the appraisal, either *task-oriented* or *self-preoccupying thoughts* will predominate; these lead to *observable behavior* indicative of either successful or unsuccessful outcomes. Sarason emphasized that too many calls to action can result in overload in the appraisal of the situation, which then interferes with effective performance. Social support is the main contextual factor described by Sarason as a resource in the appraisal process. Emphasis on these contextual variables is consistent with the stress-buffering role hypothesized for social support (Cassel, 1976; Cobb, 1976).

Pregnancy is an event with demands, constraints, opportunities, and an uncertain outcome. Although pregnancy itself is considered to constitute a stressful experience, it is not uniformly stressful among women or for the same woman at different times in her life. Instead, the context of other life events and the availability of social support were regarded as the variables of central importance to the appraisal process in this study, and two hypotheses were tested:

Hypothesis 1: Life stress (negative life events) will be positively related and social support will be negatively related to emotional disequilibrium (self-preoccupying thoughts).

Hypothesis 2: High life-stress, low social support, and high emotional disequilibrium will be positively related to complications of pregnancy.

The following sections describe the rationale for the operationalization of life stress, social support, and emotional disequilibrium as variables predictive of complications of pregnancy.

Life Stress

Methodological inadequacies of life-events or life-stress measures have been discussed extensively and several key issues remain unresolved (Rabkin and Struening, 1976; Tausig, 1982). The rationale for operationalizing life stress in our study was based on clinical research with pregnant women. Helper et al. (1968) found that stress during pregnancy is highly nonspecific and that it is based on the woman's idiosyncratic perception of events as negative at this special juncture of her life course, e.g., events thought to have potential damage to her fetus.

Thus, rather than using predetermined definitions or weightings for life events, life stress in this study was measured by a method that allows each respondent to rate the quality (good vs. bad) and impact of the life events that have occurred in the recent past (Sarason et al., 1978). We calculated scores for negative life events by adding the impact ratings for the events that the respondent rated as bad events in her life. Post hoc analysis of the life events indicated by the women who had complications of gestation confirmed that the events were spread over diverse categories.

Social Support

Although social support has been described as a moderator of life stress in both theoretical and empirical literature (Cassel, 1976; Cobb, 1976; Wilcox, 1981), what constitutes social support has not been determined. Two main factors common to most definitions of social support are some form(s) of psychological support and of tangible support. The instrument used in our study measured two types of psychological support: informational and emotional, and items were created to measure tangible support.

Emotional Disequilibrium

As extensive literature documents clinical and research findings of emotional disequilibrium during pregnancy, including heightened anxiety, ambivalence, lability, introversion, depression, and mood disturbance (Colman and Colman, 1973; Glazer, 1980; Leifer, 1977; Lubin et al., 1975; Shereshefsky and Yarrow, 1973; Standley et al., 1979). Zajicek and Wolkind (1978) found a high incidence (81%) of development of disabling emotional difficulty during pregnancy among women previously identified as psychosocially stressed and a moderate incidence (25%) among women who had been screened as mentally healthy and well-adjusted.

Among the emotional state variables that have shown a relationship to complications of pregnancy are anxiety, depression, and low self-esteem (see Table 1). We selected these variables to represent the construct of self-preoccupying thoughts (vs. task-oriented thoughts) that are postulated to lead to complications of pregnancy.

The purpose of this study was to examine the effects of these selected psychosocial variables on pregnancy complications in a naturally-occurring population of medically normal women from various racial, marital, and socio-economic groups. A secondary goal of this study was to explore the differential effects of psychosocial variables on specific types of complications, categorized as difficulties during gestation, problems of labor and delivery, and infant-condition complications.

METHODS

Sample

The setting for recruitment and monitoring of subjects was a large, urban, university medical center. The obstetric clinic included a regular clinic, plus specialty clinics for adolescents, high-risk patients, and private patients. Only the regular clinic was used in this study.

To obtain a sample of pregnant women without preexisting medial risk factors, the following criteria were used in reviewing charts: (a) age between 20 and 39 years; (b) obstetric history free from a second-trimester therapeutic abortion, fetal death after 16 weeks, cesarean section or uterine surgery, premature labor between 16 to 36 weeks, prolonged premature rupture of the membranes, delivery of a small-for-gestational-age neonate, Rh negative blood type untreated with RhoGAM following a delivery or abortion, and/or multiple gestation in the current pregnancy; (c) medical history free from diabetes, cardiac disease, hypertension, renal disease, collagen disease, malignant tumors, severely abnormal Pap smears, and/or other serious diseases; and (d) current health status free from severe maternal malnourishment or drug abuse. An additional criterion for the research design was that the woman was between 12 and 20 weeks of gestation at the time of recruitment into the study.

Every eligible woman enrolled for care in the regular obstetric clinic during a period of four and one-half months was invited to participate in the study. Eighty-four percent agreed to participate, resulting in a sample of 117 women. The mean age of the sample was 26.2 years (SD 4.21, range 20 to 37), and the mean education level attained was 13.8 years (SD 1.98, range 9 to 18). Only 6 percent had not completed high school, and 61 percent had some education beyond high school.

Although the majority of the women were married (77%), 15 percent were single, and 9 percent were divorced or separated. The ethnic composition of the group was Caucasian (61%), Black (14%), Hispanic (11%), Filipino (5%), Chinese or Japanese (4%), and other (5%). Religious preference was stated as Catholic (41%), Protestant (36%), Jewish (1%), other (6%), and none (16%). At the time of recruitment, 59 percent of the women were employed; of those, most had level 3 (semi-professional, 25%) and level 4 (clerical, 57%) occupations (mean 3.75) (Hollingshead, 1977). Occupational level for women, particularly at childbearing ages, may not be a valid indicator of social class. On the basis of education, the sample was considered primarily middle class.

Although 52 percent of the women were having their first baby, only 35 percent were pregnant for the first time, and 32 percent had had one or more therapeutic abortions. This abortion rate is comparable to the 1978 rate of 345 abortions per 1000 live births for women through age 39 in the United States (U. S. Bureau of Census, 1981). The mean number of prior births for the 56 multiparas was 1.32. The mean number of weeks of gestation at the time of testing was 16.2 (SD 2.15, range 12 to 20).

Participation in the study involved one testing session in the clinic, a mailed follow-up questionnaire, and permission for the researchers to review the obstetrical chart following postpartum discharge. Subjects were informed about all aspects of the study, signed consent forms, and were paid five dollars as partial compensation for their time or expenses; payment was made after the initial battery of questionnaires was completed.

Instruments

Five instruments were used in the study: (a) The Sarason Life Experiences Survey (LES) is a 60-item self-report questionnaire that allows respondents to indicate events that they have experienced during the past year and to rate the desirability and impact of those events (Sarason et al., 1978). The negative change score has been found to be more predictive than the total change score. Test-retest reliability for a five- to six-week period ranged from .56 to .88; validity has been shown through significant correlations with other stress-related measures. (b) Part Two from the Cohen and Lazarus Social Support Questionnaire (SSQ) was used to obtain measures of informational and emotional support from spouse or partner, friends, work or school associates, relatives, and neighbors (Schaefer et al., 1981). Test-retest reliability for a nine-month interval was .58 for informational support and .66 for emotional support. Emotional support was shown to be a significant predictor of depression. (c) The Spielberger State-Trait Anxiety Inventory (STAI) is a 40-item self-report instrument that provides separate measures for trait and anxiety (Spielberger et al., 1970). High test-retest reliability (range .73 to .86) was reported for trait anxiety, but for state anxiety reliability was low (as would be expected for this fluctuating affect). Concurrent validity has been shown with other well-known anxiety measures. (d) The Lubin Depression Adjective Checklist (DACL) Form C is a 32-item measure of affective state, as distinguished from clinical, psychophysiologic depression (Lubin, 1965, 1967). The split-half reliability for Form C was .92. Concurrent validity with the Beck Depression Inventory was .50. This instrument avoids somatic indices of depression, which may be invalid during pregnancy, and has been used previously with pregnant women (Lubin et al., 1975). (e) The Rosenberg Self-Esteem Scale (SE) is a ten-item self-report measure of the self-acceptance aspect of self-esteem (Robinson and Shaver, 1973). Test-retest reliability over a two-week period was .85. Mean concurrent validity with other self-esteem measures was .57.

We developed a three-item measure of tangible support for this study as a second approach to measuring social support. The items are: "If you had an emergency and needed a ride to the clinic or needed to borrow $10, who could you call on for this help? If you should become ill and need to be in bed for several weeks, who could you call on to help you? Please indicate how much you could rely on someone from each category for practical help." A five-point scale ranging from "not at all" to "would do everything possible" is provided. The response categories for these items consists of the same support categories used in the SSQ. For the first two questions, the number of categories checked as available is totaled (possible score for each item: zero to five). The third question is a matrix of the five support categories by the five-point scale (scored zero to four); thus, the possible score for this item is zero to 20.

Finally, a one-page demographic data checksheet was used to supplement chart records for obtaining educational level, religious preference, and marital status.

Outcome Measures

Pregnancy complications were scored from chart review. The list of complications used by Nuckolls et al. (1972) was updated through consultation with the vice-chairman of the obstetrical department of the university. The resulting definitions of complications are listed in Table 2, along with their frequency of occurrence in this sample. The figures for long labor represent one standard deviation from the mean for primiparas and multiparas (Friedman, 1978).

Procedure

The subjects were recruited at their regularly scheduled clinic visit. Following recruitment, a research assistant explained the directions for the questionnaires to the woman and supplied the subject with a notebook containing the instruments for self-administration in the clinic waiting room. The average time required to complete the set of questionnaires was 30 minutes. The research assistant was available to answer questions during the testing and to check the questionnaires for completeness while the woman was still present to supply missing data if needed.

Approximately six weeks prior to each woman's expected delivery date, a second LES questionnaire was mailed to her, to obtain data on events that occurred in the four- to five-month period between the first testing and the end of the pregnancy. Of the letters that were returned by the post office, it was not possible to obtain an updated address for six subjects. One subject returned her questionnaire unanswered because she had delivered early. Of the remaining 110 subjects, 74 percent returned completed follow-up questionnaires; the full-sample return rate was 69 percent.

After the entire sample delivered, chart review

Table 2
Definitions of Complications Used as Outcome Measures and Frequency of Occurrence (N = 117)

Definition	%
Gestation Complications	
1. Systolic blood pressure during pregnancy over 139 mm or diastolic blood pressure over 89 mm on two occasions past 28th week, associated with at least 1+ proteinuria; or admission to hospital for preeclampsia	3.4
2. Hemoglobin less than 11 grams between 28th to 36th week	6.8
3. Labor (with or without delivery) prior to 37th week	6.8
Labor, Delivery and Postpartum Complications	
1. Prolonged ruptured membranes for more than 24 hours before delivery	6.8
2. Systolic blood pressure over 139 mm or diastolic blood pressure over 89 mm on three occasions over period of at least two hours during labor or postpartum periods	13.7
3. Prolonged labor in absence of cephalopelvic disproportion:	19.7
a. Primiparas with first stage longer than 22.9 hours or second stage longer than 105 minutes	
b. Multiparas with first stage longer than 13.1 hours or second stage longer than 32 minutes	
4. Delivered by cesarean section, midforceps, or vacuum in absence of cephalopelvic disproportion	22.2
Infant-Condition Complications	
1. Apgar rating at 5 minutes of less than 7	4.3
2. Time to sustain respiration greater than 89 seconds	8.5
3. Admission to intensive care nursery	5.1
4. Birth weight less than 2,500 grams	3.4
5. Stillborn or neonatal death within first 3 days	2.6

was done by a research assistant who did not have previous contact with the subjects. Two reviewers assessed the charts of the first 25 cases independently. The inter-rater agreement was very high (97%), so only one reviewer completed the rest of the sample.

Data were analyzed with programs from the Statistical Package for the Social Sciences (Nie et al., 1975).

RESULTS

Preliminary Data Analyses

Preliminary analyses were conducted to: (a) test the representativeness of the participants in relation to the eligible clinic population; (b) test for differences between the responders and nonresponders on the follow-up life-events measure; (c) select among highly similar variables, such as parity over gravida; (d) develop composite variables for certain constructs; and (e) validate the method chosen for considering outcome scores.

To determine whether the participants differed from patients who refused, the obstetric history and demographic data obtained from their charts were compared. The only significant difference between the groups was a lower occupational level for the refusal group, Mann-Whitney $z = -3.73$, $p < .001$. The two groups did not differ on age, race, gravida, parity, or therapeutic or spontaneous abortions. Thus, the sample was considered representative of the clinic population.

To rule out bias from differences between responders (N = 81) and nonresponders (N = 36) to the follow-up questionnaire, every obstetric, demographic, and psychosocial variable was tested for differences between the two groups. The responder group was significantly older, $t(115) = -2.31$, $p = .023$ and more educated, $t(115) = -2.78$, $p = .006$, and a higher proportion of the responders were white, $\chi^2(1) = 9.076$, $p = .003$. There was no significant difference between the two groups in marital status nor in any obstetric or psychosocial variable.

Correlations between the obstetric history variable and the outcome measures were examined to determine which obstetric variables should be controlled. There were no significant relationships between complications and therapeutic or spontaneous abortions. Both gravida and parity were significantly related to labor and delivery complications and to overall complications. The correlation between gravida and parity was .70. Since the correlations between parity and outcomes were higher than between gravida and outcomes, parity was selected for further analysis and was treated as a dichotomous variable to distinguish between primiparas and multiparas.

The Pearson correlations among the emotional-state measures of state anxiety, depression, and self-esteem showed that these variables were highly intercorrelated and had a similar pattern

Table 3
Intercorrelations of Emotional State and Outcome Variables (N = 117)

	State Anxiety	Depression	Self-Esteem	Gestation	Labor	Infant	Overall	X	SD
State Anxiety	1.00 —	.73 (.00)	−.38 (.00)	.07 (.48)	.04 (.68)	.23 (.01)	.06 (.49)	38.01	11.07
Depression		1.00 —	−.52 (.00)	.07 (.46)	−.07 (.44)	.20 (.03)	.00 (.99)	7.47	4.32
Self-Esteem			1.00 —	−.12 (.21)	−.10 (.29)	−.28 (.00)	−.14 (.13)	8.58	1.72

Note: The zero-order correlation coefficients are shown on the first line, the two-tailed level of significance on the second.
[a] Dichotomized: uncomplicated (0), complicated (1).

of relationship to outcome measures (see Table 3). A principal-components factor analysis was used for data reduction (see Appendix A). The resulting factor had an eigenvalue greater than 1. The items were combined into a weighted factor by multiplying factor score coefficients by z-scores for each variable.

To cluster the social-support measures into empirically derived combinations, a principal-components factor analysis was done on the two measures (informational and emotional support) from the SSQ and the three tangible-support items developed for this study. Two distinct factors emerged with a varimax rotation (see Appendix B). The Tangible-Support Factor, consisting of the three tangible-support items, had an eigenvalue of 2.915 and accounted for 58.3 percent of the variance. The Emotional-Support Factor, consisting of the informational- and emotional-support measures from the SSQ, had an eigenvalue of 1.136 and accounted for 22.7 percent of the variance. No other factor had an eigenvalue greater than 1. Weighted factors were created by multiplying factor score coefficients by z-scores from the appropriate items.

Table 4 shows the frequencies for numbers of complications for each type of complication. Similar to the complication rate found by Nuckolls et al. (1972), 48.7 percent of the cases were classified as complicated. Although it was possible to view a number of complications as an interval scale, complications were treated as a dichotomous variable for several reasons: Complications of pregnancy have been treated dichotomously in prior studies; the scaling of complications as interval may be confounded by differing severity among the complications and the potential for redundancy among certain complications; and the correlations between predictor variables (obstetric, demographic, and psychosocial) and outcome measures were essentially the same whether total number of complications or the dichotomy was used.

Hypothesis-Testing

The Pearson correlations, means, and standard deviations for all variables to be considered in the multivariate analyses are in Appendix C. A hierarchical model was used to test the impact of psychosocial variables, first on emotional disequilibrium and then on pregnancy complications, while controlling for obstetric and demographic variables.

Hypothesis 1. In the multiple regression on Emotional Disequilibrium, Parity and Age were entered simultaneously in the first set to partial out the effects of these medically relevant variables. Race, Marital Status, and Social Class (represented by educational level) were entered together in the second set to control for these demographic characteristics; Life Stress (Prior Year) was entered next, followed by a set including the Emotional-Support factor and the Tangible-Support factor. Finally, two interaction terms were entered: The product of Life Stress and Emotional Support and the product of Life Stress and Tangible Support. Only when the set was significant were the variables within the set further tested for significance. Table 5 shows that Life Stress accounted for 21.4 percent ($\beta = .442$) of the variance in Emotional Disequilibrium, and Social Support accounted for 6.5 percent ($\beta = -.239$). Thus, Hypothesis 1 was supported.

Hypothesis 2: Overall Complications. Hypothesis 2 was tested first with a discriminant analysis of overall complications (see Table 6). The hier-

Table 4
Frequencies for Number of Complications
(N = 117)

	0	1	2	3	4	5	6	7
Gestation Complications[a]	99	16	2					
Labor & Delivery Complications[b]	71	25	15	6				
Infant-Condition Complications[c]	104	7	2	1	1	2		
Total Complications[d]	60	26	14	10	1	2	3	1

[a]Possible range: 0-3.
[b]Possible range: 0-4.
[c]Possible range: 0-5.
[d]Possible range: 0-12.

Table 5
Relation of Life Stress and Social Support to Emotional Disequilibrium in Pregnant Women With Medical and Demographic Variables Controlled (N = 117)

Source of Variation[a]	DF	RSQ Increment	F	P
Control Variables:				
Medical	2	.025	2.04	ns
Parity	1	.000	—	—
Age	1	.025	—	—
Control Variables:				
Demographic	3	.039	2.12	ns
Race	1	.000	—	—
Marital Status	1	.020	—	—
Education (Social Class)	1	.020	—	—
Life Stress, Prior Year	1	.214	34.67	.01
Moderator Variables	2	.065	5.30	.01
Emotional Support Factor	1	.055	8.85	.01
Tangible Support Factor	1	.011	.00	ns
Interactions	2	.003	2.77	ns
Life Stress × Emotional Support	1	.002	—	—
Life Stress × Tangible Support	1	.002	—	—
Entire Model	10	.347	5.62	.01
Error	106	.653		

[a]All variables were forced into the model.

archical model just described was used again, except that Emotional Disequilibrium was added to the model before the interaction terms. Because the interactions were not significant in the multiple regression, they were entered but not forced into the discriminant analysis. Only Parity and Life Stress (Prior Year) were significantly related to complications of pregnancy: Life Stress accounted for 4.9 percent of the variance. Thus, Hypothesis 2 was only partially supported for overall complications.

A second analysis of overall complications was done to test the effect of Life Stress during the last half of the pregnancy. The Follow-Up Life Stress measure from the 81 respondents who returned the mailed questionnaire was entered after Emotional Disequilibrium. This relationship was not significant, nor were its interactions with social support.

Hypothesis 2: Types of Complications. The same hierarchical model was used to test the significance of predictor variables on types of complications (see Table 6). In the analysis of complications of gestation, Life Stress accounted for 6.6 percent of the variance; however, the discriminant function was not significant. In labor and delivery complications, only the two medical control variables were significant. Although the moderator variable set was not significant, Tangible Support and the interaction of Life Stress and Tangible Support accounted for 5.3 percent of the variance. In infant-condition complications, Emotional Disequilibrium accounted for 8.2 percent of the variance.

Analysis of the types of complications was repeated as before, except that this time, the Follow-Up Life-Stress measure was added to the model (see Table 7). In no case was the effect of the second Life-Stress measure significant over and above the effects of the variables, including the first Life-Stress measure, that were already in the model. However, the interaction of Life Stress during pregnancy and the Tangible-Support factor was significant for each type of complication. This interaction accounted for 7.4 percent of the vari-

Table 6
Relation of Life Stress, Social Support and Emotional Disequilibrium to Complications of Pregnancy with Medical and Demographic Variables Controlled (N = 117)

Source of Variation[a]	Overall Complications DF	↓ in Wilks' lambda[b]	F	P	Gestation Complications DF	↓ in Wilks' lambda	F	P	Labor Complications DF	↓ in Wilks' lambda	F	P	Infant Complications DF	↓ in Wilks' lambda	F	P
Control Variables:																
Medical	2	.092	5.79	.004	2	.022	1.31	ns	2	.080	4.98	.008	2	.029	1.71	ns
Parity	1	.080	11.54	.01	1	.015	1.00	—	1	.044	8.28	.01	1	.015	2.71	—
Age	1	.012	1.48	ns	1	.007	.82	—	1	.036	4.46	.05	1	.015	1.70	—
Control variables:																
Demographic	3	.050	2.16	ns	3	.018	.71	ns	3	.049	2.08	ns	3	.005	.19	ns
Race	1	.032	4.62	—	1	.017	1.95	—	1	.018	2.75	—	1	.002	.26	—
Marital Status	1	.005	1.05	—	1	.001	.09	—	1	.004	.11	—	1	.002	.28	—
Education (Social Class)	1	.013	1.68	—	1	.000	.00	—	1	.027	3.48	—	1	.001	.13	—
Life Stress, Prior Year	1	.049	6.72	.05	1	.066	8.06	.01	1	.022	2.88	ns	1	.011	1.32	ns
Moderator Variables	2	.008	.53	ns	2	.021	1.28	ns	2	.042	2.78	ns	2	.031	1.84	ns
Emotional Support Factor	1	.002	.27	—	1	.006	.76	—	1	.010	1.36	—	1	.001	.08	—
Tangible Support Factor	1	.006	1.05	—	1	.015	.72	—	1	.031	5.52	—	1	.031	3.37	—
Emotional Disequilibrium Factor	1	.000	.00	ns	1	.000	.00	ns	1	.001	.86	ns	1	.082	10.46	.01
Interactions[a]	1	.019	2.53	ns	2	.020	1.24	ns	1	.022	.294	ns	0	not entered	—	—
Life Stress × Emotional Support	1	.019	2.53	—	1	.008	1.02	—	0	not entered	—	—	0	"	—	—
Life Stress × Tangible Support	0	not entered	—	—	1	.012	1.46	—	1	.022	2.94	—	0	"	—	—
Entire Model	10	.218	2.96	.003	11	.147	1.64	.097	10	.216	2.91	.003	9	.159	2.25	.024
Error	106	.782			105	.853			106	.784			107	.841		

[a]Except for the interaction terms, all variables were forced into the model. The interactions were entered if the F-to-enter was at least 1.0.
[b]In discriminant analysis, the cumulative 1 minus Wilks' lambda is equivalent to R^2 and represents the percent of the variance explained.

ance in gestation complications, 5.7 percent in labor and delivery complications, and 9.1 percent in infant-condition complications. Thus, additional support was shown for Hypothesis 2. For both gestation and infant complications, subjects in the high-stress/low-support quadrant had the highest rate of complications as expected. For labor and delivery complications, low support was related to higher rates of complications only in the low-stress cells.

DISCUSSION

Hypothisis 1 was supported by the results of this study. High life-stress and low social support were significantly related to high emotional disequilibrium; however, the interactions between life stress and the two social-support variables were not significant. In contrast, other studies of life stress, social support, and emotion-state variables have shown both main effects and interaction effects for life stress and social support (Lin

Table 7
Relation of Life Stress at Two Time Periods, Social Support, and Emotional Disequilibrium to Types of Complications of Pregnancy with Medical and Demographic Variables Controlled (N = 81)

Source of Variation[a]	Gestation Complications DF	↓ in Wilks' lambda[b]	F	P	Labor Complications DF	↓ in Wilks' lambda	F	P	Infant Complications DF	↓ in Wilks' lambda	F	P
Control Variables:												
Medical	2	.003	.11	ns	2	.098	4.25	.05	2	.016	.64	ns
Parity	1	.002	.21	—	1	.061	7.54	.01	1	.014	1.28	—
Age	1	.001	.05	—	1	.038	3.25	ns	1	.002	.14	—
Control Variables:												
Demographic	3	.029	.74	ns	3	.083	2.54	ns	3	.031	.89	ns
Race	1	.023	1.80	—	1	.043	4.49	—	1	.020	1.47	—
Marital Status	1	.006	.43	—	1	.019	.80	—	1	.010	.68	—
Education	1	.000	.00	—	1	.021	1.91	—	1	.000	.03	—
Life Stress, Prior Year (1)	1	.146	13.17	.01	1	.011	.98	ns	1	.007	.52	ns
Moderator Variables	2	.042	1.93	ns	2	.029	1.36	ns	2	.026	1.01	ns
Emotional Support Factor	1	.032	2.99	—	1	.029	2.67	—	1	.017	1.33	—
Tangible Support Factor	1	.009	.00	—	1	.000	.38	—	1	.009	1.66	—
Emotional Disequilibrium Factor	1	.000	.02	ns	1	.000	.02	ns	1	.049	3.96	.05
Life Stress, During Pregnancy (2)	1	.015	1.34	ns	1	.007	.61	ns	1	.031	2.57	ns
Interactions[a]	2	.074	3.63	.05	1	.057	5.50	.05	1	.091	8.34	.01
Life Stress 2 × Emotional Support	1	.012	1.18	ns	0	not entered	—	—	0	not entered	—	—
Life Stress 2 × Tangible Support	1	.062	6.06	.05	1	.057	5.50	.05	1	.091	8.34	.01
Entire Model	12	.308	2.52	.01	11	.285	2.50	.01	11	.250	2.09	.03
Error	68	.692			69	.715			69	.750		

[a]Except for the interaction terms, all variables were forced into the model. The interactions were entered if the F-to-enter was at least 1.0.
[b]In discriminant analysis, the cumulative 1 minus Wilks' lambda is equivalent to R^2 and represents the percent of the variance explained.

et al., 1979; Wilcox, 1981). In the present study, emotional support was significantly related to emotional disequilibrium, but tangible support was not. Since the variables for Hypothesis 1 were measured simultaneously, no causal statement can be made about the direction of effect.

Hypothesis 2 was only partially supported in the analysis of overall complications; however, when types of complications were examined, psychosocial variable, high life-stress from the Hypothesis 2 was more fully supported. One prior year, was significantly related to overall complications. Among the types of complications, significant main effects were found: High life-stress from the prior year predicted gestation complications, and high emotional disequilibrium predicted infant-condition complications. Although the main effects were not significant, the interaction of life stress during pregnancy and tangible support was a significant predictor of each type of complication.

The design of this study most closely resembles the Nuckolls et al. (1972) study because the predictor variables were measured in the first half of the pregnancy; two life-stress measures were taken; and "psychosocial assets" (social-support and ego-functioning variables) were measured and tested alone and in interaction with life stress. Findings from our study are consistent with the stress-buffering effect found for "psychosocial assets" in the small subsample of military wives who had high life-stress at both time periods.

Although the stress-buffering effects in our research are markedly smaller than those found in the Nuckolls et al. study, greater generalizability and interpretability of the findings are possible because: (a) The sample was drawn from the general population; (b) The smallest sample size under consideration in any analysis was 81; (c) The theoretical constructs of social support and ego-functioning—emotional disequilibrium—were measured and analyzed as separate variables; and (d) The psychometric properties of the measurement instruments were stronger. As mentioned previously, the inclusion of adolescents in the Nuckolls et al. sample, the lack of complete control for preexisting medical risk factors, or the unique properties of a sample of military dependents may account for the differences in effect-size between the two studies.

Theoretical Implications

Findings that support Hypothesis 1 are conceptualized in relation to the theoretical model: Those subjects who experienced high life-stress in the preceding year (too many calls to action) and low emotional support (a sense of low personal resources) demonstrated greater emotional disequilibrium (self-preoccupying thoughts).

The theoretical model underlying Hypothesis 2 was only partially supported because the intervening variable of emotional disequilibrium was significant only in one type of complication. Thus, either the construct of emotional disequilibrium inadequately operationalizes the theory, or the model does not accurately depict the stress process in pregnancy. Although each of the psychosocial variables operationalized from the theoretical model had significant main or interaction effects on at least one type of complication, a coherent pattern did not emerge.

Pearlin et al. (1981) reported findings from longitudinal data that support a more elaborate model of the stress process in which mediating variables, such as social support, appear to exert their effects indirectly by dampening antecedent processes. In the case of pregnancy, it may be that mediating variables exert an effect on certain intervening variables that influence important self-care behaviors, e.g., diet and exercise, which in turn affect complications. Predictive power will be enhanced by the use of models that lead to a more complete specification of variables and relationships.

The significant interaction of life stress and social support is consistent with the stress-buffering effect of social support described in the literature. It is interesting to note that while emotional support was the social-support variable significantly related to emotional disequilibrium (Hypothesis 1), tangible support was the social-support variable that was significant in interaction with life stress in predicting complications of pregnancy (Hypothesis 2). The sequence of measurement of these variables may help account for these differences.

Thoits (1982) has argued for the necessity of a longitudinal design in which all three constructs of life stress, social support, and psychological distress are measured at two time periods, to avoid inevitable confounding among these variables. In this study, the three variables of Hypothesis 1 were measured at Time 1, but life stress during the pregnancy was measured at Time 2. The level of social support measured initially was presumed to be the level available to the individual for prior and current life events—an assumption likely to be false (Thoits, 1982). The evidence from the study supports the validity of the stress-buffering role hypothesized for social support in the area of pregnancy complications, but future studies in this area should adopt the measurement and analytical strategy proposed by Thoits (1982), to obtain a sound test of the theoretical relationships.

Life Stress

The pattern of significance for the negative life-events measures and their interactions were not similar to previous studies. In this study, main effects for life stress were found for life events from the previous year for overall and gestation complications. Neither Gorsuch and Key (1974) nor Nuckolls et al. (1972) found main effects for life stress preceding the pregnancy.

The significant interaction between life stress during the pregnancy and social support is basically consistent with the Nuckolls et al. study. Gorsuch and Key found a significant main effect for life stress during pregnancy and complications; however, their measurement of life events was done after delivery when the subjects already knew whether or not they had experienced complications.

Social Support

The significant relationship between life stress and social support in predicting emotional-state variables is similar to other studies in the social-support field (Lin et al., 1979; Wilcox, 1981), except that the interactions were not significant and the effect-size for social support was much smaller. The effect-size for the interaction of social support and life stress was also smaller than that found for "psychosocial assets" by Nuckolls et al. (1972). In the social-support field, there is still no consensus on what constitutes social support or how social support or its components should be measured. Thus, the true effect-size for social support on pregnancy complications cannot be determined from this study because the measurement instruments may not have been adequately sensitive or refined.

Emotional Disequilibrium

The three emotion-state variables selected for this study—state anxiety, depression, and self-esteem—were highly related and formed a single construct. Several studies presented in Table 1 have pointed to significant relationships between these variables and overall complications of pregnancy; however, in our study, emotional disequilibrium was significantly related only to infant-condition complications.

Many of the earlier studies measured predictor variables very late in the pregnancy; however, Gorsuch and Key (1974) used a repeated measures design and found that only in the first trimester was anxiety significantly related to complications of pregnancy. Since pregnancy is a dynamic time physiologically, psychologically, and socially, a repeated measure design is necessary to determine the effect of changing emotional states on various types of complications. With regard to the present study, one might speculate that since critical embryonic development occurs during the first three to four months of pregnancy, the time of measurement coincided with this phenomenon and pointed to a relationship between the mother's emotional state and subsequent infant-condition.

Methodological Issues

Previous studies have used different criteria for defining complications, and each of the three categories of complications was not used in every study. In this study, different patterns of predictor variables were related to various types of complications, which suggests that discrepancies among past studies may be partially attributable to combining heterogeneous complications into a single construct.

Appendix A
Structure Coefficients, Communalities, and Factor Score Coefficients for the Emotional Disequilibrium Factor

Measures	Structure Coefficients	Communalities	Factor Score Coefficients
State Anxiety	.855	.731	.407
Depression	.914	.835	.435
Self-Esteem	−.731	.534	−.348

The significant effects found for parity and age in this sample point to the necessity of controlling these variables in further research on pregnancy complications. In this study, age was controlled through sampling, to eliminate the high-risk adolescent and persons over 40, yet a significant effect for age was still found in labor and delivery complications.

Conclusion

This study provides evidence for significant, but modest, relationships between certain psychosocial variables and specific types of complications of pregnancy. In addition, methodological findings can be used to guide the design of further studies in this field. This study also supports the

Appendix B
Structure Coefficients, Communalities, and Factor Score Coefficients for the Two Social Support Factors

Measures	Structure Coefficients[a] Factor 1	Factor 2	Communalities	Factor Score Coefficients Factor 1	Factor 2
Informational Support Score[b]	.148	−.605	.920	.148	.948
Emotional Support Score[b]	.268	−.507	.925	.268	.924
Short-term Aid Item[c]	.906	.526	.832	.906	.108
Long-term Aid Item[c]	.880	.458	.806	.880	.177
Overall Aid Item[c]	.656	.163	.568	.656	.372

[a] Varimax rotated factor matrix.
[b] Emotional Support Factor elements.
[c] Tangible Support Factor elements.

Appendix C
Pairwise Correlations, Means, and Standard Deviations of Variables in Analysis

	1	2	3	4	5	6	7	8	9	10	11	12	13	14	Mean	SD
1. Parity (117)	100														.48	.50
2. Age (117)	30	100													26.15	4.21
3. Race (117)	−07	−05	100												.39	.49
4. Marital Status (117)	−16	−03	02	100											.23	.42
5. Education (social class) (117)	−24	33	−07	−13	100										13.77	1.98
6. Life Stress, Prior Year (117)	−04	−13	03	27	08	100									8.24	7.02
7. Life Stress, Follow-up (81)	−07	−002	22	03	−16	51	100								9.46	9.04
8. Emotional Support Factor (117)	05	−11	−08	−07	−03	−07	−006	100							0.00	1.05
9. Tangible Support Factor (117)	−01	−03	−26	−04	−03	−28	−29	43	100						0.00	1.08
10. Emotional Disequilibrium (117)	01	−15	−001	13	21	50	47	−27	−22	100					0.00	1.00
11. Gestation Complications (117)	−12	−12	14	05	−02	27	14	10	008	10	100				0.15	.36
12. Labor Complications (117)	−21	12	14	−03	27	12	05	−03	−25	02	09	100			0.39	.49
13. Infant Complications (117)	−12	08	05	06	10	10	29	−09	−21	27	30	22	100		0.11	.32
14. Overall Complications (117)	−28	02	20	12	18	23	13	−05	−19	08	44	83	36	100	0.49	.50

Note: N's are presented parenthetically; decimals have been omitted.
Variable values: Parity—0 = primipara, 1 = multipara. Race—0 = white, 1 = non-white. Marital status—0 = married, 1 = nonmarried. Complications—0 = uncomplicated, 1 = complicated.

clinical goal of identifying, early in the pregnancy, patients who may benefit from interventions designed to reduce the deleterious effects of life stress, low social support, and emotional distress.

REFERENCES

Beck, N. C., Siegel, L. J., Davidson, N. P., Kormeier, A., Breitenstein, A., & Hall, D. G. (1980). The prediction of pregnancy outcome: Maternal preparation, anxiety and attitudinal sets. *Journal of Psychosomatic Research, 24*, 343–351.

Cassel, J. (1976). The contribution of the social environment to host resistance. *American Journal of Epidemiology, 104*, 107–123.

Cobb, S. (1976). Social support as a moderator of life stress, *Psychosomatic Medicine, 38*, 300–314.

Colman, A., & Colman, L. (1973). Pregnancy as an altered state of consciousness. *Birth and the Family Journal, 1*(1), 7–11.

Crandon, A. J. (1979a). Maternal anxiety and obstetric complications. *Journal of Psychosomatic Research, 23*, 109–111.

Crandon, A. J. (1979b). Maternal anxiety and neonatal wellbeing. *Journal of Psychosomatic Research, 23*, 113–115.

Davids, A., & DeVault, S. (1962). Maternal anxiety during pregnancy and childbirth abnormalities. *Psychosomatic Medicine, 24*, 464–470.

Davids, A., S. De Vault, & Talmadge, M. (1961). Psychological study of emotional factors in pregnancy: A preliminary report. *Psychosomatic Medicine, 23*, 93–103.

Friedman, E. A. (1978). *Labor: Clinical evaluation and management* (2nd ed.). New York: Appleton-Century-Crofts.

Glazer, G. (1980). Anxiety levels and concerns among pregnant women. *Research in Nursing and Health, 3*, 107–113.

Gorsuch, R. L., & Key, M. K. (1974). Abnormalities of pregnancy as a function of anxiety and life stress. *Psychosomatic Medicine, 36*, 352–362.

Helper, M. M., Cohen, R. L., Beitenman, E. T., & Eaton, L. F. (1968). Life events and acceptance of pregnancy. *Journal of Psychosomatic Research, 12*, 183–188.

Hollingshead, A. B. (1977). Two-factor index of social position. In D. C. Miller (Ed.), *Handbook of research design and social measurement* (3rd ed.). New York: McKay.

Jones, A. C. (1978). Life change and psychological distress as predictors of pregnancy outcome. *Psychosomatic Medicine, 40*, 402–412.

Langlie, J. K. (1977). Social networks, health beliefs, and preventive health behavior. *Journal of Health and Social Behavior, 18*, 244–260.

La Rocco, J. M., House, J. S., & French, J. R. P. (1980). Social support, occupational stress, and health. *Journal of Health and Social Behavior, 21*, 202–218.

Leifer, M. (1977). Psychological changes accompanying pregnancy and motherhood. *Genetic Psychology Monographs, 95*, 55–96.

Lin, N., Ensel, W. M., Simeone, R. S., & Kuo, W. (1979). Social support, stressful life events, and illness: A model and an empirical test. *Journal of Health and Social Behavior, 20*, 108–119.

Lubin, B. (1965). Adjective check list for measurement of depression. *Archives of General Psychiatry, 12*, 57–62.

Lubin, B. (1967). *Manual for the depression adjective lists*. San Diego: Educational and Industrial Testing Service.

Lubin, B., Gardener, S. H., & Roth, A. (1975). Mood and somatic symptoms during pregnancy. *Psychosomatic Medicine, 37*, 136–146.

McDonald, R. L. (1968). The role of emotional factors in obstetric complications: A review. *Psychosomatic Medicine, 30*, 222–237.

McDonald, R. L., & Christakos, A. C. (1963). Relationship of emotional adjustment during pregnancy to obstetric complications. *American Journal of Obstetrics and Gynecology, 86*, 341–348.

McDonald, R. L., & Parham, K. J. (1964). Relation of emotional changes during pregnancy to obstetric complications in unmarried primigravidas. *American Journal of Obstetrics and Gynecology, 90*, 195–201.

Nie, N. H., Hull, C. H., Jenkins, J. G., Steinbrenner, K., & Brent, D. H. (1975). *Statistical pack-*

age for the social sciences (2nd ed.). New York: McGraw-Hill.

Nuckolls, K. B., Cassel, J., & Kaplan, B. H. (1972). Psychosocial assets, life crisis, and the prognosis of pregnancy. *American Journal of Epidemiology, 95,* 431–441.

Pearlin, L. I., Lieberman, M. A., Menaghan, E. G., & Mullan, J. T. (1981). The stress process. *Journal of Health and Social Behavior, 22,* 337–356.

Rabkin, J. G., & Struening, E. L. (1976). Life events, stress, and illness. *Science, 194,* 1013–1020.

Robinson, J. P., & Shaver, P. R. (1973). *Measures of social psychological attitudes* (rev. ed.). Ann Arbor: Institute of Social Research.

Sarason, I. G. (1979). *Life stress, self-preoccupation, and social supports.* Technical Report #SCS-LS-008, Office of Naval Research, Washington, DC: U. S. Government Printing Office.

Sarason, I. G., Johnson, J. H., & Siegel, J. M. (1978). Assessing the impact of life changes: Development of the life experiences survey. *Journal of Consulting and Clinical Psychology, 46,* 932–946.

Schaefer, C., Coyne, J. C., & Lazarus, R. (1981). The health related functions of social support. *Journal of Behavioral Medicine, 4,* 381–406.

Shereshefsky, P. M., & Yarrow, L. J. (Eds.). (1973). *Psychological aspects of a first pregnancy and early postnatal adaptation.* New York: Raven Press.

Spielberger, C. D., Gorsuch, R. L., & Lushene, R. E. (1970). *Manual for the state-trait anxiety inventory,* Palo Alto, CA: Consulting Psychologists Press.

Standley, K., Soule, B., & Copans, S. (1979). Dimensions of prenatal anxiety and their influence on pregnancy outcome. *American Journal of Obstetrics and Gynecology, 135,* 22–26.

Tausig, M. (1982). Measuring life events. *Journal of Health and Social Behavior, 23,* 52–64.

Thoits, P. A. (1982). Conceptual, methodological, and theoretical problems in studying social support as a buffer against life stress. *Journal of Health and Social Behavior, 23,* 145–159.

U. S. Bureau of the Census (1981). *Statistical abstract of the United States 1981* (102d ed.). Washington, DC: U. S. Government Printing Office.

Wilcox, B. L. (1981). Social support, life stress, and psychological adjustment: A test of the buffering hypothesis. *American Journal of Community Psychology, 9,* 371–386.

Zajicek, E., & Wolkind, S. (1978). Emotional difficulties in married women during and after the first pregnancy. *British Journal of Medical Psychology, 51,* 379–385.

This article is printed with permission of *Journal of Health and Social Behavior.*

Copyright © 1983 American Sociological Association.

Original article:
Norbeck, J. S., & Tilden, V. P. (1983). Life stress, social support, and emotional disequilibrium in complications of pregnancy: A prospective, multivariate study. *Journal of Health and Social Behavior, 24*, 30–46.

CRITIQUE BY: JENNIFER CARLEY-ROE, BSN, RN

This critique is presented from the perspective of a newly graduated BSN labor and delivery nurse who has been practicing for just over two months. The clinical setting is a hospital that serves a population of over 90,000 and averages 250–300 births per month.

Part I: Clinical Relevance

Norbeck and Tilden's study investigated the relationships between certain psychosocial variables and complications of pregnancy. The specific theory tested by this research concerns the relationship between life stress, social support, and emotional disequilibrium as well as the relationship of these variables to physiological complications of pregnancy. If this link is substantiated by a reliable and valid study, there are implications for practice that are of relevance to the antenatal care nurse, the labor and delivery nurse, and the postpartum/neonatal nurse.

The implications for practice in using this study are greatest for the antenatal caregiver. This nurse has the opportunity to assess specific psychosocial areas of the client and to plan and implement appropriate interventions. Intervention may be aimed towards management of life stress, increasing type and quality of social support, or supporting and reinforcing positive client behaviors or networks already in place. These points of intervention are of high interest to nurses, who generally feel strong responsibility for including the psychosocial realm in providing holistic care. Interventions regarding stress management and social support also are becoming more accepted by the health care community as well as the general public.

Implications for use of this study in the labor and delivery setting include assessment of specific factors in the psychosocial realm for determination of the pregnant woman's risk profile. The nurse also should note the relevance of these factors in review of the prenatal history. This information can influence decisions regarding feasibility of different birth plan options (birthing center, labor, delivery, recovery rooms or the traditonal labor room with transport to the delivery room) as well as decisions regarding use of continuous or intermittent fetal monitoring. Anticipating possible complications allows for better preparedness in the event of actual occurrence; and knowledge of additional risk factors allows for this. This information also is of benefit to the postpartum/neonatal caregiver, who can be forewarned of impending patient care needs.

Credible demonstration of a relationship between psychosocial variables and physiological complications may strengthen the resolve of the nurse to place more emphasis on the psychosocial aspect of practice. The nurse may increase the priority value of these types of diagnoses and treat them more vigorously, using this study as rationale.

Evaluation of the plan of care and its implementation is essential to the nursing process. An aspect to be considered in evaluating this study is if the interventions implied can be evaluated using the same method of measurement used in the study.

Investigation of complications was accomplished through postpartum chart review, a suitable way to evaluate in regard to complications. However, outcome criteria chosen when treating a psychosocial diagnosis are not usually listed on the chart. Usual outcome goals are directly related to the problem (e.g., for a social support deficit, patient will contact two friends this week). If this study (and others) substantiates this theory, then perhaps nurses can view complications as a way to measure effectiveness in treating psychosocial diagnoses. However, if the nurse has set a goal in relation to complications, chart review is a possible means of evaluation. Nonetheless, the labor and delivery nurse will have immediate feedback and will, in fact, be the person documenting on the chart.

The antenatal caregiver, who may find chart review helpful, also can evaluate based on the client's subjective appraisal of the pregnancy and birth experience. The problem with chart review is accessibility of charts to previous caregivers and willingness of the nurse to track down and read charts for this purpose.

A valuable aspect of this study is the attention it calls to client appraisal of a situation. In fact, life stress was defined and measured from this perspective. This study reminds us to take client perspective seriously and to appreciate and give priority to client concerns.

This study contributes, most significantly, to the theoretical base of nursing knowledge. As an exploratory study, it seeks to relate certain psychosocial factors to specific phenomenon of complications in pregnancy. Substantial evidence in support of this concept is valuable to nursing because of the credence it lends to treatment of psychosocial diagnoses in the pregnant woman.

The investigators do not address directly any specific application to practice. However, the theoretical link must be demonstrated before interventions can be employed in modification of the variables studied. Although this study implies directing intervention towards this end, salient information addressing intervention is not offered. However, this study does imply the importance of assessment of the specific variables of life stress, social support, and emotional disequilibrium. Other research studies may focus on efficacy of interventon aimed at modification of these variables.

Part II: Conceptualization and Internal Consistency

In general, this study is impressive for the soundness of its theoretical and conceptual framework and for the way in which methods are based upon this framework. Norbeck and Tilden clearly state the purpose of the study as being "(1) to examine the effects of selected psychosocial variables on pregnancy complications in a naturally occurring population of medically normal women and (2) to examine differential effects of variables on specific complicatons." The operational definitions were all satisfactorily outlined and measurements seemed appropriate for each variable. The framework made sense and the study fit well with this model.

The justification for this study consisted of the lack of control for medical risk factors and for age in subjects previously studied by other researchers. These are major risk factors in pregnancy and their control gives further merit to this study. Knowledge of factors affecting complications is always applicable and the study questions relate well to this justification.

The second hypothesis poses a more specific problem: the theoretical leap made between emotional disequilibrium and complications in pregnancy as an observable behavior. However, this idea has been supported by previous studies cited by the investigators, and this lends credence to the hypothesis. Further research may address the question of why the factors studied influence appearance of complications.

Norbeck and Tilden outline Sarason's theoretical model of stress as an individual's appraisal of a situation and ability to successfully handle it. According to Sarason, the main contextual factor seen as a resource in this process is that of social support. This model supports the study of the independent variables, life stress and social support, and their effect on emotional disequilibrium. The methods used in this study reflect this strength.

Norbeck and Tilden chose subjects for their study from a university prenatal clinic that specifically excluded high-risk patients. By excluding medical and age-related risk subjects, Norbeck and Tilden exerted an appropriate control. The subjects, between 12 and 20 weeks pregnant when selected, comprised a successful target sample of the desired population. The sample size was 117.

The instruments used to measure variables were all satisfactorily reliable and valid according to the figures given by the investigators, with the exception of that used for tangible support. Norbeck and Tilden constructed this tool themselves. Unfortunately, they provided no figures to establish reliability and validity.

Norbeck and Tilden collected data by methods of self-report with the exception of measurement of the dependent variable, complications in pregnancy. Self-report techniques are vulnerable to problems with subjects' honesty and possible desire to skew answers to please the investigator. However, the basis of this study was client appraisal of situations as stressful. Therefore, self-report is the best method for obtaining such information. The investigators measured the variable of complications in pregnancy by chart review in comparison to an updated list of specific complications. Interrater reliability was high.

The strength of the conceptual framework and the consistency of methodology with the framework give this study merit for further examination.

Part III: Believability of Results

Norbeck and Tilden purported to test the relationship between the independent variables—life stress, social support, and emotional disequilibrium—and the dependent variable—complications of pregnancy. The information provided primarily described this phenomenon in terms of effects of independent variables. No intervention was tested. The resulting data are quantitative.

Norbeck and Tilden selected their subjects through invitation to all patients in a university medical prenatal clinic. Stated criteria specified that the subjects be between 20 and 39 years of age and that obstetric history be free of specific selected complications. In addition, medical history should be free from abnormalities that would affect the pregnancy. The women also had to be between 12 and 20 weeks gestation. This was a nonprobability sample, a sample of convenience. The investigators took this weakness into consideration in the statistical evaluation of data which compared demographic data of participants to nonparticipants. The investigators then concluded that their sample was representative of the clinic population. Differences between those who chose a clinic for health care versus those who chose an alternate health care setting cannot be ascertained from this study.

Norbeck and Tilden discussed the measures used to operationalize definitions and to collect data in terms of reliability and validity with inclusion of statistics related to these considerations. In this respect, the tools Norbeck and Tilden used were satisfactory, with reliability ranging from .56 to .92, and validity ranging from .50 to .57. The only tool not tested for these aspects was a tool developed by the investigators to measure tangible support.

Norbeck and Tilden tested for interrater agreement (consistency in data collection) by reviewing charts for complications of pregnancy. The figure for interrater agreement was very high and only one research assistant carried out the review of the final 92 charts. However, it is unclear how many assistants administered the initial questionnaires and, therefore, how consistent the methods of administration were.

The measures and methods used for collection of data were appropriate for obtaining the desired information. The initial time spent on filling out tools by subjects was reasonable; an average of 30 minutes. Considerations were made for the fact that the subjects were pregnant and certain tools were not utilized because of this. The follow-up questionnaires were administered by mail, making participation more convenient for the subjects. This method decreased response rate but did consider the women's needs for convenience. The measures and methods were well within the boundaries indicated by the subjects.

Because of the nature of this study, it was not necessary to have a control and an experimental group. The investigators had to proceed by taking the group as it naturally occurred and evaluating the differences through the use of statistical analysis. In addition, the investigators thoroughly reported results and included several tables for scrutiny by the reader. However, to evaluate appropriateness of the statistics used, I would need to consult with someone who has greater expertise with statistics than I.

In the presentation of data results, I also would have liked to know how many women experienced stress during the time studied and the sorts of events perceived as stressful by the women. I cannot ascertain this information from the data presented.

Significant correlation was found between high life stress, low social support, and emotional disequilibrium, although the interaction of life stress and social support was not significant. The investigators attributed this lack of correlation to their having measured emotional and tangible support simultaneously.

The proposed relationship between high life stress, low social support, high emotional disequilibrium, and complications of pregnancy was only partially supported. However, high life stress was significantly related to overall complications and specific complications could be predicted based on either life stress or emotional disequilibrium. Life stress and tangible support were significant predictors of each type of complication. The investigators attribute the finding of only partial support for Hypothesis 2 to inadequate operationalization of the construct of emotional disequilibrium or to inaccurate depiction of the stress process in pregnancy. They also suppose that self-care behaviors may be affected by intervening variables which influence complications in pregnancy. They suggest that models with more complete specification of variables and relationships will enhance the predictive power of future studies.

Part IV: Generalizability of Results

In this sample, the obviously high-risk patients were factored out. According to Toffel, Placek, and Liss (1987), the percentage of complicated delivery of babies in the United States increased from 51.2 percent in 1980 to 64 percent in 1985. This is a high number of all deliveries. Therefore, it is difficult to apply the statistics presented to the general public because so many people do experience complications.

In my clinical setting, we serve the majority of all pregnant women in the geographic area who choose hospital birth. Many high-risk women are served, making generalizability of this study to my population difficult. However, it may be applicable to those women who have no other identifiable risk factors.

In addition, this study found that complications in labor and delivery were more significantly related to age and parity rather than the variables under scutiny. Therefore, I would use this research with caution, refraining from placing too much emphasis on the factors studied. However, these are valuable concepts to consider in assessing and planning patient care.

The general conclusions drawn by this study were that life stress accounted for 21.4 percent of the variance in emotional disequilibrium while social support accounted for 6.5 percent, granting support to Hypothesis 1.

Only parity and life stress were related to complications of pregnancy. Life stress accounts for 4.9 percent of the variance. The conclusion was drawn that Hypothesis 2 was only partially supported. However, types of complications were analyzed and life stress was found to account for 6.6 percent of the variance in gestation complications. In infant condition complications, emotional disequilibrium accounted for 8.2 percent of the variance. The interaction of life stress during pregnancy and the tangible support factor was significant for each kind of complication.

The other research related to this study was reported in the literature review. The investigators satisfactorily compared their study to other studies by explicating differences in findings and to what they attributed them.

Based on this study, I do not suggest nonutilization, nor lack of generalizability to any setting. I would consider the variables studied in my nursing assessment and keep their significance in mind while planning the care to be given the laboring woman and her unborn baby.

Part V: Other Factors to Consider in Utilization

The decision to use this research in labor and delivery would involve including a more detailed and specific assessment of the psychosocial aspect of the patient. To do this systematically would involve: (1) reworking the admit form to include specific information; and (2) documenting how this information changed or affected the plan of care. Outcomes could then be evaluated in terms of complications. The feasibility of making such a systematic change is minimal at my institution at this time. Priorities for making changes to improve patient care are aimed at aspects of care in which intervention makes an obvious difference. Intervention was not tested by this study and, therefore, its implications for intervention are not yet research supported.

There is no risk in doing a more thorough assessment, however. In not assessing these aspects of the person's life, we risk not giving the finest holistic care we are capable of giving.

The greatest cost incurred from using this research is that of the nurse's time spent with these issues, or in changing assessment forms to include this information. Nurses elicit such information from patients easily and can do so in the labor and delivery setting during routine contact wih the patient. On busy days, however, this sort of information may be seen as a luxury and priorities would dictate attending to other patient care issues first.

I do not know what the cost of changing forms is, but, at this time, this study would not be enough to convince my administration to go to that expense.

Nonetheless, I would recommend use of this research in practice based on its solid groundwork, demonstration of significance of the factors studied, and virtually no risk to utilization. Psychosocial outcomes are difficult to evaluate directly but patient by patient evaluation is achievable with careful attention to the aspects considered in this study. Specifically, I recommend use of the study through inclusion of life stress and social support in assessment of the patient. Appropriate psychosocial intervention may be planned in consideration of the risk each patient is carrying. I would recommend including life stress and social support assessments in antenatal histories for early intervention and for consideration by the labor and delivery and neonatal nurses.

REFERENCES

Taffel, S. M., Placek, P. J., & Liss, T. (1987). Trends in the United States caesarean section rate and reasons for the 1980–85 rise. *American Journal of Public Health*, 77, 955–959.

Original article:
Norbeck, J. S., & Tilden, V. P. (1983). Life stress, social support, and emotional disequilibrium in complications of pregnancy: A prospective, multivariate study. *Journal of Health and Social Behavior, 24,* 30–46.

CRITIQUE BY: CAROL HOWE, DNSc, RN, CNM

This study was selected for critique because it exemplifies the sophistication and complexity which increasingly characterizes nursing research. Because of nursing's emphasis on the total patient, including his or her emotional, family, and social environment, the purity of the laboratory experiment is often impossible. The utility of many physiologic measurements for our research questions is rare. Consequently, nursing research must often use multivariate analysis techniques and develop creative ways of measuring constructs that do not lend themselves easily to precise quantification.

Part I: Clinical Relevance

Norbeck and Tilden's study is one of many that have attempted to explicate the relationship of stress and illness, in this case the relationship of stress and complications of pregnancy. This relationship has been appreciated intuitively for years, and has received modest support from the research literature. However, the complexity of the relationship with all of its potential intervening and interacting variables has tainted the results with methodological questions. This study represents an effort to clarify some methodological concerns and provide further understanding of the relationship of life stress and pregnancy complications. Its specific contribution is to explore the mediating effect of social support and to begin to clarify the nature of the stress and the types of support that exert the most influence. Furthermore, this study is one of the few that have attempted to define the theoretical basis for the relationship of life stress and poor pregnancy outcome.

It is unlikely that this study will significantly alter the clinical practice of individual nurses. Psychosocial assessment and attempts to enhance family and social support systems already characterize nursing practice. Clarification of the most efficacious types of support may help to guide nursing efforts. However, the most important potential contribution of this study will be to enhance policy-related activities of nursing that encourage access to care and availability of a broad spectrum of supportive services in addition to more traditional prenatal care, including: counseling services, social services, WIC, prenatal education, and so forth. Use of these services characterize the prenatal management of many nurses, including nurse-midwives and women's health care nurse practitioners.

Unlike other similar studies, this research also attempted to test a theoretical model that would explain the interaction of stress, social support, and pregnancy outcome. Again, this particular model is unlikely to significantly influence individual nursing care, but may serve to assist nurse researchers as they further explicate specific interactions. The broader links, the relationship of stress to pregnancy outcome and the mediating effect of social support, serve as the primary guide to nursing practice.

Outcome variables in the study were common pregnancy complications, including: anemia, pregnancy induced hypertension, prolonged labor, preterm labor, low birth weight, and so forth. These are variables measured in every pregnancy and available in every standard data base. In this study, the predictor variables (life stress and social support) are measured in a manner not easily incorporated by the practicing nurse. An exception to such difficulty does appear, however, in the measure of tangible support, which consisted of three short questions that could easily become a standard component of the nursing history.

In summary, while this study may not significantly alter individual nursing practice, it does serve to support a basic nursing approach and provides data and a perspective appropriate for policies that nurses continue to advocate for the benefit of their clients. Patient support has a nebulous quality that often seems to be interpreted as "being nice" or reassuring the patient—a behavior that is considered worthy but hardly researchable or with measurable impact. Its importance often seems diminished in the face of new technology and treatments to cure pathology. Nursing continues to emphasize the value of support in the prevention of and adaptation to disease states, but it must also be prepared to define support, to quantify it, and to demonstrate its efficacy—the major contribution of this study. A specific clinical contribution is the implication that tangible support questions should be incorporated into nursing assessment of pregnant clients.

Part II: Conceptualization and Internal Consistency

A strong conceptual base supports this study. Relationships between each section of the research process are succinctly outlined. The literature review is consistent with the justification for the study. The conceptual framework flows from the literature review. The hypotheses emerge from the conceptual framework. The variables and measures are consistent with the hypotheses. The overall analysis is congruent with the conceptual base, and the interpretation is consistent with the overall analysis. Each aspect of the study is explicated clearly and related to the other components. Few research reports are characterized by the clarity and consistency found in this study.

Part III: Believability of Results

This study purported to test the effect of an independent or predictor variable, life stress, on the dependent variable, complications of pregnancy. The interactive effect of an intervening variable, social support, was also examined. The design was ex post facto and correlational. The data were quantitative.

Subjects were essentially middle class low-risk gravidas attending a university-based obstetrical clinic for their prenatal care. All potentially eligible subjects between 6 and 20 weeks gestation within the two-month recruitment period were asked to participate. Subjects were asked to fill out a demographic form, the Sarason Life Experiences Survey (LES), the Cohen and Lazarus Social Support Questionnaire (Part II) (SSQ), the Spielberger State-Trait Anxiety Inventory (STAI), the Lubin Depression Adjective Checklist (DACL), and the Rosenberg Self-Esteem Scale (SE) at their initial clinic contact. Approximately six weeks prior to delivery a second LES was mailed to provide information on life events during the pregnancy. Researchers were given permission to examine the subjects' obstetrical chart after delivery to obtain data on obstetrical complications. A major strength of this approach is the prospective assessment of life events. Recall after the experience of a pregnancy complication could influence perception of life experiences.

The sample for this study was somewhat unusual, however. University clinics frequently serve a high proportion of medically indigent clients. However, by age (mean 26.2 years), by education (mean 13.8 years), and by occupation (59 percent semi-professional/clerical), this sample was clearly more middle class. Whether any particular bias exists as a result of this composition is unclear. However, a middle class population typically carries less obstetrical risk. Thus, some control may exist for medical risk factors more typical of an indigent population, potentially providing "cleaner" data on the relationship of stress and complications. On the other hand, both stress and complications may be more prevalent among the poor, providing the researcher a richer data base for analysis. It is interesting to note that at each level of potential subject attrition (refusal to participate, failure to return follow-up questionnaire) the sample became progressively more white and middle class.

Several sources of bias were acknowledged by the investigators and controlled either through sample selection or in the analysis. For instance, women with known medical risk factors were excluded from the sample. Factors known to influence complication rates, such as parity and age, were addressed through use of a hierarchical model in both regression and discriminant analysis.

The measures, particularly for the predictor variables, were instruments that had been previously validated and tested for reliability. These data were reported consistently except for the tangible support items developed by the investigators and the measures of pregnancy complications. The tangible support items possess face and content validity. Factor analysis of all of the support items (emotional, informational, and tangible) reinforced the cohesion of the tangible support items.

The measure of pregnancy complications is somewhat more complex. It was developed by adapting and updating the measure used by Nuckolls, Cassel, and Kaplan (1972), and consists of common pregnancy complications occurring during three distinct periods: (1) antepartum or "gestation"; (2) labor, delivery, and postpartum; and (3) neonatal or "infant-conditions." Results of the study classified 48.7 percent of the cases as complicated, an extraordinarily high proportion by any estimate, especially considering that patients at medical risk were excluded. These results raise questions regarding both the risk status of the sample as well as the validity of the measures. For instance, the occurrence of preeclampsia reported in the literature varies from 5–7 percent (Pritchard, McDonald, & Gant, 1985; Anderson & Sibai, 1986). However, this study reports an incidence of 17.1 percent (3.4 percent antepartum and 13.7 percent intrapartum and postpartum), a rate that would be consistent only with the most high-risk population. Furthermore, the operative birth rate (cesarean, forceps, or vacuum extraction) in this sample was extraordinary, reported at 22.2 percent in the absence of cephalo-pelvic disproportion, the most common reason for operative delivery. Current cesarean birth rates in the most aggressive of hospitals run 20–25 percent for all indications, including fetal distress and elective repeat cesarean birth. Forceps and vacuum extraction rates vary among institutions, however, the incidence has decreased markedly in recent years (O'Brien & Cephalo, 1986) and in this author's institution averages 8 percent. The nurse-midwifery practice averages a combined cesarean, forceps, and vacuum extraction rate, including cephalo-pelvic disproportion, of 10–12 percent.

A further concern is the definition used in this study for prolonged labor. Subjects were considered to have experienced a prolonged labor if they exceeded one standard deviation beyond the mean for either the first or second stage of labor (Friedman, 1978). While this definition may be statistically sound, in clinical practice a significant deviation requiring intervention is usually not identified until the labor has exceeded two standard deviations beyond the mean. For example, in common clinical practice, a second stage of labor that exceeds 32 minutes for a multipara would not be considered complicated.

The measures used in this study, while valid and reliable for research, may be open to criticism. The measures of predictor variables are excellent, but not easily incorporated into general nursing assessment. The outcome variables may have been defined so broadly and liberally as to produce vague or spurious relationships.

The study results are thoroughly reported. In addition, the analyses are exquisitely designed to tease out relationships among many interacting variables. Data reduction was accomplished using principal-components factor analysis. Multiple-regression analysis was used to test the first hypothesis, that life stress would be positively related and social support would be negatively related to emotional disequilibrium. Discriminant analysis was used to test the second hypothesis that increased life stress, decreased support, and increased emotional disequilibrium would be positively related to obstetrical complications. In each case, a hierarchical model was appropriately used to force medically relevant variables into the first set, thus controlling for the impact of these variables and looking for significance only beyond the variance accounted for by these variables.

The first hypothesis was supported by the data. High life stress and low social support were clearly related to emotional disequilibrium. The second hypothesis, however, was only partially supported. High life stress during the preceding year was significantly related to overall complications and specifically to gestational complications. Infant-condition complications were significantly associated with high emotional disequilibrium. Although tangible support did not directly predict complications (a main effect), in interaction with life stress during pregnancy, a significant relationship was noted.

The analyses are presented extensively and are interpreted cautiously and appropriately. No attempt is made to extend the data beyond the limits of the analyses nor to imply a theoretical or clinical significance that is not there.

In fact, the only difficulty with the analyses lies in their very elegance and complexity. From the perspective of research utilization in everyday nursing practice, it is clear that the average nurse without doctoral preparation does not have the background to interpret these analyses. Most readers would be left to trust the knowledge and judgment of the investigators, and would be unable to interpret the report critically. This is not to imply that nursing research must be conducted with simplistic analyses, but to call attention to the need to clearly interpret complex analyses when writing for a population less sophisticated in research methods.

The results are consistent with previous research and are in concert with the underlying conceptualization of the study. The lack of complete support of the second hypothesis may be explored from several perspectives. One might speculate that what relationship existed was due to the inordinately high "complication rate." Perhaps if complications were less liberally defined, and thus not as common, little if any relationship would remain. On the other hand, perhaps the broad definition of complications obscured some more discrete relationships that might have emerged if complications had been defined according to a model that specifically accounted for the physiological manifestations of stress and anxiety.

In this study, Sarason's theory of stress was used. In this model, a situation, such as pregnancy, results in a call to action which is influenced by life events. An appraisal of resources (support) in relation to demands results in either self-preoccupying thoughts (emotional disequilibrium) or task-oriented thoughts (low emotional disequilibrium) and is manifested by an observed behavior (pregnancy complications). In some respects, it is difficult to conceptualize pregnancy complications as a behavior. A model that acknowledges the specific manifestations of stress might allow one to more clearly predict the type of expected pregnancy complications. For instance, the release of epinephrine could be expected to have impact on complications related to vascular problems, such as hypertension induced by pregnancy, or low birth weight. Prolonged labor (more conservatively operationalized) might be expected due to the inhibitory effect of catecholamines on uterine contractions. Anemia, however, does not seem to lend itself particularly to the stress–illness relationship.

This study is methodologically sound. Although some concern is warrented regarding the measures used, methodological problems encountered in some previous studies have been addressed. Additional support for the mediating influence of support (particularly, tangible support) and the beginning of a theoretical model also are provided.

Part IV: Generalizability of Results

The study results are generalizable to an essentially low-risk population delivering their infants in a high-risk setting. The measures of stress and support are applicable to any pregnant woman. However, the results would be further clarified by additional data on lower-income higher-risk gravidas and by testing in a setting in which routine intervention may be less likely.

Application of the concepts of this study may be generalized to any setting. However, the specific assessments made in this study are not practical for clinical application. A useful extension of this study would be to determine how nurses can best assess life stress and social support in practice.

Part V: Other Factors to Consider in Utilization

This study would be difficult to replicate in a typical practice situation. As noted earlier, the measures (with the exception of outcome measures) are not a typical component of patient assessment, at least in the form used for this study. In addition, the analyses are so complex as to require the participation of experienced researchers and statisticians. However, research using concepts from this study, such as testing a particular support intervention, could be easily accomplished.

Little risk can be found in incorporating the concepts tested here into nursing practice. Benefits, if the relationships hold, would be a decrease in pregnancy complications. The cost of implementation is variable. For minimal cost, nurses could make a greater attempt to assess life stress and social support. However, if tangible support exerts the most influence on the relationship, the cost of providing it could be enormous. Providing tangible support (food, housing, transportation, home health care) is central to much of the controversy in health policy today. However, those who would argue in favor of such a policy point to the equally enormous cost attributable to pregnancy complications, particularly to preterm birth and the cesarean section rate. Even a minor decrease in preterm birth or cesarean delivery might justify economically the increased expenditure that might be required.

REFERENCES

Anderson, G., & Sibai, B. (1986). Hypertension in pregnancy. In S. Gabbe, J. Niebyl, & J. Simpson (Eds.), *Obstetrics: Normal and problem pregnancies*. New York: Churchill Livingstone.

O'Brien, W., & Cephalo, R. (1986). Labor and delivery. In S. Gabbe, J. Niebyl, & J. Simpson (Eds.), *Obstetrics: Normal and problem pregnancies*. New York: Churchill Livingstone.

Pritchard, J., MacDonald, P., & Gant, N. (1985). *Williams obstetrics*. Norwalk, CT: Appleton-Century-Crofts.

Identity of Self as Infertile:
An Example of Theory-Generating Research

Ellen Frances Olshansky, DNSc, RNC
Assistant Professor
University of Washington
Seattle, WA

This article presents results of a study using grounded-theory methodology to explore the meaning of infertility to those persons experiencing it. Thirty-two persons were interviewed, including 15 married couples and two married women whose husbands were either unable or unwilling to participate in the study. Forty-five semistructured interviews were conducted, as each person was interviewed separately and 13 couples were interviewed conjointly. Through the ongoing process of data collection and analysis, a substantive grounded theory was generated, with a core concept being that as persons experience unwanted infertility they take on a central identity of themselves as infertile. The process of taking on and managing this identity is described.

The continuing development of the discipline of nursing requires a variety of ways of knowing.[1] One such way is to generate theory through an inductive mode of inquiry. In a recent presentation, Melia[2] stated that nursing is in need of theories that are generated from inductive research and grounded in the data obtained through such research.

This article presents results of an inductive research study that was conducted to better understand the human responses to infertility and to generate a substantive grounded theory that helps explain some of these responses. This study has relevance for the discipline of nursing for two primary reasons. First, nursing is concerned with the diagnosis and treatment of human responses to actual or potential health problems, and understanding the human responses to infertility contributes to nursing knowledge.[3] Second, theory-generating research is an important aspect of scholarly inquiry that contributes to nursing knowledge and to the discipline of nursing.[2]

LITERATURE REVIEW

Approximately 20% of US couples experience difficulty trying to have a child.[4] While research on infertility is predominantly medically oriented, a growing body of literature exists pertaining to psychosocial and emotional aspects of infertility. Until recently, this literature only examined psychosocial antecedents of infertility, searching for causes of infertility, with the focus being on females almost to the exclusion of males. Rarely did researchers emphasize the psychosocial consequences of infertility or how infertility influences the lives of those experiencing it, or focus on both females and males. Recently, however, interest has heightened regarding the influence of infertility on the lives of infertile persons. Menning[5-10] noted that the process of resolving the emotional conflicts surrounding infertility involves several stages. Wiehe[11] discussed similar findings, and Sawatsky[12] discussed psychological tasks through which infertile couples must work in order to resolve their conflicts. Others[13-25] have addressed the emotional impact of infertility, emphasizing the need for sensitivity in those providing health care for infertile persons. The research presented in this article represents a new understanding of the consequences of infertility, adding to existing literature by exploring the meaning of infertility from the perspective of infertile persons themselves.

STUDY METHODOLOGY

The sample consisted of 32 informants, including 15 married couples and two married women whose husbands were either unable or unwilling to participate in the study. Informants were recruited from a large university infertility clinic on the West Coast as well as from RESOLVE, an infertility support organization. A total of 45 interviews was conducted, as each person was interviewed separately and 13 couple units were interviewed conjointly. Two couple units were not available for the conjoint interview. The women ranged in age from 28 to 41, and the men from 29 to 47. All were Caucasian from various religious backgrounds, and most were employed in professional occupations. The characteristics of the sample indicated an important limitation to the ability to generalize this study since persons from lower socioeconomic backgrounds and various ethnic groups were not represented. Infertility treatment is expensive, and the question arises concerning whether this limitation related to the study sample may, in fact, represent a larger societal problem of inaccessibility to infertility treatment by a significant portion of the population. This issue deserves further attention.

The sample was not limited to a particular kind of infertility problem. Couples who were infertile due to a physiological problem in the female, in the male, or a combined physiological problem, and those infertile due to unknown causes were included in the study. The key factor was the couples themselves perceiving that they had an infertility problem. They were at various stages of an infertility workup, including those beginning a medical workup and those actively seeking alternative solutions.

STUDY PROCEDURES

Grounded-theory methodology was used in collecting and analyzing data.[26,27] In conducting an inductive research study, the goal of the research is to generate theory that explains the phenomenon in question. Thus, a theoretical framework is not determined a priori to be tested. Inductive research is not atheoretical, however, as it is guided by certain philosophical underpinnings. Grounded-theory methodology is rooted in the theoretical perspective of symbolic interactionism. The basic premise of symbolic interactionism is that persons construct meanings for phenomena based on their interpretations of interactions that they have with one another within a social context.[28] Thus, the interactions of infertile persons will influence the meaning they attach to infertility.

With grounded-theory methodology, qualitative data are collected through observation and interviews "in the field," meaning the natural environment of the informants being studied. In this case, data were collected in the homes of infertile persons. Data were analyzed according to the technique of "constant comparative analysis," in which "slices of data" were constantly compared against other "slices of data," and each informant was compared against other informants.[26,27]

Data collection and analysis are not two discrete processes, but rather they are related in a circular fashion. Data are analyzed as they are collected, and this initial analysis guides further data collection, leading to more refined data analysis and more focused data collection. In this study, data were collected using broad, open-ended questions. The interviews were tape-recorded and transcribed for data analysis. The researcher constructed codes, or words, that captured the meanings of the transcripts, a process referred to as open coding.[27] Eventually several codes were grouped into categories that subsumed these codes. These categories guided further data collection, providing focus for subsequent interviews, as questions became directed toward understanding and verifying these categories. The initial interview questions were

- How would you say that infertility has affected your life?
- How has infertility affected your relationships with significant others in your life?
- In what ways do you deal with the feelings you have about infertility?

The interview questions used toward the end of the study after data were analyzed from the majority of informants were more focused.

- Does it seem accurate to you to describe the treatments and procedures surrounding infertility as "work"?
- Do you feel that infertility has taken a central focus in your life?
- In what ways are you able to carry on with other important things in your life while experiencing infertility?
- How do you view the various options available to you in dealing with infertility?

As data analysis continued, certain categories became more evident and the researcher focused on them, a process referred to as selective coding.[27] Eventually certain categories emerged consistently with less and less new information elicited, a point at which the researcher had reached theoretical saturation.[27] In this research, the categories that emerged consistently were "the work of fertility" and "the central identity of self as infertile." The categories and their subcategories were linked, a process termed theoretical integration, to form a substantive theory.[26,27]

As stated, the goal of this methodology is to generate substantive theory that is grounded in the data collected and explains the phenomenon in question. Ultimately, the goal is to generate formal theory in which the substantive theory has application to other substantive areas, thus becoming more formalized. Melia,[2] in advocating this kind of theory in nursing, describes substantive and formal theory as theories of the second and third kind, respectively, with theory of the first kind being that derived by the logico-deductive method.[2] The analysis in this study led to the generation of a substantive theory, or theory of the second kind, that provides an explanation and understanding of the meaning of infertility to those experiencing it.

STUDY FINDINGS

The findings of this study consist of an organizing scheme constructed from the data that represented a beginning substantive theory explaining the process of taking on and managing an identity of self as infertile. Before presenting this organizing scheme, it is important to indicate that an underlying assumption in this study, derived from symbolic interactionism (the framework guiding grounded-theory methodology), is that self is conceptualized as being composed of multiple identities.[29] These identities are dynamic, constantly shifting their positions within the self, with some identities taking on a central position and others taking on a peripheral position. The positions assumed by the various identities can and do change under differing circumstances.

Figure 1
Conceptualization of the Central Identity of Self as Infertile.

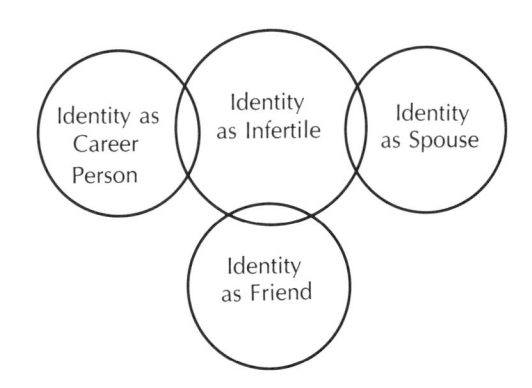

Maternity Nursing 147

Findings of this study suggest that infertile persons who are distressed by their infertility undergo a process of "taking on" an identity of self as infertile. This identity becomes central. They eventually attempt to "shed," "push," or "diminish" this identity to the periphery and "get on with their lives." For these individuals, infertility becomes all-encompassing, taking on a central focus in their lives as they "work" actively to intervene in this problem. Other important identities and their related activities, such as career identity, are "pushed" to the periphery (Figure 1).

Paradoxically, in contrast to those for whom infertility is relatively unimportant, the infertile couples in this study had to confront directly their identities as infertile in order to make these identities less central. The paradox is that in order to rid themselves of the central identity as infertile and make this identity peripheral, infertile persons must initially take on this identity centrally.

Figure 2 conceptualizes the process of taking on and managing an identity of self as infertile.[30] This process is highly interrelated with and influenced by biological, sociocultural, and

Figure 2
The Work of Taking on and Managing an Identity of Self as Infertile.

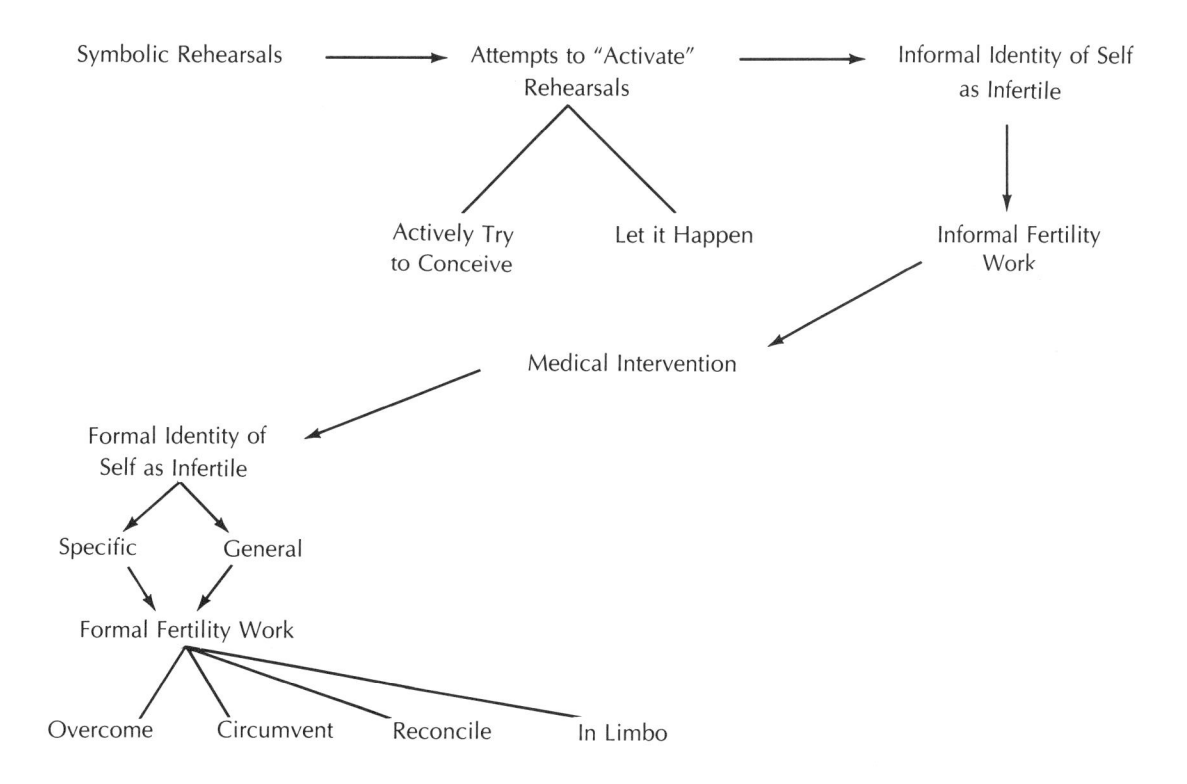

```
Symbolic Rehearsals ──→ Attempts to "Activate" ──→ Informal Identity of Self
                            Rehearsals                    as Infertile
                          ╱          ╲                         │
                         ╱            ╲                        ▼
                Actively Try        Let it Happen       Informal Fertility
                to Conceive                                   Work

                            Medical Intervention
                           ╱
Formal Identity of  ←─────
Self as Infertile
    ╱      ╲
Specific  General
    ╲      ╱
Formal Fertility Work
   ╱    │    ╲       ╲
Overcome  Circumvent  Reconcile  In Limbo
```

Reprinted with permission from E. F. Olshansky: *The Work of Taking on and Managing an Identity of Self as Infertile*, dissertation. University of California, San Francisco, CA, 1985.

psychological processes in the infertile person's life. Many variations occur as a result of individual experiences, strategies employed, and consequences experienced. The commonality, however, is the taking on and focusing on the identity of self as infertile to deemphasize this identity. This process is key in the larger process of managing infertility.

TAKING ON AN IDENTITY OF SELF AS INFERTILE

Symbolic Rehearsals

Initially there are symbolic rehearsals of becoming pregnant or becoming a parent. These symbolic rehearsals refer to a period of imagining what it would be like to be pregnant or to be a parent, imagining such specific instances as holding a baby, feeding a baby, clothing a baby. These symbolic rehearsals occur under the influence of sociocultural factors. Symbolic rehearsals may have begun years before, often during childhood play. Some examples of symbolic rehearsals are seen in the following quotes from informants in this study:

I think I have really come down to a very basic, very primitive idea that this (having children) is the way life is supposed to be, and you do it because it's natural to do, because not doing it feels very unnatural.

I think we've all grown up with the idea that pregnancy is what a woman does, it's the most natural thing, and we have a whole 2,000 years of literature and culture that have always pointed in that direction. So there has been this tradition, and it's very hard at times to redefine oneself as a woman.

I figured I could sit in the backyard and make quilts and do handwork that I love to do, which in some ways I haven't done because now I see no purpose—it is more something to do if you're pregnant. There are some things I still haven't done, like fix up the patio with astro turf, which would be nice for a child to play in. And some things I would do in the house that now really aren't needed since there are no kids. I had images and plans of things I would do.

Such critical rehearsals of identity in relation to pregnancy and child rearing most frequently lead to a decision to "activate" these rehearsals by becoming parents, either by "letting it happen" or by "trying" to conceive. That is, some people decide only to discontinue contraceptive use, while others decide to discontinue contraception and consciously "time" sexual intercourse around the expected ovulatory phase of the woman's menstrual cycle. How couples choose to try to "activate" these rehearsals may be related to how they perceive their infertility's effect on their lives.

Informal Identity of Self as Infertile

After a period of letting it happen or trying to conceive with no resulting pregnancy, the couple (or at least one member of the couple) may begin to suspect a problem. There is a persistent "thwarting" of attempts to realize the symbolic rehearsals; the couple then begins a process of "reluctant acceptance" of an identity of self as infertile. This identity is cast upon them biologically and socially. Initially this identity is of an informal nature, as it has not been "confirmed" and "formalized" through medical diagnosis. This informal identity leads to "informal work" of attempting to push aside the identity. This informal "fertility work" includes strategies related to "playing probabilities" by modifying their diets, changing positions and timing of sexual intercourse, and generally following suggestions they have received informally from friends, literature, or media.

The following example from the data illustrates this concept:

You kind of have this anticipation; and when it doesn't happen, you get tired of it and you figure you can't live the rest of your life like this. So just in general reading about it, you realize that something might be wrong and that you have to work on it.

Formal Identity of Self as Infertile

As a result of the reluctant acceptance of self as infertile, the couple (or one member of the couple) takes on the role of self as infertile, acting on it by making a commitment to "work" on deemphasizing this identity. This fertility work involves strategies of searching for a cause as well as a remedy for the infertility. Through the process of searching, these couples seek medical intervention for diagnosis and treatment. As a result of the medical diagnosis and the clinical confirmation, they take on a more formal identity of self as infertile. This formal identity can be either specific, referring to explained infertility (diagnosed cause), or general, referring to unexplained infertility (no specific diagnosed cause).

Each of these types of formal identity has its own consequences. Once clinically confirmed as infertile, the individual or couple undertakes "formal fertility work." This formal work involves following the medical regimen prescribed, such as undergoing specific treatments or taking certain drugs. The formal fertility work often has profound effects on the lives of infertile couples. A poignant example of this is evidenced in the following quote from an informant:

Our sex life hasn't recovered yet. When I finally failed the last time with Pergonal, I was so depressed that I didn't want to have anything to do with sex at all, and he was so depressed that he had been through all of this for nothing that he didn't want to have anything to do with sex. Sex was a pain. Pleasure? Are you kidding me? I'd rather go take a shot of Pergonal rather than have sex, which was so rife with emotion. So we just decided let's not even do it, if we never do it again, it's O.K. Let's just forget about it and take this negative aspect away from it, and we went for many months with no sex, and I didn't miss it at all and he didn't miss it at all either. Slowly, it's coming back, very, very slowly. Sometimes I think it's never going to be the same because of my association with it. I don't know when there is ever going to be a time in our lives when we can be relaxed enough to get back into sex as a pleasure. It became a focus for all of our rage and anxiety and fears.

Expansion of the Identity of Self as Infertile

Taking on a formal identity and role of self as infertile leads to a greater commitment to this fertility work. With greater commitment comes a greater focus on this identity. The identity as infertile eventually takes on a greater focus in the lives of infertile couples, thus their identity of self as infertile is expanded. Paradoxically, their infertility becomes all-encompassing as couples become more absorbed in the work of letting go of this identity. The following quote offers an example:

It could be getting my period, or it could be finding out that somebody else is pregnant, or it could be having to do a test that I just didn't feel like thinking about and I was just feeling sorry for myself, like that time around my birthday and finishing the second year of trying to become pregnant. Now that I'm spending such an inordinate amount of time noticing my temperature and all that other stuff, I feel like everything is under a microscope.

MANAGING THE IDENTITY OF SELF AS INFERTILE

As the identity of self as infertile is taken on centrally, the search for remedies escalates. The search for causes continues for those identified as falling into the category of "unexplained-general" infertility. In analyzing the data, it was apparent that the desired results of this search were to resolve the infertility, allowing other identities to regain a central focus as the infertile identity assumed a peripheral position. The data revealed that the infertile couples used three distinct modes of managing infertility: overcoming infertility, circumventing infertility, and reconciling infertility. Regardless of the mode of managing infertility, varying degrees of success were achieved by the couples in this study. The infertile identity began to assume a greater or lesser peripheral position for various individuals as they resolved their feelings and conflicts surrounding infertility to a greater or lesser degree.

Overcoming the Identity of Self as Infertile

Some people managed infertility by becoming pregnant, either as a direct result of, or in spite of, medical intervention. This process is viewed conceptually as "overcoming" infertility as this identity is "shed" to the periphery, while the underlying cause of the infertility is corrected, allowing pregnancy to occur. Two couples in this study fell into this category.

Circumventing the Identity of Self as Infertile

Some manage infertility through technological means such as in vitro fertilization or artificial insemination, thus circumventing the underlying cause, but still achieving pregnancy. In this case, the identity as infertile is "pushed" to the periphery, with pregnancy occurring though the underlying cause is still present. Two couples in this study fell into this category, with one couple achieving pregnancy through in vitro fertilization, and another couple currently attempting to conceive through artificial insemination. Two other couples were in the process of trying to overcome infertility. A woman in this study who became pregnant as a result of in vitro fertilization described herself as "an infertile fertile woman."

Reconciling the Identity of Self as Infertile

A third group of persons managed infertility by choosing alternative measures such as adopting, or choosing to be child-free. These strategies represent methods of reconciling infertility because the underlying cause of the infertility is not corrected nor is pregnancy achieved through technological means. These people, however, are able to come to terms with their inability to have biologically linked children. This reconciliation process allows the identity as infertile to "diminish," taking on a peripheral position in their lives. Six couples fell into this category, with three adopting children, two in the process of adopting, and one choosing to be without children.

Remaining in Limbo

A fourth mode observed does not represent a way of managing successfully the identity of self as infertile. Some infertile persons remained "in limbo" as they continued unsuccessfully to try to conceive, without attempting other strategies described above. This group of people persistently tried to overcome infertility, though they were unsuccessful. Some persons in this group discontinued actively trying to overcome infertility but had not resolved their feelings about infertility. Five couples in this study fell into this group. This group requires further study.

An initial substantive grounded theory, referred to as the work of taking on and managing an identity of self as infertile, was generated from data collected and analyzed using grounded-theory methodology. Such a theory contributes to nursing knowledge and the discipline of nursing in that it provides an understanding of the human response to infertility from the perspective of those persons experiencing it. More study is needed to build on this substantive theory in order to better understand the phenomenon of infertility, as well as to attempt to formalize this theory by testing it in other substantive areas that are relevant to nursing. In addition, other areas of infertility deserve study, such as the influence of infertility on a marital relationship, as well as on the larger family unit. This study represents an initial effort at understanding and explaining the human response to infertility.

REFERENCES

1. Carper, B. A. (1978). Fundamental patterns of knowing in nursing. *Advances in Nursing Science*, *1*, 13–23.
2. Melia, K. (1986, May 8). *Theories of the second and third kind*. Paper presented at the second International Nursing Research Conference, Edmonton, Alberta, Canada.
3. American Nurses' Association (1980). *A Social Policy Statement*. Kansas City, MO: The author.
4. Peindl, C. (1985). The expanding nursing role in infertility. In *Insights into infertility*. Serono Symposia Publishers.
5. Menning, B. E. (1982). The psychosocial impact of infertility. *Nursing Clinics in North America*, *17*, 155–163.
6. Menning, B. E. (1980). The emotional needs of infertile couples. *Fertility and Sterility*, *34*, 313–319.

7. Menning, B. E. (1979). Counseling infertile couples. *Contemporary Obstetrics and Gynecology, 13,* 101–108.
8. Menning, B. E. (1977). *Infertility: A Guide for the Childless Couple.* Englewood Cliffs, NJ: Prentice-Hall.
9. Menning, B. E. (1976). RESOLVE: A support group for infertile couples. *American Journal of Nursing, 76,* 258–259.
10. Menning, B. E. (1975). The infertile couple: A plea for advocacy. *Child Welfare, 54,* 454–460.
11. Wiehe, V. (1976). Psychosocial reactions to infertility: Implications for nursing in resolving feelings of disappointment and inadequacy. *Journal of Obstetric, Gynecological, and Neonatal Nursing, 5,* 28–32.
12. Sawatsky, M. (1981). Tasks of infertile couples. *Journal of Obstetric, Gynecological, and Neonatal Nursing, 10,* 132–133.
13. Bernstein, J., & Mattox, J. H. (1982). An overview of infertility. *Journal of Obstetric, Gynecological, and Neonatal Nursing, 11,* 309–314.
14. Frideman, B. M. (1981). Infertility workup. *American Journal of Nursing, 81,* 2040–2046.
15. Kraft, A. D., Palombo, M. A., & Mitchell, D. et al. (1980). The psychological dimensions of infertility. *American Journal of Orthopsychiatry, 50,* 618–628.
16. Mazor, M. D. (1984). Emotional reactions to infertility. In M. D. Mazor (Ed.), *Infertility: Medical, emotional and social considerations.* New York: Human Sciences Press.
17. Mazor, M. D. (1978). The problem of infertility. In M. Notman, & C. Nadelson (Eds.), *The woman patient.* New York: Plenum Press.
18. Mocarski, V. (1977). The nurse's role in helping infertile couples. *American Journal of Maternal Child Nursing, 2,* 264–266.
19. McCormick, T. M. (1980). Out of control: One aspect of infertility. *Journal of Obstetric, Gynecological, and Neonatal Nursing, 9,* 205–206.
20. McCusker, M. R. (1982). The subfertile couple. *Journal of Obstetric, Gynecological, and Neonatal Nursing, 11,* 157–162.
21. Rosenfeld, D. L., & Mitchell, E. (1979). Treating the emotional aspects of infertility: Counseling services in an infertility clinic. *American Journal of Obstetrics and Gynecology, 135,* 177–180.
22. Williams, L. S., & Power, P. W. (1977). The emotional impact of infertility in single women: Some implications for counseling. *Journal of the American Medical Women's Association, 32,* 327–333.
23. Wilson, E. A. (1979). Sequence of emotional responses induced by infertility. *Journal of the Kentucky Medical Association, 77,* 229–233.
24. Woods, N. F. (1981). Infertility. In I. Fogel & N. F. Woods (Eds.), *Health care of women: A nursing perspective.* St. Louis: C. V. Mosby.
25. Woods, N. F. (1979). *Human sexuality in health and illness.* St. Louis: C. V. Mosby.
26. Glaser, B., & Strauss, A. L. (1967). *The discovery of grounded theory.* Hawthorne, NY: Aldine.
27. Glaser, B. (1978). *Theoretical sensitivity.* Mill Valley, CA: Sociology Press.
28. Blumer, H. (1969). *Symbolic interactionism: Perspective and method.* Englewood Cliffs, NJ: Prentice-Hall.
29. Mead, G. H. (1934). *Mind, self, and society.* Chicago: University of Chicago Press.
30. Olshansky, E. F. (1985). *The work of taking on and managing an identity of self as infertile.* Dissertation, University of California, San Francisco.

This article is printed with permission of *Advances in Nursing Science.* Copyright 1987 Aspen Publishers, Inc.

6

Nursing Care of Children

Sheila Kodadek, PhD, RN
Tim Massmann, MA, BSN, RN
Charlyn Wilson, BSN, BA, RN

INTRODUCTION BY: SHEILA KODADEK, PhD, RN

Nursing of children and their families is a challenging, complex, and rewarding area of practice. Clinically relevant research to support that practice is equally challenging, complex, and rewarding. The three studies chosen for review in this chapter represent some of the best research available to help guide practice with children.

The studies chosen are both clinically relevant and conceptually and methodologically sound. The investigators paid rigorous attention to conceptualization, design, and conduct of their studies. In addition, they all were grounded in practice, taking into account nursing practice needs and realities throughout the planning and implementation of the research.

All three studies are linked to hospital-based care of children. However, in an era when children's health care is predominantly oriented to health promotion in settings other than hospitals, this presents a certain limitation.

Further limitation of this selection of studies is that they did not address issues of nursing care with very sick children in high acuity, high technology settings, such as neonatal intensive care units (NICU). Equally significant is that they do not address nursing care of chronically ill or handicapped children and their families, a population which requires knowledge and skills applicable both to care during illness and to health promotion. Research is being done in these areas and will need to continue as demands for nursing care increase with these children and their families.

The first study reviewed in this chapter is Wolfer and Visintainer's "Pediatric Surgical Patients' and Parents' Stress Responses and Adjustment as a Function of Psychologic Preparation and Stresspoint Nursing Care." This study, which is a classic in the field, addressed a continuing need in the nursing of children, ways nurses could help reduce or eliminate distress associated with hospitalization and surgery. This intervention study has influenced nursing practice with children and their parents since its publication, and it is referred to implicitly or explicitly in virtually every pediatric nursing textbook.

The second study reviewed is Savedra and Tesler's "Coping Strategies of Hospitalized School-Age Children." This is another carefully designed study which addressed the question of what strategies school-age children use to cope with hospitalization. This study was built on a strong clinical and research base (including Wolfer and Visintainer's study) and is a good example of a clinical observation matrix. Another strength of the work is the focus on school-age children, a population generally neglected in the literature.

The third study is Johnson, Kirchhoff, and Endress' "Altering Children's Distress Behavior During Orthopedic Cast Removal." This classic intervention study focused on the use of sensory information to reduce distress during a procedure. Again, this study, like the two described above, was conceived and designed with application to nursing practice in mind. This study also is distinguished for being part of a program of nursing research designed to test a theory in multiple practice situations.

All three of these studies have had an impact on practice. In the case of the two intervention studies, the impact is so generally accepted in nursing practice with children that the fact that there was ever a question about the effectiveness of the interventions comes as a surprise to some.

There are other equally exciting and well-designed studies in the literature which are relevant to nursing practice with children and their families. To choose only three studies for this text was not easy, but this is good news. In the past 10 to 15 years, there has been a significant increase in research for practicing nurses which meets the dual criteria of clinical relevance and methodological rigor. While there are still gaps, such as in health promotion of children, there are also areas of high productivity which hold great promise for the future.

Pediatric Surgical Patients' and Parents' Stress Responses and Adjustment as a Function of Psychologic Preparation and Stress-Point Nursing Care

John A. Wolfer, PhD
Chairman of Nursing Research Program
Assistant Professor
School of Nursing
Yale University
New Haven, CT

Madelon A. Visintainer, MSN
Instructor
School of Nursing
Yale University
New Haven, CT

The purpose of this study was to test the hypotheses that children who receive systematic psychologic preparation and continued supportive care, in contrast to those who do not, would show less upset behavior and more cooperation in the hospital and fewer posthospital adjustment problems and that their parents would be less anxious and more satisfied with information and care received. Eighty children scheduled for minor surgery and their parents were randomly assigned to experimental and control conditions. The experimental intervention consisted of accurate information about sequences of events, sensory experiences, role expectations and appropriate responses, previews of procedures through play techniques, and supportive care given at critical points pre- and postoperatively. Significant differences between experimental and control children and parents on ratings of upset behavior, cooperation with procedures, pulse before and after painful procedures, resistance to induction, time to first voiding, posthospital adjustment, and parental anxiety and satisfaction with information and care consistently supported the hypotheses. Results were also analyzed in relation to the age and sex of the children and whether parents roomed with the children.

Many children show adverse reactions to the stressful experience of hospitalization and surgery, both immediate reactions while in the hospital and once they have returned home (Blom, 1958; Chapman et al., 1956; Deutsch, 1942; Fagin, 1964; Gellert, 1958; Jackson et al., 1953; Jessner and Kaplan, 1949; Levy, 1945; Prugh et al., 1953). The term, "psychologic upset," has been used to refer to a variety of these immediate and longer lasting behavioral problems (Chapman et al., 1956; Gellert, 1958).

BACKGROUND

Mitigation of Hospital Stress

That the stress of hospitalization and surgery can be mitigated by appropriate psychologic preparation and supportive care has been an assumption underlying many clinical practices for several decades (Beverly, 1936; Francis and Cutler, 1957; Godfrey, 1955; Jackson, 1951; Oremland and Oremland, 1973; Plank and Ritchie,

1971) and partially documented by descriptive and experimental studies (Cassell, 1963; Coleman, 1952; Jackson, 1951; Jessner et al., 1952; Mahaffy, 1965; Prugh et al., 1953; Scahill, 1969; Skipper et al., 1968; Vaughan, 1957; Weinick, 1958).

The popularity of the idea is reflected in the wide use of preparatory booklets. Clinical research in medicine and nursing in this area over the past 20 years has helped to delineate relevant variables, develop methods of measuring adverse reactions, demonstrate the apparent beneficial effects of various types of special preparation and continued care, and, in a few instances, articulate the theoretic basis for these special practices. Although much as been learned and many changes have been made in pediatric care, few of the practices have been tested systematically for their effectiveness, and much of the underlying theory is obscure or superficial. The published work in this area contains little sustained research where critical variables regarding psychologic preparation, special care, and outcome are taken into account from one study to the next under similar conditions. Moreover, there has been virtually no replication. In addition, although some of the studies are highly suggestive of what should be done to improve the preparation and care of pediatric patients, the clinical circumstances under which the investigations were conducted may not be appropriate or feasible for normal operations where practice must be congruent with the availability of scarce human and material resources. For example, in a number of studies the caregiver who provided the special preparation and care was a highly trained person whose only responsibility on a floor was to give the time-limited special care.

As far as possible, clinical experiments designed to test the stress-reducing effects of special procedures should be conducted in such a way that effective procedures have a chance of being implemented. Finally, although there has been a proliferation of techniques and subspecialties for giving hospitalized children special preparation and supportive care in the last two decades, there have been no published attempts to implement and evaluate systematically coordinated programs for psychologic preparation and supportive care since a study by Prugh et al. in 1953.

In 1965, under the title, *The Psychological Responses of Children to Hospitalization and Illness: A Review of the Literature*, Vernon et al. provided an excellent comprehensive review of over 200 articles and books dealing with theories and data concerning why hospitalization is psychologically upsetting for children and what has been done to mitigate the problem. Only six of the studies reviewed were some form of clinical experiment where preparation was given to children or their parents along with an attempt to determine if the preparatory communication had a positive outcome (Cassell, 1963; Jackson et al., 1953; Jessner et al., 1952; Prugh et al., 1953; Vaughan, 1957; Weinick, 1958). Outcome variables were either immediate responses, meaning indications of psychological upset while the children were in the hospital, or posthospital responses, referring to indications of psychologic upset occurring after the children returned home. Discussions of psychologic preparation focused on three major themes: the factual information given to the child or parent, encouraging emotional expression, and establishing trust and confidence with hospital staff. The beneficial effects of information were assumed to result because vague, undefined threats are more upsetting than threats which are known and understood, and unexpected stress is more upsetting than expected stress.

Methodologic limitations in these studies, combined with the fact that they were not comparable in terms of design, type of preparation, measurement techniques, and outcome variables, allow only tentative conclusions about the positive effects of psychologic preparation and other supposedly beneficial procedures. As Vernon et al. (1965) noted, there is some support for the hypothesis that unfamiliarity with the hospital setting is a determinant of the level of psychologic upset experienced following hospitalization. Four of the six studies provided some findings to the effect that psychologic preparation either reduced the incidence of posthospital upset or increased the incidence of posthospital benefit.

With regard to measures of psychologic upset during hospitalization, of the three studies that provided data on psychologic preparation and immediate upset, two showed no positive findings and one had mixed findings. Again, methodologic limitations prevented definitive conclusions. In addition, these studies combined different aspects of the process of preparation, such as the provision of factual information, the establishment of a trusting relationship with a staff member, and the provision of other supportive care measures following surgery and other threatening procedures. Consequently, it is impossible to determine the relative contribution of these different sets of treatment variables.

Effect of Psychologic Preparation

A review of the medical, nursing, psychiatric, and psychologic literature from 1965 to the present revealed only three further experimental investigations of the effect of psychologic preparation and special supportive care procedures on hospitalized children's stress reactions and adjustment. In a related series of experiments, Mahaffy (1965) and Skipper et al. (1968) took a different approach from the previous investigations by concentrating the preparatory and supportive efforts on the mothers rather than the children who were having minor surgery.

The basis for the preparatory and supportive intervention was social interaction theory, the emotional contagion hypothesis (Campbell, 1957; VanderVeer, 1949), which holds that a parent's emotional state may be transmitted to a young child, and the clinical observation that uninformed or emotionally upset parents are often unable to assist their children in coping with stress. The research nurse saw mothers randomly assigned to the experimental group at admission in order to determine their emotional states, concerns, and need for information. The nurse then provided the necessary information, emotional support, and assisted them in participating meaningfully in the care of their children. Further nurse-mother contacts occurred at several points during the hospitalization: twice during the evening before surgery, when the child returned from the recovery room, twice during the first evening after surgery, and at discharge. Hence, the treatment variable consisted of a combination of advanced preparatory information and continued supportive care at potential stress points throughout the hospitalization. Mothers randomly assigned to the control group did not receive these preparatory communications and supportive attention.

It was predicted that mothers in the experimental group would experience less emotional distress, would be more satisfied with the information and medical and nursing care they received, and would feel more helpful to their child than control mothers. In turn, it was predicted that experimental group children would experience less emotional distress and evidence better adaptation and recovery in the hospital and upon returning home than control children. Outcome measures were staff nurses' observations of mothers' anxiety and adaptation, mothers' questionnaire responses regarding their level of anxiety at key points, their need for information, their trust and confidence in the staff, and their general satisfaction with the hospital experience. The children's temperature, blood pressure, and pulse were recorded at four potential stress points during the hospitalization as indicators of emotional arousal. Time to first voiding and incidence of emesis in the recovery room and amount of fluid intake were also recorded. Posthospital adjustment was determined from a questionnaire mothers completed eight days later. Results based on 80 patients in the three studies significantly and consistently supported the hypotheses on all outcome variables. A subgroup of the experimental group mothers and their children who were seen only at admission showed almost as much stress reduction and improved adaptation as those who were seen by the research nurse at six other critical points throughout the hospitalization. This finding suggested that admission is the crucial time and place to initiate stress-reduction interaction. However, the distinction between admission-only and admission-plus-follow-up interventions may have been confounded by the fact that the admission-only intervention was done by a female nurse, while the admission-plus subsequent interaction was made by a male nurse.

In these studies, consistent with the hypotheses being tested, the major focus of the preparation and supportive care was the parent. It is not clear how or to what extent children were included in the nurse-mother transactions, particularly at admission. Consequently, it cannot be determined if some of the positive effects for the children may have resulted from the preparation and support they received directly from the experimental nurse rather than, or in addition to, the indirect effects of mothers' lowered distress and improved coping.

From a theoretical point of view, it would be valuable to determine the possible independent and relative effects of parent preparation and support as distinct from child preparation and support. On the other hand, in the light of the suspected and known undesirable effects of separating young children from their parents, particularly during stressful events (Vernon et al., 1967), it would be questionable procedure. In addition, it is awkward and impractical to separate a child from his parents shortly after admission up until the evening meal because separate rooms and additional personnel would be necessary in most pediatric units.

If the patient and his immediate family are taken as a dynamic unit in the planning of care, rather than the individual patient, it is illogical to separate them in order to give them different types of interventions. Further, when the nurse works with both parent and child, they learn from each other during the three-way transaction. This is particularly true of the parent who may see, for the first time, what his child knows and doesn't know about what is going to happen as the nurse interacts with the child. Therefore, it did not seem desirable to attempt to differentiate the parent and child components of the preparation and support procedures.

Another consideration in this line of research is who should provide the special preparation and supportive care. In the Mahaffy (1965) and Skipper et al. (1968) studies, the research nurses who gave the special care were essentially visitors on the unit with highly specialized and limited functions. They were not responsible for or involved in other nursing care activities over and above what they did for the purpose of their studies. This raises the question of whether the special psychologic preparation and continued supportive care can be given with the same beneficial effects when the "research" nurse is actively involved in general nursing care on the unit and functions more as a regular member of the staff.

Finally, except for Prugh et al. (1953), none of the experimental investigations reviewed above systematically examined the effect of psychologic preparation and supportive care as a function of age or sex of the children or in relation to whether the parent roomed in. Are the apparent benefits of reduced emotional distress and a lower incidence of behavioral upset the same for younger and older male and female patients? Vernon et al. (1967) did not find a relationship between age or sex and children's degree of upset behavior at admission or at the time of induction. However, the admission procedure in the study was not found to be very distressing and the age range was restricted to two to five years. Because of the major differences in children's behavior associated with developmental level, it is especially important to take age (as an approximate indication of developmental level) into account. Whether the parent remains with the child overnight, i.e., rooms in, especially for younger children, may make an important difference in how the child responds.

PURPOSE

The purpose of this investigation as the first of a planned series of studies was to: provide a partial replication of the Mahaffy (1965) and Skipper et al. (1965) studies; operationalize the independent variable, psychologic preparation and supportive care for parent and child, in the form of a more complete nursing role on a pediatric unit; consider and explicate the transactional process of communicating with both the mother and the child; and examine the effects of the experimental preparatory and supportive transactions in relation to the age and sex of the child and whether the mother roomed in.

HYPOTHESIS

It was hypothesized that children and parents who receive special psychologic preparation and continued supportive care, in contrast to control children and mothers, would show less upset behavior and better coping and adjustment as indicated on the following ten dependent variables: blind observer ratings of the children's upset behavior and cooperation with procedures at five potential stress points; pulse rates at admission and before and after the blood test and preoperative injections; resistance to induction; recovery room medications; ease of fluid intake; time to first voiding; posthospital adjustment; mother's self-ratings of anxiety at potential stress points throughout the hospitalization; mother's rated satisfaction with various aspects of the nursing and medical care they received; and mother's ratings of the adequacy of information they received.

These dependent variables were operationalized in a similar fashion to the dependent variables in the Mahaffy (1965) and Skipper et al. (1968) studies. It was also expected that older children (seven to 14) would generally show less upset behavior and better coping and adjustment than younger children (three to six) on the first six variables.

There was no strong basis for making a hypothesis regarding sex.

METHOD

Design

A two-group experimental design was used with random assignment of children and parents to either a control or an experimental group. The control group received regular nursing care. The experimental group received special preparation and supportive care which was provided by the same nurse at six different times during the hospitalization. Children's pulse rates, which were taken at admission and before and after the blood test and the preoperative injections, were treated as repeated measures. The upset behavior and cooperation ratings were analyzed separately for each of the four events when they were made (admission examination, blood test, preoperative injection, and transport to the operating room).

Setting

The clinical setting for the study was the 30-bed pediatric unit in a 400-bed Catholic, general hospital located in a metropolitan area of 60,000. The pediatric unit admits children from infancy to 16 years of age. Over 90 percent of the elective surgical procedures in pediatrics are private cases admitted by the surgeon in the particular specialty. Children who have minor elective surgery are admitted from Sunday through Thursday, are scheduled for the operating room on the day following admission, and are discharged the day after surgery.

The nursing staff on the unit consists of ten registered nurses (RNs), four licensed practical nurses (LPNs) and ten nurses' aides (NAs), full- and part-time, divided over three eight-hour shifts. In a foster grandmother program, 17 grandmothers rotate through the day shift to escort children and their parents to their rooms and to provide comfort and support, especially for children hospitalized for extended periods of time. LPN students rotate through the pediatric service for six-week periods and are responsible for the care of one to three patients a day during the six hours they are on the ward. They were not assigned to study patients. A play therapist supervises the playroom on the ward and organizes school activities and arts and crafts for the children. She did not engage in special preparation or supportive activities or play therapy during the study.

Routine (Control) Procedures

On admission to the ward the parents and child saw the admission nurse (a part-time LPN who does admission procedure for all patients throughout the hospital). The child was weighed and measured and his vital signs recorded. The child then waited with his parents until the hospital pediatrician examined him, after which he was assigned to a room. In the afternoon a laboratory technician, accompanied by a pediatric nurses' aide, took a blood sample via vena puncture.

During the afternoon, an anesthesiologist reviewed the child's chart and wrote orders for medication. He did not routinely see the parents or child unless the child had a physical or developmental problem that might complicate surgery. No specific nursing contact, expect during change of shift, was made with the child or parent unless a problem arose. No preoperative instruction was given. Vital signs were taken twice during the evening, and one parent was allowed to stay overnight on a cot beside the child's bed.

In the morning all children scheduled for surgery had their temperature taken, were dressed in hospital pajamas, and received the preoperative medication (intramuscular Demerol® and Vistaril® or Seconal® and Atropine® given 45-60 minutes prior to induction).

The child was taken to the operating room on a stretcher by a surgical technician and was accompanied as far as the operating suite by a pediatric aide or nurse. Parents were not allowed to go with the children.

Until the operating room was ready, the child, often awake, waited with the technician in the hall of the surgical suite. Induction for children under 12 was usually by inhalation of halothane or Fluothane®. Older children frequently received intravenous Pentothol®. After the recovery period, the child was returned to the ward by the recovery room aide.

Contact between the parents and the surgeon occurred late in the afternoon after surgery. Overall, the nursing contact, except for answering call lights and special requests by parents, was limited for the control patient. In general, the nurses were friendly, courteous, and concerned in their interactions with parents and children. However, there was no formal preparation nor systematic attempt to determine parents' and children's information or emotional needs.

Sample

During the data collection period, 80 children met the following criteria and were included in the study. They: 1) were between the ages of three and 14, 2) had had no previous hospitalization within the past year, 3) were English-speaking, 4) were free from chronic diseases, 5) had no medical or psychologic condition that required consultation or special care, and 6) were admitted for elective tonsillectomy, adenoidectomy, myringotomy, polyethylene tubes (and any combination of these), or inguinal or umbilical herniorraphy. Informed consent was obtained from all parents. There were no refusals to participate in the study.

Group Assignments

With random assignment of individual children to the experimental or control conditions, some children and their parents who received different nursing interventions could have been placed in adjacent beds. Consequently, there might have been the possibility of some interaction between control and experimental subjects. Furthermore, some children or parents might have been concerned or disturbed by experiencing a type of nursing care different from that given a child in the next bed. To reduce this possibility, all children and parents admitted to the study on a given day who were assigned to the same room received the same treatment, either the control or the experimental nursing regimen. Treatment given each of the six rooms on the ward each day was determined randomly. Room assignment was made in advance by the admission office roughly on the basis of the age and sex of the child without knowledge of the experimental conditions. Forty-five children were assigned to the experimental group and 35 to the control.

Experimental Preparation and Stress-Point Supportive Care

Hospitalization and surgery create a series of real, imagined, or potential threats for the child. The exact nature of the threats depends on many factors, such as the age and development level of the child, his previous experience with similar threats, amount and type of relevant information he possesses, and amount and type of support from parents and others. The threats can be classified into five general categories, each of which assumes a need or a cluster of needs: 1) physical harm or bodily injury in the form of discomfort, pain, mutilation, death; 2) separation from parents and the absence of trusted adults (especially for preschool children); 3) the strange, the unknown, the possibility of surprise; 4) uncertainty about limits and expected "acceptable" behavior; and 5) relative loss of control, autonomy, and competence. To the extent these threats are not removed, minimized, or coped with more or less effectively, the child is under varying degrees of stress. The purpose of the experimental preparation and stress-point supportive care was to remove or minimize stress and assist the child in coping through the provision of information, instruction, and support from a single nurse who was present at critical times. The exact content of the information and the manner in which it was given depended on the child's intellectual and cognitive development following Piaget's (1958) formulations. Generally, there was a greater use of play techniques for preschool children (three to six) and more direct verbal interactions for the older children (seven to 14), depending on the individual child's ability and willingness to interact and communicate in a given way. Throughout the preparatory communications, a distinction was made between external events and sensations the children would experience in order to maximize their understanding of what would happen, when, how long it would last, and how it would feel (Johnson, 1972).

The experimental condition was a combination of psychologic preparation and supportive care provided at six points: admission, shortly before the blood test, late in the afternoon the day before the operation, shortly before the preoperative medications, before transport to the operating room (OR), and upon return from the recovery room (RR). Admission, the blood test, preoperative medication, transport to the OR, and return from the RR are stressful events for many children. The provision of information about what to expect and how to respond shortly before these events, along with support and reassurance during the events, constitutes stresspoint nursing care. The preparation and support was integrated for the parent and child, and the parental component followed the rationale and procedure used by Mahaffy (1965) and Skipper et al. (1968) and the theory and process of deliberative nursing (Orlando, 1961; Wiedenbach, 1964). During all interactions the preparation attempted to provide individualized attention to the mothers, to explore and clarify their feelings and thoughts, to provide accurate information and appropriate reassurance, and to explain how the mother could help care for her child. The preparation stressed the parent's importance to the child, her continued control over him during hospitalization, and the importance of her approval of his being in the hospital and reassuring him that she would return if she left.

The child component of the preparation included information, sensory expectations, role identification, rehearsals, and support. The initial contact with the child at admission was used to establish a relationship through an expression of interest in home or school activities and likes and dislikes. During all interactions the child's fears and concerns were explored and his understanding of and past experience with the procedures assessed. The child was asked to present his impressions of what was happening and how it involved him. Any misconceptions were clarified by using his own terms whenever possible or by asking his parents to express what the nurse had said in more familiar words. Information included the time of the procedure, who would do it and how, why it was done, how it would begin and end, and what could be expected after it was completed. The sensations and emotions he would or might experience were described and demonstrated whenever possible; for example, the cold sensation and smell of the alcohol, the pressure and smell of the anesthesia mask, and a dizzy feeling after the medication was given. For the younger child the information and sensations were presented in story form using a doll and the hospital equipment. The child was encouraged, through play, to exchange roles with the nurse and to conduct the procedure on the doll, himself, while the story was repeated. For the older child the equipment and the doll were also used; the child's curiosity about the mechanics of the procedure was recognized and more detail was given, but not in story form.

The identification of the child's role and the expected behaviors was considered essential to increasing his feelings of control and involvement in the procedure. After the information was given, the child was encouraged to express his feeling about the event. The child was then helped to identify goals and to recognize those which were obtainable. It was believed that this would direct his effort away from activities that would only lead to frustration and failure. For example, he was helped to recognize that avoiding the blood test was impossible, but shortening the length of time it would take to do it was something he could control.

After identifying the goal, the child was shown the behavior he would need to attain it. For example, for a short blood test, he would need to hold his arm still; for a fast induction, he would have to blow up the "balloon" (anesthesia bag) using the mask. The specific behaviors were then rehearsed and the child was assured of help if he needed it.

Because children have different expectations of themselves, either because of age or experience, after the prescribed behavior was determined, other actions were decided upon by the child himself. For example, holding still for the preoperative medication was essential, however, the verbal response during the test could vary within certain limits. The child was told that crying was permissible and something that even adults do during the same procedure. If the child rejected crying as unacceptable behavior, or if crying did not seem appropriate for a particular age level, alternatives were offered, such as counting or giving verbal command to the nurse, i.e., repeating the words, "hurry up." Older children did not have to focus on verbal response, but could concentrate on muscle relaxation instead. In each case, the child's choice of behavior was supported, and the behaviors practiced during the preparation period. This preparation format was followed during the interactions prior to the blood test, preoperative medication, and transport to surgery.

During the interaction on the afternoon of admission, the nurse explained in detail what would happen the next day. This contact was considered important because of the short period of time available the morning of surgery. Doll play was used for the younger children to demonstrate equipment, sequence of events, and perceptions.

A simple explanation of the surgical procedure was given, including the point that no incision would be made and no other part of the body would be touched. The sequence of events from transport to the operating room to return to the room was described in detail in terms of what the child would experience through this period.

During the interaction after surgery, the nurse reassured the child the operation was over, that he was doing fine, and that he should take fluids. She also discussed with the mother her role after surgery, what she could expect for the remainder of the recovery period, and from whom to seek help.

A brief predischarge visit was made for the purpose of explaining that the child was ready to go home, he had done very well, he would feel the same as usual in a few days, and what the mother could expect for the next few days.

Role of the Research Nurse

Before the study began the research nurse spent approximately a month on the unit, participating in all aspects of direct patient care. Throughout the study she was present on the unit from 7:00 A.M. to 4:00 P.M., six days a week, and provided direct care and supervision of care for many nonstudy patients. Typically, she played a key role in conjunction with the head nurse and team leader in the management of care for the more seriously ill cases. Essentially, she functioned as a clinical specialist in such a way that the special preparation and supportive care she provided the experimental group patients was an integral part of her overall role.

Outcome Variables

Behavioral Ratings. Two ratings of the child's emotional state and cooperation were made. 1) The manifest upset scale is a five-point scale designed to reflect the emotional state of a child at a given point in time, primarily in terms of verbal and nonverbal expressions of fear, anxiety, or anger. A rating of one indicates little or no fear or anxiety (calm appearance, no crying, no verbal protest). A rating of three, a moderate amount (some temporary whimpering and/or mild verbal protest), and a rating of five indicates extreme emotional distress (agitated, hard crying or screaming and/or strong verbal protest). 2) The cooperation scale is a five-point scale for indicating the degree to which a child cooperates with a procedure. A rating of one indicates complete cooperation including active participation in and assistance with the procedure. A rating of three indicates mild or initial resistance or passive participation without assistance. A rating of five indicates extreme resistance, strong avoidance, and the necessity to restrain the child.

The children's manifest upset and cooperating rating scales were completed by a nurse observer for five different events: admission examination, blood test, preoperative medication, transport to the operating suite, and while waiting in the hall in the operating suite. The observer also noted whether there was resistance to induction in the form of attempts to get off the operating table, verbal protest, refusing to hold the mask, fighting the mask, squirming and restlessness once the mask was applied. This observation was coded simply "yes" or "no."

All rating scales were repeatedly field tested by the investigators and the nurse observer until there was essential agreement on what types of observable behaviors were to correspond to the scale points. After the final revisions, the second author and the nurse observer made independent simultaneous ratings of a small sample of children at each of the observation points. The mean percentage of agreement between the two raters over 123 separate ratings for seven children and their parents was 90 percent. On only three individual scales was the agreement less than 80 percent— 60 percent in each case. Interrater reliability was considered adequate. The nurse observer was unaware of whether parents and children were in the experimental or control groups.

Ease of Fluid Intake. When the child first took fluids following the operation, a rating of ease of fluid intake was made by the observer on a four-point scale: one, great ease; two, ease; three, difficulty; four, great difficulty.

Pulse Rates. An indication of physiologic arousal accompanying fear, anxiety, or general emotional distress, pulse rates were recorded by the nurse observer at admission before any contact with the research nurse, before and after the blood test, and before and after the preoperative injections. The admission pulse (along with the admission upset and cooperation ratings) permitted a before-treatment comparison of subjects.

Recovery Room Medication. A further measure of upset was indicated by the way the child recovered from anesthesia in the recovery room. The first reaction to sensations of pain and fears about the surgery may vary from a quiet awakening to thrashing, uncontrolled movements, and crying. Because there was routinely an order for medication to relieve pain and reduce the restlessness, if needed, the administration of pro re nata medication in the recovery room indicated the presence of upset behavior. Although it depended upon the nurse's subjective evaluation of the child's upset, the recovery room staff were completely blind to the groups to which the children were assigned.

Time to First Voiding. A final outcome measure in the hospital was time to first voiding following surgery. This has been considered a recovery measure which reflects a patient's emotional state; the more emotionally upset a patient is, the longer before he voids (Elman, 1951, p. 42; Hollender, 1958). In the Mahaffy (1965) and Skipper et al. (1968) studies, children whose parents received the special preparation and supportive care had a significantly shorter time to first voiding than did control children.

Posthospital Adjustment. This variable was measured with the Vernon et al. (1966) Posthospital Behavior questionnaire, a list of 27 behavioral items most frequently cited in the literature as occurring in children following hospitalization. For each item the parent compares the child's typical behavior before hospitalization with his behavior during the first week after hospitalization. Five response alternatives are provided: "much less than before"—score one; "less than before"—two; "same as before"—three; "more than before"—four; and "much more than before"—five. Vernon et al. performed a factor analysis of the questionnaires of 387 hospitalized children which revealed six orthogonal factors: 1) general anxiety and regression; 2) separation anxiety; 3) anxiety about sleep; 4) eating disturbance; 5) aggression toward authority; and 6) apathy-withdrawal. Comparison of the mean factor and total scores for the full sample with the levels indicative of no overall change indicated that the combination of illness and hospitalization is a psychologically upsetting experience for children in general, resulting in increased separation anxiety, increased sleep anxiety, and increased aggression toward authority. Vernon et al. (1966) also reported a test-retest reliability coefficient of .65 for 37 children, along with a significant correlation between questionnaire responses and a psychiatric interview intended to get at the same information. Further evidence of the predictive validity of the questionnaire came from its detection of changes as predicted in studies by Vernon et al. (1966, 1967).

The Posthospital Behavior questionnaire was given to parents along with detailed instructions on how and when to complete it at the time of discharge. On the eighth day postdischarge they were contacted by phone and reminded to complete the questionnaire and return it by mail. This procedure resulted in an 87 percent return rate.

Parental Measures. Five aspects of parental experience during the hospitalization were assessed. During the admission examination, an independent observer, blind to conditions, rated each parent on two separate scales: 1) manifest upset, a five-point scale designed to indicate the degree of anxiety, apprehension, nervousness, or general emotional distress as expressed in the mother's verbal and nonverbal behavior (a rating of one indicates no signs of emotional distress; of three, a moderate degree of anxiety; of five, a high degree of emotional distress); and 2) coping and cooperation, a five-point scale designed to reflect the degree to which the mother was dealing effectively with the immediate situation as expressed in her verbal and nonverbal behavior while she interacted with the admissions nurse and her child (a rating of one indicates that the mother was in complete control in appropriately assisting with the examination, answering the nurse's questions, as well as asking questions, and appropriately supporting her child, while a rating of five indicates a complete loss of control, inappropriate and/or ineffective interaction with the nurse and her child).

Three other measures for parents were obtained from a questionnaire which was administered shortly before discharge. One assessment was the parent's self-rating of anxiety experienced at eight different points: at admission, immediately after the admission examination, during the blood test, bedtime the night before surgery, any other time during that night, before the child was taken to the operating room, during the operation, and when the child first took fluids. Each was a five-point scale with one indicating no anxiety and five an extreme degree of anxiety. The nine scales were summed to give an overall mean rating of anxiety.

Table 1
Sample Characteristics of Experimental and Control Subjects (N = 80)

Characteristics	Experimental (N = 45)	Control (N = 25)	χ^2
Female	16	14	.16
Male	29	21	
Age			
3-6	22	20	
7-14	23	15	.26
Mean age	7.1 years	7.1 years	
Birth order			
Only child	7	6	
First child	22	10	3.64
Later born	16	19	
Parent stayed			
Yes	17	17	.94
No	28	18	
Type of nursery			
Tonsillectomy	35	25	
Ear	6	5	.63
Hernia	4	5	

A final rating obtained from the questionnaire was a satisfaction with care score which was based on 20 items that covered nursing and medical procedures and the quality and effectiveness of nurse-child transactions. Each item had a four-point scale: needs much improvement—one; needs improvement—two; satisfactory—three; very good—four; and a "did not observe" box. A mean overall satisfaction score was obtained from these items.

Another score from the questionnaire was an indication of the adequacy of the information received. This consisted of items regarding whether mothers considered they were adequately informed about 18 points such as the type of operation, expected length of stay, general hospital routines, reasons for various procedures, what they could do to help. The items were coded "yes" or "no" to indicate whether mothers were adequately informed. A score of 18 indicated adequate information on all 18 items. Each item also asked from whom the information was received, including the project nurse. This not only provided a check on whether mothers received more information from the research nurse than from other sources but also indicated the number of items of information (of a possible total of 18) the mother received from only the research nurse.

RESULTS

Table 1 shows sample characteristics for experimental and control groups. As the chi-square analysis revealed, the two groups did not differ significantly in terms of sex, age, birth order, whether the parent stayed overnight, or type of surgery. Thus, the groups appeared to be comparable on these variables. For the remaining analyses, the total number of subjects in each of the groups fluctuated somewhat from variable to variable because of missing observations.

During the admission examination, before they were seen by the research nurse, all children were rated on manifest upset behavior and cooperation; all parents were also rated on manifest upset behavior and coping-cooperation. The means for these ratings were: upset behavior—children (experimental) 1.73, (control) 1.82; parents (experimental) 1.57, (control) 1.71; cooperation—children (experimental), 1.28, (control) 1.48; parents (experimental) 1.42, (control) 1.46. Comparison of the group means with t-tests showed no significant difference between experimental and control children and parents on these variables before the experimental nursing intervention began.

The results on each child's outcome measures were subjected to a three-way analysis of variance (treatment condition by age and sex) (Table 2). Upset behavior and cooperation ratings were analyzed separately for each of the four events (blood test, preoperative injections, transport to the operating suite, and waiting in the hall in the operating suite). There were no significant main effects for sex on any of these variables. Therefore, there were no consistent differences between girls and boys on these measures.

As predicted, children in the experimental group were significantly less upset and more cooperative than control children for all four events. They also had significantly lower ease of fluid intake ratings, fewer minutes to first voiding, and lower posthospital adjustment scores than the control group, again as predicted. A significant F was also obtained for age on all the behavioral ratings except upset and cooperation while waiting in the operating room and ease of fluid intake. This reflected the general tendency for older children to exhibit less upset and more cooperation than younger children as expected.

The results of the analysis of variance indicted there were no significant treatment by age interactions on any of the children's outcome variables. There were, however, three significant age by sex interactions for the transport cooperation rating, the upset rating, and the cooperation rating while waiting in the operating suite. For each of these three ratings, three- to six-year-old males had relatively lower ratings than the same age females independent of the treatment condition. This difference was reversed for the seven- to 14-year-old males versus females. This age by sex pattern did not appear on other outcome measures.

The results for the resistance to induction indicated that five of 43 children (two observations were missed) in the experimental group showed

Table 2
Mean Scores and Significance Levels for Children's Dependent Variables

Variable	Children's Age	N E	N C	Experimental	Control	Total	Effect	df	F	p
Blood test Upset	3-6	22	20	2.01	3.10	2.55	Treatment:	1	8.88	.005
	7-14	20	11	1.33	1.93	1.63	Age:	1	10.46	.002
Total				1.67	2.52					
Cooperation	3-6	22	20	1.60	2.88	2.24	Treatment:	1	6.36	.001
	7-14	20	11	1.04	1.27	1.15	Age:	1	13.25	.01
Total				1.32	2.07					
Preoperative medication Upset	3-6	22	20	2.07	3.62	2.85	Treatment:	1	25.55	.001
	7-14	20	11	1.16	2.48	2.06	Age:	1	11.08	.002
Total				1.86	3.05					
Cooperation	3-6	22	20	1.41	3.49	2.45	Treatment:	1	24.07	.001
	7-14	20	11	1.15	2.12	1.63	Age:	1	6.95	.01
Total				1.28	2.81					
Transport Upset	3-6	22	20	1.61	2.14	1.88	Treatment:	1	4.89	.03
	7-14	20	11	0.81	1.65	1.23	Age:	1	4.36	.04
Total				1.21	1.70					
Cooperation	3-6	22	20	1.48	2.14	1.81	Treatment:	1	4.58	.04
	7-14	20	11	0.81	1.40	1.11	Age:	1	5.87	.02
Total				1.15	1.77					
Waiting in operating suite Upset	3-6	22	20	1.64	1.87	1.76	Treatment:	1	6.05	.02
	7-14	20	11	.95	2.22	1.59	Age:	1	0.31	—
Total				1.30	2.04					
Cooperation	3-6	22	20	1.38	1.65	1.52	Treatment:	1	7.06	.01
	7-14	20	11	0.85	1.97	1.41	Age:	1	0.17	—
Total				1.12	1.81					
Ease of fluid intake	3-6	22	20	1.69	2.07		Treatment:	1	3.34	.07
	7-14	20	11	1.52	1.97		Age:	1	0.37	—
Total				1.61	2.02					
Minutes to first voiding	3-6	20	17	226.3	343.6		Treatment:	1	10.91	.001
	7-14	19	8	248.1	366.0		Age:	1	0.38	—
Total				237.2	354.8					
Posthospital adjustment score	3-6	19	18	79.6	85.5		Treatment:	1	12.31	.001
	7-14	15	9	80.8	87.7		Age:	1	1.22	—
Total				79.8	84.9					

resistance, compared to 11 of the 35 control children. A chi square of 4.64 indicated that significantly fewer children in the experimental group resisted induction ($p < .05$).

Table 3 shows the mean pulse rates for experimental and control children classified by sex and age, and time of measurement: at admission, before, and after the blood test. A two (treatments) by two (age groups) by two (sex) analysis of variance was performed on the pulse rates across the three measurement times (repeated measures). An unweighted-means analysis for unequal cell entries was used (Winer, 1962). The summary of the analysis of variance in Table 4 contains only significant ($p \leq .05$) or near significant ($p < .10$) effects. There was no overall significant effect for the treatment condition. The significant effects for age and sex indicated a reliable tendency of younger children to have higher pulse rates than older children and for girls to have higher pulse rates than boys, independent of the treatment condition. The significant age by sex interaction resulted largely from the younger girls' having substantially higher pulse rates at, before, and after the blood test than the other groups. The significant effect for measurement times indicated a significant ($p < .001$) overall change in mean pulse rates from the time of admission to immediately before and after the blood test. These three means (91.4, 114.8, and 104.7) were significantly ($p < .001$) different from each other, indicating that independent of age, sex, and the treatment condition, there was a significant increase in pulse from admission to before the blood test ($t = 12.0$), and a significant decrease from admission to after ($t = 6.8$) and from before to after the blood test ($t = 5.2$) as would be expected if changes in heart rate reflect changes in physiologic arousal accompanying threatening events. In addition, there was no significant difference between the experimental and control means at admission before the experimental intervention began (91.2 versus 91.6). Before the blood test the experimental group had a lower pulse than the control, but not significantly so (113.4 versus 116.2), but had a highly significantly lower pulse after the blood test (98.8 versus 109.3; $t = 5.38$, $p < .001$).

The remaining significant interactions in Table 4 for combinations of repeated measures for pulse in relation to age, sex, and treatment indicated there were complicated differential heart rate changes across measurement times which were related to the age, sex, and type of experience or preparation of the child. However, these interactions did not occur with the preoperative medication heart rates.

Table 3
Mean Pulse Rates for Experimental and Control Groups at Admission and before and after the Blood Test (N = 70)

Sex	Age	Experimental N	Admission	Before	After	Control N	Admission	Before	After
Male	3-6	17	91.3	111.2	104.1	11	91.7	112.9	106.1
	7-14	13	85.4	103.3	84.7	5	90.8	117.6	107.2
Female	3-6	4	102.0	133.0	112.0	7	88.0	134.3	129.4
	7-14	7	86.0	106.3	94.6	5	96.0	100.0	94.4
Total		41	91.2	113.4	98.8	28	91.6	116.2	109.3

Table 4
Summary of Analysis of Variance for Blood Test Pulse Rates (Significant or Near-Significant Fs Only)

Source	df	F	p
Age	1	14.81	.001
Sex	1	3.19	.079
Age × sex	1	5.73	.020
Time	2	56.56	.001
Time × treatment	2	2.82	.064
Time × age	2	6.04	.004
Time × age × sex	2	5.18	.007
Treatment × age × sex × time	2	5.49	.006

Table 5 contains the mean pulse rates at admission and before and after the preoperative medication injections. Table 6 presents the results of the analysis of variance of these data which was the same type as for the blood test pulses. In this case there was a near significant ($p = .057$) tendency for experimental group children to have an overall lower mean pulse rate than controls. Again, the main effects for age and sex indicated that overall the younger children and girls tended to have higher pulse rates independent of the treatment condition. The significant treatment-by-sex interaction resulted largely from much lower means before and after the injections for the experimental males compared to the other three groups. There was a significant ($p < .001$) F for pulse rates across the three measurement times, and the individual t-tests indicated, as with the blood test pulse rates, a significant mean pulse rate increase from admission (91.9) to before the injection (115.8), followed by a significant decrease after the injection was completed (108.7). Admission versus before mean rate showed $t = 13.0$, admission to after, $t = 9.2$; before and after, $t = 3.9$. The experimental children had a significantly lower pulse before (111.5 versus 120.0; $t = 4.84, p < .001$) and after (104.9 versus 112.5; $t = 4.42, p < .001$) the preoperative medications. The nearly significant treatment by pulse interaction indicated that the changes in mean pulse rate across the three measurement times tended to be different for the two groups, which resulted largely from the much smaller increase from admission to before the injection for the experimental children (92.0 to 111.5 = 19.5) compared to the controls (91.8 to 120.0 = 28.2). The decreases in pulse from before to after the injections was of about the same magnitude for both groups (111.5 to 104.9 = 6.6 versus 120.0 to 112.5 = 7.5). The significant age by pulse interactions resulted from the younger children's exhibiting a relatively greater increase in mean pulse rate from admission to before the injections and a relatively smaller decrease from before to after the injections than the older children.

Results of parents' ratings of anxiety, adequacy of information received, and satisfaction with care—analyzed in separate two (treatments) by two (age) by two (sex) analyses of variance—indicated no significant effects for sex of the child (Table 7). Experimental group parents had significantly lower self-ratings of anxiety, rated information received significantly higher in adequacy, and were significantly more satisfied with their care. Except for the anxiety rating where parents of younger children had significantly higher anxiety ratings, there were no significant interactions between the treatment and the age of the child. The mean number of information items (out of a possible 18) parents in experimental and control groups indicated they received from only the research nurse were 11.1 and 1.3, respectively. A t of 11.7 indicated that parents in the experimental

Table 6
Summary of Analysis of Variance for Preoperative Medication Pulses (Significant or Near-Significant Fs Only)

Source	df	F	p
Treatment	1	3.77	.057
Age	1	17.20	.001
Sex	1	3.93	.052
Treatment × age	1	5.26	.026
Time	2	71.77	.001
Treatment × time	2	2.72	.070
Age × time	2	5.35	.006

Table 5
Mean Pulse Rates for Experimental and Control Groups at Admission and Before and After Preoperative Medication (N = 70)

Sex	Age	\multicolumn{4}{c}{Experimental}	\multicolumn{4}{c}{Control}
		N	Admission	Before	After	N	Admission	Before	After
Male	3-6	17	91.3	113.1	107.5	13	91.7	125.8	119.5
	7-14	11	85.4	95.6	88.9	5	90.8	114.8	108.4
Female	3-6	4	102.0	122.5	119.0	6	90.0	129.3	121.3
	7-14	8	89.2	115.0	104.0	6	94.7	110.0	100.7
Total		40	92.0	111.5	104.9	30	91.8	120.0	112.5

Table 7
Mean Ratings and Significant Fs for the Three Parents' Dependent Variables

Variable	Children's Age	\multicolumn{2}{c}{Experimental}	\multicolumn{2}{c}{Control}	\multicolumn{2}{c}{Total}	\multicolumn{4}{c}{ANOVA}
		N	X̄	N	X̄	N	X̄	Effect	df	F	p
Self-rating anxiety	3-6	22	2.51	19	3.27	41	2.89	Treatment:	1	9.03	.004
	7-14	20	2.27	11	2.62	31	2.44	Age:	1	5.78	.02
Total			2.39		2.94						
Adequacy of information received	3-6	22	16.20	19	6.00	41	11.72	Treatment:	1	84.82	.001
	7-14	20	17.00	11	7.50	31	11.63				
Total			15.84		7.40						
Satisfaction with care	3-6	22	3.74	17	2.65	39	3.19	Treatment:	1	17.99	.001
	7-14	20	3.68	8	2.95	28	3.32				
Total			3.71		2.80						

group received significantly more information from the research nurse only than control group parents ($p < .001$).

DISCUSSION

The results of the study supported the hypothesis that children and parents who received systematic psychologic preparation and continued supportive care, in contrast to those who did not, would show less upset behavior and more cooperation in the hospital and fewer posthospital adjustment problems. The experimental group had significantly lower mean upset ratings and higher mean cooperation ratings at each of the stress points than the control group. Children in the experimental condition demonstrated nearly significantly greater ease of fluid intake, significantly less time to first voiding, had significantly lower heart rates after the blood test and before and after the preoperative medication, had a significantly lower incidence of resistance to induction, and obtained significantly lower posthospital adjustment scores. Children between the ages of three and six, compared with those between seven and 14, consistently demonstrated greater upset and less cooperation, but did not differ significantly in terms of ease of fluid intake, minutes to first voiding, or posthospital adjustment scores. Except for heart rate where girls tended to have higher pulses than boys before and after the blood test and preoperative medication, there were no significant sex differences on the outcome measures.

Parents in the experimental group had significantly lower self-ratings of anxiety, higher ratings of the adequacy of the information received, and greater satisfaction with care than parents in the control group.

Taken at face value and in conjunction with the positive findings of other preparation studies, these results seemed to provide strong support for the beneficial effect of systematic preparation and support for hospitalized children and parents. Apparently, the treatment condition which consists of preparatory communications designed to impart accurate information about events, procedures, sensations, and role expectations, combined with supportive care in the form of encouragement, reassurance, and reinforcement from a single care-giver who attends to the child and parent throughout the hospitalization, and especially at critical points, enables children to cope more effectively with and adjust to the various stresses encountered. The treatment condition seems also to result in less anxiety and great satisfaction for parents. The exact causal sequence of this involved process is complex and unknown. Presumably the preparatory instruction and rehearsal produce accurate expectations about the nature and sequence of events which in turn create an enhanced sense of control and capability for both children and parents (Miller et al., 1960). Part of this preparation, especially for the young child, is the emotional support which comes from having a sustained relationship with a consistent danger control figure who communicates in a manner appropriate for the child's developmental level. The net effect of the preparation and supportive care can be described as stress reducing. However, the precise nature of this dynamic cognitive and affective process remains to be determined.

Limitations and Suggestions for Further Study

Before the present results can be taken as conclusive, a number of questions need further investigation. First, there is the question of the possibility of observer bias. Although every attempt was made to keep the nurse observer blind to conditions while she made her behavioral ratings, possibly, part of the time, at least, there may have been cues regarding which group a particular child and parent were in. The observer was free to move about the unit and had no other responsibilities during the observation periods. When she was to make an observation, she entered the room immediately before the rating was to be made and left immediately after. Since the experimental nurse was present at each of these times for both experimental and control patients, her presence or absence was not a sign of which group a child was in. Throughout the study the observation nurse was aware of the possibility of bias and made a deliberate attempt to keep herself blind to group assignment. Nevertheless, at times it was unavoidable for her to witness some interactions between the experimental nurse and the patients which would indicate their group assignment. She reported this happened only in a few cases and for some of the ratings. Most of the time she reported she was either clearly unaware or uncertain of which group the patients were in. To the extent there was observer bias in the direction of the hypothesized effects, this was a limitation of the methodology. In further studies, it would be better if, at the very least, observers were uninformed of the purpose of the study and the nature of the experimental conditions.

There is also a possibility of bias on the part of the parents in the experimental group. Although the control parents clearly knew they were participating in a study, were given the same instructions in the use of the questionnaires at the time of discharge, and saw the experimental nurse throughout their hospital stay, the research nurse was much more involved with the experimental parents. Consequently, there is the possibility that in order to please the nurse for her extra effort, they may have been inclined to rate themselves as being less anxious and more satisfied with the information and care they received. It seems much less likely that this type of bias would be present ten days later when they rated their children's behavior at home. In a future study this possible source of bias might be controlled by having an additional condition where a single nurse spent approximately as much time with the child and parent as under the experimental condition but without providing the systematic preparation. Whether participation in a study along with special attention would produce a positive effect on parents' ratings could then be ascertained.

Another question which can be raised is whether the positive effects of the experimental condition resulted from the process and content of the preparation and supportive care as such, or from the personality and interpersonal style of the experimental nurse, or both. That is, something about the characteristics of the particular nurse might have been responsible or largely responsible for the positive effects. The answer to this requires a replication of the experimental treatment with one or more different nurses following the same principles and techniques of preparation and supportive care for stressful events can be implemented effectively by other nurses.

Closely associated is the possibility that the obtained effects resulted from the establishment of a warm, trusting relationship with a single nurse who was present at critical times throughout the hospitalization, independent of the special preparation and communication techniques. Again, to test this possibility the experimental treatment needs to be compared to a condition where a single nurse establishes a warm relationship with the child and is present at the same points throughout the hospitalization, but does not provide the systematic preparation.

Finally, assuming the positive effects on the outcome measures are primarily the result of psychologic preparation and supportive care, there is the question of whether this type of preparation and care can be given as a regular part of the nursing care in a pediatric service. The attempt in the current study was to incorporate the treatment condition into a full nursing role.

Nevertheless, the research nurse functioned more in the capacity of a clinical specialist with special responsibilities for difficult cases and for preparation and support rather than as a staff nurse. Ideally, following a primary nursing organizational plan, it would seem that each staff nurse with primary assignments to individual patients should include stress-point preparation and support for child and parent as an integral part of the care. Further research is necessary in order to determine if this is clinically and administratively feasible.

REFERENCES

Beverly, B. I. (1936). The effects of illness upon emotional development. *Journal of Pediatrics, 8,* 533–543.

Blom, G. E. (1958). The reactions of hospitalized children to illness. *Pediatrics, 22,* 590–600.

Campbell, E. H. (1957). *Effects of mothers' anxiety on infants' behavior.* Unpublished doctoral dissertation, Yale University, New Haven.

Cassell, S. E. (1963). *The effect of brief puppet therapy upon the emotional responses of children undergoing cardiac catheterization.* Unpublished doctoral dissertation, Northwestern University, Evanston.

Chapman, A. H., et al. (1956). Psychiatric aspects of hospitalizing children. *Archives of Pediatrics, 73,* 77–88.

Coleman, L. L. (1952). Children need preparation for tonsillectomy. *Child Study Journal, 29,* 18–19.

Deutsch, H. (1942). Some psychoanalytic observations in surgery. *Psychosomatic Medicine, 4,* 105–115.

Elman, R. (1951). *Surgical care: A practical physiologic guide.* New York: Appleton-Century-Crofts.

Fagin, Claire (1964). The case for rooming in when young children are hospitalized. *Nursing Science, 2,* 324–333.

Francis, L., & Cutler, R. (1957). Psychological preparation and premedication for pediatric anesthesia. *Anesthesiology, 18,* 106–109.

Gellert, E. (1958). Reducing the emotional stresses of hospitalization for children. *American Journal of Occupational Therapy, 12,* 125–129.

Godfrey, A. E. (1955). Study of nursing care designed to assist hospitalized children and their parents in their separation. *Nursing Research, 4,* 52–70

Hollender, M. (1958). *Psychology of medical practice.* Philadelphia: W. B. Saunders.

Jackson, K. (1951). Psychologic preparation as a method of reducing the emotional trauma of anesthesia in children. *Anesthesiology, 12,* 293–300.

Jackson, K., et al. (1953). Behavior changes indicating emotional trauma in tonsillectomized children. *Pediatrics, 12,* 23–27.

Jessner, L., & Kaplan, S. (1949). Observations of the emotional reactions of children to tonsillectomy and adenoidectomy. In M. J. E. Seen (Ed.), *Problems of infancy and childhood: Transactions of the third conference.* New York: Josiah Macy, Jr. Foundation.

Jessner, L., et al. (1952). Emotional implications of tonsillectomy and adenoidectomy on children. In R. S. Eissler (Ed.), *The psychoanalytic study of the child.* New York: International Universities Press, 126–169.

Johnson, J. E. (1972). Effects of structuring patients' expectations on their reactions to threatening events. *Nursing Research, 21,* 499–504.

Levy, D. M. (1945). Psychic trauma of operations in children. *American Journal of Diseases of Children, 69,* 7–25.

Mahaffy, P. R., Jr. (1965). Effects of hospitalization on children admitted for tonsillectomy and adenoidectomy. *Nursing Research, 14,* 12–19.

Miller, G. A., et al. (1960). *Plans and the structure of behavior.* New York: Holt, Rinehart and Winston.

Oremland, E., & Oremland, J. D. (1973). *The effects of hospitalization on children: Models for their care.* Springfield, Ill., Charles C. Thomas, Publisher.

Orlando, I. J. (1961). *The dynamic nurse-patient relationships.* New York: Putnam.

Piaget, J. (1958). *The growth of logical thinking from childhood to adolescence,* A. Parsons and S. Seagren, (Trans.). New York: Basic Books.

Plank, E. N., & Ritchie, M. A. (1971). *Working with children in hospitals* (2nd ed.). Cleveland: Case Western Reserve University Press.

Prugh, D. G., et al. (1953). A study of the emotional reactions of children and families to hospitalization and illness. *American Journal of Orthopsychiatry, 23,* 70–106.

Scahill, M. (1968). Preparing children for procedures and operations. *Nursing Outlook, 17,* 35–38.

Skipper, J. K., et al. (1968). Child hospitalization and social interaction: An experimental study of mothers' feelings of stress, adaptation and satisfaction. *Medical Care, 6,* 496–506.

Vander Veer, A. H. (1949). The psychopathology of physical illness and hospital residence. *Quarterly Journal of Child Behavior, 1,* 55–71.

Vaughan, G. F. (1957). Children in hospital. *Lancet, 272,* 1117–1120.

Vernon, D. T. A., et al. (1965). *The psychological responses of children to hospitalization and illness.* Springfield, IL: Charles C. Thomas, Publisher.

Vernon, D. T. A., et al. (1966). Changes in children's behavior after hospitalization. *American Journal of Diseases of Children, 111,* 561–593.

Vernon, D. T. A., et al. (1967). Effects of mother-child separation and birth order on young children's responses to two potentially stressful experiences. *Journal of Personality and Social Psychology, 5,* 462–474.

Weinick, H. M. (1958). *Psychological study of emotional reactions of children to tonsillectomy.* Unpublished doctoral dissertation, New York University, New York.

Wiedenbach, E. (1964). *Clinical nursing: A helping art.* New York: Springer.

Winer, B. J. (1962). *Statistical principles in experimental design.* New York: McGraw-Hill.

This article is printed with permission of *Nursing Research.* Copyright 1975 American Journal of Nursing Company.

Original article:
Wolfer, J. A., & Visintainer, M. A. (1975). Pediatric surgical patients' and parents' stress responses and adjustment as a function of psychologic preparation and stress-point nursing care. *Nursing Research, 24*(4), 244–255.

CRITIQUE BY: TIM MASSMANN, MA, BSN, RN

Part I: Clinical Relevance

Wolfer and Visintainer have investigated interventions designed to mitigate the adverse reactions children often experience with hospitalization, surgery, and post-hospitalization adjustment. Since a key nursing focus has long been assisting clients in responding to and coping with the biopsychosocial dimensions of illness and treatment, this work appears to have potential in influencing clinicians' thoughts and interventions in these commonplace situations. The intervention strategies critiqued here, psychological preparation and supportive care, would seem to have potential for broad applicability in providing a care planning foundation from which to work collaboratively with patients and their families during periods of high stress, anxiety, and uncertainty. We often use the nursing diagnosis of "anxiety" in a variety of medical–surgical contexts; for example, with pre open-heart surgery patients or those experiencing acute exacerbation of chronic disease. One could profitably employ the investigators' outcome measures to increase precision of what we mean by anxiety and how to evaluate our success in dealing with or mitigating this problem.

Wolfer and Visintainer's work is rich with instruments and concepts applicable to practice, and reaffirms the effectiveness of systematic preoperative preparation and supportive care as well as the necessity of viewing, holistically, the family as the client. Also, the intervention strategy of working with children at various stress points to establish and attain short-term goals to foster their sense of control can be seen as early evidence of the effectiveness of "mutual goal-setting." That this process (elaborated and researched by Crane & Horsley, 1980) can be used with *pediatric* patients is somewhat of a revelation.

There would appear to be four specific instrumental uses from this research. First, the parent scales on manifest upset and coping/cooperation can yield accurate assessment data from which to plan goals and formulate interventions. Second, the investigators employed an excellent variety of behavioral, physiological, and psychosocial outcome measures that could be used to evaluate the effectiveness of pre-, peri-, and postoperative interventions. Third and relatedly, the Posthospital Adjustment scale can also be used for evaluating long-range outcomes and for building or revising comprehensive surgical programs. Finally, the categories of threat to children — real, imagined, or potential — can guide clinicians as they struggle to assess and respond to psychological and developmental variables that may impact on ultimate outcomes. Assessing the presence or absence of threats of physical harm, separation, fear of the unknown, and loss of control and autonomy gives focus to care planning. It also can indicate the extent to which a patient is at risk for perioperative and posthospital complications. Knowing the extent of an often primary diagnosis like anxiety can facilitate the timely, focused, and tailored care planning essential in the current context of cost containment, diagnosis related groups (DRGs), and decreasing length of stays.

However, this reviewer had a problem in determining the underlying theory being tested. The investigators discuss and critique at length the studies by Mahaffy (1965) and Skipper et al. (1968) that they intend to partially replicate. The basis for this previous work was a social interaction theory employing an emotional contagion hypothesis. This hypothesis specifies that a parent's emotional state can be transmitted to a young child. If the parent is distraught, he or she will be unable to assist the child to cope with stress. One can readily appreciate, at least intuitively, the types of clinical decisions and practice styles guided by this broad theory. Limiting anxious family members' visits to a new post-myocardial infarction (MI) presents one example of application of the emotional contagion hypothesis. Remaining calm in the face of serious complications and sudden changes in a patient's status presents a second example.

Notwithstanding the commonality of such conditions both for the child and parents, the investigators do not explicitly endorse or state an intention to test their theory. A discussion of this and of possible competing theoretical frameworks would have strengthened their report.

The investigators do state that the theory and process of "deliberative nursing," put forth by Orlando (1961) and Weidenbach (1964), was the basis for the preparation and support provided by the research nurse to the parents and children. This choice seems to rest on a solid psychosocial foundation that fosters a productive therapeutic relationship. It includes providing attention to concerns the family may have, exploring and clarifying feelings, and providing accurate information and appropriate reassurance, especially during the stress points discussed later. Again, one would have liked a brief discussion of other plausible frameworks: Travelbees' existential focus or Roys' adaptation model, for example.

After discussing the threats children may perceive, the investigators detail the stress-point preparation interventions (both nursing and psychological) that are designed to counter the threats. Specifically, the experimental condition was a combination of preparation and supportive care provided at six stress points: at admission, shortly before the blood test, late in the afternoon before the operation, shortly before the administration of the preoperative medication, before transport to the operating room, and upon return from the recovery room. A research nurse provided the patient with information, sensory expectations, role identification, rehearsals, and support before each of the stress points. Providing attention to the mothers' concerns, feelings, and questions, as well as providing them with suggestions on how best to assist their child also was a critical component.

Because such interventions are primary nursing (a single care provider working closely with the family unit), teaching, planning, and supportive roles were underscored. In nursing practice, to assess the potential for utilization of an intervention, we must consider if it is an independent and feasible action a nurse can choose to implement. Concerning the former, energetic and idealistic new nursing graduates may encounter resistance to expanded roles the profession consensually wishes to take responsibility for. Complete freedom to tailor a preoperative teaching plan for an open-heart surgical patient is not always and everywhere an independent nursing function.

The investigators measured the impact of the interventions on four sets of dependent variables/outcome measures. In regard to the children, the investigators examined behavioral variables (manifest upset, cooperation, ease of fluid intake, recovery room medications, and time to first voiding), a physiological variable (pulse rates), and a psychosocial variable (posthospital adjustment). Data on the mothers' experience during the hospitalization was also collected utilizing five instruments: manifest upset and coping/cooperation scales as well as self-ratings of anxiety, satisfaction with care, and adequacy of information received questionnaires. As mentioned earlier, these outcome measures have considerable instrumental value. The variety and breadth of measures also strengthens the confidence we can place in their results. The behavioral ratings would appear to be useful in initial assessment: gathering a data base that would facilitate individualized care planning. The parental scales would be similarly useful. The posthospital adjustment scores could be valuable given the preponderance of research on stages of separation anxiety and, often, the difficulty in re-establishing the mother–child relationship on a basis of trust and intimacy after discharge. Also, it is a useful evaluation tool of the long-term efficacy of the intervention strategies. Finally, the parental measures, particularly satisfaction with care received and adequacy of information, can be seen as proxy measures of consumer satisfaction that can guide future intervention strategies or programs.

Part II: Conceptualization and Internal Consistency

In general, the report expresses cohesion and consistency. The investigators state the commonplace reality of adverse reactions to hospitalization, surgery, and posthospital adjustment experienced by pediatric patients. They provide a brief review of the previous use of psychological preparation and supportive care to mitigate this problem, highlighting what they perceive to be deficiencies in previous research: obscure underlying theory, lack of replication, and problems with the clinical environment. The purposes and hypotheses of this study are stated with concision. Independent variables, operationalized adequately, seem logically related to dependent variables.

Although the investigators can be commended for a well-designed study, there remains one primary concern with the children's behavior rating scales. Although the investigators state that the scales were repeatedly field tested, they also state that interrater agreement was "considered adequate" and that on three scales the interrater agreement was only 60 percent. What was the criteria for adequate agreement and what scales provoked a less than adequate consensus in terms of validity of the measurement tool?

Part III: Believability of Results

The investigators chose 80 children and their mothers and randomly assigned them to two groups: experimental and control. They set the following criteria for selecting the children: (1) English-speaking children between the ages of 3 and 14 with no previous hospitalizations within the past year; (2) children who were free from chronic disease; (3) children who had no medical or psychological condition requiring consultation or special care; and (4) children who were admitted for relatively minor surgery (tonsillectomy, myringotomy, etc.). The rationale for these criteria was not shared, however.

The random assignment resulted in comparable groups of both children and mothers in terms of sex, age, birth order, whether the parent stayed overnight, as well as parental manifest upset and coping/cooperation scales. Repeatedly, the investigators used the term "parent" but made no mention of fathers or other relatives in the background and conceptualization sections of the study.

On the other hand, the investigators took painstaking efforts to assure randomization in group assignments. Specifically, they prevented experimental and control families from occupying adjacent beds. In this way, they prevented the possibility of a control group parent observing a nurse provide a different type of care to a child in the next bed. All families admitted to the study on a given day were assigned to the same room and received the same treatment/nursing regimen.

Control group families did indeed receive a different type of care. The nurses were friendly, courteous, and concerned in their interactions with the parents and children but no formal preparation or systematic attempts to determine their informational and emotional needs was made. In regard to such care, several questions arise. Was this an acceptable standard of care? Would a systematic nursing process approach have contaminated the experimental and control conditions? What about the role of the physician with the study's families? Other than a brief mention of the anesthesiologist, there is not one sentence about attending physicians in the entire report. Did the investigators collaborate with the physicians? If not, can we be sure that some form of psychological preparation was not provided by the physicians to thus jeopardize the reliability of the results?

Nonetheless, the investigators' hypotheses were confirmed. Children in the experimental group were significantly less upset and more cooperative than control children at all stress points. Postoperatively, the children in the experimental group demonstrated "nearly" significantly greater ease of fluid intake, significantly less time to first voiding, significantly lower heart rates after the blood test and before and after preoperative medication, significantly lower incidence of resistance to induction of anesthesia, and significantly better posthospital adjustment scores.

Also as predicted, younger children (aged three to six) demonstrated more upset and less cooperation but did not differ in terms of ease of fluid intake, minutes to first voiding, or posthospital adjustment scores. There were no significant sex differences on outcome measures except heart rates: girls tended to have higher pulses before and after the blood test and preoperative medications.

Finally, parents in the experimental group had significantly lower self-ratings of anxiety, higher ratings of adequacy of information received, and greater satisfaction with care than parents in the control groups.

The following methodological concerns and reservations need to be considered. First, the investigators offer no explanation for the ostensibly contradictory finding that younger children did not differ significantly in terms of ease of fluid intake, minutes to first voiding, or, most surprisingly, posthospital adjustment scores. Second, administration of recovery room medications, a prima facie indicator of upset and coping and an outcome measure, was not reported in the results. Finally, the investigators state that 87 percent of the parents returned the Posthospital Behavior Questionnaire (one would have liked the investigators to have placed this in the appendix of the report). There is no indication of a more concerted effort to contact the other 13 percent. Were those families experiencing adjustment difficulties? If so, the reliability and confidence in this outcome measure is compromised.

Nursing Care of Children 177

The investigators employed three statistical techniques in their report. They used a chi square analysis to determine if there were significant differences in characteristics between the children in the two groups. This choice of technique was appropriate because it enabled the investigators to state with confidence that any subsequent differences in outcomes was not a result of differences between groups. Next, investigators employed a three-way analysis of variance and treatment condition by age and sex. This multifactorial ANOVA is a useful method to answer the crucial question of whether or not the variability in scores from the two groups of children can be attributed to independent variables. Also, it allows the investigators to determine any interactions between treatment and age and between treatment and sex on the outcome variables. Finally, the investigators used a comparison of group means with t-tests to determine if parents and children in the two groups differed on the manifest upset and coping/cooperation scales. They found no significant differences on these variables before the experimental nursing interventions began.

In summary, the investigators' choice of statistical techniques is sufficiently thorough to foster confidence in their findings.

The investigators conclude that their findings strongly support the beneficial effect of systematic preparation and support for hospitalized children and their mothers. Providing accurate information about the events, procedures, sensations, and role expectations, combined with supportive care from a single caregiver, especially at crucial stress points, enables the families to cope more effectively with and adjust to the various stresses encountered. In addition, the investigators correctly caution the reader that the exact causal sequence and dynamics in the above process remains unknown. Indeed, much subsequent research in this area has focused on, for example, locus of control as a key variable in how children cope with stress (LaMontagne, 1987).

In regard to the study's limitations, the investigators are to be commended for an excellent discussion. First, they identify the possibility of observer bias—that the nurse observer witnessed interactions between the experimental nurse and patients which would indicate their group assignment. Frankly acknowledging this possibility and being vigilant may mitigate the probability of bias yet the investigators correctly state that observers should have been uninformed of the purpose of the study and the nature of the experimental conditions.

Second, they identify the possibility of parent bias. The research nurse was more involved with the experimental parents. Perhaps the parents, in wanting to "please" the nurse for his or her extra effort, may have expressed greater inclination to rate themselves more satisfied and less anxious with the care received. Future replication of this study would, as the investigators state, benefit from having a single nurse spend approximately as much time with the control families but without providing the systematic preparation.

Third, the investigators ask whether the positive effects of the experimental conditions resulted from the process and content of the two intervention strategies or from the personality and style of the experimental nurse or both. Replicating the experimental treatment with more than one nurse following the same principles and techniques of psychological preparation and supportive care seems reasonable.

Finally, and regardless of special preparation, could the investigators have obtained positive results because of the warm, trusting relationship of a single nurse present throughout the hospitalization? The investigators raise the possibility that a primary nursing method of care, in and of itself, may have been the crucial variable.

Part IV: Generalizability of Results

Regarding this study, there is one critical reservation: its generalizability. First, the selection criteria used is problematic. Is it reasonable to assume that the accessible population is representative of the current target population of preoperative pediatric inpatients? No. The current reality reveals that hospitals care for a much sicker, complex clientele. Patients are most often admitted for acute exacerbations of existing chronic illnesses or in critical danger. Today, the children selected in this study would be treated on an ambulatory surgery basis. A rhetorical question can underscore this concern. If the proposed intervention strategies are conceptually sound and clinically efficacious, could they impact on a Hispanic child of a welfare-supported teenaged mother with a congenital heart defect admitted for a third open-heart surgery? The ultimate scope of generalizability of Wolfer and Visintainers' work depends on successful replication with a more diverse and "real" clientele.

REFERENCES

LaMontagne, L. L. (1987). Children's preoperative coping: replication and extension. *Nursing Research*, *36*(3), 163–167.

Original article:
Wolfer, J. A., & Visintainer, M. A. (1975). Pediatric surgical patients' and parents' stress responses and adjustment as a function of psychologic preparation and stress-point nursing care. Nursing Research, 24(4), 244–255.

CRITIQUE BY: SHEILA KODADEK, PhD, RN

Part I: Clinical Relevance

Can "psychologic preparation and stress-point nursing care" reduce distress associated with hospitalization and surgery during childhood? This is a clinically relevant question for nurses who care for children and their families in hospitals. Pediatric nurses are concerned with providing care which is not only technically safe, but also sensitive to the psychosocial needs of children at different developmental stages, as well as to the needs of their parents.

Wolfer and Visintainer's study demonstrated that children and parents who received systematic psychologic preparation and supportive care showed less upset behavior and more cooperation in the hospital and fewer posthospital adjustment problems than did children and parents who did not receive this care. In this carefully designed and executed study, the investigators provide information on timing and strategies of care that can guide clinical practice.

The intervention in this study was a combination of psychologic preparation and supportive care provided at six points considered critical during hospitalization: admission, shortly before the routine preoperation blood test, late in the afternoon the day before the operation, shortly before the preoperative medications, before transport to the operating room, and upon return from the recovery room. The determination of critical points came from an examination of clinical practice and research literature. The experimental intervention itself included providing accurate information about events, procedures, sensations, role expectations and appropriate responses, and providing supportive care, including encouragement, reassurance and reinforcement, by a single caregiver at the critical points.

That this intervention is feasible for a nurse in practice is not an accident. Wolfer and Visintainer designed the study with nursing practice in mind. While the research nurse functioned essentially as a clinical specialist in the setting, the investigators intended that the study intervention be such that it could be readily incorporated by the staff nurse in his or her practice. The choice of an intervention as the independent variable within nursing's control is perhaps the best example of this attention to practice.

In summary, this study receives high marks for its attention to direct application in practice, from its conceptualization through design, methods, and conclusions. That the study has direct relevance for nursing practice with children and parents adds further merit to its claims.

Part II: Conceptualization and Internal Consistency

From the introduction to the concluding suggestions for further study, a logical and consistent clarity emerges. Wolfer and Visintainer initiate their text by stating and documenting a pertinent concern: what forms adverse reactions children show in response to hospitalization and surgery, both within the hospital and after they return home? The investigators then reviewed literature about ways nurses and other researchers had addressed the question of mitigating stress related to hospitalization and surgery, and also examined literature about the effect of psychologic preparation and special supportive care in reducing or eliminating adverse reactions. They concluded that a study was needed to address both strengths and limitations of previous studies. Their study purpose and hypothesis, therefore, derived from their stated concerns.

The sample and method used also provide evidence of internal consistency. For example, characteristics of the children in the sample were consistent with the population of concern described in the conceptualization of the study; that is, hospitalized children admitted for elective surgery. The investigators also justified their choices of independent and dependent variables in terms of prior research and their knowledge of clinical nursing practice. The discussion of results explicitly linked study outcomes to initial conceptualization and to practice.

Part III: Believability of Results

This study purported to test a nursing intervention, defined as psychologic preparation and stress point nursing care, with a sample of hospitalized children and their parents. The data collected were primarily quantitative.

The 80 children in the study sample were between the ages of 3 and 14 years, were English speaking, did not have chronic or other serious health problems, and were admitted for elective tonsillectomy, adenoidectomy, myringotomy, polyethylene tubes or herniorrhaphy. The sample characteristics chosen reflect a significant population of pediatric surgery patients in the United States. At the time of the study, this was an appropriate sample on which to test the intervention.

The investigators were aware of the complexity of the variables involved and attempted to address this complexity in the report. For example, if the investigators had daily randomly assigned individual children to experimental and control (routine care) groups, children and parents receiving different nursing interventions could have been in adjacent beds. Interaction between the two groups could give rise to potential distress for families observing different care. An even more likely possibility would be the contamination of the study groups. The investigators addressed this problem by randomly assigning all children to the same study group who were admitted on a given day to the same room. (There were six rooms on the unit and treatment in the rooms was determined randomly each day.) While this was not a perfect solution, it represents an attempt to work within given realities to protect the integrity of the study.

The investigators adequately discussed the reliability and validity of the measures of dependent variables. Where appropriate, they also addressed procedures for assuring reliability. For example, two observational rating scales were used to measure the children's behavior, a manifest upset scale and a cooperation scale. The investigators stated the purpose and described the rating criteria for each scale. They indicated when the nurse observer completed the scales. They stated that all rating scales in the study were field tested repeatedly prior to the study until there was agreement by the investigators and the nurse observer on what types of observable behaviors corresponded to points on the rating scales. In essence, they were defining behavior and rules for assigning ratings to behaviors explicitly, an important issue in observation research.

When the scales were refined and prior to the study, one investigator and the nurse observer made independent simultaneous observations of a sample of children at each of the observation points and compared their ratings. The mean percentage of agreement across all scales was 90 percent, a respectable level of agreement. However, this is deceptive and the investigators report that there were three individual scales where agreement was below 80 percent (60 percent in each case). The investigators accepted this level of agreement as adequate evidence of interrater reliability. It would have been helpful to know the range of agreement across scales and the specific scales in which agreement was lowest. Also, it would have been helpful to know if further training and checks were done to increase agreement on the three scales. By inference it appears that the investigators judged as appropriate the reliabilities they reported. Additional information as described above would have made it possible for the reader to make an informed judgment as well.

It is important to know if the experimental and control groups differed significantly on sample characteristics. Chi square analysis was used to determine if the groups were comparable on characteristic including age, sex, birth-order, whether the parent stayed overnight, and type of surgery. The investigators reported that the groups appeared to be comparable on these variables and provided the chi square statistics in a table. It would have been helpful had they included levels of statistical significance to support their statement that the groups appeared comparable.

In general, the results were clearly and thoroughly reported and were related to the research hypothesis. Tables were provided for inspection of data and, in most cases, sufficient statistical information was provided to understand how the investigators determined statistical significance. In addition, the choices of statistical procedures consistently were appropriate to the data analyzed.

In the discussion and conclusions, the investigators examined the results and their meaning with logical concision. The hypothesis was supported; there appeared to be strong support for the benefits of systematic preparation and support for hospitalized children and their parents. However, the investigators acknowledged that they did not know precisely why the intervention worked, and that there were gaps in the theoretical explanation.

That the investigators did not stop here, but examined explanations for results that competed with what they had hypothesized, adds further merit to their efforts. In addition to raising alternative explanations for why the intervention worked, they also offered suggestions for how future studies might deal with potential problems.

For example, the investigators raised concerns about the potential in the study for observer bias. They described the efforts they had made to ensure that the nurse observer was blind to which children were in the experimental and which were in the control groups. Despite such efforts, they reported that in a few instances the nurse observer did know.

Another concern raised was the possibility that the parents in the experimental group may have been biased positively because of their increased involvement with the research nurse. They may have wanted to please the nurse and consequently rated their experience more satisfactory than it was.

Still another example of a competing explanation offered by the investigators was that the research nurse may have effected an intervention alone. In other words, either characteristics of the particular nurse or the fact that there was a warm, caring relationship with a consistent individual throughout the experience may have been more significant than what the nurse actually did.

Part IV: Generalizability of Findings

Wolfer and Visintainer provided ample information about the setting, routine care, and sample for a nurse reading the study to make decisions about the generalizability of findings. While some specifics may differ, the information suggests that the findings would be generalizable at minimum to children between the ages of 3 and 14 years admitted for elective surgery in urban hospitals with pediatric units.

Of note is an omission which is clinically significant and has implications for generalizability. There is an absence of information about the ethnicity of children and parents in the study and their socioeconomic status. There is some evidence in the literature that these characteristics can make a difference in care perceptions of families.

A legitimate concern may be raised about how the types of surgery chosen for the study and length of hospitalization associated with them translate to care more than a decade later. Today, the trend is for surgeries chosen in this study to be done in a day-surgery setting, with no overnight stay. Where this is not the case, generalizability of the findings would hold. Where this is the case, it would seem that a new study is warranted that would test the intervention in the day-surgery setting. However, clinically it would seem that some of the same child and parent needs for information and support would exist. In fact, perhaps some of the relief at not having to deal with an inpatient hospitalization is mitigated by the responsibility of the parent for postsurgical care.

The research nurse functioned essentially as a clinical nurse specialist in the study setting. Both the research nurse and nurse observer were trained in the specifics of the study relevant to their roles. The report also states that the research nurse, who implemented the intervention, used her clinical judgment and skills in the delivery of the preparation and supportive care. She was not reading from a script; her care was not "canned." While this could be seen as a drawback or a limitation of the study, it can also be seen as a strength. Because the nurse was able to individualize care, the intervention may seem more clinically relevant to the practicing nurse who would find a script unacceptable.

In summary, the investigators specify that what the research nurse did could be done by staff nurses who have clinical expertise in the nursing of children and their parents.

Part V: Other Factors to Consider in Utilization

Wolfer and Visintainer's study builds explicitly on prior research. They described relevant studies and stated how their study was compatible to this previous work. Such compatibility enhances the confidence one can have in using this research in practice.

Given the evidence presented in this study report and the clinical and research base on which it rests, it would appear that the real risk would be in *not* modifying practice based on the study results. The costs are few, risks fewer, and benefits substantial.

Coping Strategies of Hospitalized School-Age Children

Marilyn Savedra, DNS, RN
Assistant Professor
School of Nursing
University of California
San Francisco, CA

Mary Tesler, MS, RN
Associate Clinical Professor
School of Nursing
University of California
San Francisco, CA

To effectively plan and implement care nurses need to know the variety of coping behaviors used by hospitalized children. Little research has documented the strategies used by the hospitalized school-age child to deal with the stresses of the experience. This study sought to answer two questions: 1) what strategies does the six to 12 year old child hospitalized for surgery use to cope with the experience; and 2) can parents provide the information on admission that will predict the strategies the child will use?

REVIEW OF LITERATURE

Coping has been defined differently by various authors. Murphy (1962, 1976) and associates who have made the most significant contribution to the knowledge of coping in children, use a broad definition that includes the concepts of mastery and response to stress. Murphy describes coping as a process, "a matter of strategy, of flexible management of different devices for dealing with challenges from the environment" (1962:273). "Both methods of managing of the environment, and devices and mechanisms for managing tension aroused by the stimulus or likely to result from a given response to it, are often involved" (1962:274).

Lazarus and Launier's (1978) definition of coping is compatible with that of Murphy. Coping is explained as an individual's efforts both action-oriented and intrapsychic, to manage environmental and internal demands. White sees coping along with defenses and mastery as components of adaptation which includes three simultaneous factors: "securing adequate information, maintaining satisfactory internal conditions, and keeping up some degree of autonomy" (1974:58). All of these components directly or indirectly identify information-seeking and maintaining autonomy as components of the coping process.

Individual children use different devices in different sequences and timing when faced with specific problems. The assessment of children's coping behaviors was facilitated by Rose (1972) who operationalized Murphy's definition of coping as a process and described categories for coding observational data. The categories were based on definitions of behaviors as levels of involvement in the coping process and included: inactive; pre-coping or orienting; active coping that included cooperation; resisting; and attempts to control.

She studied the effects of hospitalization on the behavior of 14 children from one and a half to seven years of age admitted for surgery or cardiac catheterization. She hypothesized that (1) children would temporarily change their coping behavior while hospitalized and return to pre-hospital patterns after discharge and that 2) those who did not return to pre-hospital patterns would either have had more stress or less capacity to adapt to change or a combination of both. Using naturalistic observation she studied the children's behavior in the home two weeks and again at one week prior to admission, twice daily in the hospital, and in the home two and four weeks after discharge. Findings showed that while in the hospital all children increased in precoping behaviors, the magnitude varied for each child; they moved less frequently to active coping. Conversational and private speech and emotionality were reduced. Following discharge, 13 out of 14 children reverted to their pre-hospitalization behavior or changed in a positive direction. The usual categories of disruptions—disturbances in sleep behavior, temper, independence—were reported for 25 percent; however, another 25 percent reported inprovement in sleep and independence behaviors. The author cautions interpretations of these findings in view of the small sample size and urges further study.

Two researchers (Bishop, 1976; Stewart, 1978) both utilizing Rose's (1972) protocol, studied two different groups of children. Bishop adapted Rose's protocol to direct coding and examined 19 children two to five years old, half of whom had had corrective cleft palate and lip repairs and were being evaluated for speech or dental problems. The others were normal controls. Children were observed four times in their homes and no differences were observed between the two groups. Children were more frequently assessed as using pre-coping or attempting to control behaviors. Both groups showed more positive emotionality and were more verbal than non-verbal.

Stewart (1978) used the Bishop (1976) direct coding adaptation and studied the coping behaviors of 11 children between two and seven years hospitalized for medical conditions. She assessed how the coping behaviors were affected by three environmental factors during hospitalization: the occurrence of interactions including treatments and nontreatments; the presence of an interactor usually the parent or health personnel; and the presence of peripheral people in the environment. Findings indicated that when the parent was present, pre-coping behaviors decreased and resistive and cooperating behaviors increased. When the health professional was with the child, there were more pre-coping behaviors and fewer attempts to control than when the parent was with the child. In comparing children during treatment vs. non-treatment, there were more attempts to control during non-treatment and more cooperating behavior during treatment.

Research on parents' ability to describe or predict their child's behavior in specific situations is scarce. The studies that do exist focus on the use of parent descriptions of behavior for development or use of diagnostic check lists (Becker 1960; Sines et al. 1959; Dreger et al. 1964). Thomas et al. (1963) used parental descriptions to assess normal behaviors in their longitudinal study of children's behaviors. They found that the assessments of a child's behavior in the home by trained observers correlated closely to the report by parents.

DESIGN OF THE STUDY

An exploratory design was used to answer the study questions. Data were collected over a seven month period by direct observation of the child, parent questionnaire, and parent interview. The protocol was approved by the Committee on Human Research of the University of California, San Francisco. Parents and children consented to participate in the study and were assured of anonymity.

Sample

The subjects were 33 children, 18 boys and 15 girls six to 12 years of age, admitted to Moffitt Hospital, University of California, San Francisco for elective surgical procedures and accompanied by one or both parents. The names of the children were obtained from the pediatric surgical schedule. All were enrolled in age-appropriate grades in school and assessed by parents to be functioning well despite the medical problem. The sample included 21 children six to nine years old and 12 who were ten to 12 years old. Twenty of the children were hospitalized for four days or less, the majority (N = 13) having eye, ear, nose, or throat surgery. Thirteen children were hospitalized from four to 19 days, with the largest number (N = 6) having renal constructive surgery, and the next largest number (N = 4) having heart surgery.

Six children had no previous hospitalization;

six had been hospitalized six or more times; 15 had been hospitalized within the previous year; and three had no hospitalizations since infancy. Seventeen had previously been hospitalized at the study site. The pattern of parent presence during hospitalization varied. Ten parents lived in, ten visited all day until bedtime, eight visited the majority of the day, and four made daily visits.

Observation of the Children

The direct coding adaptation of the Rose (1972) protocol was used for recording the children's behaviors. Three categories of data were collected: 1) level of involvement in the process of coping, 2) communication style, and 3) emotions. (See Table I.) Notations were made that described

Table 1
Definitions of Levels of Involvement in the Coping Process

INACTIVE	Subject is silent and non-participating in any way, sitting, or lying motionless or nearly so. This includes vacant staring, blank facial expression, and apathy.		doing something to him. Accepts, agrees with, compliments, returns in kind, rewards, thanks, congratulates.
		Resists	Person may resist by withdrawing, by leaving or leaning or stepping or turning away. Implies he is leaving situation because it is undesirable.
PRE-COPING or ORIENTING	Pre-Coping or orienting behavior refers to the process by which a person familiarizes himself with the environment. The behavior may be non-verbal and non-mobile, such as looking and listening for information; mobile, such as manipulating and exploring; verbal, such as asking questions; or combinations of these activities.		
		Suspends	Person avoids situation. Physically or verbally circumventing problem by sensory withdrawal or by accepting or rejecting the resource conditionally or tentatively.
		Ignores	Does not respond to requests, offers or resources. Continues current activity ignoring person who is attempting interaction. Action seems deliberate rather than because stimulus is not perceived.
ACTIVE COPING	Processes by which a person deals with threatening, frustrating or challenging situations by:		
Attempts to Control	Offers, expresses, suggests, gives. This may be verbal such as "You could do it this way," or non-verbal such as holding out food or toy for someone to take if he wishes to. Acts autonomously. This involves action which has not been suggested or directed by another.		
		Negates	Rejects, denies, disagrees with another person. Active response. May reject by saying "No," shaking head or by pushing hand or object away.
		Attack	Attempted or actual physical attack, such as hitting, kicking, biting or verbal attack such as screaming, cursing, "bawling out."
Cooperates	Complies, allows, or accepts. Offers no resistance to someone		

Rose, 1972 (Operational definitions revised by Rose for WICHIE Study, 1977.)

the child's appearance, the environment, and what was happening during the observation.

Observations of the children were done by three research assistants, graduate nursing students specializing in pediatrics. They were trained by first observing and recording a videotape of children's play, then observing and recording children's behavior on the pediatric unit. Interrater reliability was calculated at the beginning and midway through the study using the Heinicke formula: $\frac{\text{percent agree}}{\text{percent agree + disagree}}$ (Heinicke, 1956). Reliability was 90 percent and 92 percent for coping behavior, 92 percent and 86 percent for emotions and 96 percent and 90 percent for media of communication.

Observers were as inconspicuous as possible while at the same time changing position as needed to adequately see and hear. Any cues to expose feelings or to encourage communication with the child were avoided. Comments or questions to the observer were ignored or answered by a brief, neutral response, whichever seemed most appropriate. If an emergency arose, the observation was to be terminated and appropriate action taken. No occasion for this arose. The observers found their presence was not disruptive to the ongoing activities. After the first few seconds, the children appeared to ignore the observer. At the completion of each observation, the subject was told it had been completed and questions that had been deferred were answered.

Observations of the children were done at specific stress points based on the work of Wolfer and Visintainer (1975) and at designated times throughout the hospitalization. The observation times were 1) admission (within the first hour of arrival on the pediatric unit), 2) first blood drawing, 3) pre-surgery, 4) four hours after return to the ward from the recovery room, 5) morning and evening of the day following surgery and 6) once a day thereafter, rotating between morning, afternoon and evening. This schedule of observations provided a wide range of behavior sampling that increased content validity of the behavior assessment. Each observation period, with the exception of blood drawing and presurgery observations, was 30 minutes. No attempt was made to assess the environmental stimuli during observation.

Each subject was observed for ten seconds followed by a ten-second period for recording. A one-minute break was scheduled following each five minutes of observation. Observers used tape recorders with an earpiece which transmitted the time pattern for observing and recording.

DATA FROM PARENTS

Questionnaire

A questionnaire developed by the researchers was administered to parents in the hospital prior to the child's admittance to the pediatric unit. Initially one-hour interviews were conducted with 15 parents of healthy school-age children, using open-ended questions regarding how their children usually behaved in new or stressful situations, and how they dealt with pain and restrictions. From the responses, a multiple choice questionnaire was developed and tested with 28 parents of healthy school-age children and further refined for clarity. The majority of parents had no difficulty selecting an answer describing their child's usual behavior in a given situation. They often stated that if they were describing one of their other children, the answers would be different.

Four questions were designed to assess the child's response to new situations and people or to potentially frightening experiences which were expected to predict responses during the pre-surgery period when the child was faced with the most new experiences. A sample question was:
Sample Question

How does X act when he/she meets someone for the first time?

1. Is reserved and holds back and doesn't warm up.
2. Needs a warm-up period to watch and listen before he can begin to relate.
3. Responds to their cues from the beginning.
4. Spontaneously initiates interactions with the person.

Ten questions attempted to elicit responses to pain, anger, boredom, frustration, that were considered more common to post surgery experiences. A sample question was:

Sample Question
How does X behave when he/she is moderately to acutely ill and/or not feeling well?

1. Does what is prescribed.
2. Resists the suggestion, becomes harder to manage.
3. Demands extra attention.
4. Just becomes listless and lies quietly around doing nothing.

Each item on the parent questionnaire was coded to correspond with the categories of the Rose protocol. Six pediatric nursing experts participated in the coding, achieving a 92 percent inter-rater reliability (Heinicke, 1956).

Interviews. The parents were interviewed shortly before leaving the hospital or by phone when the discharge occurred too rapidly for the interviewer to make contact. In four instances when phone contact with the parent was impossible, an interview guide was mailed to the parent. The primary purpose was to determine if the behavior exhibited by the child was what had been expected by the parent. The intent was to provide a reliability check on the parent questionnaire. Additional information was obtained about the parents' assessment of the hospitalization.

RESULTS AND DISCUSSION

The results of the study are reported in two parts. The first presents findings related to the descriptions and statistical analysis of the children's coping strategies, emotional expression, and communication style. The second section reports the findings on the relationship between the coping approaches identified by the parent questionnaire and the child's observed behavior in the hospital. Data submitted for analysis consisted of a minimum of six separate observations per child totaling 1,093 five-minute intervals and the answers to 18 questions on the parent questionnaire.

Level of Involvement in the Coping Process

The level of involvement in the coping process was determined by adding the number of ten-second incidences of behavior for each five-minute interval and for the total observation period. When the majority of the behaviors fell into a given category such as inactive, pre-coping, attempts to control, resists or cooperates, that category of behavior was designated as the dominant coping style for the five-minute interval. The dominant behavior for the total observation period was based on behavior in the five-minute intervals. When the highest number of observations fell equally within two strategies, the style was designated as mixed. This identified the pattern of coping strategies as well as identifying the dominant strategy for each observation.

A tally of the dominant coping style of the subjects indicated that although behaviors fell across three or four categories in each observation period, there was a dominant pattern of response for all periods except admission and blood drawing. (See Table II.) The predominant coping style for the pre-surgery period was compared with the post-surgery period. Nineteen children used pre-coping and 11 used attempts to control behaviors pre-surgery. All of the children used attempts to control behaviors post-surgery except one, who was inactive.

Chi square analysis for independence (Issac and Michael, 1972) for age (6-9, 10-12), grade in school, ordinal position, parents' socio-economic status, parents' education, previous hospitalization, and amount of time parent was present and length of hospitalization revealed no statistically significant patterns in coping strategies. Chi square analysis of the pre-surgery behavior indicated a statistically significant difference between coping behaviors of boys and girls ($P < .01$, $x^2 = 7.35$, 1 degree of freedom). Boys used attempts to control, and girls, pre-coping behaviors.

Patterns of Coping Strategies Used

Though a predominant coping style characterized all but the admission and blood-drawing procedures such a summary does not truly reflect

Table 2
Frequency of Five-Minute Behavior Segments by Level of Involvement for each Observation Period

Observation	Inactive	Pre-coping	Active Coping			
			Cooperates	Control	Resists	Mixed
Pre-Surgery						
Admission	0	72	23	87	0	7
Blood Drawing	0	6	13	9	1	4
Pre-Op	7	60	6	19	1	6
Post-Surgery						
1st 4 hrs. post-surg.	20	11	5	90	0	4
Subsequent post-surg.	37	57	25	506	3	14
TOTAL	64	206	72	711	5	35

the dynamic nature of children's coping approaches. Of the 1,093 five-minute intervals of observations only 233 were characterized by a single coping strategy. During 355 intervals children used two approaches, and 349 included three levels of coping during a single five-minute interval. The remainder included a panorama of four and five strategies during the five-minute interval. Eleven children, on the other hand, demonstrated a remarkable consistency in their coping; they used only two strategies for at least 70 percent of their total five-minute intervals.

Attempts to control behaviors accounted for 711 five-minute intervals, more than three times as many as for pre-coping (N = 206), the next most common approach. Resistive behavior was infrequent and short-lived. Although there were 215 ten-second assessments of resistive behavior recorded, only five of the five-minute intervals were assessed as resisting. Only one total observation, during blood drawing, was recorded as resisting.

Cooperative and inactive behaviors were more common and occurred with almost equal frequency when measured by five-minute intervals. They occurred, however, at different times during the hospitalization. Cooperative behavior was more common before surgery. Forty-two of the 72 five-minute intervals occurred during the three pre-operative periods, most during admission and blood drawing. Inactive behavior on the other hand was seen almost exclusively post-surgery, 57 of the 64 five-minute intervals occurred either during the first post-operative observation or during the subsequent days. A comparison of the ten-second distribution of these behaviors reveals quite a different picture since there were 977 assessed ten-second recordings of inactive behaviors and slightly more than 200 of cooperative behaviors. Inactive behavior, though fleeting, was interspersed throughout the hospitalization of all the children with the exception of 10, all of whom had short hospitalizations.

Children's Emotions

The emotional score was determined by assigning a numerical value to each category of emotion, very positive +2, moderately positive +1, neutral 0, moderately negative -1, and negative -2. All children demonstrated neutral emotions during the hospitalization with slight tendencies toward moderately positive or negative. Over half the children showed negative emotion during blood-drawing and the predominant emotion post-surgery was moderately negative. There were 30 five-minute moderately negative intervals and eight children had one or more ten-second episodes of very negative emotion. The emotional tone, however, was not as flat as this indicates.

Children demonstrated transient episodes of different emotions within a five-minute interval. Twenty-eight children demonstrated three levels of emotion within a five-minute interval and one showed four levels.

Children's Communication Media

The communication behavior was overwhelmingly non-verbal. Eight of the 33 children used no dominant communication pattern other than nonverbal with 25 showing one or more verbal or mixed five-minute time intervals. One child stood out with 20 five-minute intervals of verbal behavior and six of mixed. The next highest was seven episodes. Crying was not frequent and when it did occur, it was for relatively brief periods as children quickly brought their crying under control.

Only five of the 33 children showed a predominantly crying communication media for a five-minute time interval, with three children having one interval each and two children two intervals. The crying was, with one exception, during blood-drawing or pre-surgery. However, a more accurate portrait of children's crying is evidenced by the number of 10-second episodes of crying; there was 201 ten-second observations involving 22 children. (See Table III.)

Parents' Responses to the Questionnaire

Parent questionnaire responses were not predictive of the children's demonstrated emotions or communication patterns. The majority of the parents (N = 29, 88 percent) assessed their child's outlook on life as very or moderately positive. This correlated negatively with the neutral emotions of all of the children during hospitalization. Thirty-one (94 percent) of the parents assessed the child as predominantly verbal but the dominant communication pattern for all children was nonverbal. Parents were more accurate in their prediction of their child's crying pattern. Most parents (N = 23, 70 percent) said their child cried occasionally and nine parents (28 percent) said their child cried rarely. This proved to be so. Of the nine children reported to cry rarely, four did

Table 3
Frequency of Behavior Segments Children's Predominant Communication Media During Specific Procedures*

	Communication Media			
Observation	Verbal	Non-Verbal	Crying	Mixed
Pre-Surgery				
Admission	14*	175	0	0
Blood drawing	9	21	2	1
Pre-Operative	11	79	5	4
Post-Surgery				
1st 4 hours post	2	127	1	0
All subsequent post-surgery	34	603	0	5
TOTAL	70	1005	8	10

*Numbers refer to five-minute intervals.

not cry at all, and five had a total of 35 ten-second episodes of crying.

Information supplied by parents was more predictive of the children's behaviors in the periods before surgery than it was for the periods after surgery. Parent answers to questions 4-7 identifying their child's usual responses to new or stressful situations were compared with the child's coping behaviors before surgery. Sixty-six percent of the total parent responses indicated pre-coping as the usual behavior and 55 percent of the children demonstrated pre-coping before surgery. Comparison of the individual parents' response with their own child's behavior revealed that for the 19 children whose dominant style was pre-coping, one set of parents identified 100 percent, 11 parents 75 percent, and five parents 50 percent pre-coping responses. Information supplied by parents was not predictive of the attempts to control behavior manifested by 13 children before surgery. While 25 percent (N = 8) of the children demonstrated attempts to control behaviors before surgery only one parent gave two of the possible four responses as control.

Parent answers to questions 8-18 identifying their child's usual response to frustration, pain and boredom were compared with the child's coping behaviors following surgery. Of the total responses (N = 320) to questions 8-18, the largest number (N = 16, 49 percent), were reported as attempts to control behavior post-surgery. Twenty parents (62 percent) identified attempts to control as the dominant style for their child and three parents (9 percent) identified a mixed coping style which included control. Twelve of the 20 parents gave attempts to control behaviors as the usual behavior to all questions in this part of the questionnaire. Nine (75 percent) of their children manifested attempts to control as the dominant style throughout hospitalization.

The parent interview revealed that 24 of the 28 parents interviewed (85 percent) said their child had behaved as they had expected. Two felt their child had behaved differently than expected and two responded "yes and no."

CONCLUSIONS

Based on findings of the study, coping strategies were identified for a group of school-age children during hospitalization. Information supplied by parents regarding the coping strategies used in daily living experiences were more predictive of the pre-surgery than the post-surgery behaviors. Information regarding communication style and emotional response was not predictive.

The children's predominant behavior before surgery was pre-coping or orienting, demonstrating the need for nursing interventions that enable the child to get the information he needs to carry out the patient role. The finding that all children, except one, demonstrated attempting to control behaviors post-surgery and that more than one-third demonstrated this behavior prior to surgery has significance for planning care. Attempting to control, while sometimes viewed by health professionals as manipulative or resistive and thus thwarting-type behavior, is the healthy response of a child who is carefully working at regulating the amount of adaptation to be made in a compromised position. For this age group, efforts at control are age-appropriate, autonomous behaviors that need to be supported and encouraged. The child who does not attempt to control and thus regulate the tremendous input of stimuli patients have to face, or the excessive demands made on the child in the short time of hospitalization, is not using energies in the best manner. This presents a special concern for nursing care. Is the child overwhelmed by the excessive stimuli and thus disengaged emotionally from the environment, thus becoming at risk for missing important messages? Is the child too sick and are all energies diverted to physical recovery? Either requires nursing surveillance and action.

The pre-surgery period showed a wider range of coping behaviors for the group as a whole than did the post surgery period. It would seem to indicate a need for skilled nursing to assess, accurately interpret behavior, and respond with appropriate actions at this time. No statistically significant difference was found pre-surgery between the coping strategies of children who had previously been hospitalized and those who had not. It raises the question of whether coping strategies are the same regardless of whether the threat is known or unknown.

That the school-age children demonstrated very little resistive behavior was not surprising. Most children this age are expected to obey and have had considerable socialization in that aspect. The decreased amount of cooperative behavior, with the exception of the blood-drawing, poses another interesting question. How many post-operative nursing interventions are designed to encourage patient cooperation, or is it easier and more efficient to go in and do a procedure or carry out a treatment on the child without eliciting cooperation? The reduced incidence of crying was also an age-appropriate finding, but one that needs special attention when it occurs, for it can mean a loss of self-esteem that might cause the child concern.

The diminished amount of verbalization was an unexpected finding for this age. It was not predicted by parents who predominantly identified their children as highly verbal. What part does hospitalization play in a school-age child's lack of verbalization? Is the child too frightened to speak...to find out? Does the child lack the vocabulary to ask appropriate questions? Or do the routines and procedures not provide the opportunity to verbalize? The study by Klinzing et al., (1977) reported a lack of verbalizing by nurses, doctors and others coming into contact with children. What role does this play in a child's non-verbalizing? How do you talk to someone who doesn't talk to you?

Parents describe their children's typical emotional status as predominantly positive. However, during the hospital experience, the child's characteristic emotional state was observed as neutral. This finding suggests an alteration in the usual emotional state as a result of hospitalization or a difference in criteria used by parents and study observers.

Findings are informative and support the previously described Rose, Bishop and Stewart studies of decreased resistive behavior, decreased verbalization, decreased crying and increased orienting and attempts to control behaviors. The sample is too small to make sex and age-specific predictions. More observations of same and different age children are needed. Since pre-surgery observations reveal the widest variability of behaviors, this period should be studied in greater detail to achieve more definitive data. Further work is required to refine the questionnaire and to establish reliability and validity. Since 95 percent of the children post-surgery showed controlling behavior, it may be that the primary value of such research would be in relation to estimations of pre-surgery behavioral status of children. Further study on outcomes of the surgery related to coping style is also needed.

REFERENCES

Becker, W. (1960). The relationship of factors in parental ratings of self, and each other to the behavior of kindergarten children as rated by mothers, fathers and teacher. *Journal of Consulting Psychology*, 24(6), 507–527.

Bishop, M. (1976). Coping behaviors of children born with a cleft lip and palate. Unpublished master's thesis, Arizona State University, Tempe, AZ.

Dreger, R. N., et al. (1964). Behavior classification project. *Journal of Consulting Psychology*, 28, 1–13.

Heinicke, C. M. (1956). Some effects of separating two-year-olds from their parents. *Human Relations*, 9, 105–176.

Klinzing, D., & Schindler, P. (1967). A preliminary report of a methodology to assess the communicative interaction between hospital personnel and hospitalized children. *American Journal of Public Health*, 67(7), 670–672.

Lazarus, R. S., & Launier, R. (1978). Stress-related transactions between person and environment. In L. A. Perviss & M. Lewis (Eds.), *Perspectives in Interactional Psychology*. New York: Plenum.

Murphy, L. B. (1962). *The widening world of childhood*. New York: Basic Books.

Murphy, L. B., & Moriarty, A. (1976). *Vulnerability, coping and growth: From infancy to adolescence*. New Haven: Yale University Press.

Issac, S., & Michael, W. (1972). *Handbook in research and evaluation*. San Diego: Robert Knopf.

Rose, M. H. (1972). The effects of hospitalization on coping behaviors of children. Unpublished doctoral dissertation, University of Chicago, Chicago.

Sines, J. O., et al. (1969). Identification of clinically relevant dimensions of children's behavior. *Journal of Consulting and Clinical Psychology*, 33, 728–734.

Stewart, C. (1978). A study of coping behaviors of hospitalized children as affected by environmental factors. Unpublished master's thesis, University of Washington, Seattle, WA.

Thomas, A., Chess, S., Birch, H., & Hertzing, M. (1963). *Behavioral individuality in early childhood*. New York: University Press.

White, R. (1970). Strategies of adaptation: An attempt at systematic description. In G. Coelho, D. Hamburg, & J. Adams (Eds.), *Coping and Adaptation*. New York: Basic Books.

Wolfer, J., & Visintainer, M. (1975). Pediatric surgical patients' and parents' stress responses and adjustment. *Nursing Research*, 24, 224–255.

This article is printed with permission of *Western Journal of Nursing Research*. Copyright 1981 Sage Publications, Inc.

Original article:
Savedra, M., & Tesler, M. (1981). Coping strategies of hospitalized school-age children. *Western Journal of Nursing Research, 3*(4), 371-384.

CRITIQUE BY: CHARLYN WILSON, BSN, BA, RN

Part I: Clinical Relevance

The research described in this paper examined methods of coping used by school-age children hospitalized for surgical procedures. It is of interest for its potential to tell more about what to expect from children I work with in the hospital.

Savedra and Tesler's study may help focus my observations of children's coping to assess whether their behaviors are situation-appropriate and constructive, or indicative of problems. The study also looked for predictors of behavior based on reports by parents. As an exploratory study, it did not generate, develop or test a theory, proposition, or intervention. However, utilization of this study may be possible. The concept of coping is explored in the literature review and the section, "Definitions of Levels of Involvement in the Coping Process," also proves useful for assessing and categorizing children's behaviors in practice.

Part II: Conceptualization and Internal Consistency

The study is sensibly written and provides the information outlined in the introduction. Because little research has been done in this area, the investigators claim immediate justification for the study. They address study questions to fit them with their conceptualization as explored in the literature review. They base operational definitions of levels of coping on past work in this area (Rose, 1972) and appropriately use an exploratory, observational design. Subjects were drawn from the population of interest; a subset of hospitalized school-age children.

The instruments used seem relevant and likely to provide the kind of information sought. Coding categories for observations of the children have precedent in the literature; however, the investigators designed the parent questionnaire and interviewed specifically for the study. Data collection procedures, as described, seem nonintrusive. In this regard, the investigators state that observers were ignored by the children "after a few seconds." However, the presence of an unfamiliar adult could have affected a child's behavior. The parent questionnaire and interview took some time for the parents as well, but presumably that was expected from the study description during recruitment of subjects.

Conclusions drawn from the research are relevant to the study questions and follow logically from the reported results. In general, the study is cohesive; the research questions are addressed in an appropriate manner; and the conclusions flow logically from the findings answering the study questions.

Part III: Believability of Results

This study purported to describe coping behaviors of hospitalized school-age children. The investigators collected qualitative data, although they did use some quantitative analysis.

The subjects consisted of 33 children ages 6 to 12 years admitted to a university hospital for elective surgery. In regard to this convenience sample, eligibility criteria are clear, although the selection procedure is not. The investigators describe the age distribution, length of hospitalization, category of surgery, previous hospitalization experience, and extent of parental presence during hospitalization to demonstrate the range of subjects' characteristics. However, the investigators do not specify what the children and parents were told or asked to gain their participation in the study, nor why there were only 33 subjects over the seven months of data collection. Therefore, those who agreed to participate might not be truly representative of the population. I would be interested in how many and for what reason parents turned down participation in the study.

For the behavioral observations, the definitions of levels of coping and the direct coding followed the Rose (1972) protocol. The study design, focussing on six stress points during hospitalization, is "based on the work of Wolfer and Visintainer (1975)." Sufficient information is provided regarding the work of these authors to assume adequate reliability and validity for this study. The investigators describe no changes in coding procedure required during data collection or analysis.

The investigators describe the observation process in detail, presenting a picture that is almost clear enough to duplicate. Assessment of interrater reliability between the three observing research assistants is outlined; reliability is confirmed. The investigators describe the development of the parent questionnaire and give examples of its content but state that "further work is required to refine the questionnaire and to establish reliability and validity."

The study methods used seem appropriate to the study questions. Reporting of results for the observations and parent questionnaire also appears thorough. The purpose of the parent interview is given, but description of the interview content and format is without detail. The interview results make up only a small paragraph, causing one to wonder if this aspect of the study turned out to be inconclusive or of diminished importance.

The investigators do not directly address potential biases. A chi square statistical analysis, which I assume was appropriate, showed that demographic and certain other potentially intervening variables had no statistical significance. The investigators also report that notations were made regarding the environment during observations of the children, but "no attempt was made to assess the environmental stimuli during observation" of each child. In this respect, there is high probability that the environment could have affected behavior. There is no mention of potential biases or intervening variables for the parent questionnaire or interviews.

The categories of coping as described and observed seem comprehensive and specific enough for this sample. Concepts related to children's emotions and communication media also were utilized. However, results related to the concepts may have been limited by the sample. If the study had included longer term, nonsurgical, emergency care or chronically ill patients, other coping mechanisms, and perhaps other concepts, might have emerged. With a broader sample, the investigators would have explored more fully the range of coping of hospitalized school-age children.

In the conclusion section, the investigators offer explanations for both the expected and unexpected results. Certain findings were not surprising, correlating with the socialization and developmental level of this age group. The investigators also raise thoughtful questions regarding unexpected findings, challenging nurses to more specific assessment and exploration of these issues.

The investigators discerned patterns of behavior distinct in the children subjects. The investigators also acknowledge "the dynamic nature of children's coping approaches" and "transient episodes of different emotions" demonstrated by children in brief intervals.

The investigators conclude that their work supports previous studies. However, they also conclude that their sample was too small to make certain predictions. They suggest further work in areas of presurgery behavior, questionnaire reliability and validity, and the relationship of coping style to surgical outcome.

Although there are unanswered questions regarding this study, the methodology seems sound and relevant to the study questions. The results are preliminary but useful and suggest further study.

Part IV: Generalizability of Results

The sample reflects a subgroup of the population in my setting, and does allow generalizability to that group and, perhaps, a broader group of that same age. I imagine that a duplicate study done in my setting would produce similar results; I have worked with hospitalized children like those in the study and have observed similar behaviors.

The individuals doing the observations were not typical of practicing nurses, however; they were "graduate nursing students specializing in pediatrics" and with specific training for this study. The investigators did not specify who enlisted the subjects, or who presented the questionnaire or interviewed parents. Undoubtedly, it was not a practicing nurse in that setting.

I have read other studies (e.g., Vipperman, & Rager, 1980) discussing coping of hospitalized children. However, those studies did not research the area as the present study did.

Although the present study offers no specific interventions or techniques for use in practice, it is useful in increasing nurses' awareness and assisting in assessment of patient behaviors.

Part V: Other Factors to Consider in Utilization

In their conclusion, the investigators describe a need for assessment, accurate interpretation of, and appropriate responses to children's varying coping behaviors. With an increased awareness that "attempting to control" behavior can become a constructive coping mechanism for this age group, nurses might be more accepting and tolerant of demanding and resistive behavior.

The benefits of this increased awareness overcome the risks. Utilization costs might only consist of the time needed for further exploration in the area of hospitalized children's coping behaviors, and, perhaps, the time to present this information in an inservice colloquium for other nurses.

In general, then, this report is conceptually useful for its categorization of coping behaviors. It increased my awareness and assessment focus. It also stimulated my interest in further exploration of hospitalized children's coping mechanisms and of nurse–child interactions.

Part VI: Additional Comments

During my evaluation of this article, I happened upon its companion article published in *Pediatric Nursing* (Tesler & Savedra, 1981). The companion article is more clinically relevant, expanding greatly on nursing implications. It includes a table with a section for each category of coping, describing the behaviors, appropriate nursing actions, and desired outcomes for each. Although this clinical article is more useful to my practice, it was interesting to compare how the same research can be written in both a research-oriented and a clinical manner.

As with previous critiques of other studies, and by the very nature of critiquing itself, I read the present study and evaluation questions with greater awareness and interest. I then distanced myself from it to reflect on its strengths and weaknesses. Certainly, an initial reading of a study provides a less clear or certain impression than that gained after repeated readings and focused evaluation.

In this process, I always remind myself that what I am actually evaluating is the report. Weaknesses and strengths of the report might not accurately reflect the quality of the research itself.

REFERENCES

Rose, M. H. (1972). *The effects of hospitalization on coping behaviors of children.* Unpublished doctoral dissertation, University of Chicago, Chicago.

Tesler, M., & Savedra, M. (1981). Coping with hospitalization: A study of school-age children. *Pediatric Nursing*, 7(2), 35–38.

Vipperman, J. F., & Rager, P. M. (1980). Childhood coping: How nurses can help. *Pediatric Nursing*, 6(2), 11–18.

Wolfer, J. A., & Visintainer, M. A. (1975). Pediatric surgical patients' and parents' stress responses and adjustment. *Nursing Research*, 24(4), 244–255.

Original article:
Savedra, M., & Tesler, M. (1981). Coping strategies of hospitalized school-age children. *Western Journal of Nursing Research*, 3(4), 371–384.

CRITIQUE BY: SHEILA KODADEK, PhD, RN

Part I: Clinical Relevance

Nurses who work with children in hospitals are faced with the challenge of identifying and interpreting children's coping behaviors. It isn't an overstatement to call this a **challenge: children's** coping behaviors are influenced by a variety of factors including temperament, cognitive and emotional development, prior coping experience, and need for defenses. Assessment can be difficult under the best of circumstances.

Savedra and Tesler addressed the coping strategies of hospitalized school-age children. While an argument can be made that additional information about how children cope with hospitalization is needed for all ages from birth through adolescence, the school-age child in particular has been neglected in the literature. The investigators' first research question, "What strategies does the 6 to 12 year old child hospitalized for surgery use to cope with the experience?" is clinically relevant and addresses a gap in the literature.

The investigators' second research question, "Can parents provide the information on admission that will predict the strategies the child will use?" is significant for nurses who work with children. Again, there is little in the literature to guide nurses in practice. Parents generally are seen as the most valid and reliable forecasters and interpreters of their children's behavior. Nurses frequently turn to parents for help in predicting and interpreting behavior. Information about the value of parents' admission information around their child's coping strategies has obvious benefit for the nurse who is planning and implementing care for a school-age child.

Part II: Conceptualization and Internal Consistency

Attention to consistency, from identification of the problem through discussion of findings and recommendations for future work, is a significant strength of this research report. Savedra and Tesler used clear and concise language to describe first the clinical problem which prompted the study and then the study itself. They used sufficient detail to provide the reader of the report with the information needed to assess the study.

For example, in their first paragraph, the investigators stated the clinical need that formed the impetus and justification for the study. In addition, they anchored their research questions, which they relate to one another, in nursing practice. To effectively plan and implement care, nurses need to know the variety of coping behaviors used by hospitalized children. The justification for the study, then, is that little research is available which documents how hospitalized school-age children deal with stress related to the experience. The two research questions also derive logically from the clinical need and justification.

Further evidence of internal consistency in the study can be found in the literature review, which includes other studies relevant to each of the two research questions. First, the investigators briefly addressed general coping literature and then elaborated on specific, relevant studies of children's coping behavior in hospitals. Second, they examined the few research studies available on parents' ability to predict or describe their child's behavior.

The choice of an exploratory design offers another example of consistency throughout the study. Given the lack of prior research in the area, this was an appropriate choice, and allowed the investigators to ask research questions that would reveal their central interest: how school-age children cope in the hospital. A final example of consistency is the investigators' use of a convenience sample of 33 children between the ages of 6 and 12 years who were admitted for elective surgical procedures. This sample fit the age and hospitalization specifications of the research questions.

Part III: Believability of Results

This study purported to describe a phenomenon of concern to nursing, strategies used by hospitalized school-age children to deal with stresses of the experience. Primarily quantitative data were collected.

The investigators used a convenience sample of 33 children admitted to a university-affiliated hospital in a large urban setting for elective surgery. The children ranged in age from 9 to 12 years, a school-age population. Since age is not necessarily an indicator of cognitive development, the investigators noted that all children were enrolled in age-appropriate grades in school. This suggests at a minimum the absence of significant developmental delays that might alter a child's coping strategies. The investigators further stated that the children were assessed by their parents as functioning well despite the medical problem which brought them to the hospital. This is an important piece of information given the range of surgeries reported, from eye, ear, nose or throat surgery to renal reconstructive and heart surgery.

Characteristics of the sample specifically thought to influence the study results included the age of the child, sex, grade in school, ordinal position, parents' socioeconomic status and education, previous hospitalization, amount of time a parent was present during the hospitalization, and length of hospitalization. Chi square analysis for independence was used to detect statistically significant differences in coping patterns related to these factors. The only statistically significant difference found was between coping behaviors of boys and girls.

The investigators collected data by observation, parent questionnaire, and parent interview. In their observation research, they satisfied concise definitions of the phenomena to be observed and explicit rules for observation, including: when observations should be made, the frequency of observations, and length of observations. The investigators used a research protocol developed by Rose (1972) to record the children's behaviors, which included written definitions of the behaviors to be observed. The investigators collected three categories of data: level of involvement in the coping process, communication style, and emotions. In addition, they included information about the data collection procedure for the observations, including rules about timing of observations.

Observations of children's behavior were made by three research assistants who were also graduate nursing students specializing in pediatrics. Because observations are subject to observer bias, it is important to use strategies to decrease that bias. Therefore, the observers attended to their effect on the children and the strategies used to diminish this effect. The observers then reported that they perceived their presence was not disruptive to ongoing activities, suggesting that this phase of data collection did not interfere with usual practice and thus bias the results.

In regard to observer bias and its effect on subjects, the investigators described the training program they used to prepare the research assistants for the observations. Also, they reported acceptable interobserver reliabilities for the three categories of data: 90 and 92 percent for coping behavior, 92 and 86 percent for emotions, and 96 and 90 percent for media of communication, respectively.

The investigators derived parent questionnaires from one-hour interviews with parents of healthy school-age children. The process of developing and testing the multiple choice questionnaire used in the study is described in sufficient detail to judge the appropriateness of procedure. The items on the parent questionnaire were coded to correspond with the categories of the Rose (1972) protocol. An acceptable 92 percent intercoder reliability was achieved when six pediatric nursing experts participated in the coding.

The parents were interviewed at discharge or shortly after discharge. In essence, parents were asked if the behavior exhibited by the child was what they had expected; the intent was to provide a reliability check on the parent questionnaire. A reliability check like this can strengthen confidence in findings because it provides another source of data for examination.

The investigators reported study results with logical concision, and linked these results explicitly to the research questions. The investigators also included their findings and the analytical procedures they used to determine the findings. They used descriptive statistics, appropriate to the data they gathered.

Savedra and Tesler found that children's predominant behavior before surgery was pre-coping or orienting, and all but one child demonstrated attempting to control behaviors postsurgery. They found resistive behavior infrequent, cooperative behavior more common presurgery, and inactive behavior almost exclusively during postsurgery observations. Communication behavior was predominantly nonverbal. Parent information about coping strategies used in everyday situations was more predictive of presurgery than postsurgery behavior, and was not predictive of emotional response or communication style.

The discussion and conclusions of this study are among its major strengths and are appropriate to the study's design and results. Of particular note is the fact that the investigators analyzed the findings in the light of other research findings *and* clinical practice.

For example, all but one child demonstrated controlling behaviors postsurgery, and more than one-third demonstrated controlling behaviors presurgery. According to the investigators, this finding suggests that efforts at control are age-appropriate behaviors which need support and encouragement. Savedra and Tesler make the observation that in clinical practice controlling behaviors may be misinterpreted as manipulative and, rather than be encouraged, be discouraged. The investigators suggest that, in fact, it may be the child who shows no evidence of controlling behaviors who is maladaptative, and they give clinical reasons why a child may not try to control his or her environment.

This kind of speculation about clinical implications of the findings is consistent throughout the conclusions. It is a rich section and gives indication of the clinical expertise of the investigators.

Part IV: Generalizability of Results

The characteristics of the sample and setting provided by the investigators suggest they would be similar to those found in relatively large pediatric services in urban hospitals. While this limits the generalizability of the results somewhat, the consolidation of pediatric services in similar settings due to demographics and economics make this a reasonable and generalizable study.

Because observers were nurses who were graduate students specializing in pediatric nursing, baccalaureate-prepared, experienced pediatric nurses would constitute a similar group of nurses likely to be found in practice. The observers did receive training in the definitions and identification of coping behavior.

Savedra and Tesler compared their findings to those of Rose (1972), Bishop (1976), and Stewart (1978). The findings among all four studies are similar with regard to children's patterns of coping behavior. This consistency across studies increases confidence in the findings of any one study.

Part V: Other Factors to Consider in Utilization

Because this was an exploratory study, Savedra and Tesler rightly do not prescribe nursing strategies on the basis of their results. However, they do raise clinical and research questions which come from the data and their own clinical experience. And they do provide a richer understanding of how school-age children cope with hospitalization.

Use of this research in practice can mean an increased sensitivity to school-age children's coping behaviors and factors which may or may not affect them. For example, Savedra and Tesler found that in their sample previous hospitalization did not make a difference in presurgery coping strategies. This is a somewhat surprising finding and may not hold up in other samples. However, it is clinically useful if it alerts nurses to the possibility that experience does not necessarily decrease perception of threat.

Use of this research in practice to increase sensitivity to both school-age children's coping strategies and nurses' responses to those strategies is a relatively low-risk venture. The benefits, on the other hand, can be more deliberative: specific observation of children and of staff response. It seems well worth the effort to take what the investigators have found and use it to enhance practice.

REFERENCES

Bishop, M. (1976). *Coping behaviors of children born with a cleft lip and palate*. Unpublished master's thesis, Arizona State University, Tempe, AZ.

Rose, M. H. (1972). *The effects of hospitalization on coping behaviors of children*. Unpublished doctoral dissertation, University of Chicago, Chicago.

Stewart, C. (1978). *A study of coping behaviors of hospitalized children as affected by environmental factors*. Unpublished master's thesis, University of Washington, Seattle, WA.

Altering Children's Distress Behavior During Orthopedic Cast Removal

Jean E. Johnson, PhD
Professor
College of Nursing
Wayne State University
Detroit, MI

Karen T. Kirchhoff
Instructor
College of Nursing
University of Illinois
Chicago, IL

M. Patricia Endress, MN
Research Assistant
Center for Health Research
Wayne State University
Detroit, MI

The hypothesis tested was that discrepancy between expected and experienced physical sensations (what is felt, seen, heard, tasted, and smelled) during a threatening experience will result in distress. The subjects were 84 children, 6 to 11 years of age, male and female. The threatening experience was orthopedic cast removal. Tape recorded preparatory information was used to vary systematically expectations about physical sensations. The children were randomly assigned to one of three information groups: 1) sensory information which described the sensory experience during cast removal, 2) procedure information which described the steps of the experience, 3) control group which heard no tape recorded information. Nonverbal and verbal signs of distress reactions and the pulse rate were observed during cast removal. Signs of distress were scaled from zero to two, with zero meaning no distress behaviors and two, high distress behavior. A two-factor analysis of variance (two levels of pre-fear and three levels of information) was used for analysis. As hypothesized, the mean distress score for the sensation group (.50) differed significantly from the control group mean (1.00, p < .025). The procedure group distress score mean (.71) fell between the sensation and control group means but did not differ significantly from the control group mean. The no pre-fear group distress score mean (.52) was significantly lower than the same pre-fear group mean (1.00, p < .02). Mean pulse rate changes for information groups for before to during cast removal were in the same order as the distress scores, but the differences were not statistically significant. The findings were similar to those from other tests of the hypothesis.

Although the need for theory to guide nursing research and practice is recognized, the primary concern to date has been the *nature* of theory relevant to nursing and not the interaction among theory, research, and practice (e.g., Dickoff and James, 1971; Ellis, 1971; Folta, 1971; Jacox, 1974; Walker, 1971; Wooldridge, 1971). There have been few attempts to use a theoretical framework to guide a program of research on a particular aspect of nursing practice. Often the theoretical frameworks chosen are so general that they do little more than give an orientation to the problem. These general theories do not provide guidance in decision making about empirical aspects of the research such as variables to be included, design of the study, and measurement techniques.

Patients' emotional reactions to events that occur during the health care processes constitute an area of concern which has been conceptualized in several different, broad theoretical terms. These emotional reactions have usually been explained and conceptualized within some model of anxiety and/or stress. The several major conceptualizations of anxiety often imply the existence of pathology or a non-health state. Because the concept of anxiety is nonspecific, the interventions recommended to reduce anxiety have also been nonspecific and have included such interventions as providing emotional support or reassurance.

THEORETICAL FRAMEWORK

During the 1960's, a number of studies supported the notion that nurse–patient interactions designed to meet the patient's emotional needs reduce anxiety (e.g., Dumas and Leonard, 1963; Elms and Leonard, 1966; Johnson, 1966; Mahaffy, 1965). The interaction process in these studies was not specifically defined in terms of content, so that replication of the studies and incorporation into practice was difficult. The study of patients' emotional needs reported in this article was guided by specific, testable psychological theory and operationalized by a direct, controlled, and replicable set of techniques.

There has recently been a proliferation of psychological research on the effects of cognitive processes on behavior. Emotional behavior has been included in this body of research. In an experiment which has become a classic, Schachter and Singer (1962) illustrated that emotional responses can be altered by cognitive processes. Basic to the cognitive view of emotions is the assumption that one's cognitive processes evaluate a stimulus, interpret its meaning, and determine its significance (Lazarus, 1968). Following Schachter and Singer's experiment, numerous studies have shown that cognitive processes can affect subjects' emotional response to threatening stimuli. However, some of the methods which have been used to influence the subjects' cognitive processes have limited utility in health care settings. For example, Nisbett and Schachter (1966) demonstrated that when subjects were led to attribute their physiological arousal to a neutral rather than a threatening source their emotional reaction was reduced. Attribution of cause of emotional response to a neutral source has limited utility in health care settings since the threatening stimuls is often so clearly identifiable that it is unlikely that patients could be convinced that their reactions resulted from some benign stimulus.

A study based on the cognitive dissonance theory (Festinger, 1957) showed that subjects were willing to tolerate strong electric shocks when they were given a free choice to participate and no justification for subjecting themselves to shock (Zimbardo et al., 1966). These notions are not readily applicable to patients. Patients probably would not consent to most unpleasant or threatening procedures without being given a justification for the need for the procedure; and, if persuaded of the need, the patient has little choice other than to consent.

These cognitive methods of influencing patients' emotional response to threatening events are specific, but they are no more helpful to the nurse who attempts to select a method to reduce patients' emotional response than the nonspecific methods of support and reassurance. There is a need for a specific method of influencing emotional response to threatening events that is applicable to various health care situations.

INVESTIGATIONS OF THREATENING EVENTS

Johnson (1973) hypothesized that the intensity of a response that reflects emotion during a threatening event may be a function of incongruency between expected and experienced sensations. The greater the incongruency the more intense the emotional response. The hypothesis was tested in two laboratory experiments with ischemic pain in the arm as the threatening event. Groups of subjects were given different types of preparatory information. As hypothesized, subjects who were given preparatory information which accurately described the sensations showed the lowest emotional response to the painful stimulus. A third experiment specifically examined the subjects' expectations about the sensations they would experience while a sphygmomanometer cuff was in place. It was found that a description of sensations given to the subject before the experience reduced inaccurate expectations about sensations to be experienced more than it affected accurate expectations. Subjects who were told to expect specifically described typical sensations judged atypical sensations as being less likely to occur than did subjects who were not given information about typical sensations. This finding suggested that a stronger basis for the emotional response to a threatening stimulus might be the expectation of atypical sensations rather than the expectation of typical sensations. If this is true, the subject who expects both typical and atypical sensations may evaluate a stimulus as being more threatening than the subject who expects only typical sensations.

To test the notion that expecting the occurrence of atypical sensations is the factor which effects emotional response, another laboratory experiment was conducted. Again ischemic pain was used as the threatening stimulus (Johnson and Rice, 1974). Preparatory information differed in the degree of accurateness and completeness of the description of sensations typically experienced. Four types of preparatory messages were used. Each subject heard one of the following types of messages: 1) a description of all five typical sensations, 2) a description of only two typical sensations, 3) a description of two atypical sensations, and 4) a procedural description with no sensory information. Description of only two typical sensations was found to be as effective in reducing emotional response as description of all five typical sensations. Description of atypical sensations and the procedural description resulted in the same degree of emotional response, which was much higher than that resulting from the typical sensations messages. Thus, the hypothesis that expectation about the occurrence of atypical sensations during a threatening event contributes to elevated emotional response more than degree of accurateness of expectations, was supported.

The finding that incomplete sensory description was effective in reducing distress is relevant to the use of description of sensory experience in patient care situations. In a health care setting it is difficult to anticipate every sensation a patient may experience during a procedure. The laboratory research suggested that in clinical settings emotional response may be reduced by using accurate descriptions of sensations, even though the descriptions do not include all the sensations the patient in fact may experience.

The repeated demonstrations in the laboratory with preparatory information provided a description of sensations subjects experience that reduced emotional response during a threatening event. This encouraged tests of the hypothesis in health care settings. Two experiments tested the hypothesis in a gastroendoscopy clinic (Johnson and Leventhal, 1974; Johnson et al., 1973). In both experiments, adult patients who received a preparatory message which described typical sensations showed lower emotional response during the endoscopy examination than patients who received other types of preparatory information. The success of these studies with adults prompted the question of whether children, given verbal descriptions of the sensations they would experience, would also find a threatening procedure less upsetting.

DESIGNING THE STUDY

The threatening event selected for study was orthopedic cast removal among children who had had a cast applied as a result of injury. Since experience with an event can affect a subject's cognitive appraisal of the event, children who had had limited experience with cast removal (as compared with those who had had health problems that required repeated cast changes) were selected for study. It was reasoned that having a cast sawed off, though not painful, can be frightening or threatening.

The method of conveying information about sensations required consideration of the subjects' level of cognitive development. To control for variation in content, voice inflection, and other subtle differences in verbal messages, the messages were tape recorded. The same woman's voice was on each type of message. Reasoning that children of school age were accustomed to and capable of understanding verbal descriptions of future events (an assumption supported by Piaget's [1971] theory of cognitive development), the investigators placed the lower age limit for subjects at six years.

The hypothesis required that emotional response during the procedure be measured. The type of behavior which conveys emotional reaction varies among different age groups of children. For example, social convention allows young children to cry when frightened, but older children are encouraged to inhibit such behavior. The upper age limit was set at 11 years to minimize the influence on the data of such restraints on behavior.

A three-group experimental design was used to test the hypothesis. Two of the groups were control groups. The experimental group of children heard a taped message which described the sensations during cast removal. One control group heard a taped message which described the general procedure of having a cast removed. This group was a control for the effect of subjects' receiving extra attention through listening to a taped message. The content of the control message was patterned after that recommended in the nursing literature and is the primary focus of books for children about casts and hospitalization (e.g., Weber, 1969; Wolff, 1969). The second control group heard no tape-recorded message.

Hypothesis

The hypothesis tested was that children who heard a preparatory message which describes physical sensations of orthopedic cast removal will display less distress during cast removal than children who receive no experimental information.

METHOD

Site and Sample

Data were collected in the orthopedic fracture clinic at Children's Hospital, Detroit, Michigan. The children and accompanying adults waited in a large room until called to be examined by a physician. Eleven resident physicians removed casts from the children studied. The nursing staff of the clinic consisted of one registered nurse and two nurses' aides. The medical and nursing staff were not informed of the design of the study or the child's group assignment.

Children were accepted into the study if they had not had a cast removed within three months, were at least six and no more than eleven years of age, and had no obvious neurological or developmental problem. The child's age group (6 to 8 or 9 to 11 years) and sex were determined. Assignment to information conditions was in a fixed order, by age and sex classification. This type of assignment allowed even distribution in information groups of younger and older children and boys and girls and removed the possibility of systematic assignment bias. A ten-month period was required to collect the data on 89 children. Five children were excluded from data analysis because of atypical experiences in cast removal. Three children (one in each group) were so uncooperative that, in an attempt to persuade them to control their behavior, a staff member found it necessary to threaten them with bodily harm by the saw; two (one in each taped-message group) received skin abrasions from the saw.

Procedure

Children who were to have their casts removed were identified in the waiting room of the clinic by a nurse on the research staff. If the child met the criteria for subjects in the study, permission for the child to participate was obtained from the accompanying adult. Only one parent refused to allow his child to participate. Information about previous hospitalizations, cause of injury, and number of previous cast removals was obtained from the adult. The children were asked how afraid they were of having a cast removed. The children were shown stick figures of four children on an equal interval continuum. It was explained that each child in the picture was having a cast removed. One child was "not at all afraid," one was "a little afraid," one was "quite a bit afraid," and one was "very, very much afraid." A radial pulse count was taken at that time.

The research nurse accompanied the child and adult to the examining room where the physician confirmed that the cast was to be removed that day. After the physician left the examining room the door was closed. A second radial pulse count was taken for children assigned to the no information control group. For children assigned to the two taped message groups the tape was explained to the adult and permission was obtained for the child to listen to the tape. The child listened to the tape through headphones. Each taped message was two and one-half minutes in length and began with the same introductory remarks. With few exceptions, the research nurse stayed in the examining room while the child listened to the tape.

The sensation group heard a message[1] which included a few seconds of the noise of the saw, told the child that the cast would be cut on two sides and that the saw would not cut her/his skin. In addition, the message told the child that when the cast was cut, she/he would feel vibrations or tingling, feel warmth, and see chalky dust fly; that her/his skin under the cast would be scaly and look dirty; and her/his arm or leg might be a little stiff when she/he first tried to move it, and that the arm or leg would seem light because the cast was heavy.

The procedure group heard a message which told the child that she/he would go to two different rooms, that she/he would sit or lie down on a large table and that the doctor would use a circular saw to cut two sides of the cast. It was emphasized that the child would not be hurt and that the saw would not cut her/him. The use of spreaders and scissors to finish removing the cast was described. The need for a roentgenogram following cast removal was explained. The child was told he could go home after the doctor had checked the roentgenogram.

After the message, the children in the sensation and procedure groups were asked how frightening the message had been. The scale with stick figures was used again for the child's report, and a radial pulse count was taken.

The research nurse directed all children in the study to the cast removal room and, when possible, introduced them to the other investigator, who observed the child during cast removal and counted the pulse rate at specific intervals. This investigator was unaware of the child's group assignment.

The pulse count was taken at four intervals: 1) from the time the saw touched the cast for 15 seconds, 2) from 30 seconds to 45 seconds after the saw touched the cast, 3) for 15 seconds during removal of the cotton padding under the cast, 4) after the cast was completely removed. The child was also observed for occurrence of minor or major signs of distress from the time the saw touched the cast until his limb was freed from the cast. The minor signs were tension in the face (grimace, frown, tension in mouth, or tightly closed eyes), hands (clenching, extension, hands in mouth or in front of face), and feet (extension, inward rotation, and holding in a tense position). The child received a score of zero for minor signs of distress if she/he showed a minor sign of distress in none or one of the body parts, i.e., face, hands, or feet. A score of one was given for minor signs of distress in two or more body parts.

The major signs were pulling away; holding

doctor's hand; kicking; hitting; whining; saying "stop," "no," or other such verbal commands; crying or screaming. The child received a score of zero for major signs of distress if she/he showed none of the signs. A score of one was given if she/he showed any one of the signs. A total distress score was formed by adding the minor and major distress scores with a possible range of zero to two. This method of scaling was used to minimize the effects of children who attempted to meet expectations about behavior appropriate to their age. Reliability of the distress scores was determined by two persons who simultaneously observed 17 children who were not experimentally prepared. There was 88.2 percent agreement for the minor distress scores, and 100 percent agreement on major distress scores.

As the child prepared to leave the cast removal room, she/he was asked how afraid she/he had been while the doctor was taking off the cast. The stick figure scale was used for the response.

RESULTS

The characteristics of the children in the sample and their group assignment are summarized in Table 1. The mean age was 8.4 years. There were more males (62 percent) than females and more later-born than first-born children. Most children

Table 1
Characteristics of the Children by Information Groups

Characteristic	Category	Control	Procedure	Sensation
Age	6–8 years old	8.4	8.5	8.4
	9–11 years old	8.6	7.8	8.5
Sex	Male	18	17	17
	Female	10	11	11
Race[1]	White	8	2	2
	Black	20	26	26
Birth order[2]	First-born	5	7	6
	Later-born	23	21	22
Type of cast[3]	Arm	16	20	17
	Leg	11	8	7
	Spica	1	0	4
Cause of fracture[4]	Simple accident	25	24	20
	Complex accident[7] (e.g., auto accident)	3	4	8
Previous cast removed[6]	No	27	26	26
	Yes[8]	1	2	2
Accompanying adult in room while cast removed[6]	Yes	26	26	24
	No	2	2	4

[1] $\chi^2 = 7.00$, 2df, $p < .05$
[2] $\chi^2 = 0.47$, 2df
[3] $\chi^2 = 6.59$, 4df
[4] $\chi^2 = 3.41$, 2df
[5] $\chi^2 = 0.42$, 2df
[6] $\chi^2 = 1.10$, 2df
[7] No children in the control group, three in the procedure group, and two in the sensation group were admitted to the hospital as inpatients at the time of the fracture
[8] The children in the control group had had a cast removed within the year; the children in the procedure and sensation groups had had casts removed more than a year previous to the current cast

were Black (86 percent). Arm casts were most common, with leg and spica casts occurring less frequently. Only five children had had a previous cast removed. The most frequent cause of the fracture was a simple accident, and most of the accompanying adults stayed with the children during cast removal.

The data were examined for relationships between the characteristics of the children and distress scores. The only characteristic found to be associated with distress scores consistently in each information group and in the whole sample was the children's report of fear prior to cast removal ($r = .38$, df = 82, $p < .001$). A two-factor (pre-fear—two levels—and experimental information—three levels) analysis of variance, least squares method, was used to analyze dependent variables. Children who reported no fear of cast removal were placed in one group and those who reported some fear of cast removal were placed in a second group. These categories were used because they allowed as nearly as possible an equal number of children in each group (46 in the no-fear group and 38 in the some-fear group).

Distress Scores

Both pre-fear and information were related to distress scores. Children who reported no fear of cast removal had lower distress scores than children who had some fear ($p < .02$) (Table 2). (See analysis of variance summary in Table 3). The main effect for information was further analyzed with Dunnett's t test which is appropriate for simultaneously comparing several means with a preselected mean (Winer, 1971, p. 201). As expected, the sensation group mean of .50 differed significantly from the control group mean of 1.00 (Dunnett's $t = 2.44$, df = 78, $p < .025$). The procedure group mean of .71 fell between the sensation and control group means but did not differ significantly from the control group mean (Dunnett's $t = 1.40$, df = 78). Comparison of fear group means within each information group showed that pre-fear had the strongest influence on distress scores in the procedure group. It was concluded that only the sensation information was found to reduce children's distress scores sig-

nificantly and that the children who reported some fear of the cast removal showed higher distress than children who reported no fear of the procedure.

Pulse Rates

Mean pulse rates for each information group were the highest on the count taken during the interval 15 to 30 seconds after the saw touched the cast. Changes in pulse rates from waiting room to 15 to 30 seconds into cast removal were not significantly related to either the children's information group assignment or their pre-fear levels. The order of the information groups' mean change in pulse rate from waiting room pulse rate to the 15 to 30 seconds into cast removal was the same as the distress scores (control mean = 12.4; pro-

Table 2
Distress Score Means for Information Groups and Prefear Levels

Character-istics	Distress Score Means						
	Information Groups						Total
	Control		Procedure		Sensation		
	X̄	N	X̄	N	X̄	N	X̄ N
Pre-fear							
None	0.83	12	0.38	18	0.44	18	0.52 48
Some	1.12	16	1.17	12	0.60	10	1.00 38
Information							
Group	1.00	28	0.71	30	0.50	28	0.74 84

Table 3
Summary of Analysis of Variance for Distress Scores

Source	df	MS	F
Information	2	1.762	3.01**
Pre-fear	1	3.527	6.02***
Information × pre-fear	2	0.755	1.29*
Error	78	0.586	

*$p = .281$
**$p = .055$
***$p = .016$

cedure mean = 9.3; sensation mean = 5.7). The mean pulse rate changes for the no pre-fear group was 6.9; for the some pre-fear group, 11.9. Analysis of variance of pulse rates while in the waiting room and 15 to 30 seconds into cast removal within each information group revealed that the pulse rate increases were significant in the control group ($F = 13.00$, df = 1,27, $p < .005$) and the procedure group ($F = 7.68$, df = 1,27, $p < .01$). The increases for the sensation group were not significant ($F = 2.62$, df = 1,27).

Fear during Cast Removal

The means of the children's report of fear during cast removal were similar for each information group (control group mean = 1.9; procedure group mean = 1.7; sensation group mean = 1.8). The slight differences did not approach an acceptable significance level ($F < 1$). There was a main effect for levels of pre-fear of cast removal for reports of fear *during* the procedure ($F = 24.24$, df = 1,78, $p < .001$). The no pre-fear group mean was 1.4 as compared to a mean of 2.3 for children with some pre-fear.

Intercorrelation of Indicators of Emotional Response

The intercorrelation of indicators of emotional response during cast removal are given in Table 4 for each information group. The indicators of emotional response are positively correlated in each information group. The correlations were more similar (range .30 to .40) in the sensation group than in either the procedure group (range .24 to .43) or the control group (range .13 to .35).

Children's Reactions to the Messages

Children's reactions to the messages were assessed by their report of how frightening the tape had been and changes in pulse rate from before to after the message. Two-factor (information—two levels—and pre-fear—two levels) analysis of variance of reports of how frightening the tape had been resulted in borderline significant effects for information ($F = 3.37$, df = 1,46, $p < .10$)

Table 4
Intercorrelation[1] of Indicators of Emotion Response by Information Groups

Group	Indicator	Distress Scores	Pulse Change From Pre to During Cast Removal
Control	Pulse change	.13	
	Report of fear during cast removal	.34*	.35*
Procedure	Pulse change	.27	
	Report of fear during cast removal	.43**	.24
Sensation	Pulse change	.40**	
	Report of fear during cast removal	.30	.31

*$p = .10$
**$p = .05$
[1]Pearson's product moment correlation coefficients

and for pre-fear ($F = 3.46$, df = 1,46, $p < .10$). The interaction F was less than 1. Children who heard the sensation tape reported that the tape was more frightening (mean = 1.58) than those who heard the procedure tape (mean = 1.25). The no pre-fear group mean (1.29) of how frightening they found the tape to be was less than the mean (1.63) for the same pre-fear group. Two-factor (information—three levels—and pre-fear—two levels) analysis of variance of changes in pulse rates from in the waiting room to after the tape for the message groups and in the examining room for the no experimental information group produced no significant F-ratios.

DISCUSSION

The hypothesis, that a preparatory message which describes the sensations children experience during orthopedic cast removal will result in reduced distress during cast removal, was supported. Observable behaviors that indicate distress occurred significantly less frequently in the sensation group than in the no-information control group. The control group that received preparatory information about the procedures of cast removal received lower distress scores than the no-information control group, but the difference was not significant. Pulse rate changes gave some support for the conclusion that the sensation group was less distressed since only the two control (no-information and procedure) groups had significant increases in pulse rates. Reported fear during the procedure was not significantly affected by preparatory information.

The children who admitted that the idea of having a cast removed was frightening had higher behavioral distress scores and reported they were more frightened during the cast removal than children who reported they were not frightened by the idea of having a cast removed.

The findings for effects of pre-fear level and information groups suggested that sensory preparatory information had its greatest effect on the indicators of distress for those children who admitted some fear of the impending procedure. However, children who reported no pre-fear also showed low amounts of distress behavior when they had been prepared with the sensation information. It can be concluded that sensory information resulted in reduced distress behavior during cast removal whether or not the child admitted fear of the procedure.

Variations among groups in the strength of the intercorrelation of the indicators of emotional response suggested that the type of preparatory information affected the degree of convergence of the indicators. There was a stronger trend for convergence in the sensation group than in the other groups. Perhaps the sensation information tended to unify behaviors indicating distress. Difference in characteristics of the children as assessed by their reported fear before the cast removal had a stronger relationship with distress scores in the procedure group than in the sensation or control groups (correlation coefficient for pre-fear and distress scores for each group were procedure, .57, $p < .01$; sensation, .31; control, .24). This suggested that procedure information tended to increase the influence of individual differences among children. Further investigation of the interrelationships among these variables would make a valuable contribution to the understanding of the effects of information on patients' responses.

The higher mean for how frightening the tape message had been for the sensation group as compared to the procedure group may have resulted from the few seconds of the sound of the saw on the sensation tape. The sound level on the recording was about the same as the unrecorded sound level of the saw cutting a cast. It also came on the tape as a burst of noise following the statement, "You will hear the buzz of the saw, like this—."

The hypothesized mechanism for the reduction of distress during a threatening experience that guided this study involves cognitive processes. Preparatory information which describes typical sensations experienced during a threatening experience increases the accuracy of expected sensations and decreases expectations that are inaccurate. The congruency between expected and experienced sensations is associated with reduced emotional response. It is important to note that the sensory preparatory information used in this and other tests of the hypothesis did *not* include statements about the intensity of the sensations. Although preliminary investigations allow determination of sensations that are experienced by the patient, it is impossible to predict accurately any given patient's perception of the magnitude of the sensations. In addition to not giving subjects cues on the magnitude of the sensations, they were not given suggestions or instruction about expected or appropriate reactions or behaviors. The behavior which results from that type of instruction is controlled by a different process than the hypothesized process offered here. Instructing children in expected behaviors during a threatening experience has been shown to affect the frequency of those specific behaviors (Hedberg and Schlong, 1973), and a film of children who modeled appropriate or expected behavior has also resulted in altering the frequency of behaviors indicating distress (Vernon, 1974). The results achieved in the instruction and modeling studies probably reflect the subjects' willingness to follow instruction or suggestion. Imitating behavior one has been instructed to perform does not necessarily reflect one's own personal evaluation, interpretation, and determination of the significance of the stimulus.

The theoretical hypothesis that congruency between expected and experienced physical sensations results in a reduction of emotional response during a threatening experience has been supported in several situations and age groups. The hypothesis has received support when the threatening experiences were ischemic pain produced in the laboratory, gastroendoscopy examination, and orthopedic cast removal. The age groups of subjects have been children 6 to 11 years, young adults 18 to 25, and adults 21 to 65. The hypothesis has received support within male and female samples.

The theoretical notions presented here have been found to be specific enough to be testable and yet broad enough to generalize to several situations. The theoretical notions form a base of support for further research and the development of theoretical notions. The research already completed on the hypothesis suggests many extensions of this line of investigation. There are measurement problems to be solved, the role of individual differences in emotional response during health care procedures has not been adequately examined, significant differences in characteristics of situations which are threatening need to be identified, and the methods of providing preparatory information require evaluation. The rudimentary theoretical notions presented here may serve to pull a body of research together so that eventually a more comprehensive theoretical structure can be developed.

The same theories often guide practice as well as research. Even the rudimentary theoretical notions presented here can influence the care patients receive. Our research reflects consideration of some of the characteristics and demands of the situations in which patient care is delivered. We gave thought to the existing patient care situation because we believe that with cautions about overgeneralizing, the research can guide aspects of patient care at this time. The low demand on health workers' time when information is transmitted to patients by mechanical methods and the demonstration of the compatibility between transmission of information by mechanical methods and ongoing care activities should increase the likelihood that the research will influence patient care. If consideration of practical aspects of patient care continues concurrently with research developments, perhaps the time lag between knowledge generated by research and application of that knowledge will be shortened.

REFERENCES

Dickoff, J., & James, P. (1971). Clarity to what end? *Nursing Research*, 20, 499–502.

Dumas, R. G., & Leonard, R. C. (1963). The effect of nursing on the incidence of postoperative vomiting. *Nursing Research*, 12, 12–15.

Ellis, R. (1971). Commentary of Walker's "Toward a clearer understanding of the concept of nursing theory." Reaction to Walker's article. *Nursing Research*, 20, 493–494.

Elms, R. R., & Leonard, R. C. (1966). Effects of nursing approaches during admission. *Nursing Research*, 15, 39–48.

Festinger, L. (1957). *A Theory of cognitive dissonance*. Stanford, CA: Stanford University Press.

Folta, J. R. (1971). Obfuscation of clarification: A reaction to Walker's concept of nursing theory. *Nursing Research*, 20, 496–499.

Hedberg, A. G., & Schlong, A. (1973). Eliminating fainting by school children during mass inoculation clinics. *Nursing Research*, 22, 352–353.

Jacox, A. (1974). Theory construction in nursing: An overview. *Nursing Research*, 23, 4–13.

Johnson, J. E. (1966). The influence of purposeful nurse-patient interaction on the patients' postoperative course. In *Exploring progress in medical-surgical nursing practice*, ANA 1965 Regional Clinical Conferences. New York, American Nurses' Association, Monograph no. 2, pp. 16–22.

Johnson, J. E. (1973). Effects of accurate expectations about sensations on the sensory and distress components of pain. *Journal of Personality and Social Psychology*, 27, 261–275.

Johnson, J. E., & Leventhal, H. (1974). Effects of accurate expectations and behavioral instructions on reactions during a noxious medical examination. *Journal of Personality and Social Psychology, 29,* 710–718.

Johnson, J. E., & Rice, V. H. (1974). Sensory and distress components of pain: Implications for the study of clinical pain. *Nursing Research, 23,* 203–209.

Johnson, J. E., et al. (1973). Psychological preparation for an endoscopic examination. *Gastrointestinal Endoscopy, 19,* 180–182.

Lazarus, R. S. (1968). Emotions and adaptation: Conceptual and empirical relations. In W. J. Arnold (Ed.), *Nebraska symposium on motivation* (pp. 175–269). Lincoln: University of Nebraska Press.

Mahaffy, P. R., Jr. (1965). The effects of hospitalization on children admitted for tonsilectomy and adenoidectomy. *Nursing Research, 14,* 12–19.

Nisbett, R. E., & Schachter, S. (1966). Cognitive manipulation of pain. *Journal of Experimental Social Psychology, 2*(3), 227–236.

Piaget, J. (1971). *The psychology of intelligence.* London: Routledge & Kegan.

Schachter, S., & Singer, J. E. (1962). Cognitive, social and physiological determinants of emotional state. *Psychological Review, 69,* 379–399.

Vernon, D. T. A. (1974). Modeling and birth order in response to painful stimuli. *Journal of Personality and Social Psychology, 29,* 794–799.

Walker, L. O. (1971). Toward a clearer understanding of the concept of nursing theory. *Nursing Research, 20,* 794–799.

Weber, A. (1969). *Elizabeth gets well.* New York: Thomas Y. Crowell.

Winer, B. J. (1971). *Statistical principles in experimental design* (2d ed.). New York: McGraw-Hill.

Wolff, A. (1969). *Mom, I broke my arm.* New York: Lion Press.

Wooldridge, P. J. (1971). Meta-theories of nursing: A commentary on Dr. Walker's article. *Nursing Research, 20,* 494–495.

Zimbardo, P. G., et al. (1966). Control of pain motivation by cognitive dissonance. *Science, 151,* 217–219.

This article is printed with permission of *Nursing Research.* Copyright 1975 American Journal of Nursing Company.

7

NURSING CARE OF ADULTS

Charold Baer, PhD, RN
Dana Diane Penilton, BSN, RN
Theresa Lerch, BSN, RN

INTRODUCTION BY: CHAROLD BAER, PhD, RN

The nursing care of adult patients involves numerous independent and interdependent activities. For many years, health care professionals have focused concern on the interdependent aspects of patient care, and have expended resources conducting research regarding the complex technologies involved. However, the current trend in nursing is shifting from an emphasis on interdependent activities to evaluating the clinical impact of independent nursing interventions. The impetus for this shift seems to parallel the development of the profession as a unique discipline in health care.

Current nursing literature is reflective of the continuing commitment of nurses to establish a research-based practice. There are increasing numbers of research reports being disseminated to assist in accumulating a body of knowledge to support and guide clinical practice. The quality and complexity of such efforts have increased concomitantly with increases in quantity. The overall emphasis seems to have shifted from describing complex, independent nursing interventions and patient responses to evaluating the effectiveness of various interventions. Thus, the types of research designs also have progressed from descriptive to experimental or quasiexperimental designs in order to provide data regarding specific clinical questions.

The research studies selected for this chapter are representative of the progress occurring in nursing research, as well as the breadth and scope of nursing interventions being studied. Schneider's research is included because it is a double-blind, crossover experimental study that involves a nursing intervention and the human responses to that intervention. More specifically, it involves a patient's physiologic responses to a nursing intervention. In addition, the operational definition of terms, hypotheses, and data analyses are all worthy of consideration. Also, the investigator's detailing of the nursing implications of this study and the recommendations for further study facilitate the reader's comprehension and potential utilization of the study results.

The Cotanch and Strum research is included because it is an example of an experimental study that involves an independent nursing action used to treat a human response to a pathologic state. The complexity of the human response of nausea and vomiting, its prevalence, and the potential intervening variables, make this an intriguing research study to critique. In addition, it is very illustrative of the progress that has occurred in research in nursing. Also, the use of a behavioral intervention to modify a physiologic response is an interesting concept that has been widely discussed, but not sufficiently tested. Additional data are necessary in order to expand the use of such interventions in clinical practice.

The Boykin and Winland-Brown study was selected for inclusion because it deals with pressure sores, which continue to be a major clinical problem in current practice. Not only does the article address the management of pressure sores, but it also focuses on associated preventative aspects. Its major contributions to practice seem to be its demonstration of: (1) how the lack of operational definitions and descriptions of an instrument can inhibit its clinical utility; (2) the importance of validating an assessment parameter; and (3) the importance of using more than one parameter to evaluate healing. In addition, the study clearly demonstrates what appears to be an overzealous interpretation of the results of the study.

The studies included in this chapter indicate the progress that is being made in establishing a research base for nursing interventions used to care for adult patients. In some respects, they also reflect the traditional, intuitive base that has been the essence of nursing care for years. Clinicians eagerly anticipate the merging of the intuitive and research bases for practice in order to define and refine prescriptive nursing theory for futuristic practice.

Effects of Caffeine Ingestion on Heart Rate, Blood Pressure, Myocardial Oxygen Consumption, and Cardiac Rhythm in Acute Myocardial Infarction Patients

Joy Rewold Schneider, MSN, RN
Fort Lauderdale, FL

The term "coronary precautions" not only exists but is practiced by many nurses in coronary care units (CCUs) nationwide.[1] This order, whether initiated by the nurse or the physician, encompasses a list of restrictions that are imposed on patients with suspected acute myocardial infarction (AMI). Currently the list of restrictions consistently includes very hot and very cold beverages, stimulant beverages, rectal temperature measurement, and, occasionally, back rubs.[2] Unfortunately, previous research has revealed that many of these widely accepted coronary precautions were established as CCU nursing practices on the basis of years of tradition, rather than scientific rationale.[1,3] In a current review of the nursing literature on the restriction of stimulant beverages in the CCUs, I confirmed it to be an example of a traditional nursing practice.

BACKGROUND INFORMATION

Stimulant beverages are considered to be all beverages that contain theophylline, theobromine, or caffeine.[2,4,5] Of these xanthine derivatives, caffeine is considered the most potent[2] and thee most frequently consumed stimulant,[4,5] In the United States, regular coffee is the single most important source of caffeien. Eight out of ten americans drink coffee, with an average daily consumption equaling 3 1/2 cups.[6]

Although the pharmacologic actions of caffeine are not clearly understood and supported, the pharmacokinetic properties of caffeine are well documented. Oral caffeine is rapidly and almost completely absorbed in the gastrointestinal tract[3-7] and is distributed throughout the body.[3-6] Food does slow down but does not reduce the absorption of caffeine.[3,5] Peak caffeine plasma levels are reached in 15 to 45 minutes after ingestion,[8-10] with a half-life of about 3 1/2 hours.[5-7] Caffeine is metabolized in the liver into monomethyl and dimethyl xanthines and uric acid.[6] Liver disease, oral contraceptives, cimetidine, and pregnancy prolong the clearance of caffeine.[8] Smoking, on the other hand, enhances the metabolism of caffeine.[8,11,12] Caffeine and its metabolites are excreted mainly by the kidney, although small amounts can be excreted in saliva, semen, and breast milk.[8]

There are some therapeutic uses for caffeine: treatment of apnea in infants,[5-8] and headaches, central nervous system depression,[5-7] and atopic dermatitis in adults.[6-8] The therapeutic dosage for oral caffeine varies considerably in the literature from 100 to 400 mg of oral caffeine every 3 to 4 hours, depending on the adult.[4-7]

Caffeine is mainly considered a central nervous system stimulant.[5,9] The pharmacologic actions of caffeine on the cardiovascular system are complex and relatively unclear. Many of the believed pharmacodynamic theories antagonize each other, which helps explain the diverse discrepancies in the literature with regard to the hemodynamic effects of caffeine. For example, caffeine has been observed to stimulant the myocardium directly, as well as the vagal and vasomotor centers in the brain. These two simultaneous actions can produce bradycardia, tachycardia, or no essential changes in the pulse rate, depending on the caffeine dose and the subjects involved.[5,13-15]

The major nursing rationale cited for restricting stimulant beverages in the CCUs was that these beverages may increase the heart rate (HR).[2] However, there is no nursing research to support this concept. In fact, there is only one nursing research study on the effect of stimulant beverages on the heart in the literature.[16] This study was conducted with healthy nursing students with various daily caffeine consumption histories. After consuming the caffeine, these subjects demonstrated a significant decrease in their HR and no significant change in the frequency of their ectopic beats.[16]

On the other hand, medical scientists have been studying the physiologic effects of caffeine on the cardiovascular system in humans for 50 years. There are several medical studies published on this topic but with inconsistent samples, methods, and findings.[12,13,17-37] Most of these studies involved noncardiac patients,[12,18-20,24-27,29,30,32,34,36] failed to distinguish between acute and habitual caffeine consumers,[13,17,23,25,26,29,33,36,37] and/or required caffeine consumption equal to two to three cups of caffeinated coffee.[12,17,18,20-22,24-35,37] The conclusions of these studies were as inconsistent as the methods: a variety of these studies reported that caffeine consumption increased, decreased, or had no effect on the HR, cardiac rhythm, and blood pressure.[12,13,17-37]

In addition, the relationship between coffee consumption and ischemic heart disease (IHD) has not been consistently and clearly established; consequently, most experts have recently concluded that coffee consumption may not be an independent risk factor for IHD.[8,10,14,38-41] Because of these conclusions, the rationale for restricting stimulant beverages in CCUs still remains unclear. Yet, a national research survey revealed that restricting coffee was identified by the CCU nurses as the seventh most important CCU nursing intervention.[1]

PURPOSE

The purpose of this study is to examine the physiologic effect of a single caffeine dose on selected cardiovascular hemodynamic variables of AMI subjects. The following two research questions were developed:

1. What is the effect of a single caffeine dose on HR, systolic blood pressure (SBP), diastolic blood pressure (DBP), rate-pressure product (RPP), and cardiac rhythm in AMI patients?
2. What is the relationship between long- and short-term caffeine use on HR, SBP, DBP, RPP, and cardiac rhythm in AMI patients?

HYPOTHESES

From these two questions, the following hypotheses were formulated and tested at the 0.05 level of significance:

1. AMI subjects who ingest one cup of caffeinated coffee will not have a significantly greater increase in HR than the same subjects who ingest one cup of decaffeinated coffee in the hospital.
2. AMI subjects who ingest one cup of caffeinated coffee will not have a significantly greater increase in their SBP than the same subjects who ingest one cup of decaffeinated coffee while in the hospital.
3. AMI subjects who ingest one cup of caffeinated coffee will not have a significantly greater increase in their DBP than the same subjects who ingest one cup of decaffeinated coffee while in the hospital.
4. AMI subjects who ingest one cup of caffeinated coffee will not have a significantly greater increase in their RPP than the same subjects who ingest one cup of decaffeinated coffee while in the hospital.
5. AMI subjects who ingest one cup of caffeinated coffee will not have a significantly greater increase in the number of cardiac arrhythmias than the same subjects who ingest one cup of decaffeinated coffee while in the hospital.
6. AMI subjects who historically have ingested more than five cups of caffeinated coffee a day will not have a significantly greater increase in their measured hemodynamic vari-

ables in this study than those AMI subjects who historically have ingested less than one cup of caffeinated coffee a day.

DEFINITION OF TERMS

1. Acute myocardial infarction (AMI) subject: a newly admitted CCU male patient between the ages of 42 to 86 years with a documented AMI in the physician's progress notes, with concurrent electrocardiographic changes and elevated cardiac isoenzymes to support the diagnosis
2. One cup of caffeinated coffee (experimental beverage): 150 ml of brewed coffee (Maxwell House) from an automatic drip type of coffee maker that had an average caffeine level of approximately 90 to 110 mg and a temperature range of 62° to 66° C[6,10,14,42]
3. One cup of decaffeinated coffee (control beverage): 150 ml of brewed coffee (Maxwell House) from an automatic drip coffee maker that had an average caffeine level of approximately 2 to 4 mg and a temperature range of 62° to 66° C[4,6,9,42]
4. Heart rate (HR): an apical pulse rate taken for 1 minute by the investigator
5. Blood pressure (BP): the second BP reading from a Dinamap 845 automatic BP recorder with the use of the subject's nondominant arm
6. Cardiac arrhythmias: all observed electrocardiographic responses that were not considered regular sinus rhythm as determined with the standardized modified chest lead (MCL_1)
7. Myocardial oxygen consumption: the product of the HR and the SBP[43,44]

METHOD

Research Design

A double-blind crossover design was implemented in this study to investigate the effects of a single dose of caffeine on the cardiovascular system of AMI subjects.[45] Each subject was his own control subject in the study; that is, each subject consumed one cup of the control beverage as well as one cup of the experimental beverage. Each subject was randomly assigned to the treatment sequence. This study noninvasively measured the hemodynamic and electrocardiographic responses of each subject to each beverage. The crossover rule was time dependent.[45] Each beverage was administered and evaluated at 24-hour intervals to allow time for the effects of one beverage to dissipate before the other beverage was administered.

Sample and Setting

The target population consisted of AMI subjects in the CCU, intermediate care unit, and/or regular cardiac floor at a 375-bed private hospital in southern Florida who consumed a single dose of caffeinated coffee. These units did not have a standard policy restricting stimulant beverages; thus some of the subjects may have been receiving caffeinated beverages during this study.

A convenience (nonprobability) sample was used in this study.[46] The sample included the first 20 male subjects admitted to the CCU with a diagnosis of AMI and who consented to be in the study. Only subjects who were hemodynamically stable and without any intravenous medications for at least 24 hours were eligible to be in the study.

Data Collection

An informed written consent was obtained from the primary physician for each eligible subject. Next, the investigator discussed the study with each potential candidate and obtained his informed written consent for participation. The investigator reviewed the medical records for those patients who consented to participate in order to obtain the necessary medical and demographic data. This information was compiled on a master sheet that was coded by subject number.

The study was conducted on each AMI subject while he was in the CCU or intermediate care unit or on the regular cardiac floor on 2 consecutive days. Each AMI subject fasted for 4 hours preceding each of the two data collection periods so that the possible influence of food and fluids on the study would be eliminated. Each day, within 30 minutes before beginning the study, each AMI subject's oscilloscope was observed for a 15-minute period for heart rhythm changes for baseline data. In addition, for each AMI subject the baseline resting HR and BP were recorded within 15 minutes before the study was begun each day. Each AMI subject then randomly received 150 ml of either the control (decaffeinated coffee) or the experimental (caffeinated coffee) beverage on day 1 and the alternate beverage on the following day. The sequence of caffeinated and decaffeinated consumption was randomly assigned; neither the investigator nor the subject knew which beverage the subject was consuming. Each subject was given each beverage between 3:30 and 4:00 P.M. and was instructed to drink each beverage within 10 minutes. The HR and BP were determined simultaneously for each subject at 30, 60, and 90 minutes after the ingestion of each beverage and recorded. However, the investigator continuously monitored each subject's heart rhythm in MCL_1 in the subject's room for the 90-minute data collection period. Each subject remained on bed rest during the data collection period so that the possible effects of exercise on the data would be reduced. After all the data were collected on the second day, a self-report questionnaire of daily caffeine consumption was completed by each subject.

DATA ANALYSIS

Sample Description

Twenty subjects who met the inclusive criteria participated in this study. The ages for the entire sample ranged from 44 to 85 years, with a mean age of 61.3 years. All 20 male subjects were white. Of these subjects, eight (40%) were Jewish, 18 (90%) were married, and a majority of the subjects were retired (80%).

Eleven of the sample (55%) were nonsmokers. Six subjects (30%) were low caffeine consumers (<50 mg of caffeine a day), seven (35%) were intermediate caffeine consumers (50 to 499 mg of caffeine a day), and seven (35%) were heavy caffeine consumers (≥500 mg of caffeine a day).

The locations of the AMIs in this sample were established to vary among the subjects. Nineteen subjects (95%) had some previous history of heart disease, with 13 (65%) having had one or more previous AMIs.

All subjects were receiving various oral medications during the study. Eighteen subjects (90%) were taking at least one antiarrhythmic agent (β-adrenergic blocking agents (four subjects), calcium-channel blocking agents (16), quinidine-like agents (seven), and/or digitalis preparations (eight).[47] Eighteen subjects (90%) were taking antianginal agents. Only one subject (5%) was receiving specific antihypertensive agents, and seven subjects (35%) were taking diuretics. Significantly, only three subjects (15%) were receiving β-adrenergic stimulating and theophylline agents during the study.

The subjects participated in this study anywhere from day 3 to day 10 of admission to the hospital ($\bar{X}$ = 6.5 days from admission) because of the difficulty of obtaining physician approval. By the time each subject had consented to the study, all subjects were classified according to the New York Heart Association's functional classification as being in class I. Table I provides a summary of the demographic data collected on the 20 subjects.

Findings Related to the Hypotheses

There were no significant differences in the baseline measures for the dependent variables (HR, SBP, DBP, RPP, and cardiac rhythm) across all groups; therefore all multivariate analysis of variance (MANOVA) statistics were determined with the use of the raw data. In addition, there was no significant order effect. Eleven subjects (55%) consumed the caffeinated coffee on day 1, whereas nine subjects (45%) consumed the caffeine on day 2. A repeated-measures MANOVA on caffeine order showed no significant differences between consuming the caffeine on day 1

Table 1
Characteristics of the Sample (n = 20)

Characteristics		f	%
Age (year)	40-49	6	30
	50-59	3	15
	60-69	5	25
	70-79	5	25
	80-89	1	5
Marital status	Single	1	5
	Married	18	90
	Divorced	1	5
Smoking history (pack years)	0	11	55
	1-25	2	10
	26-50	3	15
	51-75	3	15
	76-100	1	5
Daily caffeine use (mg)	0-49	6	30
	50-499	7	35
	≥500	7	35
Location of AMIs	Anterolateral	3	15
	Anteroseptal	4	20
	Anterior wall	3	15
	Inferior wall	5	25
	Inferolateral	3	15
	Lateral wall	1	5
	Subendocardial	1	5
History of heart disease	None	1	5
	Hypertension	3	15
	Permanent pacemaker	2	10
	Coronary artery bypass	1	5
	Previous MI—1	10	50
	Previous MIs—2-3	2	10
	More than 3 previous MIs	1	5
Medications received during study	β-Adrenergic blocking agents	4	20
	Calcium-channel blocking agents	16	80
	Quindine-like agents	7	35
	Digitalis preparations	8	40
	Antianginal agents	18	90
	Antihypertensive agents	1	5
	Diuretics	7	35
	Antiulcer agents	7	35
	Psychotherapeutic agents	10	50
	Antibiotics	2	10
	Bronchodilators	3	15
First day in study from admission (days)	2-4	6	30
	5-7	7	35
	8-10	7	35

Legend: MI, myocardial infarction.

Table 2
Mean Hemodynamic Variables Over Time

Group	HR	ARR	SBP	DBP	RPP
Caffeine (n = 20)	73.1	2.1	122.0	73.0	9037.1
No caffeine (n = 20)	73.1	1.4	119.0	71.6	8955.0

Legend: ARR, cardiac arrhythmias.

or day 2 for HR, SBP, DBP, RPP, and cardiac arrhythmias.

Hypotheses 1 to 5

A repeated-measures MANOVA on the caffeine group (n = 20) versus the no-caffeine group (n = 20) showed no significant differences between the groups for HR, SBP, DBP, RPP, and cardiac arrhythmias. Table 2 shows the mean measurements for each of these hemodynamic variables over time.

Hypotheses 6

The sample was divided into high ($\geq$500 mg of caffeine a day), intermediate (50 to 499 mg of caffeine a day), and low (<50 mg of caffeine a day) caffeine-use groups according to the self-report questionnaire on daily caffeine consumption. A repeated-measures MANOVA between high (n = 7), intermediate (n = 7), and low (n = 6) caffeine-use groups showed no significant differences between these groups, whether they did or did not use caffeine, for HR, SBP, DBP, RPP, and cardiac arrhythmias. Table 3 shows the mean hemodynamic variables for the low (occasional) caffeine-use groups and the high (habitual) caffeine-use groups over time.

Additional Findings

The sample was divided into three age groups: young (38 to 53 years; n = 6), middle-aged (54 to 69 years; n = 8), and elderly (70 to 85 years; n = 6). A repeated-measures MANOVA of these age groups also was performed to determine the dependent variables. No significant differences were found between the age groups, whether they received caffeine or no caffeine, for HR, SBP, DBP, RPP, and cardiac arrhythmias.

A repeated-measures MANOVA of smokers (n = 9) versus nonsmokers (n = 11) also showed no significant differences between these groups, whether they received caffeine or not, for HR, SBP, DBP, RPP, and cardiac arrhythmias.

LIMITATIONS

One major limitation of the study was the sample size. With the inclusion of more patients, significant caffeine trends may have been apparent. In addition, because of the nonprobability sampl-

Table 3
Mean Hemodynamic Variables Over Time

Group	HR	ARR	SBP	DBP	RPP
Low use					
Caffeine (n = 6)	68.2	2.3	122.6	70.7	8325.2
No caffeine (n = 6)	68.2	0.5	116.4	68.1	7843.2
High use					
Caffeine (n = 7)	78.0	2.2	122.0	74.1	9110.2
No caffeine (n = 7)	79.2	0.3	121.1	75.1	9507.3

Legend: ARR, cardiac arrhythmias.

ing procedure, the results of the study could not be generalized to include the entire population.

Another major limitation of the study was that the caffeine dosages were not correlated with scientifically predetermined caffeine content values or serum caffeine levels. Therefore the results of the study could not be correlated with specific caffeine dosages or serum caffeine levels. The caffeine dosages were standardized only in how the caffeinated coffee was prepared with one brand of coffee (Maxwell House). Because the study used only one brand of coffee, the results may not be applicable to coffees produced by a different roasting technique.

Probably the most important limitation of this study was the confounding effects of the prescribed cardiac drugs, which were not investigated because of the small sample size.

Finally, the study was limited by the potential for human error. There is the possibility of bias in the frequency-of-use questionnaire by each subject. Further, there is a possibility that the investigator missed cardiac arrhythmias while occupied in collecting other data.

DISCUSSION

This study supports the investigator's six null hypotheses. In addition, the findings in this study support previous findings reported in the literature, especially in studies where (1) low doses of caffeine were used, (2) caffeinated and decaffeinated coffee beverages were consumed, (3) cardiac patients were investigated, and (4) habitual and occasional caffeine consumers were identified. A majority of the studies reviewed by this investigator revealed that small doses of caffeine (less than approximately 200 mg) in normal subjects, as well as in cardiac subjects, did not significantly affect the HR,[13,19,23,25,36] BP,[13,23] and/or cardiac rhythm.[13,16] Furthermore, the findings of previous studies in which caffeinated and decaffeinated coffee beverages were consumed were similar to those found in this study.[13,16,17,22,23,25,28,32,35,37]

In addition to the caffeine dosage and source, the presence of IHD may be a factor in this study and may therefore have influenced the HR and BP results. Only one cardiac study that investigated the effects of caffeine on the HR and BP of cardiac patients revealed a positive finding.[17] Therefore this study supports the general findings that cardiac patients do not respond significantly to various dosages of caffeine according to these hemodynamic measurements.[13,23,28,33,35,37]

With regard to the finding that there were no significant differences in the number of ectopic beats between caffeine and no caffeine, 90% of the subjects in this study were receiving some type of antiarrhythmic therapy. Specifically, 90% of the subjects were taking either β-adrenergic blocking agents, calcium-channel blocking agents, and/or quinidine-like agents that could have decreased the potential for ventricular arrhythmias.[47] However, only one study conducted with cardiac patients reported all subjects to be free of cardiac drugs for 24 hours before the study.[21] This study revealed a potential for the consumption of 200 mg of caffeine to electrically induce cardiac arrhythmias in both healthy volunteers and cardiac patients.[21] Conversely, other studies have reported that even large doses of caffeine (3 or 4 cups of caffeinated coffee) did not significantly increase the frequency of arrhythmias in cardiac patients.[17,37] Still other studies reported in the literature further confirm[13,16,28] or contradict[29,33,35] the heart rhythm findings of this study. All these discrepancies lead one to conclude that the relationship between caffeine consumption and cardiac arrhythmias is exceedingly complex.

The null hypothesis that there would not be a significant difference in the measured hemodynamic variables between the high-consumption and the low-consumption groups was also accepted in this study. This finding is supported in the literature. Only two previous studies demonstrated a significant difference in the HR between habitual and occasional caffeine consumers.[16,19] All the other studies in the literature that distinguished between occasional and habitual caffeine consumers found no significant difference in the HR.[12,24,31] Unfortunately, even fewer studies reported in the literature investigated the effect of caffeine consumption on the BP and heart rhythm between occasional and habitual caffeine consumers. Two studies reported a significant increase in the BP of both their habitual and their occasional caffeine groups,[12,24] whereas two other studies showed an initial significant increase in the SBP in their caffeine groups at the start of their 2-week caffeine protocol.[31,32] Furthermore, only one study in the literature showed no significant correlation between the daily caffeine intake and the incidence of ectopic beats observed over time.[16]

In addition, it is important to note the differences in the mean HRs between the high ($\bar{X}$ = 78.6), and low ($\bar{X}$ = 68.2) caffeine use groups. An explanation for this difference could be that four subjects (67%) in the low-use groups were taking digitalis preparations, whereas only one subject (14%) in the high-use group was doing so. However, the difference in the baseline means and the use of digitalis agents between the groups does not appear to affect the null hypothesis. Additionally, the slight difference in the mean BPs between these two groups may, again, be due to their prescribed cardiac medications. One subject (17%) in the low-use group was taking an antihypertensive agent, whereas none was prescribed for the high use group. In addition, four subjects (67%) in the low-use group were taking diuretics, whereas only one subject (14%) in the high-use group was doing so. Again, though, this difference in the mean BPs and the use of various medications between the two groups does not appear to affect the null hypothesis.

In conclusion, several factors may have affected the findings of this study. First, the sample size may have been too small for a significant effect to arise. Second, the caffeine dose may have been too low for any potential pharmacologic responses. Third, because 95% of the subjects had a history of IHD, they may have demonstrated fewer hemodynamic responses to the caffeine because of their disease process. Fourth, all the subjects were studies while receiving cardiac medications, which may have masked the effects of caffeine on their cardiovascular system. Fifth, the results of this study may be due to the fact that a majority of the sample (70%) were habitual caffeine consumers, and these subjects may have developed a tolerance to caffeine. Finally, the findings of this study could represent the ability of the body to adapt to the various pharmacologic actions of low doses of caffeine.

NURSING IMPLICATIONS

The findings of this study have several implications for nursing education, research, and practice. The scientific rationale for restricting stimulant beverages in AMI subjects was investigated in this study. The results of this study reveal that this widely accepted coronary care precaution appears to be based on years of tradition rather than scientific knowledge. Therefore it appears that the nursing profession needs to educate itself and the community on the documented effects of caffeine on the cardiovascular system and the need for more nursing research in this area.

In conclusion, the results of this study may have clinical importance because it strictly involved AMI patients, who are generally more prone to cardiac irregularities. This study is a beginning in the needed scientific investigation of a coronary care precaution that has traditionally been practiced by many coronary care nurses nationwide. The ethical and legal implications of not following the traditional norm and of allowing stimulant beverages in the CCUs in individual cases may have been reduced because of the results of this study. Once the nurse has obtained a social as well as a medical history of an AMI patient, the nurse may decide to administer a one-time average dose of a stimulant beverage while closely monitoring the patient in the CCU to alter this coronary care precaution in individual cases safely.

RECOMMENDATIONS

Further study of the effects of caffeine on the human cardiovascular system is necessary. The specific recommendations for future caffeine studies are as follows:

1. The sample size needs to be increased to allow for the numerous independent variables (such as medications) that cannot be controlled.

2. The caffeine dose needs to be scientifically determined through chemical content analysis or determination of serum caffeine levels.
3. The study needs to be replicated with documented AMI subjects.
4. A study needs to be performed in which more than one dose of caffeine is administered to AMI subjects.
5. A study needs to be performed to investigate the psychologic effects of restricting stimulant beverages in AMI patients.

REFERENCES

1. Kirchhoff, K. T. (1982). A diffusion survey of coronary precautions. *Nursing Research, 31,* 196.
2. Kirchhoff, K. T. (1981). An examination of the physiologic basis for coronary precautions. *Heart Lung, 10,* 874.
3. Dews, P. B. (1982). Caffeine. *Annual Review of Nursing, 2,* 323.
4. Graham, D. M. (1978). Caffeine: Its identity, dietary sources, intake and biological effects. *Nutrition Reviews, 36,* 97.
5. Rall, T. W. (1980). Central nervous system stimulants: The xanthines. In L. Goodman & A. Gilman (Eds.), *The pharmacological basis of therapeutics.* New York: Macmillan.
6. Raebel, M. A., & Black, J. (1984). The caffeine controversy: What are the facts. *Hospital Pharmacy, 19,* 257.
7. United States Pharmacopoeial Convention (1984). USP dispensing information, vol. 1. *Drug information for the health care provider.* Rockville, MD: The Author, p. 266.
8. Curatolo, P. W., & Robertson, D. (1983). The health consequences of caffeine. *Annals of Internal Medicine, 98,* 641.
9. Greden, J. F. (1979). Coffee, tea and you. *Sciences, 19,* 6.
10. Mathewson, M. (1984). Rule: Give only decaffeinated coffee to cardiac patients...fact or myth? *Critical Care Nurse, 4,* 12.
11. Parsons, W. D., & Neims, A. H. (1978). Effect of smoking on caffeine clearance. *Clinical Pharmacology and Therapeutics, 24,* 40.
12. Whitsett, T. L., Manion, C. V., & Christensen, H. D. (1984). Cardiovascular effects of coffee and caffeine. *American Journal of Cardiology, 53,* 918.
13. Gould, L., Venkataraman, F., Goswami, M., & Gomprecht, R. (1973). The cardiac effects of coffee. *Angiology, 24,* 455.
14. MacCornack, F. A. (1977). The effects of coffee drinking on the cardiovascular system: Experimental and epidemiological research. *Preventive Medicine, 6,* 104.
15. Victor, B. S., Lubetsky, M., & Greden, J. F. (1981). Somatic manifestations of caffeinism. *The Journal of Clinical Psychiatry, 42,* 185.
16. Newberg, S. (1984). The effects of a single caffeine dose on heart rate and rhythm [abstract]. *Heart Lung, 13,* 309.
17. Brink, L. S., McKirnan, M. D., O'Connell, S. R., Motto, R. E., & Froelicher, V. F. (1980). Caffeine ingestion by cardiac patients prior to ECG-monitored exercise training [abstract]. *Medical Science Sports, 12,* 111.
18. Charney, D. S., Galloway, M. P., & Heniger, G. R. (1984). The effects of caffeine on plasma MHPG, subjective anxiety, autonomic symptoms and blood pressure in healthy humans. *Life Sciences, 35,* 135.
19. Colton, T., Gosselin, R., Smith, R. P. (1967). The tolerance of coffee drinkers to caffeine. *Clinical Pharmacology and Therapeutics, 9,* 31.
20. Conrad, K. A., Blanchard, J., & Trang, J. M. (1982). Cardiovascular effects of caffeine in elderly men. *Journal American Geriatrics Society, 30,* 267.
21. Dobmeyer, D. J., Stine, R. A., Leier, C. V., Greengberg, R., & Schaal, S. F. (1983). The arrhythmogenic effects of caffeine in human beings. *New England Journal of Medicine, 308,* 814.
22. Freestone, S., & Ramsey, L. E. (1982). Effect of coffee and cigarette smoking on the blood pressure of untreated and diuretic-treated hypertensive patients. *American Journal of Medicine, 73,* 348.
23. Gould, L., Reddy, C. V., Oh, K. C., Kim, S. G., & Becker, W. (1979). Electrophysiologic properties of coffee in man. *Journal of Clinical Pharmacology, 19,* 46.

24. Izzo, J. L., Ghosal, A., Kwong, T., Freeman, R. B., & Jaenike, J. R. (1983). Age and prior caffeine use alter the cardiovascular and adrenomedullary responses to oral caffeine. *American Journal of Cardiology, 52*, 769.

25. Johnson, J., Prakash, R., Kaushek, V., et al. (1982). Effect of regular and decaffeinated coffee on cardiovascular function in normal subjects [abstract]. *Circulation, 66* (suppl. II), 99.

26. Onrot, J., Goldberg, M. R., Biaggioni, L., Hollister, A. S., Kincaid, D., & Robertson, D. (1985). Hemodynamic and humoral effects of caffeine in autonomic failure. *New England Journal of Medicine, 313*, 549.

27. Pincomb, G. A., Lovallo, W. R., Passey, R. B., Whitsett, T. L., Silverstein, S. M., & Wilson, M. F. (1985). Effects of caffeine on vascular resistance, cardiac output and myocardial contractility in young men. *American Journal of Cardiology, 56*, 119.

28. Piters, K. M., Colombo, A., Olson, H. G., & Butman, S. M. (1985). Effect of coffee on exercise-induced angina pectoris due to coronary artery disease in habitual coffee drinkers. *American Journal of Cardiology, 55*, 277.

29. Prineas, R. J., Jacobs, D. R., Crow, R. S., & Blackburn, H. (1980). Coffee, tea and VPB. *Journal of Chronic Disease, 33*, 67.

30. Robertson, D., Frolich, J. C., Carr, R. K., et al. (1978). Effects of caffeine on plasma renin activity catecholamines and blood pressure. *New England Journal of Medicine, 298*, 181.

31. Robertson, D., Hollister, A. S., Kincaid, D., et al. (1984). Caffeine and hypertension. *American Journal of Medicine, 77*, 54.

32. Robertson, D., Wade, D., Workman, R., Woosley, R. L., & Oates, J. A. (1981). Tolerance to the humoral and hemodynamic effects of caffeine in man. *Journal of Clinical Investigation, 67*, 1111.

33. Sarma, R. J., Prakash, R., & Prakash, S. Cardiac effects of caffeine in normal and post-myocardial infarction patients at rest and during exercise [abstract]. *Clinical Research, 32*, 203.

34. Smits, P., Hoffman, H., Thien, T., Houben, H. & van't Laar, A. (1983). Hemodynamic and humoral effects of coffee after β_1-selective and nonselective β-blockade. *Clinical Pharmacology and Therapeutics, 34*, 153.

35. Sutherland, D. J., McPherson, D. D., Renton, K. W., Spencer, C. A., & Montague, T. J. (1985). The effect of caffeine on cardiac rate, rhythm, and ventricular repolarization. *Chest, 87*, 319.

36. Svenson, E., Persson, L., & Sjoberg, L. (1980). Mood effects of diazepam and caffeine. *Psychopharmacology, 67*, 73.

37. Zeldis, S., & Katz, S. (1982). Caffeinated or decaffeinated coffee? Does it really make a difference [abstract]? *Clincial Research, 30*, 680.

38. Aro, A. (1985). Coffee and the heart. *Annals of Clinical Research, 17*, 1.

39. Kannel, W., & Schatzkin, A. (1984). Risk factor analysis. *Prognosis of Cardiovascular Disease, 26*, 309.

40. Klatsky, A. L., Petitti, D. B., Armstrong, M. A., & Friedman, G. D. (1985). Coffee, tea and cholesterol. *American Journal of Cardiology, 55*, 577.

41. Levy, R. I., & Feinleib, M. (1980). Risk factors for coronary artery disease and their management. In E. Braunwald (Ed.), *Heart disease: A textbook of cardiovascular medicine.* Philadelphia: Saunders, 1246.

42. Macaulay, T., Gallant, C. J., Hooper, S. N., & Chandler, R. F. (1984). Caffeine content of herbal and fast-food beverages. *Journal of Canadian Dietetic Association, 45*, 150.

43. Amsterdam, E. A., Hughes, J. L., DeMaria, A. N., Zelis, R., & Mason, D. T. (1974). Indirect assessment of myocardial oxygen consumption in the evaluation of mechanisms and therapy of angina pectoris. *American Journal of Cardiology, 33*, 737.

44. Gobel, F. L., Nordstrom, L. A., Nelson, R. R., Jorgenson, C. R., & Wang, Y. (1978). The rate-pressure product as an index of myocardial oxygen consumption during exercise in patients with angina pectoris. *Circulation, 57*, 549.

45. Louis, T., Lavori, P., Bailer III, J., & Polansky, M. (1984). Statistics in practice. *New England Journal of Medicine, 310,* 24.
46. Polit, D. F., & Hungler, B. P., (Eds.). (1983). *Nursing research: Principles and methods.* Philadelphia: Lippincott, 409.
47. Kienzle, M. G., Williams, P. D., Zygmont, D., Doherty, J. U., & Josephson, M. E. (1984). Antiarrhythmic drug therapy for sustained ventricular tachycardia. *Heart Lung, 13,* 614.

This article is printed with permission of *Heart and Lung.* Copyright © 1987 C.V. Mosby.

Original article:
Schneider, J. R. (1987). Effects of caffeine ingestion on heart rate, blood pressure, myocardial oxygen consumption, and cardiac rhythm in acute myocardial infarction patients. *Heart & Lung, 16(2), 167–174.*

CRITIQUE BY: DANA DIANE PENILTON, BSN, RN

Part I: Clinical Relevance

The problem Schneider studied was whether or not caffeine ingestion affected heart rate, blood pressure, myocardial oxygen consumption, and cardiac rhythm in patients who had an acute myocardial infarction (AMI). This investigation holds relevance to practice because it offers rationale for making the decision of whether or not to withhold caffeine from patients that have a diagnosis of myocardial infarction.

This study has the potential to assist with two types of nursing decisions. The first decision deals with determining appropriate assessment parameters when an AMI patient is allowed to have caffeinated beverages. Schneider utilized specific measurements (heart rate, blood pressure, EKG rhythms, and myocardial oxygen consumption) to determine patient response to caffeine; these measures also can be utilized to evaluate patient response in the clinical situation. This study helps one decide what to do when faced with the clinical problem of whether or not to allow the AMI patient to ingest caffeine. This second decision confronts the widely accepted protocols of coronary care precautions, such as withholding caffeine and ice water from AMI patients. Schneider is convinced that the theory of coronary care precautions was established on the basis of tradition rather than scientific study.

The study does not identify characteristics that might be useful for determining which AMI patient's are at risk for complications after the use of caffeine, however. Schneider's demographic data and results indicate no difference between varying patient characteristics or the amount of daily caffeine consumption. Therefore, these traits are not helpful for identifying or preventing undesirable outcomes after the use of caffeine by AMI patients.

Schneider did test an intervention in this study. The independent variable manipulated and compared was the AMI client's response to caffeinated and decaffeinated coffee. In my practice, at least, the potential exists to utilize this intervention. Since caffeine use is not included in our AMI care protocols, whether or not to allow caffeine ingestion is a nursing decision, except when a physician specifically orders that a patient not be allowed caffeinated beverages. Several nurses on my unit are reluctant to allow the AMI patient to have caffeinated coffee due to the possible side effects of increased heart rate and arrhythmias.

The investigator measured dependent variables by comparing baseline heart rate (HR), systolic blood pressure (SBP), diastolic blood pressure (DBP), rate-pressure product (RPP), and cardiac arrhythmias to measures of these parameters after the patient consumed caffeinated and decaffeinated coffee. She also evaluated the effect of a history of high versus low caffeine use utilizing the same hemodynamic parameters. In my practice, it would be very simple to utilize these same measures to evaluate patient response to caffeinated beverages. Patient HR and BP measurements are obtained every one to four hours or more often depending on the patient's status, and arrythmia monitoring is continuous via an EKG machine. A patient's baseline data are readily available to all nurses via the nursing care record. Assessment of these parameters is dictated by patient status, doctor's orders, and nursing discretion.

Part II: Conceptualization and Internal Consistency

In general, the report is easy to read and logically organized. The investigator includes her hypotheses and definitions of terms. She explains the research design and includes clear details of interventions and data collection protocols. Data analysis is straight forward, logical, and correlated with each of the hypotheses. The study also includes a nursing implications section which is helpful for putting the study into perspective with one's own practice.

Schneider utilized the literature review to focus justification for her study. Since nursing research is scant in this area, she cited several medical studies that indicate that the relationship between coffee consumption and ischemic heart disease has not been consistently or clearly established. Citing a national research survey (Kirchhoff, 1982), Schneider noted that CCU nurses identified restricting coffee as the seventh most important CCU intervention. The concept underlying the rationale for this study is that nursing practice needs to be based on scientific rationale rather than on tradition.

Schneider poses two study questions. The first deals with the effect of a single caffeine dose on HR, SBP, DBP, RPP, and cardiac rhythm in AMI patients. The second examines the relationship between long- and short-term caffeine use on HR, SBP, DBP, RPP, and cardiac rhythm in the AMI patient. These two questions relate directly to her study justification, since they potentially contribute information that would justify nursing intervention with a scientific rationale rather than a rationale of tradition.

Schneider uses methods appropriate for conducting the study. She chooses her sample from the target population: AMI subjects in the CCU, intermediate care unit, or regular cardiac floor of a private hospital in Florida. She used a convenience, nonprobability sample, and included in the study the first 20 males admitted to the CCU with a diagnosis of AMI. However, if Schneider also had included women in the study sample, generalizability of results would have increased. Nonetheless, she utilized instruments for data collection that were easily accessible and the information derived related directed to the hemodynamic measures under study. In addition, she carefully outlined the procedures of coffee preparation to ensure that each cup of coffee had approximately the same dose of caffeine. Finally, in her analysis, Schneider organized all data and information together into logically derived and useful conclusions.

In her study, Schneider posed reasonable questions but only answered the first. The second question deals with the relationship between long- and short-term use of caffeine "on HR, SBP, DBP, RPP, and cardiac rhythm in the AMI patient." In the sixth null hypothesis, which related to this question, Schneider focused on patients' history of caffeine use and compared the amount of coffee ingested per day (more than five cups or less than one cup). She divided patients into two categories, those who have historically ingested more than five cups of caffeinated coffee per day and those who have historically ingested less than one cup of caffeinated coffee per day. The word *historically* is not included in the definition of terms, however, leading the reader to question how long a coffee drinker consumes coffee before he or she has a history of drinking coffee. Therefore, I am uncertain whether the question posed (long- versus short-term use of coffee) can be answered with the hypothesis format utilized (amount of caffeine consumed per day). This appears to be worthy of two questions and two separate hypotheses, since answers to both are relevant to the study.

However, this discrepancy does not jeopardize the practical usefulness of this study; it should be considered further.

Part III: Believability of Results

Schneider selected her study sample from the target population which consisted of patients diagnosed as having an acute myocardial infarction. By utilizing criteria for sample selection, the sample became more homogeneous with regard to critical attributes. Specifically, for inclusion in the study, the subjects needed to be admitted to the CCU with a diagnosis of AMI, consent to be in the study, be hemodynamically stable, and not have received any intravenous medications for at least 24 hours. In this regard, Schneider tempered her use of a nonprobability sample by her care in sample selection, conservative interpretation of results, and suggestion that the study required replication.

Schneider designed the study as a double-blind crossover. She applied the intervention to the treatment group; the subjects themselves served as the control group. Then she randomly assigned each subject to the treatment sequence. The crossover was time dependent, allowing 24 hours to pass in order to allow the effects of each beverage to dissipate before the other beverage was tested. By utilizing experimental control with randomization, Schneider increasingly eliminated systematic bias from her rescarch design.

Schneider studied the hemodynamic effects of caffeine on AMI patients by measuring HR, SBP, DBP, RPP, and cardiac rhythm. She determined heart rate by counting the apical pulse for one minute; assessed blood pressure with the Dinamap 845 automatic BP recorder; defined cardiac arrhythmias as all electrocardiographic responses not considered regular sinus rhythm; and calculated myocardial oxygen consumption by multiplying HR by SBP.

It is inferred from the study that the investigator obtained each of the measurements personally. Unfortunately, the study does not discuss the reliability or validity of the measures themselves or whether the measurements actually evaluate cardiovascular hemodynamic response to caffeine. Since the investigator did not address these issues, the reader cannot be certain of their degree of consistency. Nor can the reader be certain of the accuracy of the measures used, thus possibly diminishing their replicability. However, in my experience, it seems that the measures used do measure hemodynamic response. In addition, if it is true that one person obtained all of the measures, then their reliability improves.

Schneider based her study conclusions on a detailed analysis of the data. She evaluated and compared patient responses to caffeinated versus noncaffeinated beverages and utilized subjects, interventions, and measures compatible with her intentions. In addition, she evaluated six null hypotheses. The first five stated that there would not be a difference in the hemodynamic parameters (HR, SBP, DBP, RPP, or cardiac arrhythmias) after one cup of caffeinated coffee. The sixth hypothesis was a comparison of AMI patients with a history of drinking more than five cups of caffeinated coffee per day to AMI patients with a history of drinking less than one cup of caffeinated coffee per day, and stated that there would not be a difference in the hemodynamic measures between these groups after consuming one cup of caffeinated coffee. The results of no significant differences in hemodynamic measures and no significant differences in hemodynamic status between the two groups supports each of the hypotheses via negative inference. The investigator suggests that these results support the "thesis" that small doses of caffeine do not affect hemodynamic variables in AMI patients. Based on my experience and knowledge, these conclusions seem reasonable.

Schneider then discusses other explanations, factors, and study limitations that may have contributed to her results. She acknowledges that her small sample size, nonprobability sampling, failure to correlate predetermined caffeine content to serum caffeine levels, possible bias in the subjects' caffeine use, self-report questionnaire, and the confounding effects of prescribed cardiac drugs may have affected her results. In general her conclusions are conservative, and this is appropriate due to the study design, limitations, and confounding variables.

Part IV: Generalizability of Results

The target population of the study is similar to the population I work with, with one exception: Schneider limited her study to male subjects; my practice deals both with males and females diagnosed with AMI. In her study, Schneider also specified several demographic characteristics evaluated in my clinical situation, specifically: age, marital status, smoking history, daily caffeine use, location of AMI, history of heart disease, and medication use. Thus, her results could be generalized to the male patient population with which I work.

Schneider provides ample information regarding previous research related to her study. She cited research on stimulant beverages, the pharmacologic and pharmacokinetic action of caffeine, and the therapeutic uses of caffeine. The nursing literature related to caffeine use addresses the rationale of CCU nurses for restricting caffeine use by their patients. The only nursing research addressing the stimulant effect of caffeine used a limited sample consisting of healthy nursing students.

Schneider notes that in pharmacodynamic theories caffeine expresses antagonizing effects, which explains the diverse discrepancies in the literature related to hemodynamic effects of caffeine. The medical studies published are inconsistent in terms of samples, methods, and findings. Conclusions drawn range from increased, decreased, and no effect on heart rate, cardiac rhythm, and blood pressure. Also, the relationship between caffeine use and ischemic heart disease has not been consistently established.

Recognizing these problems, Schneider included a comparison of her study with previous medical research that focused on similar details. Specifically, she compared her study to studies that utilized low doses of caffeine, compared caffeinated versus decaffeinated beverages, and investigated cardiac patient responses to caffeine as categorized by habitual and occasional caffeine use. Schneider's results support the findings of the majority of studies reviewed.

There is considerable similarity between Schneider's work and previous medical research. Nursing research on this subject is negligible and further research and replication of this study are needed.

Part V: Other Factors to Consider in Utilization

Before a clinician decides to utilize the interventions in clinical practice, two concepts concerning feasibility must be addressed: (1) the patients must have similar characteristics to the study sample and (2) a clinically significant improvement in patient status must be expected. Since the patients in my practice are similar to the patients in Schneider's study, the use of the interventions tested is expected to yield positive results. Therefore, a systematic evaluation of this research can be done in practice with either an individual or institution-wide approach.

The main risk of changing practice is related to unexpected or unwanted patient responses. The risk of not changing practice is to continue practicing nursing based on tradition rather than utilizing reasonable, applicable research. One way to minimize obscure results is for nurses to document carefully when, where, and how interventions were applied and the exact results obtained.

The cost of changing practice in this instance is minimal since supplies, equipment, and patient data are readily available. Nurses have access to patient data including diagnoses, age, and history of caffeine use. They also can provide caffeinated and decaffeinated beverages for patients. The hemodynamic parameters evaluated in the study are parameters normally monitored in the CCU environment.

In this instance, the benefit of changing practice outweighs the cost of not changing practice. By evaluating and utilizing research in the clinical area a precedent is established for nurses to base their practice on research rather than tradition.

Original article:
Schneider, J. R. (1987). Effects of caffeine ingestion on heart rate, blood pressure, myocardial oxygen consumption, and cardiac rhythm in acute myocardial infarction patients. *Heart & Lung, 16*(2), 167–174.

CRITIQUE BY: CHAROLD BAER, PhD, RN

Part I: Clinical Relevance

The clinical problem Schneider studied concerned the physiologic effect of a single caffeine dose, and long- and short-term caffeine use on selected cardiovascular hemodynamic variables of patients who had experienced an acute myocardial infarction (AMI). Study findings could have significant implications for patient care, not only during the acute phase of cardiac insult, but also in the rehabilitative and health maintenance phases. Such findings could add to the knowledge already accumulated and provide a basis for determining whether a patient who has had an AMI should ingest caffeinated beverages or substances. The findings also could assist the clinician in making decisions about the specific intervention of permitting the patient to ingest caffeinated beverages and which specific parameters to monitor for a patient, as well as guide the formulation of patient education content. These types of clinical decisions could result in a decreased incidence of complications experienced by the patient.

The investigator elected to study one component of a set of interventions ("coronary precautions"), which are often implemented by nurses in coronary care units. The component studied was the effect of 150 ml of caffeinated coffee, containing 90 to 110 mg of caffeine, on the heart rate, blood pressure, myocardial oxygen consumption, and cardiac rhythm of a patient who had experienced an AMI. The investigator also analyzed the effect of self-reported long- and short-term caffeine use on the same physiologic parameters. In many institutions, nurses decide whether or not to institute coronary precautions, including restricting caffeine intake, as part of the plan of care. In other institutions, however, such clinical decisions are either physician prescribed, or mutually determined by the nurse and physician. Thus, whether or not a nurse can decide to permit a patient to ingest caffeine containing beverages and substances, is dependent upon the degree of autonomy granted by the institution and physicians. Nurses possess the physiologic knowledge base to support making such decisions, but lack the research base to substantiate the decisions made.

Dependent variables in the study included cardiovascular responses of heart rate, blood pressure, myocardial oxygen consumption, and cardiac rhythm. Each of these variables was measured according to the parameter stated in the operational definition of the variable. For example, Schneider measured heart rate by counting the apical pulse for one minute; measured blood pressure as the second reading obtained from a Dinamap 845 automatic blood pressure recorder using the patient's nondominant upper extremity; measured myocardial oxygen consumption by multiplying the patient's heart rate by the systolic blood pressure; and assessed cardiac rhythm by observing all electrocardiographic responses that deviated from normal sinus rhythm while using the standardized modified chest lead. All of these measures are frequently used by nurses in various clinical settings to assess patient responses. In most situations, it is within the scope of nursing practice to determine which of these measures are appropriate for assessing a patient's state. In some institutions, however, the nurse's decision making is complicated by the need for a physician's order to justify the use of expensive, technical monitoring equipment. Even in those instances, nurse–physician collaboration usually results in supporting the nurse's decision regarding continuing patient assessment.

In general, this study has the potential for contributing to a body of research knowledge that can influence a nurse's decision making in clinical practice. The possible impact on patient care mandates that this study be further evaluated for utilization by the clinician.

Part II: Conceptualization and Internal Consistency

This study is clearly articulated, logically sequenced, and conceptually consistent. However, there is one component based on the study justification that was unexpected. The inclusion of the second research question regarding the relationship between long- and short-term caffeine use on specified hemodynamic variables for patients who had experienced an AMI seems inappropriate. In addition, the variable did not seem to be appropriately defined. The hypothesis related to this question states, "AMI subjects who historically have ingested more than five cups of caffeinated coffee a day will not have a significantly greater increase in their measured hemodynamic variables in this study than those AMI subjects who historically have ingested less than one cup of caffeinated coffee a day." However, the number of cups of caffeinated coffee ingested per day does not seem an accurate measure of long- or short-term caffeine consumption. One would expect a quantification of caffeine consumption over a specified length of time for a more appropriate definition of this variable.

The investigator clearly delineated justification for her study from clinical practice observations, knowledge from pharmacology and physiology, and numerous conflicting research reports. In addition, her conceptualization of the study is clear, with the exception of those comments previously made regarding the second research question and its variable definition. She logically relates the independent and dependent variables, as supported by previous research and knowledge. The subjects are consistent with the population of interest, but are not reflective of the entire composition of the population of interest because of the inclusion criteria used by the investigator. The measurements selected are appropriate for assessing the phenomena of interest and are currently components of the standard of practice for patient care. Thus, the data collection procedures constitute usual nursing practice and should not introduce bias into the study. The conclusions drawn from the results of this study are consistent with the conceptualization.

In general, even with the inclusion of the second research question, this study is conceptually clear and consistent and has the potential to contribute to nursing practice. Thus, it merits further evaluation for utilization by clinicians.

Part III: Believability of Results

This study purported to determine the effect of an independent variable, caffeine, on patient hemodynamic variables. The data collected were all quantitative in nature. The subjects studied were a convenience sample comprised of the first 20 consenting male subjects admitted to the CCU with a diagnosis of AMI. Additional inclusion criteria used to screen subjects were hemodynamic stability and having received no intravenous medications for at least 24 hours. The subjects were not representative of the population at large because all of them were male caucasians.

The investigator used a double-blind crossover study design with each subject serving as his own control. The investigator used this design because neither she nor the subject were aware of the type of beverage being consumed, nor in what sequence. Also the investigator used a crossover design because each subject consumed one cup of the control beverage and one cup of the experimental beverage, separated by a 24-hour time interval. Thus, the crossover was governed by time, to allow for the effects of one beverage to dissipate before the second beverage was consumed. The investigator randomly assigned subjects to the treatment sequences. She collected baseline data for each subject prior to the consumption of each type of beverage in order to make appropriate comparisons. In addition, she required subjects to fast for four hours prior to each data collection period in order to eliminate the influence of food and fluids on the findings. Unfortunately, however, while she documented medication ingestion, she did not provide controls.

Schneider discusses the limitations of the study, and cites the following: (1) small sample size; (2) use of nonprobability sampling for selecting subjects; (3) failure to correlate caffeine dosages with scientifically predetermined caffeine content values or serum caffeine levels; (4) use of only one brand of coffee for the experimental beverage; (5) confounding effects of prescribed oral medications; (6) human error in the subject's self-reporting of caffeine use; and (7) human error by the investigator resulting in missed data, such as cardiac dysrhythmias. However, she made no attempt to explain why she deemed such limitations acceptable within the study design.

The investigator does not discuss the reliability and validity of measures used to assess dependent variables. Perhaps Schneider made this choice because she assumed the measures reliable and valid based on the frequency of their use as normal assessment techniques in patient care situations. Unfortunately, the frequency of use does not necessarily substantiate the reliability and validity of a measure. Thus, concrete supporting data would have been helpful. One also would question the validity of a self-report questionnaire regarding daily caffeine consumption as a measure of long- and short-term caffeine use. Also, Schneider does not mention anything about the number of data collectors or interrater reliability. Therefore, one assumes that the investigator collected data alone.

Although Schneider reported study results with the appropriate clarity, she included numerous descriptive characteristics of the sample without stating a rationale or explanation. For example, she reported the age, marital status, smoking history, infarction location, history of heart disease, and medications ingested for the sample, but did not discuss such characteristics as related components of the conceptual framework of the study. While those data are interesting, one wonders how some of them relate to the current study. Also, the investigator chose to report both frequencies and percentages for the various characteristics—one wonders why, when the sample is so small. In some respects, the percentages tend to inflate, and perhaps overstate, the point. For example, a characteristic that appears in 50 percent of the sample still only relates to 10 people because the sample size was only 20. On the other hand, the investigator's use of repeated measures of multivariate analysis of variance to analyze data is appropriate because the data are interval or ratio level and from dependent or related samples that have received more than one treatment. In this study, the treatments were the control and the experimental beverages. In addition, such an analysis provides appropriate answers in relation to the stated hypotheses.

Based on the statistical analysis, Schneider appropriately drew conclusions related to the first five hypotheses. Hypothesis six, which related to the effects of long-and short-term caffeine use, however, cannot be addressed using the defined variable. Thus, the conclusion of no difference is not relevant to the specific hypothesis. Schneider notes that the study supported all six of the null hypotheses and that these findings are consistent with previous studies. However, she does point out several factors that may have significantly influenced study findings, including: (1) the sample size may have been too small; (2) the caffeine dose may have been too low; (3) the disease processes of the subjects may have limited their hemodynamic responses; (4) oral medications may have masked the effects of the caffeine; (5) subjects may have developed a tolerance to caffeine; and (6) the body may be able to adapt to the pharmacologic effects of low doses of caffeine. All of these potential influencing factors tend to decrease the credibility of the results of the study. Because there are so many possible alternative factors that could be responsible for producing the results, the clinician must exercise caution in continuing to evaluate the results of this study for utilization in clinical practice.

Part IV: Generalizability of Results

Schneider conducted this study in a setting representative of coronary care units in most institutions. The sample, however, was not representative of the target population. The use of inclusion criteria that limited the sample of the first 20 males admitted with a diagnosis of an AMI eliminated half of the target population of interest—females—and resulted in an age range of 44 to 85 years, which is not necessarily representative of the entire target population.

While the investigator is a master's prepared nurse with clinical experience, she has no specific additional education in relation to the study. The measures she used to collect data regarding the dependent variable all find frequent use in clinical practice. Thus, it is likely that staff nurses could implement the results of this study without additional education.

Numerous studies have been conducted regarding the effect of caffeine on the human body. As the investigator notes, each of these studies accesses a different target population, has a different design, uses different measures to assess the specified dependent variables, and results in different findings and conclusions. Therefore, some support this study's findings and others refute them. There still seems to be no clearly defined body of knowledge regarding the complexities of caffeine use on the human body, and, more specifically, on hemodynamic variables.

All of the concerns regarding this study, from design to conclusions, suggest only limited generalizability of findings. As a result, one should exercise caution when deciding whether or not to utilize the findings in the clinical setting.

Part V: Other Factors to Consider in Utilization

Since this study involves activities which are components of standard nursing practice, it would be feasible to implement its results and systematically evaluate outcomes. However, one must first determine whether the benefits outweigh the risks of implementation. If practice is altered based on this study, and the results really were due to one of the alternative factors, a patient could experience potentially devastating increases in all of the specified hemodynamic parameters. One would need to determine what level of increases in those parameters are acceptable for a patient with an AMI and how willing the clinician is to risk such increases. In addition, what does implementing these findings really mean? Does it mean that a patient could receive 90 to 100 mg of caffeine every 3.5 hours in accordance with its half-life, or just once a day?

On the other hand, the benefits of implementation could increase patient satisfaction and decrease anxiety. Yet, in many respects, the risks seem to outweigh the benefits of changing practice, particularly when in most institutions maintaining current practice involves minimal patient risks. Certainly patients could experience additional anxiety in relation to having caffeine consumption curtailed, but it would probably be difficult to assess because of the anxiety generated by the myocardial infarction.

The costs involved in implementing the study results would be minimal. Implementation would not involve additional equipment, other material resources, or personnel time or education. The costs resulting from adverse patient effects due to the implementation, however, could be expensive.

In general, it seems that there is insufficient evidence to support the utilization of the study findings in clinical practice. There are still too many questions that remain unanswered in relation to the complexities involved in the effects of caffeine on a patient's hemodynamic status. In addition to the minor design faults and nonrepresentative sample, there remain all of the other possible alternative explanations for the findings. All of these factors tend to decrease one's confidence in the findings and result in a decision not to utilize them in clinical practice. Additional research is mandatory before utilization can be recommended.

Progressive Muscle Relaxation as Antiemetic Therapy for Cancer Patients

Patricia H. Cotanch, PhD, RN
Associate Professor of Nursing
Assistant Professor of Psychiatry
Duke University Medical Center
Durham, NC

Suzanne Strum, MFA
Research Assistant
Duke University Medical Center
Durham, NC

Is progressive muscle relaxation (PMR) an effective antiemetic therapy for patients receiving highly emetogenic cancer chemotherapy? To study this question, 60 patients beginning multiple course, inpatient chemotherapy infusions were randomized into: an experimental group (trained in PMR), a placebo control group (listened to relaxing music), or a true control group (no study intervention). Patients were studied serially for one baseline and three or four follow-up chemotherapy courses. The results show that PMR was most effective in decreasing frequency and duration of vomiting, general anxiety, and physiological arousal, and in improving caloric intake in patients 48 hours following drug infusion. Evidence suggests that PMR may be effective in reducing side effects of nausea, vomiting, anorexia and emotional distress that frequently accompany chemotherapy.

Recent advances in cancer chemotherapy treatment have resulted in improved prognosis for many cancer patients. Unfortunately, the improved prognosis is often accompanied by uncomfortable chemotherapy-related side effects. For many patients the most adverse side effects are prolonged nausea and vomiting that frequently accompany treatments. Indeed, many patients cannot tolerate drug-related nausea and vomiting, and terminate potentially curative drug treatment. Such a decision may drastically shorten their life expectancy.

BACKGROUND

Because nausea and vomiting are major problems in cancer management, many antiemetic drug trials have been undertaken. Although substantial progress has been made, no antiemetic or combination of antiemetics has been found completely effective. Also, all antiemetics have side effects that may be troublesome to patients. Overall, many patients and health professionals are disappointed with the effectiveness of antiemetic drugs.

The limitations of these pharmacologic antiemetics have prompted researchers to investigate behavioral strategies for reducing chemotherapy-related nausea and vomiting. The behavioral interventions have included hypnosis with guided imagery, multiple muscle site electromyographic (EMG) biofeedback combined with relaxation, systematic desensitization, and progressive muscle relaxation (PMR).[1-6]

Four controlled studies have been conducted

and consistently support the usefulness of these techniques in reducing adverse side effects associated with chemotherapy.[1,3,4,7] To date, all the studies have concentrated on the phenomenon of anticipatory nausea and vomiting (ANV) as the dependent variable. ANV, a learned conditioned response, develops in approximately 33% of patients and usually occurs after the third or fourth chemotherapy course.[8,9] An excellent review of previous studies using behavioral intervention, including PMR, is published elsewhere.[10]

PURPOSE

This study's purpose was to determine the efficacy of an early intervention PMR technique as compared to a placebo control intervention and a no study intervention in decreasing drug-related nausea and vomiting in patients beginning a highly emetogenic course of chemotherapy. The rationale for the early intervention was to offer patients a coping strategy that would allow for psychological distraction during chemotherapy administration and improve their sense of control by developing skill in eliciting an anti-stress response.

CONCEPTUAL FRAMEWORK

In addition to the anti-stress response that PMR elicits, cognitive psychologists suggest an additional mode of action to explain the usefulness of relaxation techniques with cancer patients. According to a system-oriented conception of the stress response, subjects' appraisals of environment stimuli will determine whether or not they feel threatened and are aroused to action. Appraisals may be realistic or distorted. Physiological arousal can be very appropriate in some circumstances; at other times it may be totally inappropriate. In this context, relaxation is a response that, when mastered, can neutralize the effects of activation for *fight or flight*; and it can also alter the appraisal of a potentially threatening situation. For example, in situations of frustration resulting from a perceived lack of control, relaxation can provide a measure of control and thus change the appraisal of a potentially threatening situation. A change of appraisal generally means a change in response as well.[6,11]

METHODS

Entry Criteria

Patients admitted to an inpatient oncology clinical research unit to receive multiple chemotherapy infusions were screened for study eligibility. Patients were required to be receiving their initial course (i.e. no previous chemotherapy) of a multiple course chemotherapy regimen which had an emetogenic potential greater than 60%. Patients with clinical evidence of metastatic brain disease or gastrointestinal obstruction were excluded.

Protocol

The study, including the three different approaches for controlling nausea and vomiting, was explained to eligible patients and their written informed consent obtained. The study plan involved a randomized three-group design consisting of the experimental group (therapist directed/taped PMR), the placebo control group (therapist present while patient listens to relaxing taped attention-getting (TAG) music), and true control group (no study intervention). Patients were followed for five consecutive (one baseline and three or four follow-up) chemotherapy courses.

Study Groups

The PMR procedure involved a 20-30 minute explanation of the technique accompanied by a descriptive pamphlet. The procedure required the patients to listen to a 22 minute instructional audio tape about tense/relax exercises for 16 muscle groups from the feet to the head. The tape also included a brief hypnotic induction of a relaxing scene and suggestions for the patient to feel alert and refreshed. Following the relaxation procedure, patients were given suggestions to have an appetite and the desire to consume nutritious foods during and after chemotherapy.

Patients were instructed to listen to the tape twice a day and again while receiving chemotherapy. They were also given schedule cards to monitor home practice and asked to mail them in weekly. After listening to the tape, patients were questioned about the degree of relaxation, feelings about the intervention, and whether they wanted to emphasize any aspects of relaxation. This emphasis was the only attempt to tailor the standard relaxation procedure to individuals. The therapist/researcher spent an average of 20 minutes with the patient during the post-relaxation session.

The control group receiving the TAG music placebo was offered a 22 minute audio tape of relaxing music. The tape was intended to *control* for the possible "non-specific" effects of the researcher's time and effort with patients. Patients were instructed to enjoy the music and think only pleasant thoughts. After listening to the tape patients were questioned about their feelings of relaxation and enjoyment. They were also encouraged to share their pleasant thoughts with the researcher.

A second, or true, control group received only standard procedure. The "no intervention" group was included to control for the potential placebo effects of the attention that result from patients' participation in a clinical investigation. These patients were required to complete some of the evaluations required of the other participants. However, the researcher spent very little time with the true control group patients. Most of the patient information was obtained from their hospital charts.

Study Measures

Patients were offered standard antiemetic therapy. They were neither advised nor encouraged to begin or discontinue use of standard antiemetics nor to increase or decrease their use of antiemetics. Patients participating in pharmacologic antiemetic investigational clinical trials were excluded from the study.

Nausea and vomiting were measured using the

Figure 1
The Duke Descriptive Scale (DDS) Used to Measure Nausea and Vomiting

Duke's Descriptive Scale (DDS)

A. Nausea: Grades I-IV
   I = None
   II = Mild: no interference with activity
   III = Moderate: interference with activity
   IV = Severe: bedridden with nausea for more than two hours

B. Vomiting: Grades I-IV
   I = No vomiting 24 hours after chemotherapy
   II = Mild: vomiting less than five times within 24 hours after chemotherapy
   III = Moderate: 5-10 times within 24 hours after chemotherapy
   IV = Severe: greater than 10 times within 24 hours; patient bedridden; possible dehydration

Duke Descriptive Scale (DDS) (Figure 1), starting with the administration of the drug infusion and for 48 hours after the infusion. This self-report assessment has the added advantage of incorporating patient activity levels as a criterion for severity of nausea and vomiting. The DDS had previously been used for pharmacologic antiemetic trials at the Duke Comprehensive Cancer Center and had acceptable reliability and validity.[6,12]

Patients were instructed to keep a diary of all foods and fluids taken by mouth for two days following chemotherapy. Caloric value was obtained using the U. S. Department of Agriculture Bulletin No. 72.

The Lange Skin Fold Caliper was used to measure patients' upper arm skin folds during every hospital admission for each chemotherapy cycle. The Lange Caliper was selected because it is used frequently in clinical research studies to measure skin fold thickness, has a high degree of accuracy, is durable, and is portable. Most important, it causes no patient discomfort and obtains measurements in several seconds.

Systolic and diastolic blood pressures were recorded from patients' brachial arteries using auscultatory method. Pulse rate was recorded by palpating the radial artery for 60 seconds. Respirations were recorded by observation for 60 seconds. Physiologic arousal measurements were obtained at each admission (cycle) on all patients before and after PMR practice or TAG procedures.

Researchers used the Speilberger's State-Trait Anxiety Inventory (STAI) to obtain data on patients' anxiety levels during chemotherapy courses. The STAI was originally developed as a research instrument for the investigation of anxiety phenomena in "normal" adults. It is composed of two 20-item subscales each with a low score of 20 and high score of 80; one measures *State* anxiety and the other measures *Trait* anxiety. Researchers were interested in both subscale measurements. The State anxiety measurements were obtained at the time of chemotherapy infusion in order to measure how patients were feeling during chemotherapy administration. Trait anxiety measurements were obtained two to three days after patients were discharged from the hospital to measure patients' general feelings between chemotherapy treatments.

Other measures included obtaining patient weights at admission and discharge. Data were obtained on demographic and clinical variables to determine potential associations and/or biases in the study or treatment interventions and to identify potential correlates.

RESULTS

Sixty-eight patients considered were eligible for the study. Six patients refused to participate and

Table 1
Patient Characteristics by Study Group

	No Treatment (N=20)	Placebo Control (N=20)	Progressive Muscle Relaxation (N=20)	Total (N=60)
Age (Years)				
Range	18-66	20-58	17-68	17-68
Median	39	38	38	38
Sex (Number of Patients)				
Female	10	12	6	28
Male	10	8	14	32
Cancer Type				
Testicular	2	3	6	11
Melanoma	2	4	4	10
Hematologic	6	6	5	17
Breast	5	3	3	11
Other	4	4	3	11

Table 2
Range of Values in Variables by Treatment Group

	Progressive Muscle Relaxation Group	Taped Attention-Getting Music Group	No Treatment Control Group
Nausea (1-4)	2-4	2-4	2-4
Vomiting (1-4)	1-4	1-4	1-4
State (20-80)	27-74	28-66	—
Trait (20-80)	24-68	26-60	—
Calories (0-3000)	0-2010	0-1600	0-1800

two patients began the study but withdrew immediately after the initial intervention training session (both withdrawals were in the TAG placebo group). The results are based on 60 patients followed over 12 months involving 282 observations in the data set. Selected characteristics of the participants are shown in Table 1.

Baseline Data Analysis

The randomization procedure appeared to balance the treatment groups for baseline measurement. No statistically significant differences were found among the groups in a two tailed T-test on the DDS, anxiety rate scores, and caloric intake.

To determine whether patients' baseline findings affected their subsequent responses (post intervention), the relationship between the two scores and each of the separate scores (baseline minus follow-up scores from subsequent sessions) was calculated for each data point using the Pearson Product Moment Correlations as recommended by Benjamin.[13] Analyses revealed no significant association between initial scores, indicating that a desirable base free measure of change was likely. Ranges for obtained values in variables across all data collection points by treatment groups are shown in Table 2.

Follow-up Data Analysis

A repeated measure analysis of variance models was used to analyze data to take into account longitudinal changes within the different treatment groups and to determine hidden interaction (if any) over time. Nonparametric correlation using the Spearman Rank Correlation Coefficient was used to test pre and post-treatment intervention (PMR, TAG placebo) findings of systolic and diastolic blood pressure, pulse and respiration. The results show a consistent pattern. There were statistically significant differences in systolic (F 51.7, p = .001) and diastolic (F 27.6, p = .001) blood pressures, and in pulse rate (F 61.1, p = .001)(Table 3). No significant difference was obtained over time in comparing treatment times sessions (Tx[×]S) for physiologic measurements.

Table 3
Difference Pre-Post Treatment Session Comparing Progressive Muscle Relaxation (PMR) and Taped Attention-Getting Group (TAG)

Vital Signs	F Value	P Value
Systolic BP	51.71	.001
Diastolic BP	27.61	.001
Pulse	41.11	.001
Respiration	31.12	.002

A statistically significant difference was obtained for the dependent variables of vomiting (p = .03), trait anxiety (p = .05), and caloric intake (p = .001). However, the differences obtained for the variables of nausea and state anxiety were not significant at the .05 level. Table 4 shows the number of patients who improved, remained the same, or became worse for nausea and vomiting, calories, and anxiety comparing baseline to final session.

Admission and discharge weights did not significantly change among the three groups. Skin caliper measurements did not change between the treatment groups. No significant interaction effect existed between the variables (e.g. greatest decrease in physiologic arousal and antiemetic effect or change in STAI-S or T). There were no changes in the amount or type of antiemetics that were administered over time to the patients in the three groups. There was no correlation between practice frequency and antiemetic PMR response.

DISCUSSION

Study results strongly suggest that PMR and positive suggestions can be effective interventions for partially ameliorating chemotherapy side effects of vomiting and anorexia. This and previous studies provide some encouraging experimental demonstrations of the efficacy of behavioral interventions for patients with cancer.

The possible mechanism by which PMR may decrease drug-related symptoms has been previ-

Table 4
Subjects Response Table Comparing Baseline to Final Session

	Improved			No Change			Worse		
	PMR	TAG	Control	PMR	TAG	Control	PMR	TAG	Control
Nausea	8	4	3	10	9	10	2	6	7
Vomiting	10	2	4	10	12	6	0	6	10
State	2	6	4	15	12	11	3	2	5
Trait	8	4	5	6	10	12	6	6	3
Calories	18	4	8	0	6	5	1	10	6

ously discussed.[1-4,6,10] All investigators believe the factors are interrelated rather than mutually exclusive. For the purpose of this paper, identified possible mechanisms are discussed briefly.

Anxiety Reduction

Achieving a state of relaxation is a desired result of all the behavioral interventions used as antiemetic therapies. It is possible that the intervention's effectiveness is in part due to the physiologic or neurochemical effects of relaxation. Relaxation techniques are known to produce a general decrease in indices of sympathetic arousal;[14] this and other studies in sympathetic physiologic arousal have shown this decrease in patients who practice relaxation techniques.[6,7] However, in this study the patients who had the most noticeable decrease in physiological arousal were not necessarily those who had the best antiemetic effect from the interventions. Several investigations have identified the strong association between the sedation and effectiveness of the pharmacologic antiemetic.[10,15-17] Indeed, all effective antiemetic drugs have noticeable sedative effects.[17] Although there is considerable agreement that a sense of relaxation or sedation plays an essential role in the effectiveness of antiemetic interventions, the association still remains speculative.

It is interesting to note that the subjects' State anxiety scores did not significantly change over the course of treatment for the subjects. Theoretically, the State (S) anxiety score should change and the Trait (T) anxiety score should remain the same. Perhaps the S and T anxiety scores are reflecting a ripple effect from the chemotherapy situation and not an actual personality trait. Another study has identified an unusual change in patients' anxiety scores associated with chemotherapy.[18]

Psychological and Physical Control

Several investigators explain that behavioral strategies may enhance a patient's perceived sense of control.[1,2,5,6,10] The feeling of increased self-control may decrease feelings of helplessness and hopelessness, promoting an improved psychologic, affective state. Unfortunately, the phenomenon of improved control is difficult to measure. To date no empirical data exists to support the hypothesis of improved control. However, it is interesting to note that recognized experts in the area of antiemetic behavioral interventions consistently mention the patient's response of "feeling better" and more "in control" after learning a behavioral strategy.

The idea of improved physical (muscle) control has been mentioned. Deep muscle relaxation (especially the abdominal muscles) accompanied with controlled steady breathing may directly inhibit the sequence of events necessary for vomiting to occur. Electromyographic and electrophysiological measurements on abdominal muscles and the act of vomiting have not been obtained but are potential areas for interesting research.[17,19] This study and three pediatric studies have shown a greater reduction in vomiting than in nausea as a result of PMR.[20-22] Two patients in this study (both young men with testicular cancer receiving a highly emetogenic drug regimen) stated they were able to control vomiting using PMR but continued to experience profound nausea. Perhaps the patients were able to interfere with the abdominal and diaphramatic muscle contractions that induce vomiting, but unable to alter the stimuli that caused nausea.

Diversion

Several investigators have reported that behavioral interventions serve to divert the patients' attentions away from the noxious stimuli and help them concentrate and recall more pleasant sensations and stimuli.[1,7,21,22] However, in this study, the patients in the TAG placebo group did not differ from the no-treatment control group. Therefore, the TAG placebo either was not as strong a cognitive distraction as PMR, or distraction is only part of the effectiveness of a behavioral intervention. Another aspect of diversion that may be responsible for the behavioral intervention's effectiveness is the patient's perception of the novelty and even humor of the intervention. Many patients in this study really enjoyed practicing relaxation therapy. They would approach the chemotherapy event with noticeable and under standable dread but they would intermittently display light-hearted, almost whimsical behavior. The use of humor and laughter as a cognitive distraction remains to be investigated.

Behavioral Intervention/Drug Interaction

Finally, a possible reason for the mechanism of action of behavioral interventions is that the relaxation technique enhances the pharmacologic effects of the antiemetic drug, possibly via some unknown neurochemical interaction. Two patients in the study reported that PMR was helpful to them because they would take their oral antiemetics, practice PMR and were able to delay vomiting for at least 45 minutes. They believed the combination allowed them to attain a better blood concentration of the antiemetic drug and therefore more sedation and antiemetic effect. This poses another potential research area as the use of effective oral antiemetics is convenient for outpatient therapy and for patients who require self-medication while at home.

SUMMARY

The findings in this and other investigations show that behavioral interventions are potentially effective in reducing chemotherapy-related side effects of nausea, vomiting, anorexia, and anxiety. The mechanisms by which relaxation or other behavioral interventions produce their effect is not known. While some mechanisms have been hypothesized, none have been adequately investigated. Issues such as mechanism of action, behavioral intervention enhancing the antiemetic drug effect and visa versa, large scale clinical feasibility, selection of the optimum behavioral intervention for each patient, and patient variables that enhance effectiveness are all questions that can only be answered by further research.

REFERENCES

1. Redd, W., Andersen, G., Minagawa, R. (1982). Hypnotic control of anticipatory emesis in patients receiving cancer chemotherapy. *Journal of Consulting and Clinical Psychology*, 50(3), 14–19.
2. Burish, T., Shartner, C., & Lyles, J. (1981). Effectiveness of multiple-site EMG biofeedback and relaxation in reducing the aversiveness of cancer chemotherapy. *Biofeedback and Self-Regulation*, 6(2), 523–533.
3. Morrow, G., & Morrell, C. (1982). Behavioral treatment for the anticipatory nausea and vomiting induced by cancer chemotherapy. *New England Journal of Medicine*, 307(24), 1476–1480.
4. Burish, T., & Lyles, J. (1981). Effectiveness of relaxation training in reducing adverse reactions to chemotherapy. *Journal of Behavioral Medicine*, 4(1), 65–68.
5. Burish, T., & Lyles, J. (1979). Effectiveness of relaxation training in reducing the aversiveness of chemotherapy in the treatment of cancer.

Behavior Treatment Experiments in Psychiatry, 10(4), 357–361.
6. Cotanch, P. (1983). Relaxation training for control of nausea and vomiting in patients receiving chemotherapy. *Cancer Nursing, 6*(4), 277–283.
7. Lyles, J., Burish, T., Krozely, M., & Oldham, R. (1982). Efficacy of relaxation training and guided imagery in reducing the aversiveness of cancer chemotherapy. *Journal of Consulting and Clinical Psychology, 50*(4), 509–529.
8. Nicholas, D. (1982). Prevalence of anticipatory nausea and emesis in cancer chemotherapy patients. *Journal of Behavioral Medicine, 5*(3), 461–463.
9. Morrow, G. (1982). Prevalences and correlates of anticipatory nausea and vomiting in chemotherapy patients. *Journal of the National Cancer Institute, 68*, 585–588.
10. Burish, T., & Corey, M. (1984). Conditioned responses to cancer chemotherapy: Etiology and treatment. In B. H. Fox & B. H. Newberry (Eds.), *Impact of psychoendocrine systems in cancer and immunity* pp. 147–178. Toronto: C. J. Hogrefe.
11. Lazarus, R., Averill, J., & Opton, T. (1974). The psychology of coping: Issues of research, and assessment. In C. Coelho, D. Hamburg, & J. Adams (Eds.), *Coping and adaptation.* New York: Basic Books.
12. Laszlo, J., Lucas, V., Hanson, D., Cronin, C., & Sallen, S. (1981). Levonantradol for chemotherapy-induced emesis: Phase I-II oral administration. *Journal of Clinical Pharmacology, 121*(8,9), 518–565.
13. Benjamin, L. (1967). Facts and artifacts in using analysis of covariance to "undo" the law of initial values. *Psychophysiology, 4*(1), 178–206.
14. Burish, T., Hendrix, E., & Frost, R. (1981). Comparison of frontal EMG biofeedback and several types of relaxation instruction in reducing multiple indices of arousal. *Psychophysiology, 18*(4), 594–602.
15. Laszlo, J. (1983). *Antiemetics and cancer chemotherapy.* Baltimore: Williams & Wilkins.
16. Scott, D., Donahue, D., Mastrovito, R., & Hokes, R. (1983). The antiemetic effect of clinical relaxation. Report of an exploratory pilot study. *Journal of Psy. Oncology, 1*(1), 71–84.
17. Stoudemire, A., Cotanch, P., & Laszlo, J. (1984). Recent advances in the pharmacologic and behavioral management of chemotherapy-induced emesis. *Archives of Internal Medicine, 144*(6), 1029–1033.
18. Rhodes, V., Watson, P., & Johnson, M. (1985). Association of chemotherapy-related nausea and vomiting with pre-treatment and post-treatment anxiety. *Oncology Nursing Forum, 13*(1), 41–47.
19. Cotanch, P. (1984). Measurement of nausea and vomiting in clinical nursing research. *Oncology Nursing Forum, 11*(3), 92–94.
20. Zelter, L., LeBaron, S., & Zelter, P. (1984). The effectiveness of behavior interventions for reducing nausea and vomiting in children receiving chemotherapy. *Journal of Clinical Oncology, 2*(3), 683–690.
21. LeBaron, S., & Zelter, L. (1982). Behavioral treatment for control of chemotherapy-related nausea and vomiting in children and adolescents with cancer. *Pediatric Research, 16*(4), 208A.
22. Cotanch, P., Hockenberry, M., & Herman, S. (1985). Self-hypnosis as antiemetic therapy in children receiving chemotherapy. *Oncology Nursing Forum, 12*(4), 41–46.

This article is printed with permission of *Oncology Nursing Forum.*

Original article:
Cotanch, P. H., & Strum, S. (1987). Progressive muscle relaxation as antiemetic therapy for cancer patients. *Oncology Nursing Forum, 14*(1), 33–37.

CRITIQUE BY: THERESA LERCH, BSN, RN

Part I: Clinical Relevance

Cotanch and Strum studied the clinical problem of whether progressive muscle relaxation (PMR), as an early intervention, could be effective in decreasing drug-related nausea and vomiting in patients beginning chemotherapy. Prolonged nausea and vomiting often are the most adverse side-effects for patients receiving chemotherapy and can impact whether or not patients choose to continue with the treatment plan. The investigators defined PMR as a behavioral intervention that can be learned by patients and later utilized as a coping strategy when the behavioral response of nausea and vomiting develops from chemotherapy. In addition, the investigators expanded the scope of their study population by suggesting that PMR is practical and applicable for any patients demonstrating interest in exploring and developing their coping strategies.

The clinical problem and interventions studied are relevant and important to the practice of nursing. The study's results demonstrated an effective alternative intervention to the commonly prescribed pharmacologic antiemetics for chemotherapy-related nausea and vomiting. In addition, the investigators suggested that the behavioral intervention of PMR could potentially promote patient participation and independence in the treatment plan, thus fostering an improved self-concept.

Stress response theory, which states that the patient's response is a product of his or her appraisal of environmental stimuli, guided this research. In this context, PMR was presented as a relaxation response to an existing stress, chemotherapy. The intervention of PMR provided the patient with a tool to alter perceptions of the stimuli and achieve the desired outcome, decreased nausea and vomiting.

The study involved a randomized three-group design consisting of an experimental group with a therapist-directed taped PMR, a placebo control group that listened to relaxing, taped music while a therapist was present, and a true control group with no intervention.

The experimental group listened to a 22-minute instructional tape about PMR that involved tensing and relaxing exercises for 16 muscle groups from head to feet. The tape also presented a brief hypnotic relaxing scene that encouraged feelings of alertness, while also suggesting ways to increase appetite during and after chemotherapy. The tape sessions involved the patient listening to the tape twice a day and again while receiving chemotherapy. The investigator served as the therapist and spent an average of 20 minutes with each patient during the post-relaxation phase at the end of the tape listening sessions.

The placebo control group also listened to a 22-minute tape that consisted of relaxing music without instruction for relaxation exercises. However, patients were instruction to think only pleasant thoughts during the tape session and later to share their thoughts with the therapist. The true control group received only the standard antiemetic procedure of the institution and therapist contact during the completion of the evaluation scales.

Standard antiemetic therapy was offered to all subjects; the therapist neither advised for nor against its use. The Duke Descriptive Scale (DDS) was used to measure nausea and vomiting at the time of drug infusion and 48 hours afterwards; the patient's activity level was the criterion for assessing severity of nausea and vomiting. When used in previous pharmacologic antiemetic trials, the DDS offered acceptable reliability and validity data.

The Speilberger State-Trait Anxiety Inventory (STAI) was used to measure the subjects' anxiety levels during chemotherapy. This measure involved the subjects' assessments of how they felt during the drug infusion. It was administered a second time two to three days after discharge to measure their feelings about chemotherapy treatments.

Each patient kept a diary of all oral foods and fluids. At each hospital admission, skin fold thickness was measured, using the Lange Skin Fold Caliper. Other measurements involved weights and vital signs at admission and discharge. These measures were used to evaluate the patient's caloric intake during the chemotherapy regimen in an attempt to correlate caloric intake with the degree of nausea and vomiting.

The DDS is a measurement tool that can be implemented by independent nursing action. The scale rates the degree of nausea and vomiting according to frequency of episodes and extent of interference with the patient's activity. The objective rating of the scale facilitates accurate measurement of the patient's condition, is clear, concise, and easily utilized without extra expense or education of the staff. However, Cotanch and Strum did not fully discuss the STAI, making it difficult to assess its usefulness and practicality for utilization by the nurse. Nonetheless, the STAI measures data that are critical to the overall utilization of the research findings and are worthy of obtaining, since the interventions are based on altering perceptions of stimuli impact on stress response. Using the Lange Skin Fold Caliper and measuring vital signs also are independent nursing actions and provide vital information regarding the patient's physiologic response to the interventions.

Part II: Conceptualization and Internal Consistency

The investigators base conceptualization and internal consistency of the study on stress response theory which supports the development of PMR intervention. The investigators also state their operational definitions and attempt to evaluate the intervention by measuring various changes in the subject who is at risk for nausea and vomiting. Independent and dependent variables are logically related, given that, if PMR is effective, there will be a noticeable decease in nausea and vomiting according to the patient's own assessment, no deterioration in the patient's feelings related to chemotherapy, and improved patient physical state as evidenced by an increase in weight, or maintenance of present weight. The measurement instruments, which appeared appropriate for the area of interest, were previously tested for reliability and validity in similar environments.

Unfortunately, the investigators neglect to state a hypothesis of response outcome for each group in the study. The lack of stated hypotheses does not weaken the study design per se, but it does present the reader with an ambiguous perception of the investigators' projected assessment of the interventions and outcomes.

The investigators presented study findings clearly and with statistical testing to determine the effectiveness of PMR intervention. The investigators also included an indepth discussion of the potentially interrelated factors that led to the success or failure of the intervention, since the actual mechanisms by which behavioral interventions produce their effect are not known. This discussion allowed the reader to conclude that the investigators made every attempt to clarify the mechanisms of action of PMR.

Part III: Believability of Results

The study purported to test the effects of PMR as a nursing intervention for decreasing the frequency and duration of nausea and vomiting related to chemotherapy. The measurements utilized in the study consisted of numerically quantified information regarding the degree of nausea and vomiting, the patient's anxiety level during and after chemotherapy, and physiologic responses.

Entry criteria for prospective subjects included being admitted to an inpatient oncology unit, and receiving an initial course of chemotherapy that included a series of infusions known to have greater than a 60 percent emetogenic effect. Clinical evidence of metastatic brain disease or gastrointestinal obstruction excluded prospective subjects. The investigators then randomized subjects into the three previously explained treatment groups and followed them for five consecutive chemotherapy courses consisting of one baseline with no application of interventions and three or four follow-up intervention sessions.

The investigators identified therapist contact with subjects of the placebo-control group as a potential intervening variable, since the therapist's time was identified as being "nonspecific" when compared with the experimental group's therapist contact. The investigators also attempted to control this intervening variable by providing a tape of relaxing music and facilitating a discussion of feelings about relaxation, enjoyment, and pleasant thoughts with the placebo-control group.

The investigators noted no statistical differences among the three groups' baselines in the DDS, the anxiety scores, and caloric intake. The investigators also determined whether the patients' baseline findings affected their subsequent responses. Statistical analysis revealed that a free measure of change was likely since there was no significant association between the initial scores.

Unfortunately, the investigators did not report reliability and validity data for the instruments utilized. Although the investigators mention that the DDS was previously used with acceptable reliability and validity, they provide no specific data. In regard to the STAI, the investigators did not report reliability and validity data, as well; they only described the instrument as having been developed to investigate anxiety phenomena in "normal adults." Accordingly, the investigators' descriptions of the instruments are vague. However, their references to prior usage lead the reader to believe that the instruments are appropriate for the study.

The investigators reported that 60 patients were followed over 12 months, comprising a total data base of 282 observations. The demographics of the 60 subjects revealed a similar median age and equal distribution of gender and types of cancer throughout the three groups.

The investigators report their results utilizing repeated measures analysis of variance models for follow-up data, the Pearson Product Moment Correlation Coefficient for determining the affect of the patients' baseline data on their subsequent responses, and the Spearman Rank Correlation Coefficient for testing the effects of the pre- and post-treatments on systolic and diastolic blood pressure, pulse, and respirations. The chosen statistical analysis appears appropriate for the study. Results indicate that there were statistically significant differences for the variables of vomiting ($p = .03$), trait anxiety ($p = .05$), and caloric intake ($p = .001$). The dependent variable of state anxiety was not statistically significant.

Systolic and diastolic blood pressures and pulse rates of the experimental and placebo-control groups also demonstrated a statistical significance of $p = .001$. Between the three groups, the patients' weight at admission and discharge did not change significantly, nor did skin caliper measurements.

In addition, the investigators found no correlation between practice frequency and the antiemetic effect of PMR. Nor did the amount or type of antiemetics administered to patients change during the study. This controlled for the possibility of an intervening variable, such as a new antiemetic with increased effectiveness for decreasing the patient's nausea and vomiting.

Unfortunately, the investigators' selection of table content to report statistical outcomes was poor. Two tables of particular importance presented data by reporting the range of patient responses on the DDS, or the raw numbers of those subjects' outcomes described as improved, no change, or worse in relation to the intervention. Such tables could have been greatly enhanced by reporting a mean or median for each group's response, since the data were objective responses on a designated scale. The use of a range to report the outcome of a scale reading that has only four values tells nothing about how the scores are dispersed or what the most frequently occurring value for each group is. It leaves the reader with a sense that the differences reported were minimal.

In this study, the investigators demonstrated that PMR and positive suggestions were effective interventions for partially decreasing the side effects of nausea and vomiting resulting from chemotherapy. They clearly acknowledged that the exact mechanisms of such behavioral interventions as PMR are not known, but go on to postulate, with support of other research studies, an explanation for the effectiveness of PMR.

The investigators identified relaxation as a technique to produce a general decrease in the sympathetic response of neurochemical and physiologic reactions. They measured this decrease by differences in systolic and diastolic blood pressure and pulse rate. They also identified the degree and effect of relaxation as potentially improving the pharmacologic effects of the antiemetic drug. However, they expressed some skepticism regarding this explanation.

The investigators also mentioned deep muscle relaxation, especially of abdominal muscles, as an explanation for PMR outcomes. They speculated that deep muscle relaxation, along with controlled steady breathing, may decrease vomiting by inhibiting the required sequence of physiologic events that precedes vomiting. This explanation is supported by the study's finding that no statistical difference was noted for nausea and state anxiety during actual chemotherapy infusions.

The investigators reported distraction as a possible mechanism for the effectiveness of behavioral interventions, as supported by several other studies. However, this study's findings did not support the mechanism of distraction. In fact, no difference was noted between the placebo-control and the control group. The investigators concluded, therefore, that either the music was not a strong enough distraction or distraction was not a significant mechanism for the effectiveness of behavioral interventions.

The last mechanism of action described by the investigators concerns enhancement of the pharmacologic effects of an antiemetic drug by relaxation techniques. The investigators speculated that some unknown neurochemical interaction occurs that produces a synergistic effect. Possibly, relaxation serves as a form of sedation which enhances the effects of the antiemetic drug.

Part IV: Generalizability of Results

The research study presented interventions that are appropriate and relevant to the current practice of nursing. Behavioral interventions are an accepted form of nursing practice. The sample and setting targeted in the research is characteristic of populations in specific environments that could benefit from the use of a behavioral intervention like PMR. The study mentions various other studies that have presented similar results in similar settings so that the reader is able to judge the degree of support for the stated hypothesis.

Part V: Other Factors to Consider in Utilization

Adapting the study's results for individual or institution-wide use is feasible. Implementation would require the teaching of the relaxation techniques of PMR to all nurses, in addition to the development of a taped explanation of the relaxation technique for viewing by patients. Use of the measurement scales would require reproducing the described objective scales. Physiologic measurements, such as vital sign changes, are already being obtained in all nursing settings. In general, then, the potential cost for implementing these interventions would be minimal; an inservice education format could easily meet the needs for nursing eduction. The major cost of the project would come from the development of the taped explanation.

Utilizing such behavioral interventions as reported would provide the patient with either an alternative or complimentary treatment for reducing the nausea and vomiting associated with chemotherapy. The addition of another possible treatment for patients' nausea and vomiting could improve the patients' comfort, quality of daily living, and make the difference between compliance with or refusal of chemotherapy. Implementation of an effective intervention, such as PMR, for related side effects of chemotherapy clearly outweighs the risk of a worsened prognosis for those patients who decline treatment because of such side effects. This fact alone and the projected minimal cost of implementation suggest that the benefits outweigh the risks of not utilizing effective behavioral interventions for related side effects of chemotherapy.

Original article:
Cotanch, P. H., & Strum, S. (1987). Progressive muscle relaxation as antiemetic therapy for cancer patients. *Oncology Nursing Forum, 14*(1), 33–37.

CRITIQUE BY: CHAROLD BAER, PhD, RN

Part I: Clinical Relevance

Cotanch and Strum state that their study focuses on a specific clinical problem: using the behavioral intervention of progressive muscle relaxation (PMR) to decrease drug-related nausea and vomiting in patients receiving their initial course of chemotherapy with highly emetogenic drugs. The study design, however, suggests that they also are interested in determining the effect of PMR, imagery, and suggestion on general anxiety, and physiologic arousal and caloric intake in relation to chemotherapy. Their study results could contribute much to clinical practice in view of the following: (1) the frequency of occurrence of nausea and vomiting in patients as signs and symptoms of physiologic, pathophysiologic, psychologic, or pharmacologic processes; (2) the interrelationship of nausea and vomiting, and anxiety, physiological arousal, and caloric intake; (3) the noninvasive nature of behavioral interventions; (4) the minimal risks accompanying the implementation of behavioral interventions; and (5) the ease of implementation of behavioral interventions. Thus, because nurses frequently assist patients in coping with nausea and vomiting and anxiety, this study is clinically relevant and its findings could enhance patient care.

The clinical value of this study rests on its ability to identify a behavioral nursing intervention that is effective in treating human responses to chemotherapy. The addition of an effective behavioral intervention to other more invasive types of interventions provides the clinician with great latitude in decision making regarding patient care. Also, if a behavioral intervention is effective, it could decrease the use of pharmacologic agents in treating nausea and vomiting and eliminate the possibility of drug-induced patient complications.

PMR technique, which involved the patient listening to a 22-minute instructional audio tape on how to perform tensing and relaxing exercises for 16 muscle groups from head to feet, was the behavioral intervention tested in this study. In addition, the tape also included a brief hypnotic induction for the patient to feel alert and refreshed and suggestions to stimulate the appetite to consume nutritious foods during and after chemotherapy. Perhaps the study would have been strengthened if the design were narrowed and the audio tape had focused only on PMR technique. The inclusion of other "suggestions" added variables that also could effect nausea and vomiting and anxiety and, thus, confound the study results. Any, and all, of the components of the behavioral intervention could, however, be implemented by the staff nurse in clinical practice. In fact, all of the components are currently used in practice for a variety of purposes, including assisting the patient in decreasing stress, anxiety, and pain. The decision to implement such interventions with patients is within the scope of nursing practice and requires no additional approval or consultations with other members of the health care hierarchy.

In this study, the investigators measured the dependent variables—nausea and vomiting, caloric intake, physiologic arousal, and general anxiety—by the Duke Descriptive Scale, a diary of oral fluids and foods ingested for two days following chemotherapy, the Lange Skin Fold Calipers, body weights, systolic and diastolic blood pressure, pulse rate, respirations, and the Speilberger State-Trait Anxiety Inventory. With the exception of the Duke Scale and the Speilberger Inventory, such measures are frequently used to assess patients in the clinical setting. However, while the Duke Scale and Speilberger Inventory could easily be used with some patients, the practicality of their use with all patients is questionable. Still, because all these measures fall within the scope of nursing practice, they could be used at the clinician's discretion.

In general, this study appears to be clinically relevant. Its results could contribute much to the body of knowledge currently used to guide nursing practice. Therefore, this study merits further evaluation for utilization in practice.

Part II: Conceptualization and Internal Consistency

The investigators have written their study with logic and some conceptual consistency. However, their introduction, which initially leads one to conclude the PMR constitutes the independent variable while nausea and vomiting constitute the dependent variables, does not parallel the study design. The study design indicates that suggestion and imagery also constitute independent variables while caloric intake, physiologic arousal, and general anxiety constitute dependent variables. Therefore, conceptual consistency depends upon the reader disregarding the introduction. However, one wonders why the investigators elected to expand the study and include other variables, rather than address the clinical problem stated in the purpose. In this regard, it may be difficult to discern exactly what is responsible for differences in the subjects, if differences are indeed found.

The investigators clearly articulated justification for their study, which is drawn from clinical practice and substantiated by previous research. However, as mentioned, their conceptual framework is too terse to support the inclusion of the additional independent and dependent variables. One develops a sense of what is involved and what the relationships are, but one cannot easily deduce the study design from the conceptual framework presented. In addition, the investigators studied several variables that they did not adequately address in their justification or conceptual framework.

The operational definitions used for variables are appropriate, but perhaps not sufficient. For example, perhaps vital signs are not the only, nor the most accurate, assessment parameters for determining physiologic arousal. Also, what is the relationship between physiologic arousal and nausea and vomiting, or between physiologic arousal and PMR? While all of these may be related, it is difficult to discern how and why they were included as part of this study design.

Again, and for the aforesaid reasons, the logical relationships among all independent and dependent variables are somewhat obscure and open to misinterpretation. On the other hand, the subjects chosen for the study are consistent with the target population of interest and the measurement instruments used are appropriate for assessing the phenomena of concern. Also, data collection procedures are consistent with usual patient care activities and processes and, thus, should not bias the results.

While there do seem to be inconsistencies or inadequacies in the conceptualization of this study, its results may still add important information to the body of knowledge currently used to guide clinical practice. Therefore, the study merits continued cautious evaluation for use in clinical settings. Perhaps the complexities of the phenomena of interest necessitate such a multivariate approach. However, one would expect all aspects to be clearly detailed in the conceptualization.

Part III: Believability of Results

This study purported to test the effects of the behavioral interventions of PMR, imagery, and suggestion through the analysis of quantitative data. The investigators selected a convenience sample of 60 subjects from patients admitted to an inpatient oncology clinical research unit for their initial course of chemotherapy. Other inclusion criteria included: (1) receiving a multiple course of chemotherapy; (2) receiving a chemotherapeutic regimen that had an emetogenic potential of greater than 60 percent; and (3) having no clinical evidence of metastatic brain disease or gastrointestinal obstruction. The investigators randomly assigned the 60 subjects to one of three treatment groups and followed them over a 12-month period. The three treatment groups—the experimental group, the placebo control group, and the actual control group—all received care reflective of the current standard of practice.

Unfortunately, the investigators neglected to discuss the potential biases and threats to the internal validity of this study. One would have expected them to acknowledge the possible threats of selection, history, and maturation. They did note that "data were obtained on demographic and clinical variables to determine potential associations and/or biases in the study or treatment interventions and to identify potential correlates." In addition, they did statistically analyze baseline data to determine that there were no statistically significant differences among the groups and no significant associations between the initial subject scores.

The investigators also were negligent in discussing reliability and validity data for measures of the dependent variables. They note that the Duke Descriptive Scale had acceptable reliability and validity in previous uses, but they never present data to support this assertion. In regard to the Speilberger State-Trait Anxiety Inventory, their study suffers from the same omission; they only note that the instrument was developed to investigate anxiety phenomena in normal adults. One wonders if this inventory also is useful for assessing anxiety in ill adults. In addition, it is questionable whether a patient's vital signs are reflective of physiologic arousal for "fight or flight." In fact, there are numerous other patient responses involved in that process that could have been selected for greater accuracy. For example, there are circulating catecholamine levels. Also, it is possible that the measurement of skin fold thickness is not appropriate for assessing caloric intake in a patient with a catabolic disease, such as cancer. Finally, the investigators did not present any data regarding interrater reliability, so one may assume that all data were collected by the same individual. If such is the case, the potential for bias is present and should be addressed.

The investigators report study results both narratively and in tabular form. However, the reporting of ranges of values in relation to the variables for each treatment group was not helpful. Perhaps including a mean would have made the data more useful. The statistical tests used to analyze the data appear to be appropriate. Yet one does wonder why the investigators specifically chose to use the Spearman Rank Correlation Coefficient rather than Kendall's Tau. Again, the investigators present no rationale for their choice.

The conclusions drawn from the study results lose some credibility because the experimental treatment included three components—PMR, imagery, and suggestion—any one of which could have been responsible for the results. The investigators briefly acknowledge the lack of strength of the conclusions and then expend much energy discussing possible mechanisms for the effectiveness of PMR. Their first summary statement, however, seems to capture the essence of their conclusions: "The findings in this and other investigations show that behavioral interventions are *potentially* effective in reducing chemotherapy-related side effects of nausea, vomiting, anorexia and anxiety." In their study, however, they found no significant differences for nausea or state anxiety.

In general, the study results provide some interesting information that should be cautiously considered while continuing evaluation for utilization occurs.

Part IV: Generalizability of Results

There are a number of similarities between the methods and procedures employed in this study and those used in current clinical practice. The sample is typical of the target population of patients admitted to any oncology unit for the first course of chemotherapy. The setting is slightly atypical because it is an inpatient oncology clinical research unit, which usually differs from a standard oncology unit. The interventions implemented were similar to those used in everyday practice and one of the individuals implementing the study was a nurse. In this regard, none of the behavioral interventions would require that a nurse receive additional education for implementation.

There are other studies that have investigated various types of behavioral interventions and their effects on anticipatory nausea and vomiting. Many of these studies have noted results similar to the current study, and thus lend support for the concept. Some studies, however, have not noted clearly delineated positive results. Thus, it appears that more research is needed prior to drawing specific conclusions regarding the effectiveness of these interventions.

In general, there are some threats to the external validity of this study, including selection, Hawthorn effect, possible experimenter bias, and novelty. Therefore, one would want to cautiously continue in evaluating the results of this study for utilization in clinical practice.

Part V: Other Factors to Consider in Utilization

Implementation of study results in clinical practice is feasible. In order for a systematic evaluation to be conducted, however, it would need to be narrowed and include more practical measurements. Staff nurses could, but are not likely to, use the Speilberger Inventory to assess anxiety states. Also, in order to be useful, physiologic arousal would need to be more specifically defined than just by alterations in vital signs.

The risks of implementing these behavioral interventions in practice are minimal. Having a patient listen to an audio tape describing PMR technique, certain relaxing images, and suggestions for increasing appetite is not likely to damage his or her psyche or result in physiologic injury. Indeed, changing practice to include these interventions might aid the patient in experiencing less nausea and vomiting associated with chemotherapy, in requiring lower doses of antiemetic agents, and in acquiring an additional strategy to use in coping with stress. In this regard, to *maintain* current practice involves its own risk: patients may continue to experience debilitating episodes of nausea and vomiting in association with chemotherapy and decide to terminate therapy. No doubt, such a decision is likely to hasten the patient's demise.

Implementing study results would not be expensive. In most institutions, staff nurses would need no additional education to initiate implementation. In fact, many nurses currently use these strategies daily in clinical practice. Thus, there would not be additional educational or personnel costs engendered by implementation. However, in order to duplicate the methods used in this study, it would be necessary to obtain a copy of the audio tape, or to produce a replica, which would necessitate some minimal expenditure of funds.

In general, the benefits of utilizing the study results in practice seem to outweigh the risks, even though the exact mechanisms of action are not clear, and several behavioral interventions seem to be combined in the treatment. These unknowns and flaws suggest that further research is necessary and that cautious utilization be recommended.

Pressure Sores Nursing Management

Anne Boykin, PhD, MSN, RN
Director and Associate Professor
Division of Nursing
Florida Atlantic University
Boca Raton, FL

Jill Winland-Brown, EdD, MS, RN
Assistant Professor
Division of Nursing
Florida Atlantic University
Boca Raton, FL

A great deal of time and energy continues to be devoted to the prevention and treatment of pressure sores. Statistics compiled by the Stop Pressure Sores in Florida campaign estimated that "500,000 persons nationally suffer from decubitus ulcers ... Some 3.5 million persons in the US are considered at risk of getting pressure sores, 165,000 in Florida alone."[1] Fowler states "an estimated 30% of nursing home residents develop pressure sores."[2] Although the literature abounds with information on preventing and treating pressure sores, there remains no simple solution to this relentless problem.

Escalating healthcare costs have resulted in heightened consumer awareness of cost for essential services. In this era of cost containment, health professionals are responsible for examining healthcare practices over which they have control or influence for cost and effectiveness. One example of such a practice is the wide variety of treatments currently used to heal pressure sores.

Both intrinsic and extrinsic factors that cause prolonged compression on an area encourage the development of pressure sores.[3] Examples of factors contributing to skin breakdown are immobility, metabolic conditions, peripheral-vascular impairment, paralysis, malnutrition, and incontinence. Nursing care of clients with potential or actual pressure sores includes prevention and management.

This study addressed both these nursing components. It was designed to *evaluate* whether adherence to prescribed prevention guidelines for clients who were determined to be at risk resulted in improvement in their risk status. The second purpose was to *compare* the effectiveness of hydrocolloid occlusive dressing with povidone-iodine therapy in the treatment of pressure sores.

REVIEW OF THE LITERATURE

Nursing literature expounds on the multiple factors that contribute to the development of pressure sores. Prevention of pressure sores depends on how well these contributing factors are eliminated, diminished, or counteracted. Localized ischemia due to pressure is the primary factor contributing to the development of pressure sores.[4] Relief of pressure on bony prominences can be accomplished by using specialized mattresses and good turning protocols.

Assessing the skin frequently, improving a client's nutritional status, maintaining clean, dry skin, and teaching prevention guidelines all facilitate the prevention of pressure sores. Tooman and Patterson[5] encouraged the use of Ensure®, a liquid nutritional supplement, three times daily for all clients who had pressure sores, and improvement in the sores was evident in 20 days. Maintenance of clean, dry skin is of utmost importance since incontinence has been identified as a factor that may increase the risk of an immobile client developing pressure sores.[2,4]

Patient education is identified, however, as one of the most important factors in the prevention of pressure sores. Prevention guidelines need to address what can be done to eliminate, diminish, or counteract the contributing factors that lead to the development of pressure sores. Subjects to be taught to clients and families include skin management activity and nutritional guidelines. Patient teaching is more effective when both verbal and written methods are used.[2,6]

An informal survey of local home health agencies in the community revealed that povidone-iodine and hydrocolloid occlusive dressing (HCD) were two of the most common treatment modalities for pressure sores. HCD is a semisynthetic, relatively oxygen impermeable occlusive dressing. It consists of a pliable, water resistant outer layer and an inner layer containing hydroactive particles that interact with wound fluid.[7] The composition of this dressing allows for prolonged use and easy application.

Studies by Galub, Friedman, and Yarkony[3,7,8] indicate a marked improvement in the healing of pressure sores through the use of HCD. It was determined that the longer the period of application, the greater the ulcer response to HCD. Galub[7] reports that a lack of oxygen may, in fact, stimulate capillary growth. The promotion of granulation tissue is cited as a distinct advantage of hydrocolloid dressing.[8]

Povidone-iodine as a treatment modality for pressure sores was selected for study because of the frequency of use in many healthcare settings in southeast Florida, despite the virtual absence of research support. Documentation of povidone-iodine as an effective treatment modality for pressure sores is limited. Studies have determined that the topical application of povidone-iodine to manage infections associated with pressure sores and burns was effective.[9,10]

STUDY METHODS AND PROCEDURES

Based on the literature review, the first hypothesis stated there would be a significant difference between the initial Norton score and the score recorded following adherence to prevention guidelines by clients identified as being at risk. The Norton scale consists of five categories measuring observable data that can be assessed in a few moments time. These categories include physical condition, mental condition, activity, mobility, and incontinence. A score of 14 or below indicates that the client is at risk for developing pressure sores. The second hypothesis tested whether there would be a significant difference in the degree of effectiveness of HCD over povidone-iodine in the treatment of pressure sores.

The sample consisted of clients from two home health agencies who met the inclusion criteria of having either a Norton score of 14 or less, or an existing pressure sore. Twenty-one subjects, 15 females and 6 males, were obtained by convenience sampling. All clients lived at home and were at least 65 years of age. Ages ranged from 67 to 96 with an average age of 83. Eleven subjects had pressure sores and the remaining 10 were at risk on the Norton scale, but did not have pressure sores.

The sample for the first hypothesis included all 21 subjects. Subgroups for the second hypothesis consisted of 5 subjects from one home health agency with a total of 11 pressure sores treated with povidone-iodine, and 6 subjects from the second agency with a total of 10 pressure sores treated with HCD. The length of time in the study ranged from 1 to 12 weeks, with an average inclusion of 6.4 weeks.

A Norton scale score was obtained on the initial visit to establish a baseline score and at 1-week intervals to assess the client's potential for developing pressure sores. After the initial Norton score was completed the nurse instructed all at-risk clients and their families in the prevention guidelines. These guidelines addressed skin management, activity, and nutrition. Instructions were both verbal and written. A pamphlet, titled "Prevention Guidelines," was developed from the literature review with input from enterostomal therapists and registered nurses at the home health agencies used in this study.

Each client was visited weekly by the same

nurse. The weekly visit included reinforcement of the teaching program and reassessment on the Norton scale. Weekly Norton scores were graphed. Data collection extended over a period of 3 months at each agency.

The treatment protocols for povidone-iodine and HCD were developed in the same manner as the prevention guidelines. Each treatment procedure was demonstrated to participating staff, and copies of the procedure were distributed and discussed.

Instructions for treatment application were written in lay terminology to facilitate proper understanding by the client and family members. The investigators made random home visits with the home health nurses to determine compliance with designated protocol.

The first step in the treatment of a pressure sore was to obtain a baseline assessment of the area. Each ulcer was identified on a flow sheet according to location, stage, appearance, size, drainage, and odor. Direct measurement of the pressure sore was done by determining the sore diameter and depth using a wound size measurement scale.

Each pressure sore was evaluated on a weekly basis. Subjects were treated with povidone-iodine or HCD depending on the home health agency involved.

Table 1
Change in Size of Pressure Sores Before and After Treatment

Group	Client Number	Ulcer Number	Weeks in Study	Ulcer Size in cm (Prestudy)	Ulcer Size in cm (Poststudy)	Change After Treatment
I: Povidone-iodine*	1	1		>10	>10	0
		2	3-4	6	6	0
		3		3	3	0
		4		3	3	0
	2	5		6	6	0
		6	3-4	4	3	+1‡
		7		>10	>10	0
		8		4	4	0
	3	9	3-4	4	<1	+3
	4	10	1-2	4	4	0
	5	11	3-4	2	<1	+1
II: HCD†	6	12		5	4	+1
		13	9-10	5	7	−2§
		14		4	4	0
	7	15	12	2	<1	+1
	8	16	3-4	7	<1	+6
		17		4	<1	+3
	9	18	1-2	2	<1	+1
		19		2	<1	+1
	10	20	1-2	4	6	−2
	11	21	1-2	3	3	0

*Group I: Mean Score = .4545 cm, N = 11
†Group II: Mean Score = .9000 cm, N = 10
‡Pressure sores that show decrease in size.
§Pressure sores that show increase in size.

F statistic = .343, P = .565

Table 2
Change in Norton Score Before and After Treatment

Group	Client Number	Weeks in Study	Number of Ulcers Each	Norton Score (Prestudy)	Norton Score (Poststudy)	Norton Change
Povidone-iodine	1	3-4	4	7	8	+1
	2	3-4	4	6	15	+9
	3	3-4	1	14	14	0
	4	1-2	1	15	5	−10*
	5	3-4	1	12	12	0
HCD	6	9-10	3	8	7	−1
	7	12	1	13	13	0
	8	3-4	2	14	14	0
	9	1-2	2	13	15	+2
	10	1-2	1	13	13	0
	11	1-2	1	9	9	0
At Risk†	12	3-4		14	14	0
	13	3-4		15	7	−8*
	14	3-4		14	14	0
	15	11-12		7	9	+2
	16	11-12		13	14	+1
	17	11-12		8	7	−1
	18	11-12		14	14	0
	19	11-12		12	12	0
	20	11-12		11	11	0
	21	11-12		12	15	+3

*Client died
†χ^2 statistic = .949, P = .917
Cramer's ϕ = .150
Pearson's r = .040, P = .430

RESULTS AND DISCUSSION

Data were analyzed using SPSS on the UNIVAC 1100. The chi-square test for contingency was used to evaluate whether there was a significant change in the Norton scale score of at-risk clients after having been taught prevention guidelines. The results did not support the research hypothesis that there would be a significant difference between the initial Norton score and the score recorded following adherence to prevention guidelines by clients identified as being at risk.

The one-way analysis of variance was used to determine if there was a significant difference in the means of the two treatment groups. Although statistical results did not support the hypothesis that there would be a significant difference in the degree of effectiveness of HCD over povidone-iodine in the treatment of pressure sores, interesting patterns did emerge.

The pressure sores treated with HCD showed a decrease in size approximately twice that of povidone-iodine. The chi-square test for contingency revealed a trend that indicated HCD was better than povidone-iodine in effecting this change.

Although the sample size was too small to generalize findings to the total population, the statistical pattern indicated a trend that HCD may be more effective in the treatment of pressure sores than povidone-iodine.

Table 1 shows the difference in the size of the pressure sores prior to treatment and at the end of the study. Three sores treated with povidone-iodine decreased in size and 8 remained the same.

Of the pressure sores treated with HCD, 6 decreased in size, 2 remained the same, and 2 increased in size.

Table 2 demonstrates the change in Norton score for all subjects: those treated with povidone-iodine, those treated with HCD, and those in the at-risk category. The trend was that the Norton score either remained the same or improved. None of the 10 at-risk subjects developed a pressure sore during the 12-week period.

The importance of client teaching cannot be overlooked. Families and clients must be taught options, costs, advantages, and disadvantages of treatments. This approach places increased responsibility for health care on the consumer, promotes independence, and enhances commitment to achieving health goals. Professional caring requires that the client be the focus of holistic care.

More than ever, healthcare professionals are being required to be more responsible and accountable for high-quality, yet economical, health care. Nurses must take advantage of opportunities to identify and market nursing resources. When the physician asks nurses for input regarding treatment modalities for pressure sores, nursing resources should not be ignored.

CONCLUSION

In early studies on pressure sores it was said, "The avoidance of pressure sores is usually considered to be the concern of nurses and the occurrence of pressure sores regarded as a serious reflection on their skill."[11] Continuing research on pressure sores has demonstrated quite clearly the complexity of this nursing problem. This study brought to light, however, the question of whether good nursing care alone could heal pressure sores. It is frequently said that good nursing care prevents pressure sores; could it also heal existing sores? The time is ripe for nursing to recognize the many nursing resources that should be used in the design and implementation of quality, cost-effective nursing care.

REFERENCES

1. Arjemi, C. (1985, February 23). Statewide drive to eradicate decubitus ulcers launched in South Florida. *Florida Nursing News, 1*, 4.
2. Fowler, E. (1982). Pressure sores: A deadly nuisance. *Journal of Gerontological Nursing, 8*(12), 680–685.
3. Yarkony, G., Lukanc, C., & Carle, T. (1984). Pressure sore management: Efficacy of a moisture reactive occlusive dressing. *Archives of Physical Medicine and Rehabilitation, 65*(10), 597–600.
4. Reddy, M. P. (1983). Decubitus ulcers: Principles of prevention and management. *Geriatrics, 38*(7), 55–61.
5. Tooman, T., & Patterson, J. (1984). Decubitus ulcer warfare: Product vs process. *Geriatric Nursing, 5*(3), 166–167.
6. Andberg, M., Rudolph, A., & Anderson, T. (1983). Improving skin care through patient and family training. *Topics in Clinical Nursing, 5*(2), 45–54.
7. Galub, J. (1983). Wound dressing technology revives old concept: Don't expose wound to air. *Nursing Homes, 32*(5), 32–35.
8. Friedman, S. J., & Su, W. P. D. (1984). Management of leg ulcers with hydrocolloid occlusive dressing. *Archives of Dermatology, 120*(10), 1329–1336.
9. Lee, B., Trainor, F. S., & Thoden, W. R. (1979). Topical application of povidone-iodine in the management of decubitus and stasis ulcers. *Journal of the American Geriatric Society, 27*(7), 302–306.
10. deKock, M. (1985). Topical burn therapy comparing povidone-iodine ointment or cream plus aserbine, and povidone-iodine cream. *Journal of Hospital Infection, 6*(supplement), 127–132.
11. Norton, D., McLaren, R., & Exton-Smith, A. N. (1962). *An Investigation of geriatric nursing problems in hospital.* London: National Corporation for the Care of Old People, p. 236.

This article is printed with permission of *Journal of Gerontological Nursing*, 1986.

8

Nursing Care of the Elderly

Judy Miller, MSN, RN
Jelene MacLean, BSN, RN
Gail Perry, BSN, RN

INTRODUCTION BY: JUDY MILLER, MSN, RN

The scope of gerontological nursing, or nursing care of the elderly, is as broad and varied as the population it serves. In the past, *gerontological nursing* was commonly used to describe nursing related to healthy elderly, the normal aging process, and issues associated with the older population, such as retirement and access to transportation. *Geriatric nursing*, on the other hand, was usually taken to mean those nursing activities involving sick elderly or the diseases associated with old age.

As the knowledge base, intervention strategies and responsibilities, and practice settings of nurses who worked with the elderly grew in breadth and depth, the definitions became inadequate to correctly describe nursing practice. During the last few years, debate has grown over whether to change the name of nursing care with elderly clients to reflect its wide base of practice. As a result, the phrase, *gerontic nursing*, received some support. However, the more current move is to recognize that gerontological nursing includes elderly individuals, families, communities, and the institutions which serve them. With this perspective, the entire health spectrum also is addressed including: primary care involving health promotion, secondary care with the management of acute illness, and tertiary care including rehabilitation, prevention activities, and terminal care. For example, a gerontological nurse can be working with a retirement center to develop an exercise program for its members or be working in an intensive care unit providing direct care to an elderly patient and family.

The selection of nursing research studies for this chapter was undertaken with this current and broad view of gerontological nursing. Even so, it is impossible with three articles to fully reflect the scope of gerontological nursing practice and research. Thus, the student should read them with the recognition that they are only examples of the exciting and complex areas encountered by a nurse who works with the elderly.

The first study by Williams et al., "Reducing Acute Confusional States in Elderly Patients with Hip Fractures," was chosen because of its classic and pivotal nature. Although published in recent years, it is considered a classic and is cited in numerous studies involving acute confusional states (delirium) and hospitalized aged. This study is an extension of the work and conceptual development in the area of nursing activities and confused elderly begun by Williams et al. in 1979. It has had a pivotal impact on nursing in several regards. With this study and earlier work, Williams et al. have helped nurses to recognize that hospitalization and the trauma of hip fracture (or any acute illness) can precipitate a marked change in an elderly patient's mental status and behavior. Delirium, a potentially serious condition, is not always correctly nor readily diagnosed by nurses. Again, the work of these investigators addresses this assessment problem and provides groundwork for the identification and testing of feasible nursing interventions for the prevention of acute confusional states. Therefore, their work has helped guide practice and stimulate research in this area of gerontological nursing.

The second study, Bowers' "Intergenerational Caregiving: Adult Caregivers and their Aging Parents," is included because of its significant target population and methodology. With the current and expected explosion in the over-85 age group, care of this frail elderly population by their children who are themselves elderly is a critical health and nursing concern. Whether nurses work in the community, hospital, or long-term care setting, they are encountering the rewards, demands, and stresses incurred by family members as they attempt to care for parents who have multiple impairments and health problems. Bowers uses a grounded theory methodology to generate a theory of intergenerational caregiving. Thus, Bowers elicits from caregivers what their perspective is on caring for elderly family members. Such an approach provides a wealth of information and a broad perspective on caregiving. Bowers proposes five categories of caregiving, only one of which includes what has been commonly associated with caregiving—actual physical care. This theoretical perspective provides an important foundation upon which nursing studies and interventions can build. Its reality-based perspective of the caregiving role increases the likelihood that nursing strategies are addressing the scope of needs and tasks involved with family caregiving and the elderly.

The third study by Kim and Grier, "Pacing Effects of Medication Instruction for the Elderly," rounds out the selections by describing an intervention which is appropriate for nurses who work with elderly in community health or institutions. Kim and Grier demonstrate how a basic knowledge of normal aging changes can be applied to nursing and result in a significant intervention. The problems experienced by the elderly in following medication regimes are complex because of multiple chronic diseases, the number and types of medications prescribed, and frequent prescription changes with multiple physician involvement. Failure to correctly follow a medication regime can result in serious complications, such as confusion and exacerbation of the medical illness. Client teaching is a major activity of nurses. This study shows how modification of the teaching approach toward greater specificity to the needs of the elderly can have positive outcomes.

Reducing Acute Confusional States in Elderly Patients with Hip Fractures

Margaret A. Williams, PhD
*Professor
School of Nursing
University of Wisconsin
Madison, WI*

William J. Raynor, PhD
*Former Director
Statistical Laboratory
University of Wisconsin
Madison, WI*

Emily B. Campbell
*Professor
School of Nursing
University of Wisconsin
Madison, WI*

Susan Mlynarczyk
Social Science Research Specialist

Sandra E. Ward
Social Science Research Specialist

The extent to which the incidence of postoperative acute confusional states could be reduced in elderly ($\geq$ age 60) patients with hip fractures was tested. Interpersonal and environmental nursing interventions were carried out with 57 patients on orthopedic units in three hospitals. The incidence of confusion was reduced from 51.5% in the comparison group (n = 170) to 43.9%. Analysis that controlled for risk factors in the two groups showed the drop in incidence to be significant (p < .02). The most effective interventions appeared to be those that provided orientation and clarification, corrected sensory deficit, and increasedd continuity of care.

Acute confusional states (or confusion, used interchangeably here) are well known to clinicians working with elderly patients in acute care settings. At times the manifestation of these states is of minor consequence; at other times safety measures are required that may enforce immobility with its attendant problems. Prolonged hospitalization from accidents and injuries incurred during severe confusional states is not unknown. Increased nursing surveillance always is indicated when persons are confused, at times to the point of constant attendance.

The incidence of acute confusion among elderly patients in hospitals is certainly high, but documentation is limited. Further, comparison is difficult because of differences in patients' diagnoses and problems in differentiating acute and chronic confusional states. Incidence rates between 10% and 50% in adult patients admitted to general hospital units have been found (Gehi, Strain, Weltz, & Jacobs, 1980; Liston, 1982). In patients aged 70 or over, rates have been 41%–50% (Seymour, Henschke, Cape, & Campbell, 1980; Warshaw et al., 1982). Lipowski (1980) estimated that nearly one-half of patients 60 years or older admitted to general hospitals are likely to exhibit symptoms.

The assumption that elderly patients with hip

fractures are at high risk for confusion was borne out in the first (nonintervention) phase of the present study where over half (51.5%) of the 170 patients (M age = 78.8), with no history of mental impairment, experienced confusion within the first 5 days following surgery (Williams et al., 1985). A hip fracture presents several conditions conducive to confusion. The injury, usually a fall, occurs suddenly, hospitalization and surgery occur in rapid sequence, and there is little or no time to "work through" the events or the potential outcome.

The extent to which acute confusion can be prevented in patients with hip fractures or in other elderly patients on general hospital units has not been tested. Two experimental studies have been reported from intensive care units in which postcardiotomy delirium was lessened by a reorientation procedure (Budd & Brown, 1974); and frequent touch, eye contact, and verbal orientation by a family member while visiting (Chatham, 1978). In a third study (Owens & Hutelmyer, 1982), preoperative instruction about the possibility of unusual postoperative sensory or cognitive experiences did not result in a significant reduction in those experiences.

Confusion is not a well understood syndrome, and the potential physiological and drug-induced causes alone are legion (Ahronheim, 1982; Libow, 1973; Lipowski, 1980; NIA Task Force, 1980; Portnoi, 1981). In addition, sensory impairments and disruption in the pattern and meaning of life experiences are important factors (Wolanin & Phillips, 1981). Unfortunately, the hospital environment itself is ill suited to the maintenance of mental clarity with its routines that seldom match those established in one's home, the unfamiliar technologic devices, and the ever changing personnel. The deleterious effects of hospitalization alone or in combination with other factors have been suggested in several studies (Carino, 1976; Gillick, Serrell, & Gillick, 1982; Morse & Litin, 1969; Roslaniec & Fitzpatrick, 1979). Confusion that cannot be linked to identifiable physical causes has been termed idiopathic (Remakus & Shelly, 1981). The assumption in the present study was that idiopathic confusion may lend itself to prevention or amelioration by the activities, interpersonal approaches, and environmental manipulations over which nurses have control. The purpose of this study, therefore, was to test whether the incidence of confusion in elderly patients with hip fractures, and with no prior history of mental impairment, could be reduced by specific nursing interventions.

Before a quasiexperimental design could be instituted to test the effect of interventions, it was necessary to develop a method of assessing risk for confusion. If positive results were obtained in an experimental group that was at low risk for confusion compared with a control group, the results would be meaningless. Since the relative contribution of the many risk factors implicated in confusion is not known, the first phase of the present study was devoted to developing a quantitative method of risk assessment.

Two models were developed for predicting confusion: (a) one in which background characteristics and hospital admission factors were examined to determine those most associated with confusion in the postoperative period; and (b) one in which day-to-day factors related to treatment and hospitalization were examined, in addition to the admission factors, to determine those that appeared to put patients increasingly at risk for confusion during the postoperative period (Williams et al., 1985).

The sample used for developing the prediction models became the comparison group in the intervention phase. The admission prediction model contributed the method for comparing probable confusion with actual confusion in both the comparison (nonintervention) and intervention groups. The second model served to identify factors that might be modified by certain nursing interventions.

METHOD

Sample

Subjects were recruited from orthopedic units in four acute care community hospitals in the upper Midwest for the nonintervention phase. In the intervention phase, three of those hospitals were used. The organization of patient care on the units was a mix of team and primary nursing. With nurse aide and/or licensed practical nurse assistance, the registered nurse to patient ratio on the day shift ranged from 1:6 to 1:9 in the four hospitals; in the three hospitals it was 1:6 and 1:7. A decline in admissions and a collective bargaining dispute prolonged data collection in the intervention phase to 20 months; the nonintervention phase was 24 months.

The nonintervention sample size was 170; the intervention sample was 57. Criteria for inclusion were: age ≥ 60 years, no validated history of mental impairment, and occurrence of the fracture by trauma. To keep the perioperative event similar, persons were not included if their time from admission to surgery exceeded 2 days. Persons who developed delirium tremens also were not included because prevention is largely dependent on medical treatment and not the type of activities we were interested in testing.

Both samples, as shown in Table 1, were similar in characteristics. The average age was 78.8 (SD = 8.6) in the nonintervention group, 80.6 (SD = 8.3) in the intervention group; females comprised, respectively, 84% and 83% of both groups. Approximately one-third of both groups had education at each of the grade school, high school, and beyond high school levels. The majority [89% (nonintervention) and 93% (intervention)] lived independently or with minor assistance in the community; only 11% (nonintervention) and 7% (intervention) of each group lived in nursing homes. Over half of both groups described themselves as moderately or very active physically. Somewhat more persons were single, widowed, or divorced in the intervention group than in the nonintervention group. The intervention group also had somewhat more combined vision and hearing problems than the nonintervention group.

Measures

Project staff collected all data in the nonintervention phase. The form used incorporated the Short Portable Mental Status Questionnaire (SPMSQ) (Pfeiffer, 1975), questions relative to background, and provision for recording laboratory data, clinical data, and confusion from admission through the fifth postoperative day. Validity and reliability data on the SPMSQ and information on the other measures, were presented elsewhere (Williams et al., 1985).

In the intervention phase, project staff recorded background and clinical progress data from the patient's record while nursing staff administered the admission interview and SPMSQ. Nurses used two flow sheets for end-of-shift recording: One for recording certain clinical observations, the second for recording the presence or absence of confusional behaviors and the nursing activities used to prevent or ameliorate confusion.

Acute confusional states were operationalized in both phases as four behaviors: (a) verbal or nonverbal manifestations of disorientation to time, place, or persons in the environment; (b) inappropriate or unusual communication such as nonsensical speech, calling out, yelling, swearing, and/or unusual silence; (c) inappropriate or unusual behavior such as attempting to get out of bed, pulling at tubes, dressings, and/or picking at bedclothes; and (d) illusions or hallucinations. These were the behaviors cited by nursing staff in a prior study as indicative of confusion and which had been correlated with tests of cognitive function (Williams et al., 1979). They also fit our theoretical definition of acute confusional states: A transient or prolonged disturbance in mental processes incorporating impaired memory, thinking, attention, and orientation to time and place. Misperceptions of persons and objects, hallucinations, hyper- or hypoactivity, and emotional changes may also be present.

The scoring of each of the four confusion behaviors was: 0, not present at any time during the 8-hour shift; 1, present at some time during the shift, but in mild form; 2, present at some time during the shift in marked form. The total shift score could thus vary from 0 to 8. In the 5-day postoperative total, scores of 1 to 15 were classified as mild confusion, scores of 16 or more as moderate/severe confusion.

Table 1
Patient Background and Hospital Admission Characteristics

Characteristic	Nonintervention Group (N = 170) n	%[a]	Intervention Group (N = 57) n	%[b]
Age				
60-69	29	17.0	6	10.5
70-79	51	30.0	17	29.8
80-89	70	41.2	27	47.4
90+	20	11.8	7	12.3
Sex				
Male	28	16.5	10	17.5
Female	142	83.5	47	82.5
Education				
Grade School	62	36.9	18	32.1
Some H.S. or H.S. grad.	55	32.7	18	32.1
Beyond H.S.	51	30.4	20	35.7
Marital Status				
Married	52	30.6	13	22.8
Single/widowed/divorced	118	69.4	44	77.2
Living Arrangement				
With spouse/other	74	43.5	25	43.9
Alone	77	45.3	28	49.1
Nursing home	19	11.2	4	7.0
Vision, Hearing				
Both V & H problems	52	30.6	26	45.6
H problem only	1	.6	0	0
V problem only	114	67.1	28	49.1
No V or H problem	3	1.8	3	5.3
Activity Level				
Restricted/sedentary	73	43.0	24	42.1
Moderately active	56	32.9	29	50.9
Very active	41	24.1	4	7.0
How Fell				
Tripped, slipped	107	65.2	35	62.5
Legs gave out, "drop attack"	57	34.8	21	37.5
SPMSQ[c] Score				
0-2 errors	116	78.4	46	81.0
3-4 errors	20	13.5	8	14.0
5+ errors	12	8.1	3	5.0

[a]Adjusted frequency percent shown when n is not 170.
[b]Adjusted frequency percent shown when n is not 57.
[c]Short Portable Mental Status Questionnaire.

Procedure

The procedures used for access, patient consent, and interrater reliability in coding behaviors have been described (Williams et al., 1985). Admission data were obtained as soon after the patient arrived on the unit as possible. The median time from unit admission to interview was 3.4 hours in the nonintervention phase and less than 1 hour in the intervention phase.

The 24-hour preventive measures for confusion were carried out by regular nursing staff. The head nurses of the orthopedic units participated in planning the approaches to be used, the in-service sessions, and the general logistics of the project. Project funds enabled modest supplementation of staffing when a study patient was on the unit. This was operationalized in different ways in the three hospitals varying from almost no use, to use of a part-time, evening shift person, to use of staff from the hospital's mobile nursing unit.

Orientation of unit personnel included meeting with staff (primarily the registered nurses) from all shifts to discuss the purpose of the study, staff responsibilities, measures to be used, and recording procedures. A videotape also was shown of a patient being admitted into the study. A booklet was kept on each unit that described in detail all procedures and approaches. A summary form of the approaches was also placed in the patient's care plan.

The nursing approaches were drawn from experience, discussion with orthopedic and gerontological nurses, results from the first phase of the study, and from the literature, particularly Wolanin and Phillips (1981), Trockman (1978), and Hahn (1980). Preventive approaches were related to six problems: strange environment, altered sensory input, loss of control and independence, disruption in life pattern, immobility and pain, and disruption in elimination patterns. Ameliorative approaches were related to five problems: mild behaviors suggestive of confusion, sundowning, unsafe behavior, hallucinations or illusions, and fright.

Throughout the intervention phase, project staff discussed each study patient with his or her primary caregiver of the day, evening, and sometimes night shift; validated the coding recorded for confusional behaviors, and served, in general, as backup resources. A nurse visitor (a clinical specialist in psychiatric nursing) was introduced after analysis of data from the first 25 patients showed a significant drop in the occurrence of confusion. This was done to test whether an even larger drop would occur from having a "constant" person who listened to patient's concerns, reflected with them on life experiences, and reinforced staff efforts in maintaining mental clarity. The role was structured so that it would be complementary to the staff nurses' role with study patients.

Whenever possible, the nurse visitor saw the patient before surgery as well as after, with daily visits ranging from 10 minutes to 1 hour. Notes on the visit were recorded and kept where caregivers on all shifts could peruse them. Her observations also were shared verbally with the caregiver on the shift during which she visited and, if warranted, approaches were modified.

In data analysis, comparison was made of the intervention patients' risk of confusion and actual occurrence with the nonintervention patients' risk of confusion and actual occurrence. Each person received a risk score indicating probability of confusion through use of the admission prediction model. The 3 risk factors (out of 21) that were significant in that model were increased errors on the admission SPMSQ, increased age, and a low level of physical activity preinjury. The scoring function of the model includes weighting of the 3 factors (Williams et al., 1985). The model is shown in Table 2.

After adjustment for risk scores a logistic regression model was fit in which both groups were required to have the same slope (for the score function), but were allowed to have different intercepts (i.e., level of confusion). A significant difference between the intercepts implies that the incidence in one group is lower than the incidence in the other group after adjustment for the difference in their risk scores.

The difference in incidence rates was tested separately for the mild confusion group and the moderate/severe group. In each case, the con-

Table 2
Model for Predicting Postoperative Confusion in Elderly Patients with Hip Fractures Using Hospital Admission Variables

Moderate/Severe Variable	Mild Confusion Beta	SE	Confusion Beta	SE	X^2
Constant	-5.160	1.919	-11.330	3.126	15.38
SPMSQ[a] Score	0.885	0.595	2.193	0.654	11.96
Age	0.051	0.025	0.104	0.038	8.62
Prehospital Activity	1.100	0.500	1.652	1.095	6.30
			Overall X^2 = 49.05		

Note: The n for model development = 148.
[a]Short Portable Mental Status Questionnaire.

fused patients were compared with the patients who did not show any confusion. The two categories of confusion also were combined to test for a difference in any confusion.

RESULTS

Incidence

The overall incidence of confusion in the intervention sample was 43.9% compared with that in the nonintervention sample of 51.5%. Incidence did not vary significantly by hospital in either phase. Mild confusion was, respectively, in the nonintervention and intervention samples, 35.5% and 35.1%; moderate/severe confusion was 16.0% and 8.8%. The intervention sample showed a significantly lower level than the nonintervention sample of both mild and moderate/severe confusion after adjustment for the score variable; p = .032 and .018, respectively. The associated Z statistics were -1.84 and -2.91. Both tests were performed as one-sided tests. The change in the intercept was -0.657 (±.357) for mild confusion and -1.337 (±.639) for moderate/severe confusion.

The version of the model using the combined category of some confusion compared with no confusion also showed a significant drop in the incidence of confusion in the intervention group, with a one-sided p value of .013. The associated Z statistic was -2.22. The change in intercept was -0.7709 (±.347).

There was no significant difference in the incidence of confusion among patients seen by the nurse visitor (n = 30) compared with those not seen by her (n = 25). The average length of stay for the intervention sample was 14.5 days. This was a day shorter than that of the nonintervention sample in the same three hospitals, 15.5 days, but the difference was not significant.

These results are based on 5-day aggregated scores that combine both severity and duration. For example, a patient was classified as having mild confusion with a score of 12, but that score could represent 1 day during the 5 when severe confusion was present or it could represent five days of mild confusion. The results, therefore, do not indicate whether interventions were more effective in preventing short, severe episodes of confusion or prolonged mild confusion. It appears, however, that interventions were most effective from admission through the third postoperative day; by postoperative Days 4 and 5, the difference in percent of patients exhibiting confusion in the two groups became less. A prevalence graph showing the above trend is shown in Figure 1.

DISCUSSION

Because the study extended over considerable time, we were concerned that organizational or personnel changes during that period might have

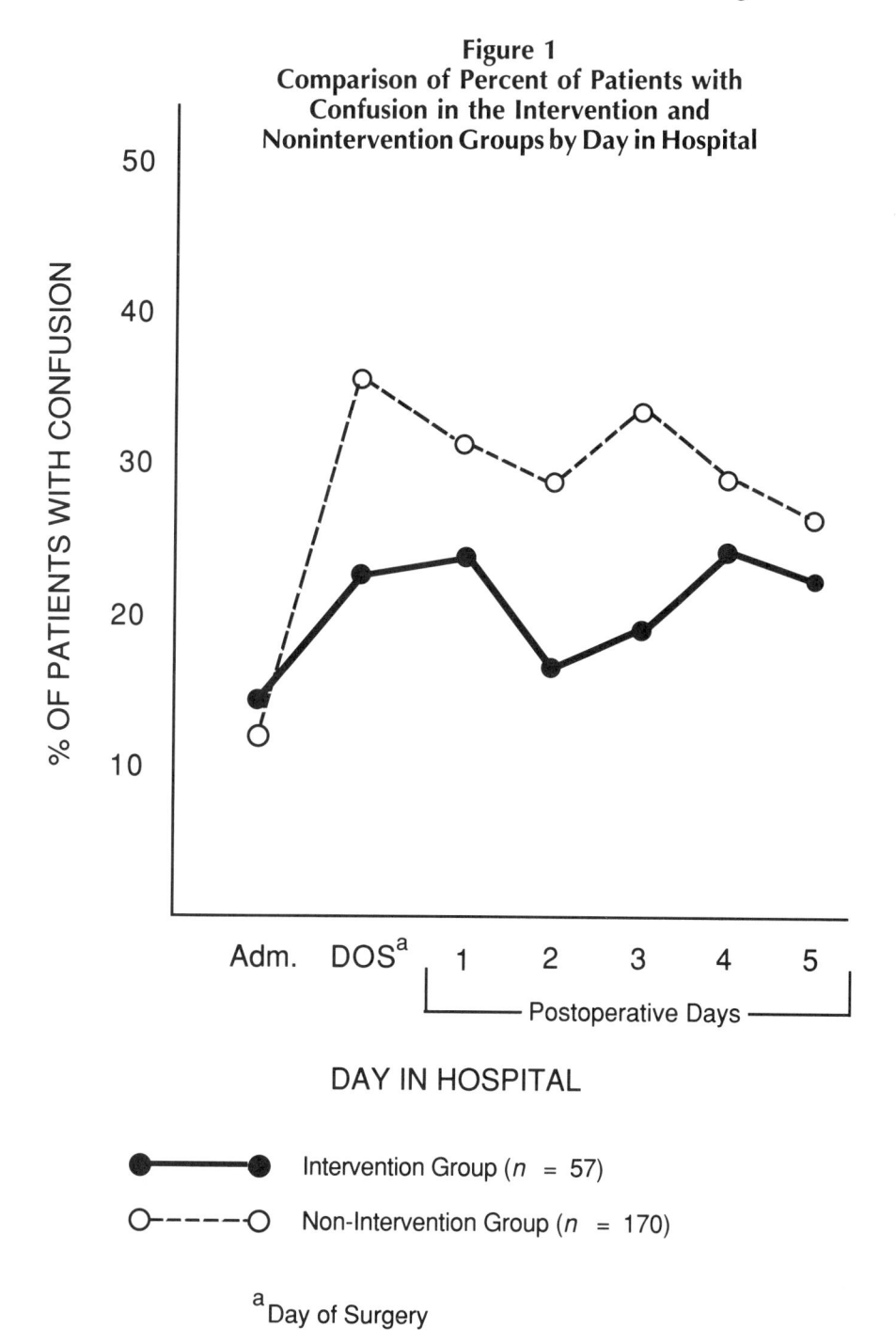

**Figure 1
Comparison of Percent of Patients with
Confusion in the Intervention and
Nonintervention Groups by Day in Hospital**

●——● Intervention Group (*n* = 57)
○------○ Non-Intervention Group (*n* = 170)

[a] Day of Surgery

affected the outcome rather than the planned interventions. This did not appear to be the case. There was departure of only one private surgeon with subsequent replacement; there was no change in orthopedic residents' rotation, or in pre- or postoperative regimens. The head nurses remained the same, and similar (moderate) turnover in staff nurses occurred in both phases. The lack of difference by hospital in incidence of confusion in both phases supports the premise that institution-specific organizational or personnel variables did not produce the difference in outcomes.

In several instances, the nurse visitor picked up early symptoms of alcohol withdrawal coupled with a more accurate history of alcohol use than had been provided. Thus, greater confusion in the nonintervention phase may have been partially due to unrecognized numbers of persons suffering from alcohol withdrawal. Reexamination on a case by case basis, however, did not produce evidence of oversight.

An overrecording of confusion might have happened in the intervention phase because nursing staff were "keyed into" its occurrence. Conversely, underrecording could have occurred because of investment in the study's outcome. Both possibilities exist although there was extensive checking and counterchecking among nursing and project staff in both phases. The ethos of accurate reporting for legal as well as clinical reasons would make substantial reporting changes unlikely, however.

The number of chronic illnesses generally was similar between the two groups. Proportionately the same (few) numbers of patients in each phase were ill enough postoperatively to be sent to the intensive care unit for several days. Thus it does not appear that changes in the population appreciably influenced the outcome.

A major limitation of statistical prediction models is that only recurrent major risk factors emerge as significant from grouped data yet certain infrequently appearing factors may be clinically significant for an individual. One has to assume that clinical factors other than those in the prediction model "evened out" over the groups. The fact that the two groups were similar in background characteristics supports that assumption.

It was also difficult to determine which activities or environmental manipulations most influenced the outcome because approaches were individualized, particularly the interpersonal ones. Certain events were suggestive, however. For example, continuity of care was greater in the intervention phase. This was calculated by dividing the number of shifts from the time of a patient's admission through the fifth postoperative day by the number of nurses who had been the responsible caregivers on those shifts (the more nurses, the lower the continuity of care score). The average continuity of care increased from 1.99 (SD = .39) in the nonintervention phase to 2.38 (SD = .52) in the intervention phase. The difference was significant: $t(208) = -5.96, p<.001$.

In the nonintervention phase only about half of the patients had a timepiece visible to them; in the intervention phase all did. Slightly more narcotics (measured in equivalences to morphine sulfate) also were given on 3 out of the 5 postoperative days in the intervention phase.

The use of the end-of-shift flow sheet for checking the nursing activities that had been carried out proved less than satisfactory. It was difficult to divide care into discrete actions and to estimate the extent to which the action had been carried out. Activities also were occasionally checked the same way as on the prior shift. However, when tallies were made of most and least-checked categories, there was correspondence with responses on an end-of-study staff questionnaire. Staff were asked to specify the degree of difficulty they had in implementing 15 specified activities. The activities presenting the least difficulty to implement, and, by implication, carried out the most consistently were: weaving orientation information into conversation; keeping patient informed about and giving rationale for treatments and procedures; and correcting sensory deficits (i.e., having glasses, hearing aids in place when needed). Interventions preventing the most difficulty were: keeping the number of hospital personnel who interact with the patient to a minimum; encouraging family members to visit; and assisting the patient in having a sense of control over what is happening.

The relative frequency of implementation of interventions also was congruent with project staff observations. Results thus indicate that the most effective activities probably were those that provided orientation and clarification, corrected sensory deficits, and increased continuity of care.

The drop in incidence of confusion in the intervention group was particularly heartening because it occurred through the efforts of nursing staff on typical orthopedic units. (The nurse visitor's influence was positive, we believe, but cannot be formally evaluated.) The supplementation of staff when study patients were on the unit was not sufficient to increase nursing time available to patients to a great extent and regular use of such supplementation occurred in only one hospital. That hospital was the one that contributed the largest number of patients to the intervention sample, however, so that one must conclude that confusion-preventive measures are most effectively implemented when there is adequate time for care. That conclusion seems patently obvious, but there is no doubt that many of the older patients who comprise the usual hip fracture population present many problems of nursing dependency, aside from orientation needs, and direct care cannot be hurried. At the same time, the type of interventions implemented in the study are not difficult and, when persons are sensitive to them, could be incorporated in the care of all elderly patients.

Even though the incidence of confusion was reducible by conscious, deliberative approaches in this study, the fact remains that over 40% of persons in the intervention group still manifested some degree of confusion. The greater extent of confusion in the nonintervention group is consistent with Lipowski's estimate that nearly half of patients 60 years or older admitted to general hospitals may exhibit some symptoms of mental impairment (1980). To what extent this figure could be reduced by more radical alteration of features of hospitalization than we employed is conjectural. Physiologic alterations that have the potential of compromising the cerebral support system are frequent accompaniments of trauma, surgery, and immobility, and attention to rapid correction of such alterations when they occur is, of course, imperative. Such attention frequently may be easier, however, than radically altering features of hospitalization. The interventions in this study, for example, did not get at the problem of multiple persons interacting with the patient (in fact, we added one person to the milieu at one point), routines far different than those at home, and the lack of usual home amenities and personal artifacts of living. At the same time, it is evident that the high incidence of confusion in elderly orthopedic patients, who have no history of chronic mental impairment but who suffer sudden injury and rapid hospitalization, can be reduced by conscious attention to interpersonal and environmental nursing approaches.

REFERENCES

Ahronhein, J. C. (1982). Acute confusional states in the elderly. *Seminars in Family Medicine, 3*, 20–25.

Budd, S. P., & Brown, W. (1974). Effect of a reorientation technique on postcardiotomy delirium. *Nursing Research, 23*, 341–348.

Carino, C. M. (1976). Behavioral responses of disoriented patients compared to oriented patients in intensive care units. *Dissertation Abstracts International, 37*, 1623B. (University Microfilms No. 76-21, 867.)

Chatham, M. A. (1978). The effect of family involvement on patients' manifestations of postcardiotomy psychosis. *Heart and Lung, 7*, 995–999.

Gehi, M., Strain, J. J., Weltz, N., & Jacobs, J. (1980). Is there a need for admission and discharge cognitive screening for the medically ill? *General Hospital Psychiatry, 2*(3), 186–191.

Gillick, M. R., Serrell, N. A., & Gillick, L. S. (1982). Adverse consequences of hospitalization in the elderly. *Social Science and Medicine, 16*, 1033–1038.

Hahn, K. (1980). Using 24-hour reality orientation. *Journal of Gerontological Nursing, 6*(3), 130–135.

Libow, L. S. (1973). Pseudosenility: Acute and reversible organic brain syndrome. *Journal of the American Geriatrics Society, 21*, 112–120.

Lipowski, Z. J. (1980). *Delirium*. Springfield, IL: Charles C. Thomas.

Liston, E. H. (1982). Delirium in the aged. *Psychiatric Clinics of North America, 5*, 49–66.

Morse, R., & Litin, E. (1969). Post-operative delirium: A study of etiologic factors. *American Journal of Psychiatry, 126*, 388–395.

National Institute on Aging Task Force (1980). Senility reconsidered: Treatment possibilities for mental impairment in the elderly. *Journal of the American Medical Association, 244*, 259–263.

Owens, J. F., & Hertelmyer, C. M. (1982). The effect of preoperative intervention on delirium in cardiac surgical patients. *Nursing Research, 31*, 60–62.

Pfeiffer, E. (1975). A short portable mental status questionnaire for the assessment of organic brain deficit in elderly patients. *Journal of the American Geriatrics Society, 23*, 433–441.

Portnoi, V. A. (1981). Diagnostic dilemma of the aged. *Archives of Internal Medicine, 141*, 734–737.

Remakus, B. L., & Shelly, R. M. (1981). How to prevent confusion in hospitalized elderly. *Geriatrics, 36*, 121–122, 125.

Roslaniec, A., & Fitzpatrick, J. J. (1979). Changes in mental status in older adults with four days of hospitalization. *Research in Nursing & Health, 2*, 177–187.

Seymour, D. G., Henschke, P. J., Cape, R. D. T., & Campbell, A. J. (1980). Acute confusional states and dementia in the elderly: The role of dehydration/volume depletion, physical illness and age. *Age and Aging, 9*(3), 137–146.

Trackman, G. (1978). Caring for the confused or delirious patient. *American Journal of Nursing, 78*, 1495–1499.

Warshaw, G. A., Moore, J. T., Friedman, W., Currie, C. T., Kennie, D. C., Kane, W. J., & Mears, P. A. (1982). Functional disability in the hospitalized elderly. *Journal of the American Medical Association, 248*, 847–850.

Williams, M. A., Campbell, E. B., Raynor, W. J., Musholt, M. M., Mlynarczyk, S. M., & Crane, L. F. (1985). Predictors of acute confusional states in elderly patients. *Research in Nursing & Health, 8*, 31–40.

Williams, M. A., Holloway, J. R., Winn, M. C., Wolanin, M. O., Lawler, M. L., Westwick, C. R., & Chin, M. H. (1979). Nursing activities and acute confusional states in elderly hip-fractured patients. *Nursing Research, 28*, 25–35.

Wolanin, M. O., & Phillips, L. R. F. (1981). *Confusion*. St. Louis: Mosby.

This article is printed with permission of *Research in Nursing & Health*.
Copyright © 1985 John Wiley & Sons.

Original article:
Williams, M. A., Campbell, E. B., Raynor, W. J., Mlynarczyk, S., & Ward, S. E. (1985). Reducing acute confusional states in elderly patients with hip fractures. *Research in Nursing and Health, 8,* 329–337.

CRITIQUE BY: JELENE MacLEAN, BSN, RN

Part I: Clinical Relevance

It is refreshing to read a research study that deals with a problem that health professionals in gerontology encounter frequently. "Reducing Acute Confusional States in Elderly Patients with Hip Fractures," by Williams et al., presents plausible evidence that the incidence of confusion can be reduced through nursing interventions. Each aspect of the study has the potential of providing assistance in identifying which elderly are at risk for developing an acute confusional state. The most effective interventions determined as a result of the study are included and could be implemented in either an acute-care or long-term care setting.

The study purported to "test whether the incidence of confusion in elderly patients with hip fractures, and with no prior history of mental impairment, could be reduced by specific nursing interventions." The investigators divided the study design into two phases: (1) a nonintervention phase where two different models for predicting confusion were developed, and (2) an intervention phase where project and nursing staff collected patient data, made clinical observations, and recorded confusional states and nursing activities utilized.

The investigators present study results in a concise and logical manner. Although a portion of the interventions suggested could be implemented by an individual nurse (those of correcting sensory deficits and providing orientation and clarification for the patient), a collaborative effort among the nursing staff as a whole would be necessary in order to achieve significant results in actual clinical practice.

The investigators eliminated subjects for their sample population if they possessed a history of mental impairment, alcoholism and potential for delirium tremens, or if time from admission to surgery exceeded two days.

In general, if adequate staffing patterns prevailed and the prediction models as well as end-of-shift recording tools for documenting both confusional states and nursing interventions were available, the theory presented in this study would have potential for use in the general hospital practice setting. More specifically, the theory has potential for use in my current practice as gerontological nurse on a medical–surgical unit.

Part II: Conceptualization and Internal Consistency

Williams et al. have written a report that flows cohesively from the introduction and literature review to the discussion and conclusion. The investigators discuss risk factors affecting the elderly not only because of the initial injury (hip fracture) but also because of the stressors presented by the hospital stay itself. Included is the acknowledgement that these risk factors can be assessed at admission, monitored throughout the hospital stay, and that nursing interventions can be initiated to correct for these factors to reduce the incidence of acute confusional states postoperatively.

Because high percentages of elderly patients admitted to general hospital units with hip fractures develop some degree of acute confusion, the justification for this study is clear. The investigators further support this justification by references cited in their literature review. In addition, my experience as clinician on a skilled Medicare unit enhances support for this study. In fact, hip fractures constituted the number one diagnosis of patients admitted from the hospital for rehabilitation. Often, the patient was admitted with a secondary diagnosis of either senile dementia or organic brain syndrome. This was usually coupled with an order for Haldol or some similar medication for use because of the patient's confused or combative nature. Upon interviewing the family or significant others, it came to our attention that the confusional state had not been present prior to hospitalization and that the medication had been prescribed because of calling out in disorientation, climbing out of bed, or pulling at intravenous tubing or indwelling catheters. Usually, the confusion seen at the time of admission for rehabilitation would clear within a week or two and orientation would return.

The present study supports my own belief that confusion following hip fractures can be short term and that the incidence of confusion can be reduced when appropriate nursing steps are taken. I also believe that nurses in hospital settings have an obligation to recognize the limited nature of this type of confusion and make every effort to avoid labeling a patient chronically confused. At the same time, nurses must encourage physicians to avoid diagnosing the patient as chronically confused. In this regard, the concepts presented in the study have major ramifications for how the subject of confusional states in the hospitalized elderly is addressed.

The quasiexperimental design of this study allows the investigators to fulfill their purpose and to answer all questions posed by their theory within the hospital setting. According to Polit and Hungler (1985), the quasiexperimental design is noted for its great strength because of its practicality and feasibility. When used as a research plan, the quasiexperimental design introduces some controls when full experimental sterility is lacking. On the other hand, disadvantages of quasiexperimental design include lack of randomization or a randomly equivalent comparison group.

The issues addressed at the beginning of the study, including the development of the quantitative method for assessing risk, are consistent with the body of the study, the results, their analysis, and conclusions. Throughout the study, the investigators also act as their own critics. They point out the strengths and weaknesses of their design so that the reader has the option of accepting or rejecting them in light of the reader's own clinical experience or practice.

In general, therefore, the investigators have presented their study cohesively, and with sufficient justification and attention to internal consistency to warrant consideration for use in care of the elderly with acute confusional states.

Part III: Believability of Results

This study purported to test the effects of specific nursing interventions on reducing the incidence of acute confusion in elderly hip fracture patients age 60 years or older. Sample size included 57 subjects in the intervention group and 170 subjects in the nonintervention group. The portion of the sample used when developing the tools for predicting confusion became the comparison group in the intervention portion of the study. However, this multistage design can cause confusion. There is reference to the use of four hospitals in the nonintervention phase of study and use of only three hospitals in the intervention phase of study. To this reader, such a discrepancy remains unclear.

The investigators described hospital staffing as a mixture of primary and team nursing where the registered nurse is assisted by a nurse aide, a licensed practical nurse, or both. The generic description of "four acute-care community hospitals in the upper Midwest" and the believability of staffing patterns contribute to the potential generalizability of this study.

In addition, the investigators paid close attention to detail in drawing up specific guidelines regarding subject selection in order to achieve internally consistent results. Criteria for inclusion consisted of specifics as to age, normal mental status, and etiology for hip impairment. The investigators excluded subjects if they exhibited signs or symptoms of delirium secondary to alcohol abuse. In order to maintain control over the perioperative period, the investigators also excluded subjects if their time from admit to time of fracture fixation exceeded 48 hours. Even though this is a convenience sampling within a quasiexperimental design, the investigators' attention to controlling for characteristics that might influence study results convinces me that this sample is representative of the typical elderly hip fracture population that could develop confusion postoperatively.

Measures used incorporated the Short Portable Mental Status Questionnaire (SPMSQ). There also are questions pertinent to background, space allowances for documenting laboratory and clinical data, and measures for indicating confusion up through the fifth postoperative day. The investigators do not discuss validity or reliability but indicate that the date on the SPMSQ and information on the other measures were presented elsewhere by Williams et al. (1985). The procedures used for access, patient consent, and interrater reliability in coding behaviors also are described as having been presented in the same previous article. Despite this reference to another article for clarification of validity and reliability, I feel certain that the information presented in chart form as derived from the interview tools can be taken at face value in determining potential use in the clinical setting.

The investigators also provide sufficient detail of information describing the statistical analysis of data and results to allow for a thorough assessment of validity of results. However, because I have only limited experience with statistics, I would have to refer to two different texts in order to understand the significance of the calculations presented. Even so, Williams et al. do acknowledge which findings are significant and which are not, which allows readers with limited exposure to statistical methods to derive some useful content without referring to other sources. In this regard, the findings between the intervention group and the nonintervention group are significant for the research questions posed.

The problem of seeing mild to severe confusional states in elderly patients with hip fracture is a serious one in my own practice. Therefore, I think this study warrants the additional effort to verify the validity and reliability of the measures.

Part IV: Generalizability of Results

The extent to which the information uncovered in this study is applicable to a general hospital setting with geriatric clientele shows its true strength. The investigators based results of the intervention component on information gathered at three generically described hospitals, using staff nurses as primary data collectors after training by project staff. Their orientation consisted of an explanation of the purpose of the study, staff responsibilities, measures and how to use them, as well as being shown a videotape of a patient being admitted to a study. Patient care plans included a summary with chosen approaches decided on after discussion with orthopedic and gerontological nurses, results from the first phase of the study, and from specified literary sources. The attention to adequate staff preparation and the experience and theory on which interventions were decided contributes to the believability and reliability of the study. The attention to meeting with primary caregivers on each of the three shifts throughout the study to validate information recorded also contributes to the validity of the findings. In addition, a consistent nurse visitor was employed to act as an objective observer to further collaborate observations made as to confusional symptoms exhibited.

In analyzing data, the investigators compared risk of confusion scores of patients in the intervention groups with the actual occurrence of confusion. This procedure presents a further strength of the study: patients were not only compared to a control group but also with themselves pre and postoperatively.

In the literature review, the investigators provided references to other studies conducted to measure confusion in hospitalized elderly patients. Strange as it may seem, however, none of these references related to hip fracture patients. Nonetheless, in analyzing the data presented, I am willing to discuss utilization of the prediction models, end-of-shift recording flowsheets, and nursing interventions of increasing orientation and clarification, correcting for sensory deficits, and increasing continuity of care with the administrators in the general hospital where I currently practice.

Part V: Other Factors to Consider in Utilization

Because the hospital in which I work has only 28 beds, feasibility exists for doing a systematic evaluation of these research-based practices. Because of the small setting and limited number of staff employed, risk and cost would be minimal and include merely the time and cost to orient hospital nurses to the use of the forms, interventions, and monitors. The benefits of instituting such research-based practices also include something more than greater patient satisfaction with their hospital experience. The increase in continuity of care used will overlap into other patient care situations involving different types of confusional states in the elderly.

In contrast, the risks of not changing current practices include financial, ethical, and health care considerations. Because of continuing confusion or combativeness, elderly patients may be kept longer in the hospital than would be warranted with more appropriate care. Or, as a result of their condition, they may suffer transfer to long-term care facilities when they could have gone home under the care of a home health agency. Similarly, there are techniques, as reported in this study, to control confusion or combativeness other than by psychoactive drugs. In the same light, there also is the chance of an incorrect and highly stigmatizing diagnosis that can follow the transiently confused patient after hospitalization.

After reading and carefully considering this study, I feel that nurses in general hospital settings dealing with geriatric hip fracture patients have everything to gain by instituting changes within their practices based on the research findings presented. Nor would such changes benefit only those patients at risk within the common target population. Enhancing quality of care here would also effect the quality of care provided institutionwide.

REFERENCES

Polit, D. F., & Hungler, B. P. (1985). *Essentials of nursing research: Methods and applications.* Philadelphia: Lippincott.

Original article:
Williams, M. A., Campbell, E. B., Raynor, W. J., Mlynarczyk, S., & Ward, S. E. (1985). Reducing acute confusional states in elderly patients with hip fractures. *Research in Nursing & Health*, 8, 329–337.

CRITIQUE BY: JUDY MILLER, MSN, RN

Part I: Clinical Relevance

With a reported incidence of 10–52 percent, depending on the study and population studied, acute confusional states (ACS) in hospitalized elderly is a significant problem for nursing. The elderly patient who is confused requires a great deal of nursing attention. Diagnosing the confusion and symptomatology associated with other medical problems is made difficult by the inability of the patient to provide reliable information. The confused, elderly patient also is at high risk for other complications and problems requiring nursing attention, such as falls and incontinence. Discharge planning is problematic because of uncertainty as to the length of time before resolution of the ACS and limited lengths of stay within the hospital. The elderly patient with ACS is at higher risk for hospital readmission secondary to problems complying with the health regime and managing in the home or institutional environment. Thus, nurses working in units throughout a hospital, from the emergency room to the home health and discharge coordinator, as well as nurses in long-term care settings and community agencies, will find this study useful to their practice.

The study, which builds on the investigators' earlier work (Williams et al., 1979, 1985), identifies:

1. Observations which are useful in the early diagnosis of ACS with elderly patients.
2. A model for predicting postoperative confusion in elderly patients which can help nurses to target their preventive interventions.
3. Interventions designed to reduce the incidence of ACS in hospitalized elderly.

4. Clinically usable measures of ACS.

The usefulness of this study for nursing practice would be greatly enhanced by providing predictive information from the Williams et al. (1985) study. Unfortunately, the study under critique presents only a summary table of the prediction model for ACS using hospital admission variables. Consequently, the nurse, seeking to determine who would be the high risk patients, would know only that increased errors on the Short Portable Mental Status Questionnaire (SPMSQ), increased age, and a low level of pre-injury physical activity were important predictors. To understand the rationale for the model, the nurse would be forced to read the predictor study and review all factors that were measured and how the predictors were defined. (For example, what is low level physical activity?) Although the SPMSQ is fairly well known to nurses working in gerontological nursing, one would not expect the nursing student or beginning staff nurse to have a working familiarity with its format and questions.

Additionally, it is difficult to determine the exact nature of all 15 nursing interventions measured in the present study. Williams et al. describe problems that the interventions are designed to address, and from this one can infer appropriate nursing actions. However, only nine of the interventions are actually mentioned and that does not occur until the discussion section. A clearer presentation of the treatment, such as a table listing and describing the 15 interventions, would be helpful and strengthen the study.

Williams et al. categorize the interventions as preventive or ameliorative approaches. Preventive approaches deal with contributory problems, including: strange environment, altered sensory input, loss of control and independence, disruption in life pattern, immobility and pain, and disruption in elimination patterns. Ameliorative approaches, on the other hand, focus on manifestations of ACS, including: mild behaviors suggestive of confusion, sundowning, unsafe behavior, hallucinations or illusions, and fright. The manner in which the nursing interventions were developed, and examples of the interventions that are given, suggest that they are independent nursing actions. Some will require more of a nursing unit and administrative change approach than others. For example, having the patient's timepiece readily available is an intervention which can be done by an individual nurse. However, controlling the number of hospital personnel who interact with the elderly patient is a nursing intervention that might require a change in the unit's philosophy and administrative discussion with physicians and department heads. Other examples of interventions include: weaving orientation information into conversation, ensuring the patient has glasses and hearing aids in place when needed, encouraging family members to visit, and assisting the patient in having a sense of control over what is happening.

In general, this study merits consideration by the practicing nurse. Its greatest potential for application is for elderly at risk for trauma and acute medical problems. Additionally, it can help to shape nursing practice in the areas of diagnosis and interventions.

Part II: Conceptualization and Internal Consistency

A clinician, seeking interventions for practice, may find the title of this study misleading. Although its content is consistent with its title and purpose, much of the study deals with preintervention work. The conceptualization of confusion and development of the quantitative method of risk assessment are critical to the soundness of the intervention portion of the study. However, the actual intervention portion of the article is limited in description and exploration.

Beginning with a statement of justification, Williams et al. have presented their concerns with clarity and concision. They explain the need for examination of ACS and nursing interventions with the hospitalized elderly based on: the high occurrence of ACS; limited existing knowledge on preventive strategies; and strong suggestion as to the iatrogenic nature of many acute confusional episodes secondary to the hospital environment.

This study is a grouping of important building blocks in addressing the research question. In their 1979 work, Williams et al. developed conceptual and operational definitions of ACS that are directly relevant to nursing practice, yet are also consistent with definitions used by other health care providers. One of the major problems for nurses who work with confused elderly has been difficulty with defining the problem or in measuring patient response to nursing measures. Previously, nurses commonly relied on one of two ways to communicate information about a confused elderly patient: measures of mental status or descriptions of behaviors. Measures of mental status, such as the Short Portable Mental Status Questionnaire, at best only indirectly reflect the behaviors that the elderly person may exhibit. Descriptions of behaviors, such as the statement, "He's confused and disoriented," are often misinterpreted because there is no clear understanding of what the terms mean. In this regard, Williams et al. provide a theoretical definition of ACS which encompasses the phenomena of delirium. They present their operational definition, which covers all aspects of the concept, in four descriptive behaviors based on their 1979 work with nurses.

The preliminary work done by the investigators in developing a quantitative method and regression model for predicting postoperative confusion in elderly patients with hip fractures was critical to the success of the present study. The regression model identifies those characteristics of elderly patients (variables) which are most highly associated with the development of postoperative confusion. These high-risk variables form the basis for comparison of the control and experimental groups. As they state, "If positive results were obtained in an experimental group that was at low risk for confusion compared with a control group, the results would be meaningless." The interventions would be considered effective if a high-risk group (as defined by the regression model) received the experimental treatment and developed a lower incidence of ACS than that predicted with the model. Williams et al. do a good job of describing and comparing the sample used for developing the prediction model with the elderly subjects used in the intervention portion of the study (refer to Table 1). Since the prediction group (nonintervention subjects) formed the basis for comparison regarding the incidence of ACS, this was very important as it constitutes the control group.

For the most part then the groups are quite similar and consistent with the population of interest. Differences on characteristics either tend to be small or balance out between the groups with regard to degree of impairment or risk for development of ACS. For example, the nonintervention group has fewer problems of vision and hearing combined, but have more patients who have at least one of the sensory deficits. There was a fairly sizeable difference with the nonintervention group having a greater number of very active subjects. A low level of pre-injury activity is a factor associated with the development of ACS according to the regression model. The investigators reduced this source of variability (an important difference between the two groups) by collapsing the three levels of activity into the two categories of moderately or very active and restrictive/sedentary. One can argue that collapsing the categories after the data are collected is an artificial manipulation of information done to strengthen the study. However, all conceptualization involving the defining and categorization of phenomena is artifical. Acceptability of the categorization is determined by its relevance to reality. The investigators' recategorization is acceptable, therefore, since it is restricted activity and immobility, such as with bedrest, that they associate with changes in mental status. The degree of mobility is less important. The nurse reading this study will find its subjects quite similar in characteristics to his or her elderly patients who are admitted with hip fractures and no history of pre-existing confusion.

For greater precision, the investigators developed an instrument likely to measure behaviors of ACS in hospitalized elderly that are observed by nurses. However, in terms of content validity, it is important to understand that the instrument measures behaviors *associated* with ACS—behaviors likely to be observed by nurses—and not ACS. Information regarding the validity and reliability of the instrument is included in another article (Williams et al. 1985). The investigators report that this instrument was correlated with other measures of mental status, which is an important indicator of construct validity. The reader would have to return to the 1985 article in order to determine how high (strong) was the correlation. A high, negative correlation would indicate that subjects exhibiting ACS behaviors in a marked form would receive low scores on tests of mental function. However, based on the information provided in this study, all that can be said is that it is probably a valid measure of behaviors observed by nurses as being associated with ACS in hospitalized elderly. Because the investigators did not provide examples or definitions, it remains unclear as to what distinguishes mild confusion from moderate to severe confusion. Even so, scores of 1 to 15 are used to define mild confusion while a score of 16 or above is used to define moderate to severe confusion. One does not know if this score reliably reflects a "type" of confused patient or was a natural break in the range of scores of subjects in the study. As identified by the investigators, the scores do not discriminate between duration of confusion and severity. Thus, a patient who suffers mild confusion for several days could obtain the same score as a patient who suffers severe confusion for one day. Since the behaviors, experiences, and effects would be different for the patients, depending on their severity and duration, the validity of the tool can be seriously questioned with regard to the measurement of type and severity of confusion. Nursing interventions would also differ, and so the clinical usability of the tool is diminished. One way of resolving these issues would be to use total shift scores to measure severity of confusion and presence or absence of behaviors within each category to measure duration.

Several other potential weaknesses occur with regard to the sensitivity of the instrument in measuring ACS. First, nurses must have enough contact and involvement with the patient to be able to note that the behaviors are occurring. Periods of low patient contact would decrease the likelihood that such behaviors would be noted unless they were extremely disruptive and noisy. Second, the elderly patient who is not very verbal or active can be very confused, but it would only be detected by a nurse who has worked with the patient and is astute to subtle behavior changes and checks mental status periodically. Third, the instrument itself relies on recall. Nurses are asked to score the four confusion behaviors as to their occurrence during the previous eight hours on an end-of-shift record. Thus, the instrument is probably much more reliable as a measure of the dramatic behaviors associated with ACS, such as yelling and attempts to get out of bed. Such behaviors would be called to the attention of the nurse, require action on his or her part, and would generally be remembered. However, the instrument which records the interventions may not reliably indicate the nurse's effectiveness in reducing or preventing confusion. As Williams et al. note, the end-of-shift flow sheet for the recording of the interventions suffered from the same problems encountered in routine nursing charting. Thus, staff either failed to report the interventions they were using, or routinely checked the same interventions that the previous shift recorded. As counterbalance, project staff did observe for the frequency of nursing actions, and there was consistency overall between what the nurses reported in a questionnaire and what the nurses recorded as to their most and least commonly implemented actions.

Despite these shortcommings, Williams et al. clearly identify the potential bias that can occur because of the data collection procedures. Administration of the admission interview and SPMSQ by staff nurses during the intervention phase certainly sensitized them to the occurrence of confusion with elderly patients, and may have served to increase their reporting of confusion and investment in carrying out the interventions. The measurements of intervention implementation and effectiveness of those interventions (e.g., increase or decrease in confusion behaviors) by the same staff nurses who are doing the interventions is definitely a source of bias, however. One agrees with Williams et al. in anticipating an underrecording of confusion behaviors as outcome measures. Nonetheless, they report that there was extensive checking among nursing and project staff during all phases of the study to minimize the over and underreporting of confusion.

In general, this study is conceptually clear and internally consistent. The investigators understand the phenomenon of concern and their measures of it are logical. While there are evident weaknesses with the instruments used, I encourage nurses to consider the study for application to practice.

Part III: Believability of Results

This study uses quantitative measures to test the effectiveness of nursing actions to reduce or prevent confusion in hospitalized elderly. Toward that end, the investigators obtained a convenience sample from four community hospitals. Criteria for subjects included: (1) patients over the age of 60; (2) patients with surgery within two days of admission for traumatic hip fractures; and (3) patients without pre-existing confusion or the development of delirium tremors.

It is important to note that the use of several hospitals increases the likelihood of generalizability of the results beyond the study sample. The systems of patient care and nurse:patient ratios in the study hospitals are similar to those throughout the country, and indicate that the interventions are feasible from a staffing perspective. On the other hand, the preoperative period was limited to two days to increase comparability of subjects: This excludes an important population of hospitalized elderly who have a lengthy preoperative period secondary to unstable medical problems, nutritional deficits, and iatrogenic illnesses. One can anticipate that the incidence and severity of confusion in this population would be even higher than that in the sample. As previously discussed, the investigators compare the pre-intervention and intervention samples on important characteristics.

In Part II of this critique, I discussed potential biases and reliability and validity issues. Of concern to the investigators was an important, potential intervening variable: the impact of time. Data collection extended over a period of 44 months, during which several historical and maturational events could have happened to bias the results. This could include such things as: changes in staffing patterns, experience, and composition; new knowledge regarding care of the confused elderly; experiences with elderly patients on units which changed the way staff viewed care; seasonal changes which would effect the incidence of hip fractures or complications, such as hypothermia during winter which could alter mental status; and eventual nursing staff disinterest in the study because of the length of time. Williams et al. examined the changes in nurse and physician personnel, care practices, and incidence of ACS among the different hospitals to correctly support their claim that time did not have a major impact as an intervening variable. Another source of potential bias with regard to the effectiveness of interventions is the effect of project staff presence and involvement with nursing staff during the intervention phase of the study. However, in this study, such potential bias did not occur. Yet it is unclear how much involvement the project staff had with nurses during the pre-intervention phase of the study. In this regard, the results could be indicative not so much of the effectiveness of the interventions, but of the effect of the attention given to the nurses by the investigators. As a result of this attention, the nurses may have felt, and, therefore, acted differently toward their practice and patients. The presence of the "nurse visitor" midway through the intervention phase could have had a similar impact or led the nurses to decrease their involvement with patients since someone else was there to help. As previously mentioned, the investigators do not discuss reliability and validity issues in any depth, but refer the reader to another article. However, based on the types of questions that the investigators raise, design, use of the SPMSQ, and safeguards, the reader can feel fairly comfortable with the internal validity of the methods and study design.

In this quasiexperimental study, the investigators did not randomly assign subjects to the treatment and control groups. Rather, they compared them on the basis of significant variables. To reduce the effect of contamination, subjects involved in the pre-intervention phase of the study served as the control group. Sources of contamination would include the presence and interaction of the investigators with patients, and attention to environmental factors and treatments which could sensitize staff. The nursing staff probably became more aware of the occurrence of confusion and, perhaps, needs of these patients because of the data collection being done by project staff. One can assume that these elderly patients received nursing care that was better than, but still comparable to, the current standard of practice.

As stated in Part I of this critique, the study could have benefited from a more detailed description of the interventions given to the treatment group. In order to judge the scope of interventions, study design, and results, Williams et al. should have provided a list of interventions under the preventive and ameliorative categories, as well as definitions and frequency and duration of the nursing activity. The reader does not know which interventions were most effective in preventing confusion or in ameloirating it with patients having mild versus moderate to severe confusion. The investigators suggest that the most frequently recorded interventions, which were also the least difficult for the nurses to implement (e.g., correcting sensory deficits, such as with eyeglasses) were the most effective in reducing acute confusional states. However, one can certainly argue with this conclusion as very effective interventions done less frequently (e.g., encouraging family members to visit) may have led to the results. In this regard, the study could have been strengthened by looking at the following dependent variables with each of the 15 nursing activities and grouping of interventions (preventive and ameliorative) as the independent variables: mild versus moderate to severe confusion, and each of the four behaviors of ACS. This would answer the clinically important question of which interventions are done and are helpful with which types of behaviors and levels of confusion. However, by breaking down the treatment into so many independent variables, the strength of the intervention and likelihood of statistical significance is markedly reduced. Only by looking at each individual subject's behaviors and their increase or decrease would the reader be able to determine which interventions were the most effective. The study results, therefore, can only be interpreted as indicating that the package of all of the interventions did reduce ACS in a group of patients.

A one-tailed z-test is an appropriate statistic for use in comparing the average between two groups of such sample sizes when the direction of the hypothesis can be stated. Results indicate that, after the adjustment for risk (based on the regression model), there was significantly less combined, mild, and moderate to severe confusion in the treatment group compared to the control group. The differences between the groups for the incidence of mild confusion would probably not be clinically significant (35.5 versus 35.1 percent), and could be attributed to the large sample size. However, the differences may have been minimized secondary to the potential measurement error previously discussed. The other differences would be quite notable to the nurse in practice. The results are clearly explained, particularly in the graph comparing the incidence of confusion by group with the day in hospital. On the day of surgery, the control group had a marked higher incidence of ACS which slowly declined over the hospital course. This is quite different from the trajectory of the experimental group in which there is less of a rise postoperatively, followed by a marked decline in ACS on day two, but then a gradual increase in ACS for the remainder of the study period. By postoperative days four and five, the groups had fairly similar occurrences of ACS (approximately 22 percent for the experimental and 25 percent for the control group). The investigators explain these results as indicating that the interventions are most effective from admission through the third postoperative day. Although this is a plausible explanation, it is also possible that some of the interventions increase confusion, particularly after the second postoperative day. One can also argue that, if one looks at the final outcome, on the fifth postoperative day, the interventions did not make much of a difference statistically or clinically. This presents the major impediment in a utilization decision and occurs because of the grouping of patient responses (control versus experimental) over and above examination of individuals. If the investigators had graphed the trajectories on a randomly selected subgroup of patients from each group with the identification of the timing of specific interventions, then the reader could feel more comfortable with the interpretation of the results.

Part IV: Generalizability of Results

The strengths of this study include a sample typical of the target population. In addition, the interventions require minimal staff development. The study population, settings, and staff are comparable to elderly patients hospitalized with hip fractures across the country and, to varying degrees, internationally. The interventions were carried out by typical practicing nurses and only limited training was necessary. Williams et al. are pioneers in the area so there is little with which to compare their results. Other studies do support their results regarding the incidence of ACS in hospitalized elderly.

Part V: Other Factors to Consider in Utilization

The utilization decision is a difficult one. Certainly, the high incidence of confusion among our elderly patients supports a need to evaluate new practices. The strengths of this study entice one to recommend utilization, but such a decision is premature. The interventions are, for the most part, neither complex nor costly, and many are routinely implemented by nurses with even a limited background in gerontological nursing. From what Williams et al. presented, the instruments do not seem complex nor time consuming, so it would be fairly easy to do a systematic evaluation of the innovation on a hospital unit. However, I would not recommend adoption of the innovation as a whole or even as a trial, given the concerns regarding the effectiveness and appropriateness of all of the interventions with elderly having various levels of confusion. I do recommend conducting some case studies, using the measures developed by Williams et al., however. Nurses who are skilled in care of the elderly would use the instruments as they work with their patients to monitor confusion and individual response to the interventions. Thus, there would not be an investment or focus in teaching new procedures. Additional important information would be the nurses' interpretation of the comprehensiveness of the tool in describing their actions to reduce or prevent confusion. From these activities, such information would provide the further specification needed before utilization and also serve to identify other interventions for study.

Intergenerational Caregiving: Adult Caregivers and their Aging Parents

Barbara J. Bowers, RN, PhD
Assistant Professor
School of Nursing
University of Wisconsin
Madison, Wisconsin

Theory-generating methodologies can be used to add to our knowledge in areas that are already well researched in addition to areas that have not been extensively studied. The study presented here demonstrates how the grounded-theory method was used to generate a new theory of intergenerational caregiving. Analysis revealed five conceptually distinct, overlapping categories of caregiving. Only one of these includes what is generally considered to be caregiving, that is, hands-on caregiving behaviors or tasks. The other four types are not observable behaviors but are processes crucial to intergenerational caregiving and to an understanding of the experience of intergenerational caregiving.

Intergenerational caregiving is becoming a significant issue for nurses practicing in a variety of settings. Nurses are in a pivotal position to provide care to both aged individuals and their family caregivers. The findings from the study presented in this article indicate that nurses and other health care professionals may lack an adequate understanding of family caregiving experience, precluding effective nursing intervention. What many family caregivers consider their most important work (protection) is often not considered at all by health care professionals. Despite the volumes of caregiving research, a theory-generating method of analysis, grounded in caregiver experience, can provide useful new insights having both practical and theoretical implications.

BACKGROUND

During the past decade, family caregiving research has experienced an explosive growth resulting in a large and diverse knowledge base. The variables investigated, the hypotheses generated, and the questions asked by researchers cover a wide range of topics but can be conceptually divided into the following general categories: (1) characteristics of those in need of care; (2) characteristics of caregivers; (3) content of caregiving; (4) impact of caregiving on the frail, elderly population; and (5) impact of caregiving on caregivers.

Based on recent US Bureau of the Census data, both the number and proportion of individuals over 65 continue to grow. In 1900, only 4% of Americans were over 65 as compared with the current 11.3%. Projections indicate continued growth of this age group to 21.8% by 2050.[1] Even more striking is the growth in the very old population. The over-85 group is expected to triple between 1980 and 2020. The significance of these data is underscored by a national study of well-being in the elderly, which reported the tremendous rise in general impairment levels corresponding to increases in age.[2] According to this report, only 6.3% of the US population under 70 is extremely impaired, while 9.3% of those between 75 and 79 and 22.5% of those over 85 are classified as extremely impaired. Many of these extremely impaired elderly can be found among the institutionalized populations. However, many more remain in their own homes with assistance from caring relatives.

Townsend's[3] recent study in Britain indicates that there are three times as many severely impaired individuals living at home than in all institutional settings combined. These data supported the findings of several other investigators, which repeatedly demonstrate the significance of family caregiving in preventing institutionalization of the elderly.[4-6] Recent government policies have increasingly been targeted at supporting or mandating family caregiving in an attempt to reduce institutionalization.[7-8] While not all of these non-institutionalized, impaired elderly have relatives to care for them at home, there is a strong positive correlation between increasing age and likelihood of moving into the home of relatives.[4,9]

Research on family caregiving has demonstrated the predominance of women, particularly wives and daughters, among the care providers for our nation's elderly.[6,9,10] These female caregivers tend, increasingly, to be participants in the paid labor force outside the home as well as being unpaid care providers within the home.[11-14] A number of recent studies[12,15,16] have documented the burden placed on these women caregivers and the stress experienced by them. Brody's well-known discussion of "women in the middle" identified the impact of simultaneously caring for one's children and one's parents or parent.[10] Other investigations have revealed increased incidences of both psychological and somatic symptoms among groups of caregivers.

The content of family caregiving has also received considerable attention. Studies of what caregivers do generally focus on the specific tasks involved in providing care and are often defined in terms of tasks such as bathing, transporting, grooming, preparing meals, giving financial assistance, etc. often referred to as activities of daily living. Caregiving can then be evaluated in relation to which tasks are being performed by whom, how often, and with what consequences for both the elderly and their caregiving relatives.[3,17-20] A comprehensive review of caregiving literature by Clark and Rakowski[21] divides caregiving into 45 separate caregiving tasks.

Overall, research on family caregiving supports or assumes a positive correlation between increasing frailty or impairment of the aged relative and caregiver stress. The assumptions are frequently made that living together is necessary for caregiving to occur and that the amount of caregiver work and stress is generally associated with performing caregiving tasks for very impaired elderly. The stress experienced by offspring of mildly impaired elderly can be easily overlooked. These caregivers are not considered at high risk and are therefore rarely included in caregiving studies. Indeed, many of these caregivers have become invisible. In order to understand this invisible caregiving and the associated stress, it is necessary to understand the world of caregiving from the perspective of the caregivers. Focusing on the tasks of caregiving effectively diverts attention from much of the work these caregivers are engaged in and renders them invisible.

STUDY OVERVIEW

Given the comprehensiveness of the caregiving literature, it seems there may be little to gain from an exploratory study. However, the current study demonstrates how a theory-generating method can add to our knowledge of an area that has already received much careful, scholarly attention. Grounding a study in the experiential world of the subjects can indicate where researchers have incorporated assumptions that are inconsistent with that world and, consequently, how those theories need to be altered. The study described here of middle-aged women caring for their aging parent(s) indicated that task-based categories are conceptually inadequate for understanding intergenerational caregiving (IGC). The study demonstrated how a reconceptualization of caregiving activities—distinguished by purpose rather than by task—is a more accurate representation of the experience, work, and stress of IGC. It also demonstrated how a task-based focus obscured an important aspect of family caregiving work.

The findings reported here represent one piece of a much larger study looking at intergenerational caregiving. This article focuses on the caregivers' perspectives rather than those of siblings, parents, or health care providers, all of whom are significant and will be discussed in future articles.

STUDY METHODS

A grounded dimensional analysis (a form of grounded theory) was used to conduct the study.[22-24] The method is grounded in a phenomenological epistemology and represents what Allen[25] described as interpretive science. The method evolved within the sociological tradition of symbolic interaction and is directed at developing a greater understanding of the experiential world of the research subject. Data collection and analysis are conducted concurrently, facilitating the discovery process by allowing research questions and hypotheses to evolve in response to the emerging theory. Consequently, the nature and focus of the initial research questions or hypotheses are often transformed during the research process, moving from very general to very focused.

A dimensional analysis was used to identify significant aspects of the caregiving experience. The constant-comparative, grounded-theory method was used to develop a sample of subjects and conditions representing various theoretical possibilities. Sixty interviews were conducted with 27 parents and 33 of their offspring. In some cases, the siblings of primary caregivers were also interviewed.

Caregivers range in age from 38 to 72. Thirty-one offspring caregivers were female and two were male; 18 caregivers were employed full time, 2 were employed part time, and 13 were unemployed. A caregiver employment level of 65% is consistent with the findings of previous studies.[11-13] Parents ranged in age from 62 to 97. One parent was below 70, 13 parents were between 70 and 79, and 11 parents were between 80 and 86. Only two parents were over 90. This sample, therefore, represents primarily elderly in the middle range rather than the very old group.

Living arrangements varied within the sample. Unlike some caregiving studies that include only families where the older parent lives with the offspring, several parents lived alone. Only 8 parents lived with caregiving offspring, 16 lived alone, and 3 lived in retirement centers.

THEORETICAL SAMPLING

Theoretical sampling was based on comparisons between cognitive and physical impairments and among levels of cognitive impairment. Analysis presented is based primarily on the sample of cognitively impaired. Theoretical sampling was also directed by a comparison of various living arrangements. Pairs of parents and offspring living together were compared with those living in separate residences. This sampling facilitated a focus on the invisible caregiving in which tasks were not of central importance and caregiving occurred from a distance.

DATA COLLECTION AND ANALYSIS

Data were collected through interviews that were taped, transcribed, and coded by the principal investigator. Interviews lasted from 20 minutes to three hours. Length of interviews varied in response to subjects' time restrictions and fatigue. Each subject was interviewed only once. Most interviews were conducted in the homes of the subjects, and caregivers and their parents were interviewed separately. Interview questions evolved during the study in response to the emerging theoretical categories, and the need to identify comparative conditions became more focused as the study proceeded. Some of the early research questions included:

- How does one become a caregiver?
- What is most stressful about being a caregiver?
- What is it like to be a caregiver of one's parent?

Later questions focused more on the consequences of failed caregiving and strategies for invisible caregiving. Later questions included:

- How does one care for an aging parent while preventing the parent from discovering that he or she is being cared for?
- How does this goal influence interactions with other offspring, other relatives, or health care providers?
- What strategies are used to respond to the parent who perceives that he or she is being cared for?
- Under what conditions are parents not upset about being cared for by offspring? How would this affect strategies for caregiving?

Analysis of the data from the early interviews offered insight into the research questions listed above and raised many new ones. Although it was not one of the initial research issues, the task-based definition of caregiving became problematic since it was clearly inconsistent with the caregivers' experiences. Analysis of these interviews revealed that the process of caregiving is much more complex than these commonly used definitions would indicate and that much of the stress associated with caregiving is unrelated to the performance of tasks. Furthermore, distinguishing among tasks may be irrelevant to understanding the experience of IGC.

DEFINING CAREGIVING

The work of caring for an aging parent, particularly in the presence of a mild cognitive defect, was discovered to be largely invisible. This invisible work is directed primarily at protecting both the parent's self-image and established parent–offspring relationships. Protective caregiving is experienced by many family caregivers as their most important work.

Caregiving is defined here by the meaning or purpose a caregiver attributes to a behavior rather than by the nature or demands of the behavior itself. Any process engaged in for the purpose of caregiving is therefore included. This method of defining caregiving has important implications.

First, both observable behaviors and mental activities are included. Plans and decisions made by caregivers are not observable tasks but may have important consequences for their lives. Second, consensus and shared understandings by parents and caregivers about the meaning of an activity are not necessary for an activity to be defined as caregiving. There are numerous instances in which a particular activity is perceived by one individual as caregiving, while others define the same activity quite differently. For example, caregivers were more likely than were parents to describe an activity as caregiving. Siblings of caregivers were also less likely than caregivers to perceive an activity as caregiving. Third, a behavior may serve more than one purpose simultaneously. When *forced* to label a particular behavior as either caregiving or something else, caregivers made purely arbitrary distinctions. Preparing a meal may be either a gesture of caring, a technical task, or both at once. A single activity such as meal preparation may be used to communicate very different messages. Frequently, the message intended by the caregiver is not the message received by the parent or others. Because caregiving is an interpretation of a situation rather than an observable event, any situation is open to multiple and conflicting understandings.

FIVE CATEGORIES OF CAREGIVING

A dimensional analysis of the data revealed five conceptually distinct but empirically overlapping categories of family caregiving. These categories include anticipatory, preventive, supervisory, instrumental, and protective care. Only the instrumental care includes the traditional definition of caregiving, that is, the hands-on caregiving behavior or tasks referred to earlier. The other four types, while not defined by or directly associated with observable behaviors such as tasks, are processes crucial to the IGC experience and to our understanding of how families care for their elderly relatives.

Analysis of the first three interviews revealed all five theoretical categories of caregiving. The 57 subsequent interviews provided considerable depth and elaboration while confirming the validity and consistency of these same five categories. Protective caregiving was experienced by these caregivers as both their most significant work and the most frequent and powerful source of stress. The centrality and invisibility of protective caregiving was repeatedly confirmed by the caregivers' experiences. Although protective caregiving was central for many caring offspring, it was a particularly critical issue when the aged parent had a mild to moderate cognitive impairment. Protective caregiving actually became less of an issue as a parent's cognitive impairment became more severe.

The following briefly outlines the five types of caregiving engaged in and then focuses on the most central category of protective caregiving.

Anticipatory Caregiving

Anticipatory caregiving includes behaviors or decisions that are based on anticipated, possible needs of a parent. It was usually observed in parent-offspring pairs who were not living together. It is a form of caregiving that often occurs from a distance. For example, as one woman explained:

> A lot of what I decide to do myself during the next few years ... I base not only on Joe, ... my son, ... but on my parents. Right now if I wanted to find a decent job, I could find it if I moved away from San Jose. But at this point, I feel that I have a certain responsibility to be here ... just in case.

"Just in case" is the key conceptual distinction of this category. This woman's decision about which city to live in is clearly, at least in part, a caregiving decision. Anticipatory caregiving is a mental event or perception that has, in situations such as this, a powerful impact on a caregiver's actions. This form of caregiving encompasses a great range of possible behaviors. Many important life decisions involve this type of anticipatory caregiving. This category cannot be defined by any associated, observable behaviors that allow it to be identified as caregiving. It is also rarely talked about openly between parents and their offspring. Many caregivers perceive an open discussion about this anticipatory care as threatening or insulting to their parent(s). It is a form of caregiving that is intentionally invisible. Shared understandings about the meanings of anticipatory caregiving behaviors are carefully avoided by offspring.

Preventive Caregiving

Preventive caregiving frequently includes activities carried out by offspring for the purpose of preventing illness, injury, complications, and physical and mental deterioration. It generally involves more active monitoring and supervising than anticipatory caregiving. Prevention includes activities such as altering the physical environment to increase safety; questioning the parent about symptoms, medications, etc; and preparing chicken soup or meals. Again, it is distinguished by its purpose rather than its associated tasks.

Supervisory Caregiving

Supervisory caregiving, the third category, is observed in situations where identifiable care is given to a parent. This type is generally experienced as an active and direct involvement of the offspring and is likely to be recognized by the parent and others as actual caregiving activity. Activities include arranging for, checking up, making sure, setting up, and checking out. They may be done with or without the parent's awareness. Archbold also identified a similar category of care, distinguishing between family care providers and care managers.[26] Again, it is the purpose that defines the category of caregiving.

Instrumental Caregiving

Instrumental caregiving includes "doing for," "assisting," "providing," and "giving." It is the hands-on caregiving more commonly recognized as caregiving. The purpose of this care is to maintain the parent's physical integrity and health status. Not surprisingly, it was most often observed in situations where the parent was ill or disabled. While this is the type of caregiving that is most often studied by social scientists, health care professionals, public health professionals, and public policy analysts, it was considered by family caregivers as the *least* important type. This perception of lesser importance is directly related to its purpose. Instrumental care is related to physical well-being and the care of the body rather than to emotional well-being and protection of the parents' identity, which are characteristic of protective care.

Protective Caregiving

Protective caregiving, the fifth category, was experienced by most caregivers as the most difficult and important type of care provided. The purpose of protective caregiving is to protect the parent from the consequences of that which was not or could not be prevented. These potential consequences were perceived by caregivers as threats to the parent's self-image rather than to their physical well-being. For example, while cognitive decline could not be prevented, the parent's altered self-image or depression resulting from the awareness of cognitive decline could be. At least caregivers believed they could affect the situation and made active attempts to do so.

A 57-year-old woman, Anne, described how her elderly mother took great pride in having dinner prepared for her each night when Anne came home from work. The mother's ability to cook was seriously affected by her mild cognitive as well as sensory impairment. This meant that Anne was frequently given meals she described as inedible (for example, salt was substituted for sugar). Rather than confront her mother with the situation, she ate what was put in front of her.

This example of protective caregiving clearly has consequences for both the parent and the caregiver. The parent's self-perception as competent and independent is protected while the daughter suffers silently over a barely edible meal. This daughter had also stopped inviting guests to dinner, fearing what her mother might serve them.

A very important aspect of protective caregiving is the caregiver's frequent attempts to protect the parent from awareness that she or he is being taken care of. While caregivers often used the language of role reversal, they also described their enormous efforts to prevent the parent from sharing this reversed role perception. Caregivers described the importance of protecting both the parent's identity and the parent–child relationship. An inordinate amount of protective caregiving work is directed toward this goal and creates much caregiver stress. This protective care was engaged in most intensely when a parent had a moderate cognitive impairment. Even the minimal loss of cognitive abilities was perceived by caregivers as very threatening to a parent's self-image and to the parent–child relationship. This perceived threat accounts for much of the stress related to mild cognitive decline and the intensity of caregiving work in response to an apparently minor problem. Many caregivers were extremely successful at providing care in a way that was not perceived by the parent as caregiving, as in the following example:

A 62-year-old daughter who was caring for her frail, 92-year-old mother discussed her mother's increasing forgetfulness and confusion. The daughter was concerned because her mother's weekly trip to the bank involved three bus transfers. The daughter was fearful that the older woman might become lost in the large inner city during one of her trips. The younger woman convinced her elderly mother that their bank was unsafe. It had been robbed recently. Both women changed all of their accounts to another bank, which, coincidentally, was only a few blocks from their home.

Several offspring described what they did for a parent and the nature of their relationship with the parent as representing a reversal of roles. They described themselves as giving care to a parent who was "like their child." However, on closer observation, several discrepancies with the role reversal model were discovered. This role reversal was, in fact, very different from a simple reversing of activities and methods of interacting. The offspring had not become "like a parent," nor was the parent treated "like a child." Two important characteristics of the situation distinguished it from a simple reversal of roles. First, the parents were not aware of the offspring's perception that roles were reversed. Thus, while the offspring might see themselves as acting like a parent, the parent never described himself or herself as feeling like a child. Preventing the parent from "discovering" a reversal of roles was an active strategy engaged in by offspring caregivers.

The second distinction is related to the first. Although *what* an offspring did may have been experienced as representing a role reversal, *the way in which* it was done was not representative of this reversal. In fact, caregivers carefully orchestrated their caregiving activities to appear as if the parent–child relationship was intact. For example, a son or daughter might claim to take care of a parent's needs, "look after" him or her, monitor health problems, etc. just as one would do for a child; however, the way in which these things were done maintained consistency of the actual parent–child relationship. Parents were checked up on or looked after in a way that was not "parental," as in the following example:

> One daughter described how she telephoned her mother's physician before and after each of her mother's clinic visits. Each time, the daughter instructed the physician to write out the mother's prescriptions and treatments on a piece of paper. The daughter also requested that information be sent to the daughter so that she could supervise her mother's care at home. Finally the daughter requested that the physician not inform the mother of the conversation between physician and daughter. This revelation, the daughter believed, would be "insulting" or "demeaning" to her mother. In this way, the daughter explained, she could supervise her mother's activity while not revealing her action to her mother. As the daughter explained, "I can suggest instead of tell her. I can't tell her what to do. She's my mother. I can suggest it."

STRATEGIES FOR PROTECTIVE CAREGIVING

Caregivers engage in three strategies of protective care. The first is to protect the parent from awareness of an *event*. The example of the salty, inedible meals represents this first strategy. The daughter's silent acceptance of an offensive meal is an instance of protective caregiving. She is protecting her mother from evidence concerning the mother's competence. Although there is no observable caregiving task, the daughter's decision has clear implications for the daughter's life and should be considered an example of protective caregiving.

A second strategy is to protect the parent from awareness of the *meaning* of a situation. This process involves acknowledging the existence of an event while reconstructing its meaning or significance. Caregivers engaged in this second strategy when the parent could not be protected from awareness of the event. An event may be acknowledged as an isolated incident, ignoring its significance as part of a larger pattern. This is done in situations where it is the pattern or consistency of an event, rather than its substance alone, that imputes the undesired meaning. Thus, forgetting is not in itself significant; however, continual forgetting has important negative implications (i.e., senility). Forgetting a pan of vegetables cooking on the stove and starting a fire and forgetting whether one has eaten breakfast have greater significance than other types of patterns of forgetting.

> One daughter explained how she was never upset by her father's forgetting dates, names, or appointments; however, she became concerned when he began to forget whether he had eaten meals. This particular forgetting was different both in its meaning and its consequences. The meaning was suddenly perceived as more serious.

Another interesting aspect of this type of protective caregiving is that siblings often disagreed about what represented "significant forgetting."

Caregivers actively reconstruct the meaning of an event or situation by rendering the event consistent with the parent's personality. Likening a developing problem to an idiosyncratic characteristic effectively neutralizes a significant event. For example, losing things may be considered an indicator of senility to the offspring but may be represented to the parent as "the way you've always been." Much of the stress associated with caregiving is related to the process of continually constructing and reconstructing the meanings of events. The sources of stress are both the amount of work related to this process and the caregivers' sense of how vulnerable this process is to the influence of outsiders.

These processes are generally used in the order in which they are listed above. Caregivers often attempt first to prevent parent awareness of an event. When this fails, strategies are aimed at careful reconstruction or control of the meaning of the event in question. Failure to control this awareness is often perceived by caregivers as having great consequences for both themselves and the parent.

One daughter described how she protects her mother from awareness of things the mother does. For example, when the mother threw out seven years of the daughter's income taxes, the daughter did not tell her mother what she had done. This daughter also did not tell her mother about how bad the mother's cooking had become because she frequently became confused and forgot ingredients. The mother was prevented from being aware that she was doing these things. When the daughter could not prevent the mother's awareness of forgetting, misplacing, etc., the daughter redefined the situation to render the meaning of the incident not threatening to the self-characterization. For example, when the mother misplaced some important papers and left part of their dinner in the oven, the daughter joked that "you've never been able to remember those things." The daughter explained, "It's lifelong (the forgetting), so therefore, it's just a continuation, only more so. She used to put things away and one of us kids would have to watch her, see where she put it so we could tell her later. So we've always teased her about it. It's worse now." Because forgetting is consistent with the mother's self-characterization, increased forgetting is interpreted as "just like Mom" rather than as representing senility. "But we can still tease her about it." As the mother became aware of the possible influence of getting older and becoming senile, she became very depressed. Once her mother became depressed, the daughter could sometimes reverse the depression with ice cream or a phone call (to siblings). That usually helped. "She's an ice cream freak."

Another strategy for neutralizing the significance of a situation is to attribute its cause to something perceived as less distressing than its "real" cause. For example, one parent who was continually breaking objects was worried that she was "losing control" of herself and developing a dreaded neurological disease. The daughter, in response, convinced her mother that the clumsiness was due to fatigue caused by her medications and did not herald the neurological disorder. The daughter was herself fearful that the mother's suspicions were correct. Because of the risk of revealing the true cause of the clumsiness, the daughter did not seek medical help for her mother. She could not trust the physician to collaborate with her protective caregiving activities. The physician was clearly perceived as a threat to successful protective caregiving work.

It was not known, in this instance, whether the mother was developing the dreaded disease. However, awareness of the disease as a possibility provided an important condition influencing the daughter's caregiving strategies. Without such awareness, the caregiving strategies might have been different.

Protective care was perceived as so crucial that, in many instances, caregivers were more willing to risk physical harm to a parent than to risk an insult to the parent's self-image or to the relationship between the parent and the caregiver. Many caregivers were clearly more concerned with protective care than with getting the tasks done or even with preventing physical injury. The successful implementation of instrumental care was often believed to conflict with protective care. The purpose of protective care was generally perceived by caregivers to be of much greater significance than the purpose of instrumental care. In fact, this dilemma and how it was solved formed the basis of most of the conflicts among family members and between caregivers and health care professionals.

The source of this conflict was most often

whether protective or preventive and instrumental care were more important. Primary caregivers overwhelmingly chose protective care, while health care professionals and less involved relatives more often considered preventive and instrumental care more important. The consequence for many caregivers was to limit or prevent the involvement of others in the care of their parents. This decision increased the isolation of caregivers and severely limited their possible use of resources, including nurses and other health professionals. Removing themselves from the health care system and sometimes from the family system was one way to maintain control of the situation.

RELEVANCE TO NURSING INTERVENTION AND RESEARCH

It is clear from the study presented that the efficacy of nursing interventions depends on the nurse's ability to assess family involvement in the care of older parents. Distinctions among the various categories of caregiving activity must be included in this assessment. Failure to recognize the occurrence and significance of protective caregiving can lead nurses to inappropriately assess a family member as uncooperative or noncompliant. Worse still, a family member engaged in protective caregiving often feels most threatened by nurses and other health care providers who focus their efforts on one of the other categories of caregiving. Consequently, family caregivers feel compelled to protect their parent from the intrusion of health care professionals. A carefully informed assessment of the caregiver's perceptions and priorities can prevent the nurse from being perceived as an adversary rather than an advocate for the patient and his or her family.

The study also demonstrated the importance of nurses pursuing the use of theory-generating methodologies such as dimensional analysis and grounded theory. Although intergenerational caregiving has been intensely studied with other more traditional methodologies, the instrumental task-based conceptualization of caregiving has gone unchallenged. Failure to ground theoretical categories in lived experience of the subjects has led to the development of an inaccurate or inadequate knowledge base. The use of theory-generating research is appropriate at all stages of knowledge development. It can be used to generate knowledge in a content area about which very little is known. It can also be used to clarify, develop, or redirect research in a content area about which much is already known, such as intergenerational caregiving.

REFERENCES

1. Biennial census of population. (1984). *Current Population Reports*. US Bureau of the Census series P-25, No. 952.
2. *Public policy and the frail elderly*. (1978). US Dept of Health, Education and Welfare, Federal Council on Aging, OHDS publication No. 79-20959. Government Printing Office.
3. Townsend, P. (1981). Elderly people with disabilities. In A. Walker & P. Townsend (Eds.), *Disability in Britain*. Oxford: Martin Robertson.
4. Shanas, E. (1977). *National survey of the aged*. Chicago: University of Chicago Circle, final report.
5. Brody, S., Poulshock, W., & Mascioachi, C. (1978). The family caring unit. *Gerontologist 18*, 556–561.
6. Young, M., & Willmott, P. (1957). *Family and kinship in east London*. London: Routledge & Kegan Paul.
7. Hatch, O. (1982). Government's impact on the family: A professional view. *The Hatch Report*, Aug 8-14.
8. U.S. wants children to help pay for elderly parents' care. *San Francisco Chronicle*, (1983, March 30), p. 10.
9. Crystal, S. (1982). *America's old age crisis*. New York: Basic Books.
10. Brody, E. (1981). Women in the middle and family help to older people. *Gerontologist, 21*, 471–480.
11. Beechey, V. (1978). Women and production: A critical analysis of some sociological theories of women's work. In A. Kuhn & A. Wolpe (Eds.), *Feminism and materialism*. London: Routledge & Kegan Paul.

12. Finch, J., & Groves, D. (1983). *A labour of love: Women, work and caring*. London, Routledge & Kegan Paul.
13. Cantor, M. J. (1983). Strain among caregivers: A study of experience in the United States. *Gerontologist, 23*, 597–604.
14. *Employment and Training Report to the President*. (1976). US Department of Labor, GPO publication No. 746-C, GDL-1-42-2. Government Printing Office. 1976.
15. Soldo, B., & Myllyluoma, J. (1983). Caregivers who live with dependent elderly. *Gerontologist, 23*, 605–611.
16. Miller, D. A. (1981). The sandwich generation, adult children of the aging. *Social Work, 26*, 419–423.
17. Shanas, E. (1968). Family help patterns and social class in three countries. In B. Neugarten (Ed.), *Middle age and aging*. Chicago: University of Chicago Press.
18. Sussman, M. & Burchinal, L. (1968). Family kin network: Unheralded structure in current conceptualization of family functioning. In B. Neugarten (Ed.), *Middle age and aging*. Chicago: University of Chicago Press.
19. Cicirelli, V. (1983). A comparison of helping behavior to elderly parents of adult children with intact and disrupted marriages. *Gerontologist, 23*, 619–625.
20. Robinson, B., & Thurner, M. (1979). Taking care of aged parents: A family transition cycle. *Gerontologist, 19*, 586–593.
21. Clark, N. M., & Rakowski, W. (1983). Family caregivers of older adults: Improving helping skills. *Gerontologist, 23*, 637–642.
22. Glaser, B., & Strauss, A. (1968). *Discovery of grounded theory*. New York: Aldine.
23. Glaser, B. (1968). *Theoretical sensitivity*. Mill Valley, CA: Sociology Press.
24. Knafl, K., & Howard, M. (1984). Interpreting and reporting qualitative research. *Research in Nursing and Health, 7*, 17–24.
25. Allen, D. (1985). Nursing research and social control: Alternative models of science that emphasize understanding and emancipation. *Image, 17*, 58–64.c.
26. Archbold, P. G. (1980). Impact of parent caring on middle-aged offspring. *Journal of Gerontology Nursing, 6*, 79–85.

This article is printed with permission of *Advances in Nursing Science*. Copyright 1987 Aspen Publishers, Inc.

Original article:
Bowers, B. J. (1987). Intergenerational caregiving: Adult caregivers and their aging parents. *Advances in Nursing Science*, 9(2), 20–31.

CRITIQUE BY: GAIL PERRY, BSN, RN

Part I: Clinical Relevance

Bowers conducts a theory-generating study of intergenerational caregiving (IGC) with the purpose of examining a well-researched topic in a fresh light. Although this study is one element of a larger project Bowers is conducting, here she develops theory relating to the content of IGC from the perspective of the caregiver.

In her study, Bowers includes areas of caregiving that have been overlooked in the past. She mentions "invisible caregivers," or those who have either a mildly impaired parent or those who do not live with their impaired parent and yet take some responsibility for that parent. She also differentiates her study from previous studies by stating that previous studies define caregiving in terms of tasks performed. In this regard, Bowers attempts to show that much of caregiving, and, therefore, much of the stress associated with caregiving, needs to be evaluated in terms of purpose rather than tasks.

New theory regarding caregiving is potentially very practical. Additional well-developed theory in this area would give nursing a greater structure in which to assess needs, define outcomes, and plan interventions for IGC family units. Given the possibility of the findings being useful in practice, the study deserves further examination.

Part II: Conceptualization and Internal Consistency

Bowers' study has internal consistency. She examines concepts of IGC from the viewpoint of the caregiver, as proposed in her opening paragraphs. Her language is clear and her logic concise.

Bowers begins to justify her study by acknowledging the important role nursing plays in providing care to elderly persons and their caregivers. She claims that if nurses do not understand the caregiving experience, they cannot intervene successfully in these nursing situations. She states that certain assumptions have been made by previous researchers of the subject, including: defining caregiving in a task-oriented framework; assuming that caregiving only occurs when the family lives together in the same residence; and that stress is linked to the tasks of caregiving. Given these assumptions, which she claims have colored much of the previous research, Bowers states that a fresh look at the experience of caregiving is needed. She also stresses that caregiving must be understood from the viewpoint of the caregiver.

As a descriptive study, the study question itself seems to ask, "What is the experience of caregiving in an IGC situation?" This fits very well with the justification, which states the need to reexamine IGC. The investigator does not begin with operational definitions or a list of concepts to be examined, as this is incompatible with her research methodology. Instead, the investigator develops these as the research progresses. The concepts and definitions that the investigator formulates from the research continue to fit with the justification and study question.

The study question posed by Bowers is a level I problem. Research at this level is intended to lead to theory development, as is done here. In terms of study methodology, Bowers states that she used grounded dimensional analysis, which is derived from phenomenological epistemology. Unfortunately, I have only a simplistic knowledge of such methods. In addition, most of my training in research is based on traditional scientific procedures, wherein credibility of a research effort is established in relationship to its adherence to the scientific principles of gathering evidence. Not all topics are able to be appropriately studied in this manner, however. One school of thought in research is built on phenomenologic approaches, in which case the traditional scientific method is not used but disclaimed. It is difficult for one trained in the traditional scientific method to fairly evaluate such phenomenologic research. I will attempt to do so, but my bias toward more traditional approaches will be apparent.

Grounded dimensional analysis provides Bowers with the specific tools she needs to accomplish her objective. As mentioned, this approach allows the investigator to explore a topic without defining in advance ideas that she hopes to find. That is, it allows one to label concepts as they emerge from the data. In exploring the experience of IGC, Bowers does so by interviewing persons who live within that setting. Therefore, her subjects are consistent with the population of interest.

For her instrument, Bowers used an unstructured interview that allowed her to explore concepts as they arose. (This is a commonly used and acceptable tool with which to explore a level I problem.) The instrument evolved from general to specific over the course of the interviews based on Bowers' analysis of data as collected. To organize the data analysis process, Bowers taped, transcribed, and coded the interviews. She categorized concepts that arose in early interviews and looked for them in following interviews. These methods provided Bowers with a vehicle for fully exploring a topic and also meeting the need for progression from general to specific, a necessary continuum in exploratory theory development. Taping an interview, while possibly making a subject nervous, would not interfere with the quality of data collected.

The conceptualization for Bowers' study appears logical, appropriate, and internally consistent throughout. To this point, this research has good credibility and is worth further examination.

Part III: Believability of Results

As discussed earlier, the purpose of Bowers' study is to describe a phenomenon of concern to nursing. The data collected are qualitative in nature.

The subjects consisted of 27 parents and 33 offspring. Caregivers were age 38 to 72 years. Most caregivers were female and varied in terms of employment and living situation. Parents were ages 62 to 97 years, with most being in the middle range. Their living situations varied. Some were cognitively impaired while others were physically impaired.

At this point, however, a question rises. Bowers states that she based her analysis on the cognitively impaired sample, but she does not state how large that portion of the sample was. However, later in the study, she states that she uses all 60 subjects in the development of her theory of the five categories of caregiving. Therefore, the actual sample size remains unclear.

In addition, Bowers does not state how she selected her sample or where she found her subjects. This leads me to assume that she used a sample of convenience. She does have a wide variety of subjects who are involved in caregiving situations as parent or offspring. Apparently, she attempted to obtain as wide a variety within her sample as possible. This has both strengths and weaknesses. For a descriptive study, a wide variety of subjects would help to gather as much diverse information from people involved in a family IGC experience as possible. Apparently, Bowers attempts to use this variety of subjects to compare subgroups of subjects, such as the caregivers who live with their parents versus those who live alone. However, it seems that there are not enough subjects in any one of the subcategories to be able to significantly compare groups. In fact, although Bowers used subgroups of the sample in the data analysis, she does not inform her readers of the number of subjects in each of the subgroups cited.

Several potentially problematic areas in Bowers' methods exist that may introduce the possibility of an unmeasurable bias. In the interviews and data analysis, concepts might be over emphasized or ignored by the investigator, based on her personal bias. The coding and analysis of data are open to her interpretation alone. Another potential bias relates to the fact that the manner in which people represent themselves and their views may be influenced by face-to-face interviewing. People want others to see them in a good light and tend to interpret facts in a way that makes them look good. In addition, although a single interview per subject is widely practiced in phenomenological research, meeting a subject only once creates the possibility of that subject having either an unusually good or bad day, which may bias his or her report of the situation.

Bowers does not discuss such possibilities, suggest they might influence the quality of results, or give ways these might be accounted for. Many investigators discuss weaknesses in their research and warn appropriately of caution in generalization or utilization of results. Bowers does not do this, and I feel that this research is weaker for lack of this perspective on Bowers' part. In addition, and because Bowers uses no quantitative measurement tool, reliability and validity are moot points in regard to her instrument.

Sampling is evidence of another weakness on Bowers' part. Her sampling, which seems too broad and shallow, is simply not adequate to cover this topic. The subjects come from many categories, but each category needs to be represented in more depth.

The data collection and analysis appears to have been a subjective task, and much detail is not given. It is stated that "a dimensional analysis was used to identify significant aspects of the caregiving experience." However, Bowers offers no further explanation. Nor does she state that interview questions changed during the study as the theoretical categories began to emerge. Is this to be taken as a given? Or did the questions become more focused on these emerging categories as the series of interviews continued?

In regard to the theoretical categories used, they seem to be separate from each other, without an overlapping of content. Aside from a few illustrations, Bowers, again, fails to report the observations that support the theoretical categories. In fact, it may be that the data Bowers gathered, which consists of the stories and lives of many people, are not readily accessible for inclusion into such a short article. Therefore, the reader is unable to examine the quality of the categorizations as they pertain to the data base. Even so, Bowers does state that she developed all five categories of caregiving from the first three interviews, and that all the following interviews supported those categories.

The methodology of this research has many problems. In addition, much of the information needed to judge the worthiness of the conclusion is not made available. While I have no training in the method Bowers uses, this shortcoming does not prevent me from questioning the completeness and reliability of Bowers' results. With the information available, however, I would have to say that, although the five theoretical categories defined by Bowers are interesting and even fascinating, too many problems are inherent in the study to accept them at face value. They are intriguing, but a sound documentation does not exist to support their believability. Caution should be practiced in the utilization of these concepts of caregiving.

Part IV: Generalizability of Results

Even without questions raised regarding quality of results, the generalizability of this study would be in question. Some aspects of the study that would determine generalizability are well done. The sample and setting are representative of the sample and setting that nursing deals with. The sample consisted of the actual caregivers and impaired elderly that are involved in IGC situations, and the setting of the home is one of the settings of current practice for nurses. In addition, the experiences of these subjects were determined by interviewing, in which nurses are thoroughly trained. But in spite of the similarity between practice and the research sample, setting, and technique, the complete lack of replication of this material at this point prevents it from being generalized to other populations. Remember, Bowers presents utterly new information. No other study has as yet replicated these findings, and Bowers cites no previous theory that would add support to this newer theory.

In general, I feel that even if the methods had been exemplary or understandable to me, the newness of this theory would urge caution in generalization and utilization. New theory must be validated by other studies.

Part V: Other Factors to Consider in Utilization

After reading this study, curiosity may prompt many nurses to assess clients involved in caregiving in order to see how their experiences fit with Bowers' theory. This would be quite appropriate and easily done through interviewing. Until further studies are done, each nurse can assess and decide for him or herself the applicability of Bowers' five categories of caregiving.

Beyond this, however, is a striking need for someone to develop a quality scientific tool that would test Bowers' theory and utilize it with a large sample of caregivers. Several investigators in several parts of the country would need to validate this before it could be accepted as theory by the nursing community and applied to general practice.

I see two risks of changing practice based on this research. First, such practice would be based on inconclusive theory. If accepted at this point, nursing would sell itself short by adopting new, inadequately investigated research. The second risk, which might never occur, would be that Bowers' theory might take attention away from the needs of caregivers who suffer the stress of 24-hour "task" caregiving. Hopefully, this would not occur. Bowers' research, therefore, would best be an addition to present theory, and not a replacement of it. I have done 24-hour a day caregiving and am aware of the stress and exhaustion it entails. The need to give respite care and assistance to caregivers who have demanding loads of physical care and 24-hour caregiving schedules should be unchanged by this study.

On the other hand, if this study is not applied, many needs will be overlooked in which nursing could otherwise intervene. Numerous "invisible caregivers" would remain invisible. In addition, Bowers cites the example of caregivers who, to protect their cognitively-impaired parent's self-esteem, also have to protect them from health care providers who, being unaware of the practice of protective caregiving, might be a threat to such parent's self-esteem. It is impossible to build trusting, therapeutic relationships with clients in situations as these.

The benefits of adopting this theory as a basis for practice include the discovery of invisible caregivers, whose needs could then be assessed and interventions planned to help them. Health care providers would be able to learn to work within the client's caregiving framework, thereby promoting therapeutic relationships with caregivers and the impaired elderly.

I see little cost involved in adopting this theory as a basis for practice once it has been adequately validated. It would involve changing a mind set among nurses regarding caregiving, however. Although this does not come easily to nursing as a whole, this change of thinking could be integrated without excessive difficulty by nurses who are patient advocates and who are concerned about giving quality care to their clients, both physically and psychosocially.

A balance needs to be found between the utilization problems related to methodology and lack of outside validation, and the benefits of adopting this theory. Until further studies can be done, nurses should keep these concepts in mind when they are dealing with caregiving families and assess the presence of these categories of caregiving and any needs related to them.

Although the critique of this study has demonstrated some weakness in methodology leading to questionable usability, this study has some impressive strengths. The justification for such a study is excellent, and the investigator's observations support the justification. Bowers proposes through her theory that a non-task-oriented theory base regarding IGC is clearly needed. This has the potential to have a major impact on future thinking on caregiving. If Bowers' theory is validated by other investigators, an expanded definition of caregiving will arise along with a new focus of assessment and new ways of intervention. Bowers' theory holds great promise.

Even though this research is inconclusive in itself, its publication was appropriate so that nursing could become aware of new and important concepts. Other nursing researchers now need to validate Bowers' study in a precise, scientific manner. Fortunately, this theory is exciting enough and promising enough that it should have no difficulty generating the necessary interest.

Original article:
Bowers, B. J. (1987). Intergenerational caregiving: Adult caregivers and their aging parents. *Advances in Nursing Science, 9*(2), 20–31.

CRITIQUE BY: JUDY MILLER, MSN, RN

Part I: Clinical Relevance

Intergenerational caregiving is the topic of research in this study. The problems of families giving care to elderly members is an important area for understanding and involvement by nurses. As aptly described by Bowers, the growth of the elderly population and particularly those over the age of 85 presents a major social challenge, much of whose responsibility is assumed by the family. Effective family caregiving can prevent institutionalization of the elderly person. However, the problems of multiple chronic diseases, physical limitations, and cognitive impairment which become more common in elderly over the age of 85 can create intense emotional stress and place a heavy, physical burden on the family. Nurses have a major responsibility in helping to promote and maintain the health of all family members as well as the family unit.

This study helps nurses to identify and begin to assess the key tasks and potential problems encountered by family caregivers. The investigator states, "the study demonstrated how a reconceptualization of caregiving activities—distinguished by purpose rather than by task—is a more accurate representation of the experience, work, and stress of IGC (intergenerational caregiving)." Bowers' study generates a new theoretical perspective on the nature of caregiving. By broadening our view of the scope of the caregiving role, it has definite potential for use in nursing practice. Areas of assessment, teaching, and counseling with families need to be tested and expanded based on this theoretical perspective.

Part II: Conceptualization and Internal Consistency

The study follows through with its stated intent of examining intergenerational caregiving with elderly parents. Its language is readable with the major exception of the study methods section. Qualitative research and use of grounded theory methodology are not common in nursing research literature. Thus, while the investigator correctly identified the need to describe this form of research, her description of it, at least for this reader, leaves much to be desired. In fact, the study methods section is a conglomeration of vocabulary that only a reader knowledgeable in grounded theory would understand. The introductory paragraph to this section, which would probably be unnecessary to such a reader, also is not helpful to the nurse new to qualitative research. The study could be strengthened, however, by using the introductory paragraph to provide basic guidelines and definitions useful in reading grounded theory research.

Justification for the study is well established, but based primarily on the findings of the study. It would be interesting to know what led the investigator to suspect that there were gaps and weaknesses in the existing wealth of information about caregiving. Bowers concludes that caregivers of mildly impaired elderly are a population who are frequently ignored, and, therefore, merit study to determine their problems.

Although not stated explicitly, this study purports to understand the world of caregiving from the perspective of the caregiver. The grounded theory approach is an appropriate methodology for obtaining such data. In this approach, the concepts and definitions develop through the study and lead to generation of theory. Unfortunately, Bowers does not present her initial definition of family caregiving which guided the literature review and early stages of the study. Based on her report of the problem that caregiving created for family members, it is apparent that Bowers' initial definition of caregiving had the commony used task orientation. However, the categorization of caregiver topics and the thorough literature review does provide some parameters for the study and is consistent with areas of interest to nurses.

Using the grounded theory approach, an investigator provides a general statement and question to subjects as a means of guiding the interview. A flaw in methods occurs when Bowers fails to present the initial study question. Subsequent questions that Bowers identifies (e.g. "What is most stressful about being a caregiver?") are valid for the purpose and justification for the study.

Study questions with grounded theory methodology are guided by continuous analysis of the data. Information from the early interviews generates the questions asked of subjects who follow. Because Bowers does not provide the initial ("grand tour") question or a conceptual framework, it is not clear as to whether she conducted the study in a way to answer the study question regarding the nature of caregiving. Bowers states that later questions focused more on the consequences of failed caregiving and invisible caregiving strategies. Even so, one still does not know if the focus of the study went in this direction because it was most important to the world of the caregiver or because it was the area which had the most gaps in a developing conceptual framework of caregiving. Presentation of even a tentative conceptual framework showing the relative importance and relationships of the categories of caregiving could be expected as a conclusion with this type of study. Nonetheless, information presented in the different sections of this study build well on each other in a logical manner consistent with the grounded theory approach.

Beyond family units where there is an elderly member, it is not clear what the population of interest is. When the investigator reports results, she does not limit the comments to the study population. The family units interviewed do not represent the population of intergenerational caregiving. It would have been helpful for the investigator to explain why she chose to focus on middle-aged daughters caring for elderly parents with cognitive impairment who were not physically frail. Is this the population of interest? Does the subject population mirror the problems of any type of family unit or elderly member with different levels or types of physical or cognitive impairments?

Although there are weaknesses in methodology and the conceptual framework for the study, they may be the result of missing pieces of information rather than major gaps in design. Since this study is an element of a larger project, it is likely that several of the problems identified would be resolved with the student reviewing the entire study. Therefore, my recommendation is to continue with a more detailed evaluation of the research study.

Part III: Believability of Results

In this study, Bowers gathered qualitative data for the purpose of describing the phenomenon of caregiving from the perspective of the caregiver. Because Bowers does not indicate how she initially recruited subjects, I assume that it was by way of convenience. A potential bias of a convenience sample is that subjects who agreed to participate did so because the caregiving situation was either very good (so they were pleased to talk about it) or very bad (and they were seeking assistance or an opportunity to ventilate). A study strength is the use of subjects who were involved in the caregiving situation as either primary caregiver, sibling of the caregiver, or carereceiver. Thus, the qualitative data obtained was generated from the reality of the caregiving situation.

Description of caregiver characteristics on age and employment indicate a good representation of age and employment level consistent with previous studies. However, the distribution by gender, with only two male subjects, seems slanted even with the predominance of female caregivers in the general population. In addition, Bowers does not explain if daughters caring for their elderly parents were the intended population of intergenerational caregiving chosen for study or were the result of convenience sampling. As she indicates, the problems of female caregivers in this country are significant and merit study.

Two findings of this study are the role reversal of the elderly parent and child (caregiver) and the importance of the protective caregiving function. The study does not explore the possible effects of the sample characteristics of gender and position in the family on these results. For example, are the patterns of role changes similar when the caregiver is a wife instead of a daughter? Does the child have a greater need to maintain the image of the parent (thus, engaging in protective caregiving functions) than the wife? A strength of this study is the variety of living arrangements represented in the sample. Unlike many studies which only include families where the elderly person lived in the same household, this study also includes elderly who live alone or in retirement homes. Purposeful sampling was used, consistent with grounded theory methodology, to obtain this representative sample for the characteristic of living arrangement. This enabled the investigator to pursue and develop the concept of invisible caregiving.

The characteristics of carereceivers (elderly parents) in the sample are not clear and problematic to interpretation of the study findings. Ages are presented but not levels of cognitive and physical impairments which certainly impact on the types and amount of care needs. Bowers states that she based her analysis primarily on the sample of cognitively impaired, and much of the results refers to those with moderate cognitive impairment. However, she does not define or describe moderate impairment, nor do we know the relative distribution of levels of impairment within the sample. With advancing age among the elderly, the prevalence of concurrent physical and cognitive impairments increases. This leads one to question whether those in the sample analyzed by Bowers had few, if any, physical problems which would be acharacteristic of the population. Because of these questions regarding sample composition, generalizability of Bowers' findings regarding invisible caregiving and the relative importance of the types of caregiving is limited. It may be that protective is the most important type of caregiving only in situations where physical care and safety needs are low, as represented in this sample. Also, the investigator does not discuss the effect of potential biases or intervening variables with sampling.

Taping of interviews, followed by transcription and coding of the data, are common means of data collection with grounded theory methodology. Unfortunately, the investigator does not discuss the reliability of these measures. Of course, taping is more reliable than notetaking during interviews. The investigator also enhanced reliability and validity by interviewing caregivers and elderly parents separately in their homes, which reduced possible interruptions and the uneasiness of subjects in an unfamiliar environment. It is more likely that subjects would report their true thoughts about the caregiving situation if other family members were not present. Since the principal investigator conducted all the interviews, interrater reliability is not at issue here. It would be important, however, for the interviewer to identify her biases and factors which could impinge on the manner in which she conducted interviews and the accuracy of transcription/coding (e.g., interviewer fatigue). The great variation in the length of the interviews leads one to question the reliability of the shorter interviews.

Validity is another area not thoroughly discussed by the investigator. Of particular concern is that the interviewer did not return to at least some of the subjects to verify the definition of caregiving and the caregiving categories derived from the interviews. Bowers reports that the five theoretical categories of caregiving developed with analysis of the first three interviews, with subsequent interviews confirming the validity and consistency of the categories. This can be viewed as a strong indicator of validity. However, the possibility exists that premature closure of study resulted from using the developing categorization too early in guiding subsequent interviews. The study also does not indicate whether Bowers asked other experts in the field of gerontology or family caregiving to review the coding of data and conceptualization. This is an important aspect of content validity. As is consistent with grounded theory method, interview questions did develop during the study in response to information obtained during early interviews.

In conclusion, with the absence of validation of the coding and categories (via return to the subjects and expert review), one cannot be assured that the investigator stayed within the boundaries indicated by the subjects. However, the following two actions by the investigator offer some reassurance: validation of the categories of caregiving in subsequent interviews; and providing examples of statements made by subjects within the categories of caregiving which support the conceptualization.

As previously noted, because Bowers does not clearly state the population of interest, questions exist regarding the sampling method. If the population of interest consists of daughters caring for elderly parents, then Bowers has good representation. The number of subjects interviewed and the inclusion of elderly living alone as well as with caregivers are particular strengths of sampling in this study. By interviewing caregivers, carereceivers, and siblings of the caregivers, Bowers obtains important viewpoints on the world of the caregiver. One could argue that it would be helpful to have interviewed health care providers to obtain their perspective on the caregiving situation for families. This could provide information regarding the nature of the caregiver–carereceiver relationship and cost of caregiving in terms of the caregiver's health. However, health care providers are not members of the family system so this would not be an important focus of the study. However, sampling leaves representation of the general concept of family caregiving to elderly members incomplete. It is unknown how the concept and categories of caregiving would develop given different caregiver relationships to the carereceiver or different physical care needs.

Bowers describes some aspects of data gathering and analysis in detail. She provides a good explanation of the problems associated with the initial task-focused, caregiving definition. For example, she shifted data gathering in order to pursue the areas of failed caregiving and strategies for invisible caregiving. However, she is not specific as to how the caregiving categories developed. It seems that they became apparent early in the data collection phase. One does not know how much coding and recategorization was necessary in developing the conceptualization. The category label of supervisory caregiving is compared to the similar research findings of Archbold (1980). The category labels are not described in relation to other research or theoretical perspectives or as coming directly from the vocabulary of subjects. Thus, it is unclear how they were derived.

Bowers provides excellent examples of observations to support each concept label. As a result, the categories of caregiving are clear, internally consistent, and representative of the group of observations. A major result of this study is the relative low importance of instrumental caregiving (physical care activities) compared to other categories of caregiving. In this regard, Bowers identifies protective caregiving as the most difficult and important type of care. However, Bowers' findings on the relative importance of caregiving activities can be criticized based on the types of subjects in the study. One can argue that the proposed relationships would be different had Bowers used a more representative sample, especially with regard to level of care needs. In clinical practice, caregivers report and exhibit many symptoms of stress as they expend a great deal of energy managing the physical care and safety needs of frail, elderly, family members. It also is not clear whether subjects were asked to rate the intensity of the categories of caregiving or whether this was determined by subject-initiated reporting. Protective caregiving is presented as a critical behavior undertaken by family caregivers to preserve the carereceiver's self-esteem, even at the cost of neglecting physical care needs and limiting involvement with health care providers. Another possible explanation, not explored by Bowers, is that the behaviors were undertaken as an attempt by caregivers to maintain the family unit and family self-view and not directly to protect the elderly carereceiver. Or, protective caregiving can be a means for the caregiver to deny the severity of the parent's problems.

There are several methodological problems with this study that support nonutilization of findings. The low risk of utilization of the results and recognition that this study is only an element of a larger project allow one to proceed with the next component of the research critique, however.

Part IV: Generalizability of Results

This study is significant and unique because it explores family caregiving of elderly members from the perspective of family members. As such, its findings have not been replicated and are different from other studies. The nurse researcher used an interview format to explore caregiving. The use of therapeutic communication, and guided and unstructured interviews, are all common to nursing practice, so that the study methods are generalizable to nursing practice. Training would be necessary in constant comparative analysis, although it is an extension of validation of assessment and diagnosis. Problems with sample generalizability have previously been discussed. This study is valuable to the nurse who works with women in the community who are caring for their fairly functional, elderly parents.

Part V: Other Factors to Consider in Utilization

There are great potential benefits in using this study to modify one's nursing practice, and no identified risks. The study results suggest that we may be ignoring major areas of effort and concern to family caregivers by our tendency to focus on the physical tasks of caregiving. In addition, caregivers may avoid contact with the health care system to protect the elderly parent from direct mention of the person's limitations. With all clients who are caring for elderly family members, regardless of the levels of cognitive or physical impairments and types of family relationships, the following changes in nursing practice should be made:

- Conduct interviews with family members individually as well as together to determine the nature of the caregiving situation, problems, and concerns.
- Avoid premature focusing on the tasks of caregiving by using a more open-ended interview format.
- Have the elderly person present his or her perspective of health needs/problems to avoid using diagnoses which may be problematic to his or her self-image.

These suggestions were listed to show how the findings of this study do not really change nursing practice as much as to emphasize and remind nurses of some of the basic communication skills and approaches that they were taught. Nurses who use these guidelines in their practice and make notes of the important areas identified by caregivers would be able to engage in a feasible, systematic evaluation of Bowers' findings, with far greater generalizability. To fail to attend to the findings of this study is to potentially ignore the needs of many family caregivers and elderly.

Pacing Effects of Medication Instruction for the Elderly

Katherine K. Kim, MSN, BSN, RN
College of Nursing
University of Illinois
Chicago, IL

Margaret R. Grier, PhD, BSN, RN
Associate Professor
College of Nursing
University of Illinois
Chicago, IL

Over the past two decades, research in learning has consistently demonstrated that the elderly perform poorly in fast-paced learning situations. Thus, for effective teaching, it is imperative that nurses slow their instruction for elderly clients. We conducted a study to examine the effect of pacing medication instruction on the learning of elderly clients, and the results confirmed the importance of slow instruction for the elderly.

Studies indicate that errors in self-administration of medication among the elderly are common and often lead to serious problems.[1-3] Medication studies that categorized types of errors found that clients make one or a combination of the following types of self-medication errors: (a) omission, (b) inaccurate knowledge, (c) incorrect dosage, (d) improper timing and sequence, and (e) medication taken but not ordered by the doctor.[4] Factors related to the occurrence of these medication errors included age, ability to cope with the environment, the number of medications prescribed, and knowledge about medications. The probability of making an error increased with age.[1-3] As the client's ability to cope with the environment increased, the tendency to make medication errors decreased.[3] The probability of error increased with the number of medications.[3,5-7] As the client's knowledge of medication increased, the tendency to make medication errors decreased.[1,2,6,8] Knowledge about medications is, thus, one factor related to the occurrence of self-medication errors, but there has been limited research documenting the effectiveness of teaching in reducing medication errors among the elderly.[1,6,9-13]

Recent research on learning in old age suggested many variables that influence learning. Learning deficits in old age are attributed to changes in sensory perception, memory, and/or intelligence; heightened arousal of the autonomic nervous system; increased cautiousness; slowed responses to environmental stimulation; and instructional variables such as pace of presentation, task relevance, and task difficulty.[14-18] While little can be done about the cognitive variables, nurses can control instructional variables. Of these, pacing, defined as speed or rate of performance, is of major importance.

A number of studies reported that when the time to study visual materials is increased, the old benefit more than the young.[19,20] The elderly also benefit from a longer time to give responses.[19,21-23] The comprehension of speech can reveal speed deficits among the aged.[24-26] Panicucci and associates[27] conducted a study on the use of slow speech and self-pacing with the aged and found that slow speech increased the aged person's ability to integrate information and respond appropriately. Thus, one way to help the older person is to slow the pacing of learning events.[15]

HYPOTHESES

1. Elderly clients who are instructed at a slow pace will have greater gain from the pretest to the posttest score than those instructed at a normal pace and those receiving no instruction.

2. Elderly clients who are instructed at a slow pace will make fewer total response errors to questions during the medication instruction than those instructed at a normal pace.

In addition to testing these hypotheses, we also examined the time the elderly clients took in giving their self-paced responses during the medication instruction.

DEFINITION OF TERMS

Normal pace: Rate of 159 words per minute. An average speaking rate of English-speaking college students was used for establishing rate.[28]

Slow pace: Rate of 106 words per minute. Thus, normal pace was 50% faster than slow pace.

Self pace: Rate controlled by the subject, an opportunity to take as much time as needed for a performance.

Gain score: Difference in the pretest and the posttest scores.

Response error: Incorrect or no responses by the subject during the medication instruction.

Self-paced response time: Number of seconds the subject used in recalling and repeating the drug information given in the instruction. In self-pacing responses, the subject was allowed to take as much time as needed within a limit of four minutes.

METHODS

Sample

The study was conducted in a 1200 bed public hospital, located in the Midwest and serving adult patients with chronic diseases. From a total of 410 patients in two units, 48 were selected. Patients 65 years of age or older with a prescription for a diuretic, antihypertensive, or digitalis drug were identified using the medication Kardex. We obtained permission from the attending physician for the patient's participation in the study. After consulting the nurse in charge as to the advisability of including the patient in the sample, one of us (KK) met with each patient to evaluate that patient's orientation to time, place, and person. If the patient met the sample selection criteria, the purpose of the study was explained and the patient's consent to participate was obtained. A number was assigned to each patient according to the order selected for the study. The patient was then assigned to one of three study groups using a block randomization method. Two of the 48 patients refused to participate; one patient became too ill to take the posttest and was replaced. Thus, a total of 45 patients was studied, 15 in each of the three groups.

Learning Materials

The medication instruction included five areas: name of the drug, purpose, frequency, dosage, and time of drug administration. The instruction was presented to the patients using audiotape and written learning material. The audiotape was used to control the presentation of learning material at a normal pace (159 words per minute) and a slow pace (106 words per minute). The tape was prepared by blocking the script into 30-second intervals: the number of words in each interval depended on the desired rate of presentation. The speaker spoke at an even pace, visually checking the end of each 30-second interval on a stop watch. The written learning material listed the five content areas of instruction, and was typed in large print.

Instruments

The measurement tools, the pretest and the posttest, were essentially the same as to content, number of items, and scoring system. The tests covered the areas included in the medication instruction. For each content area one recall and two recognition items were developed, resulting in a total of 15 items for each test. Content validity was established in accordance with the opinion of experts. Reliability of the instruments was tested using a test-retest procedure ($r = .84$, $p < .05$).

Procedure

A pretest-posttest control group design[29] was used in the study. The research design included two experimental groups, the normal-paced and the slow-paced groups, and a control group. The pretest was administered to all three groups individually, in a private room. The first author read each question slowly and loudly for the patient and recorded the patient's answers on a prearranged recording sheet. The tests took 10 to 20 minutes and were administered during one day.

Immediately following the pretest, one experimental group received the medication instruction at the normal pace, while the second group was given the instruction at the slow pace. Each patient received instruction for one prescribed medication. The control group was not given the medication instruction. All patients received individual instruction from the first author in a private room. The instruction took approximately 5 to 10 minutes.

Before presenting the medication instruction the volume of the audiotape recording was adjusted to the patients' hearing level; this volume was maintained throughout the instruction. First, the patients were told the name of drug, its purpose, frequency, dosage, and time of drug administration. The patients then were asked to recall these five items of drug information. They were told to take as much time as needed to answer the questions. It should be noted that the written learning material was presented to the patients during the first part of the instruction, but was removed from the patients when they were responding to the questions. The instructor gave correct answers to the questions immediately after the responses.

During the medication instruction, patients' responses to questions were recorded on tape. Response errors used to test the second hypothesis were measured from these responses, and were not taken from the posttest. The tape recording was used later with a stop watch to measure the time it took a patient to give each response. The time interval between asking the question and the patient's verbal response was used as a measure of the self-paced response time.

Approximately 24 hours after giving the medication instruction, the posttest was administered to the two experimental groups. The control group also was given the posttest at a comparable time but without the medication instruction. For ethical reasons, the control group was given slow-paced instruction after the posttest.

Results

The 45 subjects ranged from 65 to 94 years, (mean 77.7 years). There were 17 men and 28 women in the sample. All subjects had at least one diagnosed medical problem. Statistical analysis showed that the three groups did not differ as to age, sex, formal education, and number of prescribed medications. To ascertain the complexity of the learning task, length of the drug name was examined. Chi-square analysis revealed that the three groups did not differ with respect to the number of letters in the drug name. The average number of letters in each drug name was seven to eight. Analysis of variance of the pretest scores revealed that the three groups also did not differ as to knowledge of drugs prior to instruction (Table 1.)

Gain Scores

The mean gain score of the slow-paced group was significantly greater than that of the normal-

Table 1
Knowledge of Medication Gained by Elderly Patients

Instruction group	M	SD
Normal-paced (n = 15)		
Pretest	4.53	4.22
Posttest	7.33	5.07
Gain	2.80	2.81
Slow-paced (n = 15)		
Pretest	4.40	3.76
Posttest	11.80	2.57
Gain	7.40*	4.17
Control (n = 15)		
Pretest	5.13	4.70
Posttest	6.40	4.78
Gain	1.27	2.74

Note: The possible range of the pretest and the posttest scores was 0-5
*$p < .01$

Table 2
Frequency of Response Errors
by Elderly Patients During Instruction

Instruction group	M	SD	Range
Normal-paced (n = 15)	3.267	1.751	0-5
Slow-paced (n = 15)	2.200	1.373	0-4

t(28) = 1.856, p < .05, one-tail test

paced group, t(28) = 3.543, and that of the control group, t(28) = 4.761, p < .01, one-tail test (Table 1). There was no significant difference in the mean gain scores of the normal-paced group and the control groups, t(28) = 4.514, p > .05. In the posttest, the number of patients *recognizing* the name of their drug was greater than those *recalling* the drug names. The ratio between the percentage of patients recognizing the drug name and recalling it in the normal-paced and the slow-paced groups was 33.3%:6.7% and 73.3%:20.0%, respectively.

Response Errors

The mean number of response errors by the slow-paced group are significantly less than those of the normal-paced group, t(28) = 1.856, p < .05, one-tail test (Table 2). The normal-paced group correctly recalled slightly more than one-third (35%) of the items during the medication instruction, while the slow-paced group recalled 56% of the items correctly. When response errors to each question were examined, recalling the name of the drug was the most difficult learning task: 77% of the 30 patients in the two instruction groups were unable to recall the name of the drug 4.5 minutes after receiving the information and 40% of these patients made response errors in the frequency of the drug administration question.

Self-Paced Response Time

Since the self-paced response time of the control group was also measured, these data are in Table 3 for comparison among the groups. The total self-paced response time was calculated by adding all response times to the five questions. The data show that the three groups did not differ significantly from each other in the total self-paced response time, $X^2(2) = 4.98$, p > .05. A chi-square test was used for this analysis because variance of the three groups were significantly different, $F_{max}(14) = 18.218$, p < .05.[30] The median was used as a measure of central tendency because of the number of extreme values. The common median of the total response time was 12.25 seconds. The self-paced response time to any one question ranged from 0.5 to 48 seconds. Some patients took as long as 40 to 48 seconds to recall drug information such as name, purpose, and frequency of drug administration.

DISCUSSION

The findings of the present study support the hypothesis that elderly patients who are instructed at a slow pace will have greater gain from the pretest to the posttest score than those instructed at a normal pace and those receiving no instruction. Furthermore, the gain score of the group receiving instruction at a normal pace did not differ significantly from that of the group who did not receive any instruction. Thus, we conclude that elderly patients learn more when the speech rate used for instruction is slowed.

The data also show that elderly patients who are instructed at a slow pace make fewer errors

Table 3
Number of Elderly Patients in Each
Medication Instruction Group
According to Self-Paced Response Times

	Instruction group			
Response time*	Normal-paced	Slow-paced	Control	Total
Shorter	10	4	8	22
Longer	5	11	7	23
Total	15	15	15	45

*The terms longer and shorter apply to more or less than the common median value of 12.25 seconds of the total time to respond to five questions.

in responding to questions during the instruction than those elderly instructed at the usual rate. This further emphasizes the importance of slowing the pace of instruction for the elderly. The results of our present study agree with those of other investigators, who found that elderly persons are at a disadvantage with insufficient study time.[19,20] The present results also agree with Panicucci and associates,[27] who found that slow speech created a difference in the aged patient's ability to integrate information and to respond appropriately.

Our study revealed that, regardless of the pace of instruction, elderly patients have difficulty recalling drug information within 1.5 minutes after receiving it. When response errors to each question were examined, recalling the name of the drug was the most difficult learning task. Less than one fourth of the patients in the experimental groups were able to recall the names of their drugs 1.5 minutes after receiving the information. The high response errors in recalling drug names may be explained partly by complexity of drug names, and the fact that with age the decline in recall is greater than the decline in recognition of learned material.[15,17] Although the average number of letters in each drug name was seven to eight, six patients had a prescription for hydrochlorothiazide (19 letters). It should be noted that all five questions that measured response errors were recall items, whereas the posttest consisted of both recall and recognition items. In the posttest, the patients had more difficulty in recalling the names of their drugs than recognizing the drug names.

Fortunately, when taking a prescribed medication at home the patients usually need to recognize rather than recall information on the drug container label. Nevertheless, this finding emphasizes the importance of written instructions in addition to verbal information for the elderly. Written information not only gives an opportunity to review information, but also encourages recognition of learned material.

Our study showed that pacing of medication instruction had no significant effect on the self-paced response time. Canestrari[21] reported that older persons used significantly more time under self-paced learning conditions than did younger persons. Our data showed the importance of recognizing a wide individual variation in self-paced response time among the elderly.

Caution should be taken in generalizing the results of this study. In addition to the uniqueness of the sample and setting, the sample size was limited to 45. Additional studies need to be done to validate the results of this study with another population. In future studies, the levels of the speed of instruction could be increased to determine the appropriate speed of instruction for the elderly. How slowly should the instruction be delivered to the elderly? Future studies should be directed to answer this question.

CONCLUSION

In summary, the findings of this study showed that slow-paced instruction benefits elderly patients in their learning. The patients in the slow-paced group had not only greater gain from the pretest to the posttest score, but also made fewer errors during the medication instruction. As evident in the literature and in our study, speed of instruction is a major variable influencing learning in the elderly. In providing drug information to elderly patients, it is important that nurses not only deliver their instruction at a slow pace, but also provide sufficient time for patients to respond to questions.

Acknowledgement

The authors wish to thank the thesis committee members, Dr. Mary Bevis and Dr. Alice Dan for their assistance during various phases of the study.

REFERENCES

1. Boyd, J. R., Covington, T. R., Stranaszek, W. F., Coussons, R. T. (1974). Drug defaulting part ii: Analysis of noncompliance patterns. *American Journal of Hospital Pharmacy, 31,* 485–491.
2. Latiolais, C. J., & Berry, C. C. (1969). Misuse of prescription medications by outpatients.

Drug Intelligence and Clinical Pharmacology, 3, 270–277.
3. Schwartz, D., Wang, M., Zeitz, L., & Goss M. F. W. (1962). Medication errors made by elderly, chronically ill patients. *American Journal of Public Health, 52,* 2018–2029.
4. Stewart, R. B., & Cluff, L. E. (1972). A review of medication errors and compliance in ambulant patients. *Clinical Pharmacology and Therapeutics, 13,* 463–468.
5. Clinite, J. C., & Kabat, H. F. (1969). Prescribed drugs, errors during self-administration. *Journal of American Pharmacy Association, NS9,* 450–452.
6. Malahy, B. (1966). The effect of instruction and labelling on the number of medication errors made by patients at home. *American Journal of Hospital Pharmacy, 23,* 283–292.
7. Neely, E., & Patrick, M. L. (1968). Problem of aged persons taking medications at home. *Nursing Research, 17,* 52-55.
8. Given, C. W., Given, B. A., & Simoni, I. E. (1978). The association of knowledge and perception of medications with compliance and health states among hypertension patients: A prospective study. *Research in Nursing and Health, 1,* 76–84.
9. Spector, R., McGrath, P., Uretsky, N., et al. (1978). Does intervention by a nurse improve medication compliance? *Archives of Internal Medicine, 138,* 36–40.
10. Gibmle, J. G. (1967). Oral medication and the older patients. In: *ANA regional clinical conferences.* New York: Appleton-Century-Crofts.
11. Hecht, A. B. (1974). Improving medication compliance by teaching outpatients. *Nursing Forum, 13,* 112–129.
12. Kelly, P. (1972). An experiment in self-medication for older people. *Canadian Nurse, 68*(2), 41–43.
13. Libow, L. S., & Mehl, B. (1970). Self-administration of medications by patients in hospitals or extended care facilities. *Journal of American Geriatrics Society, 18,* 81–85.
14. Arenberg, D., & Robertson-Tchabo, E. A. (1977). Learning and aging. In J. E. Birren & K. W. Schaie (Eds.), *Handbook of the psychology of aging.* New York: Van Nostrand Reinhold.
15. Botwinick, J. (1978). *Aging and behavior* (2nd ed.). New York: Springer.
16. Corso, J. F. (1971). Sensory processes and age effects in normal adults. *Journal of Gerontology, 26,* 90–105.
17. Craik, F. (1977). Age differences in human memory. In J. E. Birren & K. W. Schaie (Eds.), *Handbook of the psychology of aging.* New York: Van Nostrand Reinhold.
18. Eisdorfer, C. (1977). Intelligence and cognition in the aged. In E. W. Busse & E. Pfeiffer (Eds.), *Behavior and adaptation in later life* (2nd ed.). Boston: Little Brown.
19. Arenberg, D. (1965). Anticipation interval and age differences in verbal learning. *Journal of Abnormal Psychology, 70,* 419–425.
20. Eisdorfer, C. (1965). Verbal learning and response time in the aged. *Journal of Genetic Psychology, 107,* 15–22.
21. Canestrari, R. E. (1963). Paced and self-paced learning in young and elderly adults. *Journal of Gerontology, 18,* 165–168.
22. Eisdorfer, C., Axelrod, S., & Wilkie, F. I. (1963). Stimulus exposure time as a factor in serial learning in an aged sample. *Journal of Abnormal Social Psychology, 67,* 594–600.
23. Monge, R. H., & Hultsch, D. F. (1971). Paired-associate learning as a function of adult age and the length of the anticipation and inspection intervals. *Journal of Gerontology, 26,* 157–162.
24. Konkle, D. F., Beasley, D. S., & Bess, F. H. (1977). Intelligibility of time-altered speech in relation to chronological aging. *Journal of Speech and Hearing Research, 20,* 108–115.
25. Schon, T. D. (1970). The effects on speech intelligibility of time-compression and expansion on normal hearing, hard of hearing, and aged males. *Journal of Auditory Research, 10,* 263–268.
26. Sticht, T. G., & Gray, B. B. (1969). The intelligibility of time compressed words as a function of age and hearing loss. *Journal of Speech and Hearing Research, 12,* 443–448.
27. Panicucci, C. L., Paul, P. B., Symonds, J. M., & Tambellini, J. L. (1968). Expanded speech and self-pacing in communication with the

aged. In *ANA clinical sessions*. New York: Appleton-Century-Crofts.
28. Kelly, J. C., & Steer, M. D. (1949). Revised concept of rate. *Journal of Speech and Hearing Disorders, 14*, 222–226.
29. Campbell, D. T., & Stanley, J. C. (1963). *Experimental and quasi-experimental designs for research*. Chicago: Rand McNally.
30. Sokal, R. R., & Rohlf, F. J. (1973). *Introduction to biostatistics*. San Francisco: Freeman.

This article is printed with permission of *Journal of Gerontological Nursing*, 1981.

9

Mental Health Nursing

Beverly Hoeffer, DNSc, RN
Laurie Beeson, BSN, RN
Valerie Gowdy, BSN, RN

INTRODUCTION BY: BEVERLY HOEFFER, DNSc, RN

Psychiatric and mental health nursing is concerned with phenomena associated with both mental health and mental illness. In this specialty, nursing practice focuses on assisting individuals and families across the life span to develop competencies and coping strategies that prevent dysfunctional responses to stressful events and transitions or that enable them to manage the effects of mental illness in their daily lives. The purpose of psychiatric and mental health nursing research is to develop theory and to test clinical approaches that enhance practicing nurses' capabilities to intervene therapeutically with clients in a variety of institutional and community settings.

The first two studies selected for inclusion in this chapter represent efforts to develop practice-relevant theory to guide nursing interventions with persons suffering from a chronic mental illness. Although all nursing specialties address psychosocial aspects of patient care, psychiatric and mental health nursing has been concerned with vulnerable individuals who are susceptible to disabling mental disorders, such as schizophrenia.

The first study, Tudor's "A Sociopsychiatric Nursing Approach to Intervention in a Problem of Mutual Withdrawal on a Mental Hospital Ward," was selected for critique because it is considered to be a classic in the field. Sills (1977) cites it as a benchmark study that represented a conceptual shift from investigating within-person to within-relationship phenomena. More recently, the study has been cited as an example of how practice-relevant theory can be generated through a process of identifying phenomena embedded in the clinical context (Hoeffer & Murphy, 1982). In 1952, the causes of mental illness were unknown and intrapersonal theories of mental illness prevailed. Patients spent years in mental hospitals where little emphasis was placed on the impact of the hospital milieu on the maintenance of their symptoms. Similarly, the definition of the role of the psychiatric and mental health nurse as an active participant in patients' treatment versus custodial caretaker and technician was in its infancy. Hence, does the study conceived and conducted in such a context have relevance for practice today? Does it have the potential to enable students and nurses on inpatient psychiatric units of the 1980s to solve current clinical problems? In my opinion, the answer is yes.

The second study, Davidhizar, Austin, and McBride's "Attitudes of Patients with Schizophrenia Toward Taking Medication," was selected because it represents current research in the field. In this study, theory borrowed from another discipline was used to explain patients' attitudes towards taking medication, a clinical phenomenon thought to be associated with compliance with prescribed psychotropic medications. Psychiatric and mental health nurses in inpatient and outpatient settings are frequently involved in teaching patients about their medications and in monitoring patients' adherence to medication regimens. Hence, knowledge about how such attitudes are related to patients' insight into their illness and treatment would be particularly useful in developing effective nursing strategies to facilitate medication management. Moreover, the study is more worthy because it emphasizes the importance of understanding illness experiences of persons with schizophrenia from their perspective in the process of planning nursing care. Also, because the study was replicated a year later (Davidhizar, 1987), it exemplifies an approach to nursing research (i.e., evaluation through replication) that enhances its utiltiy for practice.

The third study, Burgess and Holmstrom's "Recovering from Rape and Prior Life Stress," was selected for inclusion in this chapter because it represents another aspect of the field. Psychiatric and mental health nursing also is concerned with developing practice-relevant theory to guide nursing interventions with persons experiencing the sequelae of an acute crisis precipitated by a traumatic life event. Women's experience of rape received considerable attention in the nursing and nonnursing literature during the 1970s. In part, this attention reflected an increased awareness and acknowledgment by clinicians and public of the adverse effect that acts of violence and abuse had on women's mental health and their lives in general. However, as Burgess and Holmstrom noted in the study presented here, studies of the long-term consequences of rape and victim's recovery from the experience were infrequently reported in the literature. Hence, the longitudinal study of female rape victims' recovery over a four to six-year period was especially timely. Since a major focus of nursing practice is restorative care (i.e., to promote recovery and optimal levels of wellness and functioning), the study continues to be relevant to mental health nurses who practice in any health care setting in which rape victims are clients.

Besides its clinical relevance, the study is noteworthy as an example of meaningful interdisciplinary research on the relationship between stress and mental health outcomes. In this case, a nurse and a sociologist with differing perspectives and expertise examined a phenomenon that cut across discipline boundaries. Such collaborative efforts have the potential to generate shared knowledge that can contribute to nursing's conceptual base for practice.

Psychiatric and mental health nursing practice encompasses a much more comprehensive range of phenomena than are reflected in these three studies, however. For example, the subjects in all three studies were experiencing a mental illness or mental health problem during adulthood. No studies were selected that focused on phenomena related to children's or older persons' experiences of acute or chronic mental health problems or to dysfunctional families, such as those at risk for family violence. Nonetheless, the three studies provide a representative sample of psychiatric and mental health nursing research that has utility for clinical practice.

REFERENCES

Davidhizar, R. E. (1987). Beliefs, feelings and insight of patients with schizophrenia about taking medication. *Journal of Advanced Nursing*, *12*, 177–182.

Hoeffer, B., & Murphy, S. (1982). The unfinished task: Development of nursing theory for psychiatric and mental health nursing practice. *Journal of Psychosocial Nursing and Mental Health Services*, *12*, 8–14.

Sills, G. (1977). Research in the field of psychiatric nursing: 1952–1977. *Nursing Research*, *26*(3), 201–207.

A Sociopsychiatric Nursing Approach to Intervention in a Problem of Mutual Withdrawal on a Mental Hospital Ward

Gwen E. Tudor, MA, BS, RN
Director of Nurses and
Assistant Professor of Psychiatric Nursing
State University of Iowa
Iowa City, IA

Psychiatric nurses in a mental hospital are increasingly expected to manifest their competence in nursing by an awareness of and an ability to handle their interpersonal relations with patients in a therapeutically useful manner. Such expertness with the patient in his daily living is oriented primarily in three directions: The nurse functions to facilitate the patient's communication. Since mental illness is, in part, a defect in communication, any understanding of the patient's nonverbal gestures or symbolizations and in turn the conveying of meaning to the patient should be of therapeutic value. Secondly, the psychiatric nurse functions to facilitate the patient's social participation. Since the predominant characteristic of the mentally ill person is his withdrawal, both physical and social, the nurse who is able to "make a contact," to convey to the patient through mutual participation that social relationships need not be frightening and anxiety-provoking, but can be both satisfying and security-giving, has enabled the patient to take the first step toward mental health. Finally, the psychiatric nurse functions to fulfill the patient's needs. The form of expression these needs take, the manner in which they are fulfilled, and the appropriateness of the fulfillment in terms of the manifest need are all matters which the nurse must consider in relating herself to the patient.

There is a growing awareness on the part of some psychiatric nurses that the traditional skills of the psychiatric nurse, although they are important, are not sufficient for fulfilling these three functions most effectively. It is the contention of this paper that the psychiatric nurse must use, to some extent, the tools of the social scientist and combine these with the skills of the nurse. It is hoped that from this liaison will emerge a new skill which will enable the nurse to function more effectively. The social context as it determines and affects the nurse-patient relationship has been insufficiently explored and taken into account in psychiatric nursing. Although a particular nurse may establish effective and satisfactory relations with a patient, this can be easily undone by what others do with the patient, by the formal and informal social structure on the ward which tends to maintain the patient in his mental illness, by the interpersonal relationships among the staff members, and by the general institutional context which orders and forbids certain activities. The social context within which the patient lives is that pattern of interpersonal relations which is the network of reciprocal activities of all those on the ward. It is this social context which both determines in large part the nurse's attitudes and modes of behavior and also facilitates or deters the patient's mental health. The first step is for the nurse to realize that she is part of this social context. She is affected by it and, in part, determines and maintains it. Thus the envelope of characteristic attitudes and activities which constitute the nurse's formal and informal participation is an integral part of the patient's living and will move him toward health or away from it. In turn, the patient also contributes to this context, resulting in a reciprocal influence between patients and personnel: both are affected by and maintain the social context, which, in our study, is the ward—which is itself imbedded in a wider social context called the hospital.

Within this general theoretical framework, our first general assumption is that *"the patient's mental illness is a mode of participation in the social process."*[1] What has ordinarily been considered a symptom—the patient's assaultiveness, incontinence, hallucinations and delusions, demandingness, withdrawal (physical and verbal), and destructiveness—we view as his characteristic pattern of relating to other people. The interpersonal situations he characteristically integrates constitute his mental illness. The second assumption follows from the first: *This mode of participation—the patient's mental illness—can be altered and influenced by the activities others direct toward him*. And the third assumption is that *an alteration in the patient's participation can come about if the nurse is aware of, and acts upon the awareness of, two sets of phenomena*: (1) the nature of the specific interpersonal situations she integrates with the patient; and (2) the nature of the general social context within which these interpersonal situations take place.

Thus not only does the psychiatric nurse need to include the perspective of the social scientist in her operations, but she also needs to become as skillful an observer as she is a participant in psychiatric nursing. Her observations must include an awareness and evaluation of as many as possible of the relevant factors in order to best work in the direction of a therapeutic social context. Without this observational ability, the nurse cannot adequately meet the needs of the patient and facilitate his communication and social participation. Thus, the nurse must become a participant observer, free to see the actualities and potentialities in patient-staff situations and, at the same time, able to deal with the current requirements of the situation. From our point of view, psychiatric nursing can be conceived of as a continuous interpersonal process consisting of these overlapping and definable components: *observation, evaluation of the observations, determination of the various alternatives possible within the situation, intervention, evaluation of the intervention with reference to the reasons for success or failure, and further intervention on the basis of the new data obtained.*

PROBLEM

The problem undertaken for study was twofold: first, to determine the social context and specific social situations with which the patient in a psychiatric unit was integrated and in which he maintained a recurrent pattern of participation, and to identify the various modes of such participation; and second, to determine the ways in which, and means whereby, appropriate intervention might be instituted so as to alter these modes of social participation in the direction of increased security, satisfaction, and higher self-esteem for the patient.

SETTING

The data were collected in a 14-bed ward for disturbed women, which was part of a 50-bed

---

[1] This framework is derived from the work done by M. S. Schwartz and A. H. Stanton. "A Social Psychological Study of Incontinence." Psychiatry (1950) 13:399–416.

private psychoanalytic hospital.[2] The patients in this ward all have the clinical diagnosis of schizophrenia, with the exception of one diagnosed manic-depressive psychosis. Data pertaining to the rest of the hospital were considered only when they seemed to be related to the patients or personnel in the selected unit. Because these patients were severely disabled by their illnesses in terms of caring for themselves or following ordinary social conventions, the personnel-patient ratio was high. The physical facilities provided for patients' living were minimal, consisting only of bare essentials.

At the beginning of the study, the ward organization was such that the investigator characterized it as authoritarian as compared to the general attitude in the hospital. It was highly organized around the ideas and wishes of the charge nurse. A rigid routine had been established, to which few exceptions were made. Rules and regulations regarding the patients' living were numerous, and maintenance of these rules was stressed repeatedly with the personnel. This allowed little spontaneity or initiative on the part of the personnel, because they were kept so rigidly in line by the charge nurse's orientation; nor did it permit the undertaking of alternative attitudes and activities on the part of the personnel with patients. Patient-personnel contacts were largely limited to essential care or occasions when requests were made by the patients. These contacts appeared to be quite stereotyped in that most activities were governed by regulation, or, if not, a decision for such an activity was made by the charge nurse in accordance with a pre-established set of ideas and characteristic prevailing attitudes. One characteristic attitude which prevailed was that a "good" nurse or aide was one who "did not have any trouble with patients."

During the second month of the study, a change in charge nurses was made. The new charge nurse was a very permissive person and the ward changed rapidly from a rigid, authoritarian constellation to one in which much disorganization and confusion existed, both among patients and personnel. However, this regime did allow for greater flexibility in dealing with patients and did permit various alternatives to be used in their care. At the end of the study, the ward organization had not crystallized into a highly organized form, but there was evidence that this might occur in the future.

From the point of view of the study, however, it should be noted that the initial period of observation occurred in the authoritarian context, whereas the final period of observation, evaluation, and intervention occurred in the more permissive context.

METHOD

A method for study was evolved through the joint planning of the sociologist[3] and the investigator, both of whom felt that merging of sociological concepts and psychiatric nursing skills might lead to a new approach—a product of both disciplines—which might be termed sociopsychiatric nursing. In addition, a new method or technique for social psychological investigation might be evolved.

The techniques used in this study were: (1) the systematic collection of data on the interpersonal situations surrounding the patients and the noting of factors indirectly related to the situations; (2) participant observation by the investigator; (3) analysis and evaluation of the data with the sociologist who was outside the situation; (4) formulation of plans for intervention in accordance with the analysis and evaluation of data.

The total length of the study was 6 months. For the first month the investigator made general ob-

---

[2] The unit selected was the same as that used in the Schwartz-Stanton studies. For a more extensive description of the setting, see reference footnote 1.

[3] It should be pointed out that the sociologist's major field of interest was social psychology and that he had training and experience in intensive psychotherapy.

servations of the ward as a whole. These were then discussed and evaluated with the sociologist. Out of this larger body of data, a particular focus of interest developed. For the rest of the time, the investigator concentrated on the problems surrounding two patients who presented similar modes of participation on the ward.

ROLES OF THE INVESTIGATOR

The investigator changed roles from time to time during the study, according to plan.

Collaborator.—Six hours each week were spent in conference with the sociologist, during which time the data were reported, discussed, and analyzed.

Observer.—During the first month the investigator attempted to maintain the role of observer without actively participating and made as complete observations of the total social situation as possible in the 34 hours which were usually spent on the ward each week.

Participating member of the staff.—For the next 2 months, the investigator made herself available to patients and staff for 34 hours each week, although she was not held responsible for nursing service. In this role the nature and amount of the data obtained were altered. By being available to patients, the investigator was able not only to observe, but also to experience their modes of participation and to evaluate more closely her own reciprocal response. Out of this role there seemed to develop another role which might be referred to as "float nurse." Because the investigator was not responsible for nursing service, and not in a position to make administrative decisions regarding patient's living, she sought out, or was sought out by, patients whose needs apparently were not being understood and or fulfilled.

Instructor.—During the last 3 months of the study definite plans for intervention were formulated, introduced, and followed through. To facilitate intervention, the investigator assumed the role of instructor to the personnel on the ward, conferring with groups and individuals in order to clarify attitudes toward patients in terms of the patients' present mode of social participation, and to stimulate the formulation of alternative attitudes and ways of dealing with patients. The investigator observed the results of the intervention and discussed this in turn with the personnel; and a continuous process of reformulation of personnel activities occurred in accordance with the changing situation.

Data

The data presented in this study are taken from the larger body of data collected. The patients who were selected for focus presented problems which revolved primarily around the fact that there was a constant tendency on the part of the personnel to *avoid* them. The patients' dominant pattern of participation was that of withdrawal. It was because of this recurrent avoidance on the part of the staff of these patients with the concomitant isolation and neglect of them and indifference toward them that these patients were chosen for study. We believe that this pattern of avoidance-withdrawal is a dominant reason for the maintenance of these patients' illnesses. It should be noted that the patients were integrated at different levels of participation in the social process. The second patient participated only on a nonverbal level and was withdrawn physically, while the first patient communicated verbally in a highly autistic manner, although in variable amounts, and was not as withdrawn physically.

The investigator's notes on each patient will be presented separately and in chronological order.

Mrs. Smith

Mrs. Smith was a 43-year-old woman who was admitted to the hospital following the death of her husband in an airplane crash. She was an attractive, feminine person. Her clinical diagnosis was paranoid schizophrenia.

At the end of the first part of the study, at which time the observations on each patient were being systematically collated, the investigator discovered that no data were recorded for Mrs. Smith. In discussing this with the sociologist, the things recalled by the investigator regarding Mrs. Smith were vague and irrelevant and no specific experiences with her could be remembered. The investigator felt, during this initial discussion with the sociologist, that this patient must not be a nursing problem and that she must take care of her own dressing, eating, and so on, although later it became apparent that this was not true. Because of the systematic approach that had been taken in making observations on *all* patients, the fact that no observations were made on Mrs. Smith suggested that the problem surrounding this patient indicated the need for further investigation and study.

The investigator quickly discovered that other personnel responded similarly to this patient, that is, they avoided her, but their withdrawal from her was in such a quiet, insidious way that they, too, were not aware of their response. Preliminary inquiry indicated that the problem surrounding this patient could be a challenging one since she was so effectively excluded from the vision of the personnel.

The following questions were formulated as guideposts: (1) Is the recurrent avoidance response a pattern with everybody, or is it peculiar to certain people? (2) Are the personnel aware that they avoid the patient? (3) What are the reasons behind the avoidance? (4) What can be done to alter the situation? (5) Can new ways of participation with the patient be conveyed to the personnel? (6) What changes in the social structure will be necessary in order to prevent this avoidance pattern?

In order to give a clear picture of the process type of approach to psychiatric nursing problems, a chronological view of the procedure followed is given below.

A plan was formulated by the investigator and the sociologist in which (1) systematic observations would be made on Mrs. Smith, in an attempt to evaluate her present mode of participation; (2) the investigator would spend considerable time with her in order that interpersonal contacts might be experienced and evaluated; (3) personnel would be observed and their responses to this patient noted by the investigator; and (4) casual conversations with personnel regarding their experiences with Mrs. Smith would be initiated, in order that existing attitudes might become clear.

At the next meeting with the sociologist, two days after the plan was formulated, the investigator presented data on various patients for evaluation. The sociologist asked about Mrs. Smith, and the investigator realized that she had made no observations on this patient, nor had she contacted the patient, even after having a conscious plan to do so. This was again discussed at length.

The next day, upon the investigator's return to the ward, the following observations were recorded:

Mrs. Smith was observed sitting on the porch. I approached and asked if I might join her. Mrs. Smith was agreeable. A conversation, about the weather's being "so hot and humid" resulted. A long silence ensued, and I became more and more uncomfortable. The patient made no further attempts at conversation, but stared fixedly at me. I finally excused myself. Later I observed the patient sitting in a far corner of the porch. Mrs. Smith coughed and spit on the floor; this was repeated at frequent intervals. There was some explosive laughter. She called loudly, "Bring me a cigarette." Aide approached with cigarette, lit it, said nothing. Another aide and student came on the porch; they sat near Mrs. Smith, not paying any attention to her. Mrs. Smith was incontinent of urine through clothing and onto floor and uttered, "Oh, gee," in loud, shrill voice. Student approached another patient on porch and started to converse. Aide looked at large pool of urine on floor and got up and walked into ward. (This type of activity is unusual. When a patient urinates, the floor is usually cleaned immediately, and the patient is changed.)

After four or five minutes, Mrs. Smith got up and went to her room. She returned shortly, having changed her clothing. "Nurse, bring me a cigarette and some milk." Student brought milk and cigarette but said nothing to Mrs. Smith, who giggled loudly, and rocked in the chair, repeating, "Jesus."

Later, I went to Mrs. Smith's room. She was on her bed, with legs apart, moving her hips. I offered her a cigarette and smoked one with her. Mrs. Smith covered up, remained still, giggling and staring at me. I had no success at conversation. I remained with her thirty minutes, at the end of which time she voided in bed. I said nothing, got dry clothing for her, changed her bed, and left.

Later, Mrs. Smith came out of her room for cigarette, and sat on hall, smoking. A nurse and an aide were present. Again she voided onto floor. Aide: "Is anything wrong, Mrs. Smith?" Mrs. Smith giggled loudly, "Oh, my." Aide walked away. Mrs. Smith sat for ten minutes, got up, went to room, crawled into bed with wet clothing on. Later I heard her shout, "Unlock my drawers." I entered room and unlocked dresser drawers. After Mrs. Smith had selected dry clothing, she stripped, put it on, and walked onto hall.

[The following day (Sunday), I planned to go to ward for a brief period only, to observe Mrs. Smith. This plan was completely forgotten.]

During the three subsequent days, although on the ward, the investigator made no observations and had no contacts with the patient. This, again, was not in keeping with the plan that had been formulated. The investigator, in discussing this with the sociologist, could give no reason for avoiding the patient. "Was very busy with other patients." "Spent time with personnel." (Mrs. Smith was not discussed with them, however.) "Seemed to forget about her."

The above makes it quite apparent that, in spite of much interest and enthusiasm of the investigator regarding this problem, and in spite of a definite plan of approach, the avoidance persisted.

During the evaluation of data with emphasis on the persisting avoidance of this patient, the sociologist speculated that the patient's behavior might have a sexual significance, of which the investigator was apparently unaware. Although the investigator experienced anxiety and discomfort with the patient, their source was not clear to the investigator, and the patient continued to be avoided. The investigator had been greatly puzzled by this and by her persisting anxiety in the presence of the patient and her inability to maintain this patient in focus, despite her curiosity about the problem.

Following several discussions with the sociologist, some understanding was reached regarding the possible meaning of this patient's symbolic mode of participation. With the discovery that the anxiety concerned itself primarily with what was felt to be a sexual appeal being made by the patient, the investigator's anxiety with this patient disappeared, and subsequent contacts with her were markedly different. Thus when the problem came into focus, the anxiety disappeared, and the investigator was able to see this patient's total behavior as an attempt to form a human relationship. The patient, in turn, seemed to become correspondingly less anxious and to notice and seek out the investigator's company.

It cannot be emphasized enough here that this sort of finding is nearly impossible to discover in day-to-day nursing care of a patient. It is only when this "process approach" (observation, evaluation, intervention, observation, and so on) is attempted, that one becomes aware of this type of recurrent response in relation to a patient's mode of participation. It also points up the importance of having this type of supervision, in which inquiry is made into minute details by a person who is far enough removed from the situation to be able to evaluate the data in a more comprehensive perspective.

Although the investigator had discovered a disturbing and separating aspect of the interpersonal situation and thus was able to alter her mode of participation with this patient, none of the other personnel had examined their participation in a similar way, so that they persisted in their usual pattern.

The following excerpts indicate the nature of the interpersonal contacts and the type of participation undertaken by the investigator and Mrs. Smith.

Mrs. Smith was on the porch, sitting in a chair. I sat down beside her. She did not respond to my greeting, but continued to stare, giggle, and spit at regular intervals. I made several attempts to converse with her, but she gave no evidence that she heard. She occasionally looked directly at me, and went into hysterical laughing. She continued to cough and spit about once per minute. I sat quietly for about thirty minutes.

Investigator: "You seem quite bothered by the cough."
Mrs. Smith: "Oh, it's nothing much, but very uncomfortable."
Investigator: "It is uncomfortable?"
Mrs. Smith: "Yes. You know what it is, don't you?"
Investigator: "No, I don't think I do."
Mrs. Smith: "I have this thing in my throat, and it makes my throat hurt and burn. The spit is not from my nose or stomach, but from the pus of this infection. The same thing is the cause of this vomiting." (Gets up and goes to her room. Returns and sits beside me. Does not speak, giggling and spitting continue, I remain for about twenty minutes.)

Mrs. Smith was in the living room with a nurse, Mary (another patient), and me. Mary was telling about her trip and dinner at the Flamingo. Mrs. Smith asked an occasional question, laughing explosively on four or five occasions. Mary continued her story. Mrs. Smith voided on the floor. There was silence for several minutes.

Mary: "You're having quite a discharge, Mrs. Smith." (Leaves the room.)
Nurse; "Do you want to change your things, Mrs. Smith?" (Mrs. Smith rushes from the room, strips her clothing off and puts on a robe, I go to her room several minutes later, sit on her bed, and attempt to chat with her for a minute. Mrs. Smith asks for a cigarette, which I give her.)
Investigator: "I was wondering how you were feeling when you urinated in the living room a little while ago."
Mrs. Smith: "Oh, I didn't urinate. That is life water, and not the same at all. You think it is urine, but it is not. It is life water."
Investigator: "You think it is life water?"
Mrs. Smith: "Certainly. Would you light my cigarette again? It has gone out."
Investigator: "Surely." (Lights cigarette.) "Do you mind talking about this life water?"
Mrs. Smith: "No, I don't mind, but I'd rather discuss it later, if it is the same to you. I'd like to have a bath before I go for a visit. You know I'm having a visitor this morning."
Investigator: "Yes, I know you are. I'll get your bath ready. What do you want to wear?"

Mrs. Smith was in her room on the bed. She was very thoughtful, and did not notice me as I came in.
Investigator: "May I come in, Mrs. Smith?"
Mrs. Smith: "Yes, of course. Did you bring my cigarettes?"
Investigator: "Yes, I did." (I light a cigarette for her. She looks in the other direction, staring at the wall, smoking in silence.) "Did you have a pleasant visit yesterday?"
Mrs. Smith: "Yes, very pleasant."
Investigator: "How long is she planning to stay here?"
Mrs. Smith: "As long as she wishes."
Investigator: "I see." (There is silence for about fifteen minutes, interrupted only by explosive giggling.)
Mrs. Smith: "May I have another cigarette?"
Investigator: "Yes. You seem very thoughtful this afternoon."
Mrs. Smith: "Yes. I have been for a while now. I was thinking of that Greek who killed her children. Do you remember that?"
Investigator: "Yes, I remember—is it Greek mythology?"
Mrs. Smith: "I'm wondering now if this idea to kill the children was really Medea's, or whether it was really her husband's. You know, because of the trouble they were having."
Investigator: "Why would it be her husband's?"
Mrs. Smith: "Oh, I don't really know. Maybe..." (Her talk is rapid and undistinguishable for several minutes.)
Investigator: "I can't understand you. I can't hear what you are saying."
Mrs. Smith: "I was just inferring that the basic

conflict is between man and woman, whether it be interpersonal, interdependent, or interaction." (She goes into a long, involved discussion about men and women, the equality of their rights, and so on. I am not able to understand most of this, or even to identify the main theme.) "Could I have another cigarette, please?"

Investigator: "Yes, Mrs. Smith, I'd like to talk to you about some things."

Mrs. Smith: "Yes, what is it?"

Investigator: "I want you to feel free to tell me if you don't want to discuss it."

Mrs. Smith: "Yes, I will tell you."

Investigator: "I was wondering if there is anything that we could do to understand more about your urinating—you know, like yesterday morning in the living room."

Mrs. Smith: "Oh, that. Well, I don't think people should make a fuss and ask you for reasons. Were you there yesterday?"

Investigator: "Yes."

Mrs. Smith: "And who else?"

Investigator: "Miss Brown and Mary."

Mrs. Smith: "Well, I didn't urinate. That is life water, and it's a lot different."

Investigator: "It is different?"

Mrs. Smith: "Yes, it is a clear, heavenly fluid. It's good. It is not urine. I want you to understand that."

Investigator: "What was going on at the time this life water came, or just before? Do you recall?"

Mrs. Smith: "Yes, I can remember Mary was talking about the Flamingo and having dinner there. Miss Brown was looking at her tangerine nail polish that matched her lipstick. You were encouraging Mary. I could see that."

Investigator: "How did that make you feel?"

Mrs. Smith: "You kept getting Mary to talk. I was wondering why, and about Mary."

Investigator: "What about Mary?"

Mrs. Smith: "Well, first I thought she was just talking and hadn't really been to the Flamingo. Then I realized she had been. She kept getting the bar, cloak room, and the ladies' room mixed up. I was trying to put together what Mary was saying—What do you think of Mary's breasts? There is a word for them. I can't think of it."

Investigator: "A word for Mary's breasts?"

Mrs. Smith: "Yes, it is like a bower, or something. I was wondering what you thought."

Investigator: "You were wondering what I thought about what?"

Mrs. Smith: "About life and the pursuit of happiness. You kept telling Mary to talk and this kept coming up in my mind. Life—life and happiness. Then I thought about the book I had told you about the other day. You kept looking at Mary."

Investigator: "How did you feel?"

Mrs. Smith: "Oh, fine, I guess."

Investigator: "You weren't upset?"

Mrs. Smith: "Oh, no, I felt wonderful—sort of floating."

Investigator: "This was when you urinated?"

Mrs. Smith: "Yes, but I told you it was not urine. It is a purer fluid."

Investigator: "Where does it comes from?"

Mrs. Smith: "I'm not just sure. But not from the bladder. From the womb, I suppose."

Investigator: "Is this different than when you go to the bathroom?"

Mrs. Smith: "My, yes. Very different."

Investigator: "How is it different?"

Mrs. Smith: "It floods, is very warm and very pleasant. When I urinate, it isn't like this. It is a sharp thing and you feel indifferent to it. Oh, it is not the same at all."

Investigator: "Is it like anything else, this feeling you have with the life water?"

Mrs. Smith: "I don't know." (Long pause.) "Oh, yes. It seems like an orgasm, just like intercourse."

Investigator: "Just the same?"

Mrs. Smith: "Well, not exactly, but nearly like it. I don't know how it is different. There is much more fluid, I guess. Do you think it comes from my womb?"

Investigator: "I can't see how it could."

Mrs. Smith: "You can't?"

Investigator: "No."

Mrs. Smith: "Well, isn't the bladder connected to the womb?"

Investigator: "No, it isn't."

Mrs. Smith: "Do you know how it is—I mean, the kidneys, bladder, and womb, and all that?"

Investigator: "Yes, I guess I do."

Mrs. Smith: "Can you tell me something about it?"

Investigator: "Yes."

Mrs. Smith: "Draw it for me. Then it will be clearer."

Investigator: "All right." (I explain, with drawings, a little about anatomy, and so on. Mrs. Smith asks many questions, requesting all the technical names.)

Mrs. Smith: "Now tell me about the ovaries, tubes, and the womb." (I tell her briefly in a very simple fashion. She asks about menses.) "Well, now if that is the way it is, I'm not so sure where this life water does come from, are you?"

Investigator: "I think that it comes from the bladder. It must be urine."

Mrs. Smith: "Yes, maybe. But it doesn't seem that way." (A nurse comes in to tell Mrs. Smith that her visitor is waiting downstairs to visit again.)

I am seated in the living room. Mrs. Smith comes in and pulls a chair up beside mine, and offers me a cigarette.

Mrs. Smith: "How are you today?"

Investigator: "Fine. And you?"

Mrs. Smith: "I'm feeling much better." (She stands up and pulls her dress up. Then she sits down again, making sure that none of her dress is underneath her.) "I was hoping you would be here, so we could have a short talk."

Investigator: "Fine." (Mrs. Smith talks rapidly in a rather disorganized fashion about various places, plays, and college days. I say very little, making listening sounds for the most part. This continues for about 45 minutes. Suddenly she leans back in her chair, laughs in an explosive fashion, stares straight ahead, and voids.)

Investigator: "Mrs. Smith—"

Mrs. Smith: "Yes, what were we talking about? Oh, yes. You say you have been in Alaska." (An aide comes in and tells Mrs. Smith that it is time for her hour. She excuses herself, goes to her room, changes her pants, and goes down to her hour.)

Mrs. Smith continues to sit for long periods, laughing, spitting, and voiding. She voids three or four times each day, usually when seated in a group or with one person. Today she voided while off the ward with a student nurse. They were seated on a bench in the yard. Later, on the ward, Mrs. Smith comes and sits by me.

Mrs. Smith: "Just what are you doing on the ward? You are a nurse, aren't you?"

Investigator: "Yes, I'm doing a study here." (Explains.)

Mrs. Smith: "That's interesting. I wondered why you always carried the notebook. You talked to all the patients. I thought maybe you were a student doing something. What did you find out about me? At first you never talked to me. I wondered why."

Investigator: "That is true. I guess I avoided you at first. I had been meaning to ask if you had noticed, and wondered why."

Mrs. Smith: "I surely did. That's the way it goes. Were you too busy—or what happened?"

Investigator: "Not entirely. I was busy, but I don't think that was the reason."

Mrs. Smith: "Well, you'll probably find out." (Conversation shifts.)

The investigator continued to spend time with the patient each day. Careful analysis of the contacts revealed that the type and level of communication changed during this period in the following ways: Periods of silence became infrequent (other than natural lags expected in any discussion). The amount of autistic thinking decreased markedly (the patient was well informed and had traveled a lot, so there were always abundant topics for conversation). The patient began to take initiative in making contact with investigator, would call to her upon hearing her come on the ward or say, "Let's have a cup of tea and talk a while." Most personnel on floor were referred to as "Nurse," "Hey," "You," but the patient always called investigator by name, sometimes Miss Tudor, and sometimes by her first name. The investigator always informed patient when she would be leaving and when she would return, and on several occasions when the time of return was altered, Mrs. Smith would ask, "What happened? I thought you were coming this morning." It became possible to include another person or personnel in our contacts, by inviting a patient to have tea with us, or by going with Mrs. Smith into a group of other patients and personnel.

The type of interpersonal contacts with Mrs. Smith ranged from participating in daily care (bathing, fixing hair, helping her with meals, taking her to her therapeutic hours), to more social activities, such as visiting, singing, reading together, and so on. An average of two and a half hours each day was spent with the patient. Because the investigator had gained this new perspective, which enabled the relationship with the patient to improve, the patient's behavior changed so markedly that the therapist was led to comment about it to the investigator, pointing out the therapeutic usefulness of this relationship to the patient.

It soon became apparent that, despite the increased patient-investigator participation, the constant personnel response was still that of avoidance. A summary of the data collected on this patient revealed that no approaches were made to this patient other than for eating, bathing, dressing, and going to her hour. Despite the fact that the patient would respond and participated freely with the investigator, she often refused to get up, eat, bathe, and so on when approached by others. The result was that much of Mrs. Smith's daily care had indirectly become the responsibility of the investigator.

In a discussion with the sociologist, the following question was raised: If the investigator were to withdraw and the personnel continued their pattern of avoiding the patient, would the withdrawal of the patient be reinforced? If the patient resumed her isolation, we would have additional evidence that the specific interpersonal relationships between patient and investigator had contributed to the change in the patient's level of participation. It would also suggest the importance of the general social context (the staff's avoidance of the patient integrates with the patient's withdrawal) in maintaining the patient's illness.

At this point in the investigation the investigator withdrew from the ward to go on vacation. The following data indicates the course of the patient's behavior:

[Prior to going on vacation, the investigator informed Mrs. Smith of her plans: the patient became interested in where the vacation would be, what the investigator would be doing, and so on. On return from vacation, the investigator asked the charge nurse for a detailed verbal report of all patients.]

Charge nurse: "Mrs. Smith has been staying in bed almost constantly, she has been incontinent four to six times per 24 hours in bed, or in her clothing, if up. She has been tearing her clothing and hospital sheets and blankets. The vomiting and spitting have increased. For the most part, she is mute, and unresponsive, 'out of contact.' Has not eaten or bathed regularly. Does come onto hall for cigarette [patients are not permitted to smoke in their rooms unless specialed] but for the most part remains in bed with her head covered. Her analyst has been coming to the ward for her hours."

[I approached patient, who was in bed with head covered, and called her name several times. There was no response. I remained seated on bed for fifteen minutes, occasionally calling her name or touching her. I then got a cup of tea and returned.]

Investigator: "Mrs. Smith, I want to talk to you. Let's have some tea and a cigarette." (She sits up in bed abruptly.)

Mrs. Smith: "Hi, how are you? How was Iowa? How was your sister's wedding? What did you wear? Tell me about everything!"

Investigator: "We have plenty of time to talk, Mrs. Smith. I'm interested in how you are, too." (The visit continues for thirty minutes. Mrs. Smith remains alert and interested, asking many questions.)

Investigator: "Mrs. Smith, are you tired?"

Mrs. Smith: "Yes, very. Mind if I go back to sleep? I've not been sleeping at all nights—just think, think, think, all night. I'll tell you about it later."

Investigator: "All right. You take a nap and I'll be back later. Maybe you'd feel like a hot bath."

Mrs. Smith: "Yes, I'd really like that." (Turns face to wall, covering head.)

After this initial response, the patient lapsed into withdrawn, autistic behavior. It was not possible to elicit responses from her as previously, and giving her care required much special ministration. The personnel response continued as before—avoidance. The following notes indicate the second phase of the interpersonal relationship between the patient and the investigator.

I have been unable to gain Mrs. Smith's attention for the past three days, even with repeated attempts. Have remained with her, mostly in silence, occasionally making a comment or calling her name. Have changed her bed and clothing as often as necessary (voiding). Have told her when I was leaving and when I would be back.

Today I began taking Mrs. Smith something every hour—juice, milk, pieces of apple, a cigarette, hot tea. She responds by accepting what I bring. No conversation. She stares into space, never looking at me, and continues to spit and vomit. She is frequently incontinent in bed. When I asked her about a bath and took her hand, she went with me. It was necessary to bathe her. She made no verbal responses, but followed simple suggestions.

Mrs. Smith continues mute and unresponsive. She has been tearing clothing and blankets, and spitting and voiding much. I continue to spend time with her and take her things periodically.

Patient began to talk a bit again today. She also giggled and said, "Oh, God," "Oh, dear," "Oh, my," and so on. Attention is difficult to maintain. It is often necessary to take her hand or arm to make her aware of my presence. Also, if I shift position, and get in line of her vision, she will then speak and remain in contact for a short period.

Data of the next several weeks show that I spent an average of one and one-half hours daily with the patient. Her communication progressed from silence to fluent conversation and became less and less autistic. Other aspects of her mode of social participation also changed. She stopped spitting and vomiting. Voiding continued, but was less frequent. Giggling persisted and was louder. She screamed, "Oh, my, oh, my," louder and more frequently throughout the day.

Thus the types of interpersonal experiences were changing. At first there was just sitting, with little conversation; then participation in her daily care; then reading together; finally singing together and with the group. Mrs. Smith learned to play the Autoharp and enjoyed playing and singing with the investigator and the group.

At this point, the patient's mode of social participation had again changed. She was spending much time out of bed, she was conversing with other patients, joining some group activity (singing and dancing), her incontinence had decreased—she was going to the bathroom sometimes on her own initiative, and sometimes at the suggestion of the investigator, frequently being continent for an entire 24-hour period. It was assumed that the interpersonal experience the patient was having with the investigator was an important contributing factor in this change. In order to validate this, and again to evaluate the effect of the ward's avoidance on this patient, a plan was formulated whereby the investigator (with much personal misgivings) would avoid the patient for a period of one week, and observe her response. The following are excerpts from the data collected during this time.

First day. Mrs. Smith remained in bed much of day. She did not respond to aide who asked about bath. She came onto hall, loudly demanding, "Nurse, get me some tea and a cigarette." (I withdrew from hall.) In p.m. she was gotten out of bed by another patient, giggled loudly, and repeated "Jesus." She voided twice in bed during day, and then once shouted, "Hey, change this bed." She was reported to have voided two times in bed during the night.

Second day. Mrs. Smith had her head covered in bed at 8 a.m. and refused breakfast. She was approached for bath at 10 and did not respond. She came onto hall on several occasions. She shouted, "Nurse, nurse, get me a cigarette." Later, "I want tea—hot tea, not lukewarm." She voided two times while sitting in hall, sat for long period in wet clothing, exposed self while on hall, and did not seem in contact except when shouting requests. She did much loud giggling and shouting, "Oh, dear!" (I remained away from patient.) She was observed to be spitting on floor.

Third day. I was not on ward. Report on patient was much the same as the previous day.

Fourth day. I was in hall outside Mrs. Smith's door, talking with another patient who was demanding to get out. Mrs. Smith got out of bed, came to hall, and said, "Gwen, let's have a cigarette. What the hell is wrong with you? So damn snooty—get us both some tea and come in here." (Very irritated.) I complied and visited with her for thirty minutes, then helped her with her bath. Later, when I was playing records on hall with group of patients, Mrs. Smith brought a chair up to mine and listened to music. She patted my hand on several occasions. In p.m. she was on bed for a while. She came to nursing station and said, "Gwen, get the harp. Let's get some singing going. You play and I'll sing. Maybe some of the rest will, too." We played harp and sang. I told her that it was time to leave. "Will you be back tomorrow?" "Yes." "What time?" "In the morning at 8:00." "All right, we will have coffee in the morning."

Fifth day. I could not avoid patient, since she made requests almost continuously as she did yesterday, until I started taking things to her before she asked. She then became less demanding.

The significance of this is that the ongoing social process may disrupt the best laid plans of investigators; that once having established a relationship with the patient, it was not easy to avoid her, even for purpose of research. From the first few days, however, it was evident that the avoidance of the patient by the investigator contributed to her withdrawal and more disturbed behavior.

In the situation of mutual withdrawal between the patient and personnel, the patient played her part by spending long hours in bed, occasionally making demands on the personnel, spitting and vomiting, which repelled them, yet at the same time forced some contact in the clean-up process. Personnel would not, however, talk to her during the cleaning. Mrs. Smith would giggle and shout, "Oh, Jesus," or some similar expression, making the personnel quite anxious, and reinforcing their need to withdraw from her. The following extract indicates a fairly typical response to it:

Investigator: "Why do you think Mrs. Smith says things like 'Oh, dear,' 'Oh, God,' 'Oh, my,' and so on? What does it mean to you?"
Aide: "I don't know. I wish she would stop."
Investigator: "How does it make you feel?"
Aide: "I really don't know. Like something is very wrong. Maybe she is laughing at me, making fun of me, I don't know, except that I get very uncomfortable. I just want to run."

The staff's avoidance was so excluded from their awareness that they were reluctant to talk about her, although this was in direct contrast with their collaborative attitude with the investigator about other patients. When the avoidance was pointed out, they refused to accept its validity. The following excerpts indicate the staff's attitude.

Investigator: "About Mrs. Smith, I was wondering what your ideas were. What has your experience with her been?"
Nurse: "What do you mean? She seems to get along all right. What is the problem?"
Investigator: "People seem to avoid her. I was wondering why."
Nurse: "I don't agree that she is avoided. She often refuses to do things, but people do make an effort to contact her."

This was discussed repeatedly with this nurse, who continually questioned the point that the patient was avoided.

Investigator: "What about Mrs. Smith's incontinence? What could we do about it?"
Nurse: "It may be just a phase."
Investigator: "I wonder if she would discuss it."
Nurse: "I don't think so. It is representative of something."

I talked to the entire ward personnel about some of the things I had been doing on the ward and asked for their cooperation in relating the experiences they had been having with three specific patients, of which Mrs. Smith was one. The other two patients were discussed fully. Mrs. Smith was not mentioned.

In a small ward conference (five personnel), I

again talked with personnel, asking for experiences with the *three* patients. The entire conference time was spent on two. Mrs. Smith was again omitted.

Investigator: "I was wondering what you thought about Mrs. Smith. What kind of experiences do you have with her?"
Aide: "I don't have any trouble with her. I like her quite a bit."
Investigator: "Have you had any chats with her?"
Aide: "Oh, yes, she is interesting to talk with. I do spend time with her."
Investigator: "What do you talk about?"
Aide: "Oh, the usual things. Let's see—Well, I can't remember any specific thing right now."
Investigator: "Do you usually initiate the experiences, or does she?"
Aide: "Oh, it's fifty-fifty, I guess."
Investigator: "When was the last time you had a five or ten-minute contact with her?"
Aide: "Well, let me think. (Pause.) I can't remember when I really talked with her that long. I take her tea and cigarettes."
Investigator: "Does she usually ask, or do you take them on your own?"
Aide: "Oh, she asks. Let's see—When did I talk to her? I guess I haven't lately. I can't really say for sure."

The above-mentioned aide was always fairly accurate in reporting her experiences with other patients. She was quite free with the investigator in expressing how she felt about patients—such as whether she liked them or not, sought them out or not. The investigator had not observed this particular aide making a single contact with Mrs. Smith other than when a demand was made of the patient, or by the patient. This is an example of the aide's not really being aware of how she functioned with this patient. She distorted at first, and when questioned more closely, could not remember. This is the sort of inquiry that may lead the personnel to really question how they do respond to patients.

With some personnel, it was found that evasion was used when this patient was mentioned:

Investigator: "I was wondering what we might do with Mrs. Smith. Tell me a little about your experiences with her."
Aide: "We get along just fine. She makes a lot of requests, but that is what I'm here for. I like all the patients, and I enjoy doing things for them—even Miss Brown." (Goes into lengthy discussion regarding this other patient. Her observations are accurate and she is free to express her feelings.)
Investigator: "To get back to Mrs. Smith. Have you visited with her lately?"
Aide: "I've noticed that she is becoming very friendly with Miss Brown. They seem to be great pals."
Investigator: "Yes, I've noticed that."
Aide: "I think it is good for Miss Brown. I'm always glad to see the patients getting on so well." [Several more unsuccessful attempts were made to bring the discussion around to Mrs. Smith.]

Investigator: "I wanted to ask you what you thought about Mrs. Smith's giggling and the way she says 'Oh, my,' 'Jesus,' and so on. What does it mean to you?"
Aide: "I think it is disturbing to the others. They get tired of it. I've heard them tell her to shut up."
Investigator: "Do you think she is amused, or what?"
Aide: "I really couldn't say. It is hard to tell."
Investigator: "How does it affect you?"
Aide: "Well, I know she can't help it." [Laughs and walks away.]

Mrs. Smith was discussed with a student nurse who had been on the ward for ten weeks. At first the student felt she had a good relationship with this patient. After further discussion, she became aware that she had not made a single contact with this patient during her entire ten weeks, other than to take her food, cigarettes, and so on. This student was an exceptionally sensitive, imaginative person, who had unusually constructive interpersonal experiences with the majority of patients on this unit.

The reaction of the patient to this avoidance and her awareness of it is indicated below.

Mrs. Smith was approached by a nurse in regard

to an appointment for an eye refraction. She did not respond, and nurse repeated her request. Mrs. Smith became very angry. "Go to the doctor, go to your appointment. I'm not going, and you can get the hell out of here. I'm sick in bed, and not getting up." Nurse left.

I later went in to talk to patient regarding this.

Investigator: "Mrs. Smith, what about your appointment for an eye refraction? You can't read with those old glasses. We should take care of it real soon."

Mrs. Smith: "Yes, I know. I want to get it done. I've got to real soon."

Investigator: "I was wondering why you got so upset when Miss Nelson asked you about it."

Mrs. Smith: "I get sick of their paying absolutely no attention for months, then, 'Get up, get up, go to the doctor.' They don't care if I'm living or dead until they want me to do something. I've got the flu, and they don't even know it." [Patient had a cold and was probably chilly and achy.]

Investigator: "I see. Well, I don't want you to let your glasses go too long."

Mrs. Smith: "I intend to go to the eye doctor. Tell them to make the appointment. It's just that I get mad when—well, you understand."

Investigator: "Yes. Want some aspirin and a water bottle?"

The incident of the appointment for an eye refraction was discussed with the nurse involved. She had been rather surprised at Mrs. Smith's reaction and stated that perhaps this "patient is being avoided." This was contrary to her previous feeling regarding this pattern.

Our interpretation of this situation was that continued avoidance of this patient by the personnel was a result of both the lack of awareness of the staff of their pattern of avoidance, and the sexual connotation of the patient's behavior—her use of the terms "Oh, my," "Oh, God," "Jesus," and so on, and her incontinence, all of which seemed to contain orgasmic qualities.

Throughout the study the investigator had frequent contacts with the therapists whose patients were living on this ward. Mrs. Smith's therapist was contacted at the point in the study where the investigator wished to begin fairly lengthy and consistent contacts with the patient.

The pattern of mutual withdrawal was discussed, emphasizing the subtle nature of this problem, including the investigator's failure to recognize this pattern initially, and the fact that this was currently true of the rest of the personnel. The therapist felt that because a strong, positive (good mother) relationship had finally been formed between the patient and the investigator, her negative feeling was beginning to come out and be worked out with the therapist. This was something that had not been accomplished previously in the therapy. Because avoidance was no longer necessary on the part of the investigator, she was free to form a relationship which focused on the healthy part of the patient. Because the patient could begin to be aware of some of her health, she could then begin to deal with her sick part with more comfort.

The therapist also felt that the investigator had been able to give an unconditional type of care to this patient, making almost no demands of her, anticipating her needs, and setting limits only as determined by the situation. This had communicated the investigator's acceptance of the patient on a level she could understand (taking her things, sitting with her for long, silent periods, bathing her, feeding her, and so on). This type of acceptance was a prominent need in this patient, and could not be conveyed on a verbal level. It was felt that the fulfillment of this need was appropriate to the patient's present level of participation.

SUMMARY

In reviewing the course of the participation with this patient, it became clear that without the *joint analysis* of the data with an outside person possessing a perspective of the social structure and who was not involved in the interaction, the subtle nature of the avoidance pattern might never have been uncovered. The following steps constituted the joint process undertaken by the sociologist and the investigator:

(1) Recognition and observation of the interpersonal situation surrounding this patient—the avoidance-withdrawal pattern.
(2) Evaluation of these observations, including the reasons for the avoidance resulting in a reduction of the anxiety of the investigator, which then permitted the problem to come into sharp focus.
(3) Recognition of the problem as one in which the staff's mode of participation maintained the patient at a withdraw, autistic level.
(4) Intervention in the process of avoidance by the investigator's providing those interpersonal experiences that both fulfilled the patient's needs and were appropriate to her present level of participation.
(5) Observation and evaluation of these interventions: it was seen that the interpersonal situation with the investigator permitted the patient to participate at a higher level.

MISS JONES

Miss Jones is a 25-year-old woman, who has been hospitalized for the past 10 years. The onset of her illness was acute, and the diagnosis at the time of admission was schizophrenia.

Miss Jones is a tall, very thin, attractive girl, with long blond hair, worn either in pigtails, or piled high on top of her head. She appears much younger than her stated years. Miss Jones' mode of social participation at the beginning of the investigation was one of almost complete physical and verbal withdrawal. The investigator's first introduction to Miss Jones and her difficulties was during the investigator's initial orientation to the unit. The following are verbatim comments made by the head nurse:

"Marian Jones has been here for 10 years. She is about 30 years old. She is mute and inactive, and for the most part, remains in bed. She will not talk to you. She has ceased being assaultive, but will blow up and attack you if you get too close to her. She cannot tolerate *closeness*. She will accept routine nursing care, like bathing and having her hair combed. She eats poorly and has to be reminded about this—or forced to eat. She sometimes refuses to go to her hours, and we do not force her to go."

Daily observations were made on Miss Jones by the investigator. The following gives a picture of Miss Jones' usual day, abstracted from observations made early in the study.

Breakfast finds Marian in bed, not asleep, but with her eyes tightly closed as if dreading the prospect of another day. The covers are pulled tightly about her, her body in a rather shrinking position, denoting in itself withdrawal from the surroundings. "Here is your tray, Marian." There is no sign of interest, the only response being that the covers are pulled more tightly about her. Her facial expression seems to combine apathy and distaste. "Now, you must eat your breakfast," continues the voice in a very automatic fashion. The tray is placed beside her. Her eyes close even more tightly, and she relaxes slightly after she hears the footsteps leaving the room. After 4 or 5 minutes, she opens her eyes and glances at the tray, reaches for her nearly cold coffee, has a few swallows and sinks back into the bed. Then, as if compelled, she eats a few bites of breakfast, swallowing hard with each bite. Turning over in bed, she assumes her former position. It is almost as though she eats just enough to keep alive, not really to satisfy her, but just to exist.

Around 9:00 or 9:30, Marian is again approached for her bath and dressing. She physically clings to the bed, but after much urging, starts toward the bathroom, being more pushed than going on her own. A hot bath with perfumed bubbles is ready. There is no pleasure in this, despite the fact that, other than eating and perhaps a silent walk, this is to constitute her day. Her clothing has been selected. Marian dresses automatically, with help, and allows her long, thick blond hair to be combed and piled attractively on top of her head. She then is led to the porch to a chair. She sits here, legs and feet outstretched on the floor. Sliding down in the chair, she rests her head and face on her right hand, carefully covering her mouth. Her gaze is directed at the floor; she does look around occasionally, but if you catch her eye, she quickly looks at the floor, as if frightened at the prospect of exchanging a smile or a glance.

Little is said to Marian, other than at meal time, or if it is time for her hour or a walk. Then, "Marian, it is time for your hour." No response. "Marian, come on, let's go to your hour." Then she is taken by the hand and led to the door. Often, she shakes her head, "No," as she goes out the door. At times she holds onto the chair and does not go. Her eyes remain on the floor. She knows that she will not be forced to go. Occasionally, persons will sit beside her for a short while and leaf through a magazine or say a few words, but they soon leave. Marian may glance quickly up as they go. In the evening, she sits in front of the television. At times she watches, but the major portion of the time her eyes are on the floor. Soon it is bedtime. Marian goes willingly, hurrying into her pajamas and toward her bed.

Periodically Miss Jones becomes upset. Over a period of time it was observed that (1) the upsets always occurred after a contact with the personnel; (2) the upsets occurred when some sort of demand had been made of the patient; and (3) the content of the verbalizations was always very similar. The following is a fairly typical upset taken from the data collected by the investigator on this patient:

Marian has remained in bed all day today, refusing her meals and her bath. At 2:00 p.m. she is approached for her hour. She refuses to get out of bed. The aide urges her, as usual, and then leaves the room. Marian begins to scream, and this continues for about twenty minutes. I can get only part of the content of this upset, since she is screaming and shouting at a very rapid rate.

Marian: "Why I put up with this, I don't know. Nothing to drink but water since I was a baby. I'm not taking it any more. I'll marry Winston Churchill or anyone else that they say. That dirty rotten whore. I never had trouble with people in my life before I came here. They try to teach us how to live and they don't know how to live themselves. Filthy whores, filthy bitches, horrible old prostitutes dressed in white satin and shoes. I was brought up by a lady, never treated like this. They will apologize or know the reason why. No one understands anything around here. I can't stand this. Eat this, do this, do that. Come on, now, Marian, you know you must do this. She yells and screams when I don't feel well. How in hell can I put up with this? Throws a fit at me. There is no reason in the world why she has to act like this. This place is a dirty, filthy whore house. It's the dirtiest filthy whore place in the country. They don't have any respect for living. They don't have manners, or live on Fifth Avenue, or pay their bills. I tell the truth, but no one will listen. They try to train me to do something I can't learn. I can't be this way. How can you walk in high heels when you haven't learned to walk yet? Most people sit up to eat. Most people do this and that. Throw her out, knock her down. I don't want her. She is filthy. She doesn't pay her bills or live on Fifth Avenue. I can't do anything about it. I can't wear high heels. I'm sick of all of this. I won't stand it any longer. Get rid of it. I can't do it any longer. They tell you how to walk. Then they say, 'Poor girl, she never got well. She can't walk. I don't want Miss Jones. I can't stand her. I can't understand why I do things wrong. Miss Jones, Miss Jones, do this, do that, do this, do that. I can't stand this. They tear up my clothes, my hair, my body. They slobber on me. Slobber all over me. I can't do it any longer. I don't want her. Her father throws her in a mental hospital and lets her rot. He can't understand. She is crazy. I can't have it. I'm sick of it. Miss Jones. She has been trying to learn how to walk in a mental hospital for years. If Miss Jones can't learn how to behave, then why doesn't she leave? I can't stand her. Her background is horrible. Wears ridiculous clothing. She hasn't a bit of taste in food. Not a nurse in the world could take care of her. She has the worst family. Her mother screams all the time. I've had enough of Miss Jones. Old, broken-down person. No one wants to help her. No on wants to know her."

Data were also collected regarding the recurrent responses of the nursing staff in their relations with Marian. The most frequent experience personnel had with Marian was that of *failure*. Because of the repetitive experience of failure, the staff became indifferent and apathetic and developed much guilt. By labeling the patient "hopeless," this guilt could, to some extent, be alleviated. Her upsets were dismissed as being caused by "too much closeness with people." In casual conversation, the personnel would point out that they did try, they did make a few approaches, but they felt that there was no hope. There was also some evidence of hostility and contempt toward Marian, probably derived in part from the repetitive failure. The following extracts from the data illustrate these attitudes on the part of the staff.

Three days out of four, Marian remains in bed the greater part of the day, and the personnel report that she refuses to get up. Her eating habits are very poor and any attempts to urge her to eat are unheeded or precipitate an upset. Verbal responses are completely absent. (The first notation in the data of any verbal response is "uh-huh," which was made 8 weeks after the study began; this was the first verbal response any of the personnel at the time had experienced other than during an upset.) Consequently, the personnel make few approaches to Marian other than those absolutely necessary for her care—that is, for baths, meals, analytic hours, and bathroom. She is frequently incontinent of urine and feces, although she usually responds to toileting when approached.

Aide: "Marian refused her breakfast tray. What should I do?"
Nurse: "Well, let it go. I don't know what we can do about it."
Aide shrugs shoulders and walks away.

Aide: "Marian, would you like a bath?" (No response.) "Come on, honey. You have to take a bath." (No response.) "Marian, do you hear?" (Aide pulls at bed covers. Marian makes no verbal response, but turns toward wall and holds tightly onto covers.) "Marian." (Aide leaves room. Marian remains in bed the entire day.)

Marian is incontinent of feces in bed. This is reported to the nurse. "Well, invite her to go to the bathroom. We can't be cleaning that stuff up all the time."

Investigator: "I noted that Marian Jones is up and dressed today. I wonder what happened. What was done differently?"
Nurse: "Oh, periodically she will. Nothing particular happens. This has been going on for ten or so years. She takes spurts and will do things but she will be back in bed tomorrow. It's the same old pattern."

Aide: "She has been sick so long. She seems to be happiest when left alone. I hate to upset her, and you know it will happen if you get too close."

Nurse: "Marian is a good example of a hopeless patient. One would never realize that she was well educated, and had traveled abroad, to see her now."

A new aide on the floor made several approaches to Marian. The aide then asked Marian to take a walk with her. Marian became upset, shouting and screaming. "This dead body of mine! Marian Jones, that crazy person. You're insane. You're crazy. Such behavior is expected of you. You'll never get well. You'll never learn how to walk. You can't be a lady. You can't act right. Do this. Do that...(and so on)." She pulled the aide's hair and beat her. The aide discussed this incident with a nurse, following the upset.
Nurse: "Marian attacked you because you got too close. This is a repetitive pattern. Marian always turns on those who are good to her."

Marian was rarely consulted as to what clothing she might like to wear or what kind of juice and sandwiches she would like for lunch. Even though she probably would not respond, most patients on the ward were given a choice in these matters.

Personnel were observed combing and brushing Marian's hair, without making any verbal approach to her.

Marian was incontinent of urine and feces in bed. The nurse cleaned her up and changed her bed. In doing this, there was no explanation made to the patient.

The above illustrations certainly would raise the question as to whether or not Miss Jones existed as a person to the personnel. In her very disturbed periods, Miss Jones did refer to "my dead body," which may have revealed how she felt about her existence as a person, and in a reciprocal fashion, personnel, too, treated her as if she were nonexistent.

New personnel soon fell into the same types of responses to Marian that were predominant on the ward.

Monday. New aide oriented today. In afternoon she was observed sitting with Marian on porch. She attempted to converse. Marian frowned and turned head. Aide withdrew.

Tuesday. Marian in bed. Aide approached Marian with a magazine. "Let's look at this, Marian." Marian frowned and turned toward wall. "Don't you want to read the magazine?" Marian made no response. Aide walked away.

Wednesday. Aide made friendly approach to Marian, who turned away. Aide asked nurse about patient. Nurse, "She can't stand you to come too close. She will turn on you and attack you if you get too close."

Thursday. Aide's interest seemed to be lessening. Today she did not give Marian her warm greeting. Made only the necessary approaches.

Friday. Aide observed to pass patient several times. Gave no evidence of seeing her.

In evaluating the data, from which the above was abstracted, the interpersonal situation, surrounding this patient could be readily visualized. Her mode of participation was withdrawal, both physical and verbal, interspersed with very disturbed upsets. Her communications, other than during upsets, were entirely on a nonverbal level. Her responses to contacts were minimal and gave evidence of much anxiety. The response of the personnel in this situation was reciprocal to the patient's mode: staff withdrawal, minimal communication of personnel when making demands on the patient, no respect for her as a person, and evidence of anxiety when contacting this patient.

The predominant attitude on the part of the personnel (and it can be assumed that this was conveyed to the patient) was *hopelessness*, which grew out of repeated failure, indifference, guilt, and hostility.

Thus, the interpersonal context, as observed, consisted of failure with regard to the patient, indifference and apathy toward her, guilt about avoiding her, labeling her as hopeless to avoid this guilt, and, finally, rationalizing the avoidance by saying that the patient could not tolerate closeness. This patterned attitude-response prevailed with such intensity that new personnel were almost immediately indoctrinated into it. If a new aide started with a different approach, he was easily persuaded, both directly and indirectly, into adopting the prevailing attitudes of both the staff and the patient.

Four main problems became apparent in attempting to formulate a method of intervention into the above described mode of social participation. (1) How does the nurse become aware of her feelings regarding the patient? The attitude that the patient was *hopeless* had blocked the personnel in their ability to engage in any interpersonal contacts other than those which maintained the present mode, or the illness of the patient. (2) What needs does the patient communicate through this type of social participation? If these needs are anticipated and fulfilled, will they foster a higher level of participation? (3) What kinds of interpersonal activities can be engaged in with this patient? (a) Does one begin with nonverbal communication? (b) What is the way of moving on from nonverbal communications? What specific forms of communication can be used? (c) What types of interpersonal situations can be structured? (4) What type of social structure will best facilitate an alteration in the staff's mode of participation regarding: (a) the staff's taking Miss Jones into their purview and moving in her direction, in contrast with their present moving away and ignoring her; (b) the staff's looking upon her mode of participation as a problem which is constantly to be grappled with; and (c) mobilization and maintenance of enthusiasm and interest on part of staff that will promote this?

The first step in this plan was to have the investigator herself experience the patient, consider the various alternative ways of responding to her, try a number of these alternatives, determine the one or ones which were most successful, continue this process, and observe the effect on or changes in the patient's behavior. As envisioned, the plan would comprise a series of steps in which the patient was responded to and with, at the level she was capable of at the time. Once having achieved an integration at this level, higher levels of integration would be attempted with the patient.

The second step was to communicate the procedure to another staff member who would then attempt to participate with the patient in the mode similar to that of the investigator. In this way, the following questions could be answered: Is the method of participation developed by the investigator intrinsic to her type of personality, unique experience, and skills, or can another staff member be trained to participate with the patient in this mode? Can a staff member maintain an attitude toward the patient counter to the general staff attitude? If this is possible, what are the consequences of maintaining the counter attitude?

This process, as it was carried out, is stated in the following abstracts from the investigator's notes:

First week. I sat with the patient for two hours—one in a.m., and one in p.m. I made very minute observations, but during this period was silent. Marian remained turned toward wall, with covers pulled tightly about her, her body tense and in curled position, her eyes tightly closed, and her fists tightly clenching the covers. Respirations were fast. If I moved, Marian frowned, closed eyes more tightly, and held onto covers. At the end of 30 minutes, Marian began to relax, straightened legs, changed position in bed, and no longer clenched the covers. After 45 minutes had passed, Marian glanced at me several times, but looked quickly away when I met her glance. At end of hour, I touched her hand and left.

In the afternoon, this was repeated. Patient began to seem comfortable at end of 15 minutes.

These interpersonal contacts were repeated on three subsequent days. The patient's response was increased, in that many glances were exchanged: she allowed the investigator to take her hand for long periods, although she did not return the grasp; she followed with her eyes when the investigator entered or left the room.

The response on the part of the investigator is also significant. The patient began to become quiet real; there was much more awareness of the patient's expression, and a real feeling that the patient was being experienced as a person.

Second week. I went to the patient, sat on her bed, and began to talk with her about the weather and other general topics. Marian frowned, her body became tense, her eyes closed tightly. I talked on, becoming more and more uncomfortable, for 30 minutes, at which time Marian turned her face to the wall and pulled the covers about her. She did not become disturbed to the point of an upset. I made no overt demands on her during the monologue.

For past two days I have been sitting with Marian, saying nothing. Her response similar to those reported during first week. At end of 40 minutes, I said, "Marian, I'm going to be going in 5 minutes." Marian looked at me and nodded, "Yes." "I will come back later. All right?" Marian nodded, "Yes."

I left and returned later that day.

I asked, "Marian, do you want me to stay with you?" Marian shakes head, "No." "O.K., I'll go now, but I will be back." Marian nodded, "Yes."

(The investigator assumes here that a demand was made on patient—to make a decision about the investigator's sitting with her. If she had said yes, she would have been assuming some responsibility for the contact, and therefore might have had to participate with the investigator.)

I returned and said, "I'd like to be with you, Marian." Marian said, "Uh-huh." (Verbal.)

As a result of the initial contacts, it was easily

determined that the first steps were merely sitting with the patient, or being with her in silence. Verbalization at this point only made her uncomfortable and succeeded in disrupting the relationship. However, after a long period of nonverbal participation had occurred, a word or two could be interjected and would be responded to by the patient. After two weeks of contact, verbalization was more readily accepted, as it indicated below.

Third week. Subsequent contacts were initiated by statements such as "I want to stay with you." "I'd like to show you this magazine." "I'd like to brush your hair." "I'll help you with your bath."

Miss Jones' response continued to be a verbal "uh-huh," nothing more, but she watched the investigator, smiled readily, and returned the investigator's grasp. The type of interpersonal activity changed from sitting with patient (with no verbal communication), to physical contacts, holding hand, brushing hair, looking at book, reading, singing with patient. This was the next step in the process. Physical contact with the investigator brought appropriate responses from the patient. Such activities at the beginning were not responded to at all.

Investigator: "Marian, I brought the Autoharp. I'd like to sing with you." Marian smiles and says, "Uh-huh." Other patients gather around and begin to sing with me. Marian smiles, is very alert, rocks in chair in time to music. (Patient does not sing, but her rocking indicates a further step in participation.)

Fourth week. Marian is spending more time out of her bed. Personnel are observed to say, "Hi" or sit beside her for a moment in the hall, or take her a magazine. Marian responds by smiling or saying, "Uh-huh."

As a result of the investigator's interest in the patient, and as a result of direct propaganda, personnel developed a greater interest and approached the patient more frequently. In addition, as a result of the investigator's interest, the patient became more active. As she became more active, personnel dealt with her more easily. Thus, the reciprocal process of staff-patient interaction started to move slowly away from the avoidance-hopelessness state. The patient, however, moved slowly, taking only minute steps—the distance yet to go was great.

Fifth week. A new student nurse approached Marian for her bath. Marian responded well. This student was observed to spend one hour sitting with patient today. She made some inquires of the investigator regarding the patient, and often observed the investigator when she was with the patient.

At this point, it was decided that the investigator would attempt to work through this student.[4] A plan was formulated in which the investigator would supervise the student in the same way that the investigator was being supervised by the sociologist. Being a new student, she had not become indoctrinated with persisting attitudes of the ward, nor was she "caught in the hopelessness" surrounding the patient. Could she be prevented from falling into the reciprocal responses to this patient's mode? If so, what type of interpersonal experience would it be necessary to structure, and what sort of direction would be necessary? What type of changes in the social organization would be necessary? If this student should experience successful interpersonal contacts with this patient, how would this be viewed by other personnel on the ward?

It was felt that much could be gained in understanding not only how to interrupt a certain mode of participation on the part of the patient, but how this skill could be transmitted to another person.

With the cooperation of the nursing service and

---

[4]Grateful acknowledgment is made to Miss Jo Ann Crisp, senior student in the Park View Hospital School of Nursing, Rocky Mount, N. C., for her participation in this study.

education departments, and agreement by the student, arrangements were made for this student to spend ten consecutive weeks on the ward, to be partially free of responsibility to the rest of the ward, and to have time for conferences with the investigator which would enable her to discuss fully her experiences with Miss Jones, and her feelings about Miss Jones' reaction to her.

The remaining data on Miss Jones consist of the investigator's and the student's observations of the experiences with this patient, the joint evaluation, and the subsequent action on the part of the student.

Sixth week. For the past three days, Miss C (the student) has spent varying lengths of time with Marian, just sitting, making an occasional comment. In conference with Miss C we have discussed these interpersonal experiences, stressing what happened, Marian's response, Miss C's feelings, and alternatives that might be considered in future contacts. The role of the therapist was discussed with Miss C and how the varying roles became integrated in the interpersonal situation.

Miss C goes to Marian, who is seated in hall.
Miss C: "I've brought some juice."
Marian: "Uh-huh."
Miss C: "Which do you want, pineapple or tomato?" (No response.) "Tell me, Marian, which do you want? Hear, Marian?—you choose."
Marian becomes upset, starts to scream: "Tomato or pineapple, grapefruit. It doesn't matter. Give the sick girl tomato or pineapple or grapefruit." (Hits and kicks Miss C.) "Men try to rape her. She keeps bleeding. It is all mixed up. Menstruation, babies, egg salad sandwiches. She will never get well. That poor insane Marian Jones. Stay away from me. Get out, get out. She'll never get well." (This continues for about 20 minutes. Miss C stays near.)

In conference between investigator and student, the upset was discussed, with emphasis on the following points: how Miss C felt, the possibility of a choice (pineapple or tomato) at this point being perceived by Marian as a demand, the positive effect of just staying near rather than leaving, and how this relates to future experiences.

The twofold significance of this incident was pointed out to the student: (1) that at this point, a choice for Miss Jones is too much of a demand upon her; and (2) that the most important thing about the upset is not that it occurred, but how it was handled. The latter point served to allay the student's guilt about the upset, and indicated a method for handling it.

Seventh week. Miss C was in another room. Heard Marian beginning one of her upsets (precipitated by another personnel, regarding eating her dinner). Miss C went to Marina, took hold of her arms.
Miss C: "Marian, I'll stay with you."
Marian: "Go away. Meat and potatoes, eat this. She doesn't know how to live. She can't even walk. Get out. Stay away."
Miss C: "Marian, do you know who this is?" (Marian continues to scream.) "Marian, I'm staying with you. It is Miss C. Hear, Marian?" (Marian becomes quiet.) "It is Miss C and I'm staying with you."
Marian: "Uh-huh." (Relaxes and sinks back on bed. Miss C remains with her, holding onto her hand.)
Miss C: "Marian, I'm going now. I'll see you tomorrow. I'll be back tomorrow. Goodnight."
Marian: "Goodnight." (Whisper.)
[Here the student put into practice the result of previous discussions—that is, staying with Miss Jones during an upset.]

Marian attended tea dance with Miss C today. They held hands and skipped over to another building on the hospital grounds. Marian was not verbal, but smiled much and was very alert. She danced two numbers with Miss C, but refused invitations of others to dance. [The student was still participating with the patient on a nonverbal level, but getting much responsiveness from the patient.]

In conference with Miss C, the attitude of a nurse on the floor was discussed. The nurse had been interrupting Miss C's interpersonal contacts with Marian by asking her to do other assignments on the ward, and had made inquires of Miss C as to why she talked to investigator so much, and criticized her for interrupting Marian's hour with the therapist (hour being held on hall, Miss C speaks to Marian as she passes.)

In discussing this situation with the head nurse, it was determined that the difficulty could be attributed to the fact that the plan had not been communicated to the nurse involved. Following a discussion between the head nurse and the nurse in question, during which she was taken in on the plan, this difficulty immediately cleared up, Miss C began (on her own intiative) to share some of her experiences with this nurse. This nurse became very interested in the situation and was observed to do a number of extra things to further the interpersonal experience of Miss C and Marian.

The above is an example of what happens when the communication between the personnel breaks down. It is also an illustration of what happens when certain members are "left out." It should be emphasized that the entire plan can be disrupted and thus the possibility of failure increased if both of these points are not considered. It poses the important question as to what type of organization must be maintained within the social structure to avoid this kind of breakdown in communication, and as to the need to bring personnel in on any special plans being carried on so that they will not disrupt them, directly or indirectly.

Eighth week. Miss C reported several more upsets during her interpersonal contacts with Marian. These were discussed and evaluated. The upsets are changing in nature: (1) they are shorter now, lasting approximately 5 minutes, in contrast to 20 or 30 minutes; (2) there is little physical striking out or kicking; (3) there is some difference in content (that is, more reference to "I" - "I don't understand," "I'm so ugly," "I can't get well,"—rather than to "that insane girl," "that Marian Jones. She can't even walk"); and (4) Miss C has little anxiety during upsets, is able to stay with Marian in relative comfort.

Here, again, it was concluded by the investigator and student that the important fact was that *an upset was successfully handled* rather than that *an upset was avoided*. In future interpersonal experiences with Miss Jones, we would not attempt to avoid all upsets, but would concern ourselves with noting the factors precipitating them, the nature of the upsets (length and content), and what we did during and immediately following the upset.

Miss C reported that she now talked fluently with Marian during her bath, combing her hair, and sitting with her. Marian looks directly at her, nods and smiles in response to her remarks. They have read together, sat looking out at the rain, watched the moon together in the evening, and Marian participates by keeping time to the music when Miss C sings. The investigator suggested that the student let her imagination "run wild" in thinking of activities in which Marian might participate more actively. In sharp contrast to a few weeks previously when participation was minimal, (when any verbalization would result in evidence of much anxiety and withdrawal), the patient's present response to verbalization is acceptance and nonverbal responsiveness. How can this type of participation be further altered?

Miss C's enthusiasm and interest was very apparent. She appeared to anticipate her contacts with Miss Jones and reported them to the investigator in detail and with much satisfaction. This enthusiasm was accompanied by a change in her role. From this point on, she began to be much more imaginative and resourceful in her relationships with the patient.

Ninth week. Miss C reports: "Today we sang for a while. Marian kept time with her hands to my singing. Her eyes were shining and she smiled. Looked me straight in the eye most of the time. Then I got the idea of the old patty-cake game— you remember—slapping your knees, then clapping your hands, and then meeting the other person's hands." (Demonstrates.) "I began, Marian giggled, watching me; then she began. She would hit her legs, then clap and hold her hands up. At first, I'd always have to meet her hands—she wouldn't come to meet mine. Finally, she did. It was really exciting. Later when I went to go, I stopped to say goodbye and tell her when I'd be back. I took her hand and actually felt her squeeze mine back. Do you suppose she will ever talk to me? I'd really be thrilled." [Here the patient has moved to another level. She now participates more actively, but is still on a nonverbal level.]

This type of contact continued. Miss C reported: "Today we listened to records. I said, 'Come on, Marian, let's be orchestra leaders.' She did, right away, keeping real good time, and laughing."

Miss C: "We were just sitting. Marian was very sober. She had her hands clasped together. I started to play with my hands. 'This is the church and this is the steeple. Open the door, and see all the people.' Marian laughed and would go through the motions with her hands as I said the words."

Miss C reported: "Marian gets up nearly every day now. She went to the patients' floor meeting. She kept looking at me and smiling."

Miss C reported: "Birthday party for Marian on the ward. She smiled and laughed when we sang happy birthday. The personnel were all so interested. The other patients, too. She wouldn't blow out the candles, but she seemed to like the cake." [Not only was the patient showing greater responsiveness to the student, but to the others on the ward.]

Tenth week. Miss C reported: "Today in the bath I said, 'Wash yourself, Marian.' She took cloth and began. I washed her back. Helped her get out of tub. 'Want to brush your teeth?' She said real plain, 'Yes.' I was so surprised I said, 'What?' Then I said, 'It feels good to brush your teeth, doesn't it?' Marian said, 'No, it doesn't feel good to brush my teeth.' 'It doesn't?' 'No, it doesn't.' She really spoke. Very calm. Her voice is different than when she is upset. I was real thrilled. When we finished, I asked if she wanted to go to the hall. 'Yes.' 'Want to sit here for a while?' 'Yes.'"

Miss C reported: "We were playing records. Marian danced with me. She seemed to enjoy it." We discussed at length the entire experience, including how Miss C felt. "I was so excited when she began to say 'Yes,' and then the time she said the whole sentence. She seems so much more like a person than she did seven weeks ago, when I first met her. I am much more aware of her every response. Another thing—I'm not apprehensive about her upsets. I was afraid at first, and dreaded them. More dread than fear, I guess. I felt I was doing something wrong, and I couldn't relax with her. Now, it's different. She knows me and I think she knows I'm really interested."

Investigator: "How do you think you maintain this feeling with her?"

Miss C: "By being with her. I always tell her I'm here when I first come to the floor, and say goodbye when I leave, and when I'll be back. I never go past her without speaking. She follows me with her eyes."

There has now been an evolving mutual relationship in which the student's continuing enthusiasm and interest in the patient is maintained by her satisfaction in direct participation with the patient, by approval and discussion with the investigator, and by feeling that she is doing a worthwhile piece of work. In turn, the patient has now reached the point where she can be asked to make a choice, and instead of "blowing up," she can respond with words. This is at the end of five weeks of contact between the two. In addition, the student is shaping time for the patient, making it more definite, announcing her arrivals and departures, and is maintaining her awareness and interest in the patient, even when not with her.

Eleventh week. During the eleventh week, Miss C was not on duty because of illness. Other students reported to her that Marian was remaining in bed. This caused great discouragement on the part of Miss C, who felt, "When I leave, everything will go back the way it was before." This was discussed, and the importance of sharing these experiences with others was emphasized. It was felt that the nature of the interpersonal relationship existing between Miss C and Marian was such that interpersonal situations which would bring

Marian and Miss C into the group should be structured. Also, both the investigator's and Miss C's activities would focus on the other personnel in an attempt to stimulate interest and enthusiasm regarding Marian's mode of living on the ward. Miss C would also continue in her contacts with the patient.

Thus as soon as the student withdraws, the patient returns to her old pattern of behavior. This may elicit and reinforce the old feeling of failure and hopelessness. Thus we see the importance of organizing the social context to provide for the simultaneous participation of several staff members, so that the absence of one person does not disrupt the increasing participation of the patient in the social process.

Twelfth week. Miss C's report: I was going to class. I said goodbye to Marian. Asked her to tell me goodbye. "No." "Come on, Marian, tell me 'bye.'" "No." "Will you tomorrow?" "Yes." Next day, when I left for class, I said, "Bye, Marian." She smiled and looked away and then said, "Bye, bye." The following conversation took place.
 Miss C: "Anything you want before I go?"
 Marian: "No." (Hesitates.) "Yes."
 Miss C: "What, Marian?" (No response.) "Want some juice?"
 Marian: "Yes."
 Miss C: "What kind?"
 Marian: "Pineapple juice." (Student brings juice.)
 Miss C: "Anything else, Marian?"
 Marian: "Yes. Do you have a little piece of cake or something?" (Student bring some crackers and jelly.)
 Miss C: "I'm going now. I'll be back after class." (Marian starts to be upset, throws some juice across hall.)
 Marian: "I don't understand. I don't understand..." (Miss C sits beside her, begins rocking chair.)
 Marian: "Go away from me. Get out."
 Miss C: "I'm going to stay with you. I'm not leaving you." (Marian relaxes and stops screaming.)
 Miss C: "You all right now, Marian?"
 Marian: "Yes."
 Miss C: "Tired?"
 Marian: "Yes."
 Miss C: "Want to take a nap?"
 Marian: "Yes."
 Miss C: "All right. I'm going to class. I'll be back in an hour and then I'll stay with you a while."
 Marian: "Yes."

In this incident, the patient was apparently objecting to the student's departure. No provision had been made for the patient to participate in this decision. When the student stayed with her for a short while the patient was then able to accept the second attempt at departure of the student.

Miss C has been talking the past few days about cutting Marian's hair. This was discussed with all the personnel. Marian smiles when this is mentioned, but does not answer. Today during bath:
 Miss C: "Want me to cut your hair, Marian?"
 Marian: "Yes."
 Miss C: "Want it parted in the middle, or on the side?" (No response.)
 Miss C: "In the middle?"
 Marian: "No."
 Miss C: "On the side?"
 Marian: "Yes."
 Miss C: "O.K. As soon as we finish your bath, we will cut your hair." (Marian gets out of tub. Miss C stars to whistle.) "Can you whistle, Marian?" (No response.) "Want me to teach you?" (Marian frowns and looks disgusted.) "Oh, you can whistle?"
 Marian: "Yes." (Begins to whistle, smiles. Someone begins to play music on ward, Miss C begins to do Charleston to music.)
 Miss C: "Come on Marian, Charleston with me." (Holds out hands. Marian takes them. Charlestons with Miss C. Much laughing and smiling. Finishes dressing, goes to room.)

This afternoon Miss C cut and fixed Marian's hair.
 Miss C: "You should have seen how everyone on the ward reacted. She looked so well. Like a different person She is so pretty. When she looked

at herself in the mirror, she was really pleased. Kept touching her hair and smiling. All the patients remarked, so did the personnel. They really seem to be interested in her. I notice everyone pays a lot of attention to her. I've noticed them sitting with her. We talk a lot about her."

Although no one has actually taken over from this student, personnel are paying more attention to the patient. The patient now talks more than she has in years; her greater response is reciprocated by a livlier interest on the part of the staff; the patient is now even making some beginning gestures to talk in the presence of other people.

Group was singing Christmas carols on the ward, Miss C and Marian joined group. Marian moved lips, but did not sing out loud. Watched everyone. Personnel remark to each other about her moving lips in singing.

Thirteenth week. Since this was to be Miss C's last week on the ward, plans for termination were formulated. Miss C would be assigned to O.T. for the last two weeks of her time at the hospital, so would be coming to the ward for short contacts. In addition to explaining this to Marian, Miss C would continue her contacts with the patient. The following are excerpts from the data collected during this week, and they give positive evidence of a constructive change in Marian's mode of social participation as well as a corresponding change in the personnel's reciprocal response:

Marian starts to bathroom with Miss C. Both bathrooms are busy, so they sit in the hall.
 Miss C: "Want me to stay, or get your things ready?"
 Marian: "You can come back."
 Later, in bathroom, tub is nearly full of water.
 Miss C: "Like this, Marian?"
 Marian: "Yes. I like lots of hot water."
 Miss C: "Want to wash yourself?"
 Marian: "Yes." (Washes self.)
 Miss C: "I'll do your back?"
 Marian: "Yes."
 Marian dresses herself without help. Combs own hair, and puts on make-up. Goes onto hall with Miss C.
 Miss C: "Would you like some coffee now?"
 Marian: "Yes."
 Miss C: "How do you want it?"
 Marian: "With cream and sugar."

Marian is dancing on hall with Miss C.

Miss C: "What do you want to wear, a dress or skirt and blouse?" (Standing at Marian's closet.)
 Marian: "A dress."
 Miss C: "Which one?"
 Marian: "A dress. Any one will do."
 Miss C: "A red one?"
 Marian: "Yes."
 Miss C: "Which?" (Has two.)
 Marian: "This one. This red dress."

Miss C and Marian attend the dance. At first Marian refuses to dance with anyone else. Later, several of the men (both patients and personnel) cut in. Marian dances every dance. At one point, ends up across room from Miss C. Looks all about, finds her, nods and smiles. Goes on dancing with one of the men. Later in dance, Miss C asks if she wants to jitterbug. "Yes." They jitterbug to "Slow Boat to China." Miss C begins to sing it softly. Marian smiles and moves lips with the words. They go to table for refreshments. Marian says, "Tea with cream and sugar."

Marian continues to say, "Bye" when Miss C leaves the ward.

The patient's participation is now spreading to others. She can now sustain a separation from the student and still participate with another person.

During Marian's bath, Miss C begins to hum "Slow Boat to China." Marian smiles.
 Miss C: "Remember this at the dance?"
 Marian: "Yes." (Simles.)
 Miss C: "Let's sing it."
 Marian: "Yes." (Sings out loud with Miss C. Marian knows all the words.)

O.T. worker came onto ward to make programs for Christmas party. Miss C and Marian join the group. Marian participates in making programs by cutting the paper.

Miss C is playing piano. Marian comes to piano and joins group who are singing. Moves lips in words of Christmas carols, occasionally singing out loud.

Group dancing on the ward. Marian joins group with Miss C. Patients are dancing alone and with group. Marian begins to tap dance after seeing Miss C tapping. Later does the hula with the group.

Marian joins group in living room. Nancy (another student) is reading aloud from a new book. She passes the book to Betty (another patient) who reads a bit, and then passes it on to Miss C. Book is then passed to Marian who takes it, reads paragraph silently, and passes it back to Nancy.

As seen in the above notes, Miss Jones is moving toward the group, whereas her participation previously has been limited to one person. The recipocal response of the group, both personnel and patients, is to begin to include her in their activity. Because of Miss Jones' constructive experiences with Miss C, Miss Jones is able to move with Miss C into a more complex interpersonal situation and begin to participate with a group.

The "whirlpool-like" interpersonal activities as seen in the events with this patient can be synoptically described as follows: The sociologist offers advice and suggestions to the inestigator in evaluating this patient; the investigator offers guidance, counsel, and suggestions to the student; the student participates in a spontaneous fashion with the patient; the patient's greater responsiveness toward the student enables her to engage in more activities with other persons on the ward. The staff personnel respond both with qualitative and quanitative differences to the patient.

Miss Jones' therapist was approached as to the types of interventions the investigator felt might be successful in altering Miss Jones' present mode of social participation. At the termination of the study, an attempt was made to evaluate with the therapist the relationship between Miss Jones' interpersonal experiences on the ward, and the progress made in the analytical hours. The therapist felt there had been three major changes in the analytical hours that could be directly related to Miss Jones' experiences on the ward:

(1) There was an increase in the capacity to follow an idea or thought from one meeting to another. Prior to the intervention on the ward, the therapist felt that between hours "Marian seemed to drop out of existence." He no longer felt this way; probably because of the more consistent environmental support she seemed no longer a person lost on the ward, but had more positive experiences in her living between therapeutic hours. There would seem to be a direct relationship between this change and the fact that Miss Jones was having experiences on the ward that enabled her to carry a thought from one day to the next—or one hour to the next. "I'll sit with you a while." "I'll be leaving in five minutes, but I'll be back tomorrow moring." "Maybe you will say 'Bye' tomorrow," and so on. This aided in shaping time for Miss Jones, and in helping her to identify people and experiences in her living.

(2) It was much easier for the therapist to deal with deep, regressed feelings and needs in the analytic hours as the patient became more comfortable in her relationships on the ward and as her participation on the ward became more socially acceptable. Miss Jones' experiences on the ward were planned to facilitate communication and participation at whatever level was possible, always watching for cues that indicated her ability for a higher level of participation. This was accomplished because of the constant observation-evaluation process.

(3) The therapist's dealings with the ward personnel had changed completely. Before, he had much hostility and resentment toward the personnel. Now he felt much backing and support. The interest and enthusiasm in the patient was very apparent to the therapist. The therapist also felt more comfortable on the ward and had little an-

xiety in leaving Miss Jones after an hour, even if she had been quite anxious during the hour.

While exploration of this is not within the scope of this study it raises some assumptions or speculations: Hopelessness on the part of the nursing personnel must be conveyed to the therapist. Either he takes on this attitude himself, or he has resentment toward the nursing staff. This could have two ramifications: (1) this hopelessness is conveyed to the patient, and reinforces her withdrawal; (2) the staff perceives this resentment and may interpret it as "the therapist feels we are no good." Thus, there is additional confirmation of their failure. The whole process of hopelessness regarding the patient is reinforced.

Thus, the significance of the *total social context*, in affecting a variety of interpersonal relationships in regard to the patient, is evident.

SUMMARY

In summarizing the data on this second patient, a progression of steps becomes clear: observation of the interpersonal situation of the patient and the relationship of this to the total social structure; evaluation and analysis of this situation; formulation of alternative interpersonal experiences; intervention; further observation and analysis of the results of the intervention; and further formulation of alernatives, in accordance with the results of the intervention. From this process, the following steps evolved in attempting to solve the problem of mutual withdrawal surrounding this patient: recognition of the pattern of avoidance-withdrawal existing between patient and personnel, with the resultant attitude-response of hopelessness on part of both; participation with patient on nonverbal level (just sitting with patient in silence); physical participation of patient in form of gestures (frowning or smiling), body tensions (rigid or relaxed), body position (turning back to wall); verbal communication to patient as she begins to respond with appropriate nonverbal gestures (shaking and nodding of head, pressure of hand); physical participation of patient in response to verbal requests (get up, take bath, and so on); hand games—patient begins to participate and to move actively; one or two-word verbal responses on part of patient which are solicited by personnel; one or two-word remarks initiated by patient; response by patient to making a choice; hesitant response by patient to participation with others in group; greater response by patient to participation with others in a group; reciprocal response of entire staff, whose approaches to patient are more frequent and of a different kind.

CONCLUSIONS

The problem of mutual withdrawal was selected for investigation because of its critical significance in the maintenance of the patient's mental illness within the ward setting. Not only does this process reinforce and stabilize the patient's mental illness, but it also enters into other problems of patient-staff interaction on the ward. Thus, the labeling of patients as "hopeless," "assaultive," "unresponsive," and "unable to tolerate closeness," serves as a convenient rationalization for avoiding the patient, and thereby perpetuating the process of mutual withdrawal. We have demonstrated that this deeply ingrained and subtle process, often running its course outside the awareness of the participants, *can be systematically observed, evaluated, and interrupted*. In order to do this, we have attempted to develop a *sociopsychiatric nursing* approach, combining the knowledge and conceptual tools of both the sociologist and the psychiatric nurse. A perspective has emerged in which the specific interpersonal relations that the nurse engages in with both patient and personnel, and the ward context with its social structure are viewed as a total interacting process; and in which this interaction is kept under constant scrutiny, in order to determine and evaluate the interventions instituted. As a guidepost for this type of approach, we have asked the following general questions in the course of the study:

(1) What is the nature of the social structure as it exists on the ward, and what are the dominant attitudes and patterns of activity which characterize this social structure?

(2) What is the relationship of this structure to the therapeutic progress of patients? What criteria can be used in evaluating this relationship?

(3) What is the role of the psychiatric nurse? What contradictions are there in this role? What alterations can be made?

(4) What is the nature of the interpersonal relations engaged in by the personnel? How do they relate to other aspects of the social structure and to the patient's progress?

(5) How can these interpersonal relations and the social structure be altered, and in what direction, to facilitate the patient's recovery?

Evidence for the value of this type of approach resides in the fact that the investigator was able not only to employ this approach herself, but also to communicate it to another nurse and to enable this nurse to utilize the approach. Through this procedure, the process of mutual withdrawal was interrupted, and significant alterations in the patient's mode of participation occurred. While the problem of maintaining and carrying forward favorable change among these mentally ill patients has not been dealt with in this study, its significance is manifest. In order to capitalize on the favorable change, it must be carried through to the eventual "cure" of the patient. Psychotherapy—the intensive investigation of the patient's difficulties in living—must be integrated and coordinated with sociopsychiatric nursing care in order to consolidate and continue the improvement.

This article is printed with permission of *Perspectives in Psychiartric Care*.

Original article:
Tudor, G. E. (1970). A sociopsychiatric nursing approach to intervention in a problem of mutual withdrawal on a mental hospital ward. *Perspectives in Psychiatric Care, 8*(1), 11–35.

CRITIQUE BY: LAURIE BEESON, BSN, RN

In the 1950s, at the advent of the integration of psychiatric/mental health nursing into nursing curriculum (Hoeffer & Murphy, 1982), Gwen Tudor became interested in the growing expectations of psychiatric nurses. She designed and carried out a single-case research study whose purpose was "to determine the social context and specific social situations with which the patient in a psychiatric unit was integrated and ... to determine the ways in which, and means whereby, appropriate interventions might be instituted." Tudor saw a need in nursing and embarked on a path to find a solution. The following paper will critique her research study.

Part I: Clinical Relevance

Tudor first provides the reader with a brief background discussion of the concern she saw for the need of consistency in the nurse–patient relationship in the psychiatric setting. Tudor argued that the traditional skills of the psychiatric nurse were insufficient to fulfill patients' needs most effectively. She set out to validate the premise that the "psychiatric nurse must use, to some extent, the tools of the social scientist and combine these with the skills of the nurse."

Tudor's study focused on the "social context within which the patient lives." She believed this social environment, by and large, determined both the nurses's attitude and the behaviors elicited by the patient. In other words, the social environment of the hospital could be either detrimental or beneficial to the patient's mental health. In addition, it is the nurse's responsibility to realize that he or she is an integral part of this social context.

Current psychiatric nursing, in a hospital setting, focuses much attention on the milieu. The milieu, the social or cultural setting, is designed to enhance the patient's social skill development. The entire premise of Tudor's research is of great value to current psychiatric nursing and its focus on milieu therapy.

Tudor's study flows logically. In her problem statement, she identified two areas that could potentially be helpful to the practicing nurse or nursing student. Initially, she set out to identify the social setting of a psychiatric unit. Observation, which provides the nurse with a framework in which he or she will be working, is of obvious value at the onset of a study. Following such observation, Tudor anticipated that she would "determine the ways in which, and means whereby, appropriate intervention might be instituted." Although Tudor's actual setting and specific interventions may seem old fashioned, the process is still of value.

In terms of theoretrical framework, Tudor felt that the social setting not only determines the nurse's attitudes and behaviors but also can facilitate or deter the patient's mental health. In view of this theoretical framework, Tudor makes three general assumptions:

1. The patient's mental illness can be a mode of socialization.
2. Participation can be influenced by the activities others direct toward the patient.
3. The patient's participation can be affected by the nurse, through the nurse–patient interpersonal relationship, and through the general social context of the unit.

Each of these assumptions could afford the nurse with various interventions carried out independently of the physician or other health professionals. However, as Tudor conducted her research, it became obvious that the cooperation and general approval by other health professionals was important to the success of the chosen nursing interventions.

Methodologically, Tudor employed a single-case study design. She measured her outcomes in a qualitative sense, by the overall decrease of mutual withdrawal between patient and personnel, as seen subjectively.

Tudor designed her study to evaluate a clinical problem and then apply appropriate interventions. In her observations, she identified mutual withdrawal as a concept in need of intervention. Mutual withdrawal is defined first by a patient whose dominant pattern of socialization is withdrawal. This characteristic is then responded to by avoidance or withdrawal by staff. Thus, the patient and nurse mutually withdraw from each other. Tudor then aimed study interventions at decreasing withdrawal by staff in hopes of decreasing withdrawal seen in patients. This research process (observation, evaluation, and intervention) is particularly valuable since it constitutes the basis of the nursing process. The nurse should employ this method not only in the psychiatric setting but in all areas of caregiving.

By observing the social setting of a medical surgical floor, for example, would the nurse become aware of sociopsychiatric practices that hinder or facilitate patient recovery?

Part II: Conceptualization and Internal Consistency

Because Tudor conducted her study over 35 years ago, a reader may construe that it has little relevance or value to current nursing practice. However, Tudor's study not only expresses conceptual unity, it is written in common language and is more than readable.

Tudor justifies her study on what she perceived as a growing demand for psychiatric nurses to have greater skills than those traditionally required. As previously stated, she felt that a psychiatric nurse needed to know how to combine social science approaches with nursing skills in order to be most effective. Tudor had no way of knowing that deinstitutionalization of the psychiatric hospitals in the 1970s would only reemphasize the need for psychiatric nurses to incorporate social science approaches into their nursing practice. Justification for the study is apparent.

At the onset of any study, it is the responsibility of the investigator to operationalize study variables. However, in this single-case, mostly descriptive study, operational definitions may not be crucial. In this study, the investigator set out to merge "sociological concepts and psychiatric nursing skills." Therefore, identification of "sociological concepts" and "psychiatric nursing skills" may be necessary. Thirty-five years after the fact, however, definitions may only be of historical interest to a reader and especially at a time when the concepts from the two disciplines are quite intimately integrated.

Tudor's data analysis further reveals "mutual withdrawal" as the end result for patients whose dominant pattern of participation was withdrawal. She defines mutual withdrawal as "recurrent avoidance on the part of staff of these patients."

The investigator set out to identify methods or techniques that would improve psychiatric nursing. By employing a participant–observer approach, she was able to apply her methodology as the study progressed. However, if Tudor was a true participant observer, one who joins a group as one who is similar, this leaves open the ethical concern of informed concent. If Tudor did not act as a participant observer, her data collection may have been biased simply because the usual ward routine would have been disrupted. Nevertheless, data collection was continuous and analysis was simultaneous with collection. In this way, Tudor was sure to measure the desired phenomenon.

Part III: Believability of Results

The investigator collected data from one area, a 14-bed ward for disturbed women, which resulted in a sample of convenience. Since the investigator was attempting to integrate psychiatric nursing skills with social science theory and techniques, the setting and sample were appropriate.

Typically, a single-case research design follows either a descriptive or an experimental approach (Holm, 1983). In Tudor's case, the design combined the descriptive with the experimental approach. Tudor described the development of mutual withdrawal in the case of Mrs. Smith. In the case of Miss Jones, Tudor applied interventions with the intent of decreasing the mutual withdrawal phenomena. In this case, Tudor did not use a control subject; essentially, this too became a descriptive approach.

By using a convenience sample , the investigator is less able to generalize results. However, as Holm (1983) has argued, in single-case research if an "effect has occured in one individual, it is logical to suppose there will be others who will exhibit similar effects."

Nonetheless, the investigator of the present study makes no attempt to discuss reliability of her tool or data. That she is the primary data collection agent, consults with a sociologist, and acts as an advisor to a nursing student are clear, but overall the experiment lacks two data collectors. Reliability measures in an observational study focus on interrater reliability, which refers to having two or more investigators observe a situation and then compare the extent of agreement between their ratings. Therefore, the means to evaluate interrater reliability are nonexistent in this study. Tudor mentions extraneous factors that could influence data collection but makes no systematic attempt to rule out their influence.

Given these shortcomings, Tudor analyzed her data as she collected it making additional interventions as necessary. In this sense, and because of the absence of interrater reliability, Tudor's evaluation was primarily subjective. Nevertheless, Tudor's study, like many others in the area of clinical psychology, served, according to Kazdin (1982), as a basis "for drawing inferences about human behavior."

Ultimately, Tudor concluded that once a process is identified (i.e., mutual withdrawal), it can be "observed, evaluated and interrupted." She labeled the method of interruption "sociopsychiatric nursing." However, the exact differentiation of psychiatric nursing skills, sociological techniques, and sociopsychiatric nursing skills is unclear.

From the information presented in Tudor's paper, it is easy to follow how she was able to draw her conclusion, even though it is hard to distinguish what constituted the sociopsychiatric techniques per se that she utilized. In addition, her solitary analysis of the data she collected could be subject to personal biases. However, in this instance, the question of biases is relatively minor because a single-case study serves as a basis for information about the uniqueness of the person.

Part IV: Generalizability of Results

The ability to generalize research results is key. Often the value of research findings is based on the degree to which the results can be generalized. In the instance of a single-case study, generalizaton is based on the assumption that other clients will respond similarly. In order to increase generalizability, the study should be replicated. If, in a replication, there are consistent results in terms of a decrease in mutual withdrawal, then the professional nursing knowledge base is broadened.

Tudor's study is particularly applicable to replication for the nursing student population. In her study, she described teaching a nursing student how to decrease withdrawal with a second patient as a way of "replicating'" results. An attempt to replicate this study today would present many obstacles, however. Current psychiatric practice is vastly different from that of 1952. With the advent of neuroleptic medications, the deluge of theories on psychodynamics, and the extensive use of milieu therapy, exact replication would be impossible. However, the process of observation, evaluation, and intervention is one that could be used in current clinical settings.

Part V: Other Factors to Consider in Utilization

Implementation of Tudor's methods to decrease mutual withdrawal could be easily accomplished. The cost of implementation would only be in time. If a nurse practicing in a psychiatric setting is dealing with a patient who exhibits withdrawal symptoms, the nurse could incorporate interventions into a working nursing care plan. Again, the cost would be low for implementation and the results could only be beneficial.

In general, and while Tudor's study design and implementation express flaws particularly evident today, her concerns can be seen in a more positive light. As a study that laid groundwork for this special nursing concern, it merits serious consideration for implementation in practice.

REFERENCES

Hoeffer, B., & Murphy, S. (1982). The unfinished task: Development of nursing theory for psychiatric and mental health nursing practice. *Journal of Psychosocial Nursing and Mental Health Services, 20*(12), 8–14.

Holm, K. (1983). Single subject research. *Nursing Research, 32*(4), 253–255.

Kazdin, A. E. (1982). *Single-case research designs, methods for clinical and applied settings.* New York: Oxford University Press.

Original article:
Tudor, G. E. (1970). A sociopsychiatric nursing approach to intervention in a problem of mutual withdrawal on a mental hospital ward. *Perspectives in Psychiatric Care, 8*(1), 11–35.

CRITIQUE BY: BEVERLY HOEFFER, DNSc, RN

Part I: Clinical Relevance

Thirty-five years ago when Tudor conducted her study, the causes of mental illness were unknown and intrapersonal theories of mental illness prevailed. Patients spent years in mental hospitals where little emphasis was placed on the impact of the hospital milieu on the maintenance of their symptoms. Similarly, the definition of the role of the psychiatric nurse as an active participant in patients' treatment versus custodial caretaker and technician was in its infancy.

The investigator embarked on the study with a general theoretical framework in mind that differed considerably from the prevailing medical model. Her position was that insufficient attention had been given to formulating how the psychiatric nurse could systematically collect and utilize data about the social context to devise interventions that would have a therapeutic effect on patients' behavior. As Tudor wrote,

> The social context within which the patient lives is the pattern of interpersonal relations which is the network of reciprocal activities of all those on the ward. It ... both determines in large part the nurses' attitudes and modes of behavior and also facilitates or deters the patients' mental health.

Tudor then set forth the following propositions (which she termed *assumptions*) to guide the study:

1. Symptoms associated with a patient's mental illness characterize the patient's pattern of relating to others on the ward.
2. This pattern can be altered by the actions of others.
3. The psychiatric nurse can have a therapeutic influence on patients' participation in the milieu through a process that includes systematic observation and analysis of specific interpersonal situations and the social context of the ward.

She proposed that the psychiatric nurse become an active participant with the patient within the milieu, and a skilled observer through borrowing techniques used by social scientists. She conceived of psychiatric nursing "as a continuous interpersonal process" consisting of overlapping steps that included observation, evaluaton of data, hypotheses about the situation, intervention, and reevaluation to determine the effectiveness of actions taken.

The clinical problem addressed was two-fold: (1) to describe the social context and specific social situations of a ward that contributed to a patient's recurrent pattern of participation; and (2) to develop and test nursing intervention strategies for their effectiveness in altering patterns of participation that maintained a patient's symptoms and dysfunctional behavior.

In the three decades since Tudor conducted her study, the impact of the social milieu on maintaining or exacerbating symptoms and dysfunctional behavior associated with mental illness is accepted as common knowledge. The process she described is the underpinning of the nursing process and clinical decision making, and is clearly evident in current accepted standards for psychiatric nursing practice (American Nurses' Association, 1982). The specific dysfunctional interpersonal pattern of participation between staff and selected patients that Tudor identified (described in the title and later in the study as "mutual withdrawal") remains a significant clinical problem. Hall (1976) reported results from a field study 20 years later documenting the same pattern of behavior. However, such a pattern may be less obvious to staff and hence more difficult to resolve in the context of today's shortened hospital stays that mitigate against the development of interpersonal relationships. Nonetheless, the ability to implement and evaluate interventions that Tudor suggested is clearly within the purview of nursing in psychiatric inpatient settings.

Part II: Conceptualization and Internal Consistency

Tudor's study develops in a logical and consistent manner from section to section. A clear fit is evident between the rationale for the study, the general theoretical framework and propositions proposed, and the nature of the clinical problem addressed. Although lengthy, the judicious use of lay language makes the study quite readable.

Unlike shorter research reports written today, Tudor presented extensive data on two female schizophrenic patients so that the reader can follow the identification of recurrent patterns of participation and testing of nursing interventions. Students or nurses who have had minimal experience working with severely disturbed psychiatric patients may be put off by some of the subjects' language and behavior reported in the data section. However, the data accurately reflected the interactions between patients and nursing staff in mental hospitals in the 1950s.

In additon, the underlying conceptualization of the study makes sense. The investigator presented a convincing rationale for carrying out the research in the clinical setting. However, one confusing aspect may appear. In the title to her study, Tudor used the concept of "mutual withdrawal" but interchanged this term with "avoidance-withdrawal" in the text to describe the interpersonal pattern of participation observed between nursing staff and the two patients. She reasoned that this recurrent pattern of staff avoidance and patient withdrawal contributed to maintaining illness behavior.

To test her hunch, Tudor used the qualitative method of participant observation to conduct the six-month study. She made detailed notes of her observation of two patients as they interacted within the social context of a 14-bed ward for mentally ill women during the first three months. After identifying the recurrent pattern of mutual withdrawal, she participated directly in the patients' care during the next three months by using interpersonal contacts as an intervention to change the patients' pattern of participation on the ward. During this phase, she continued to collect and analyze data on the impact of her interventions. However, another more pressing issue regarding reliability appears here. Tudor served both as the vehicle for the intervention as well as the instrument of data collection for the first patient. In response to this issue, Tudor recognized the inherent difficulty in undertaking clinician and researcher role simultaneously. For example, to minimize the effect of her subjective responses on the data collection and analysis, she reviewed her field notes with an outside methodological expert on a regular basis. This enabled her to guard against biases that may have affected the conclusions she drew when addressing the research questions outlined for each patient. Subsequently, she taught the interventions she had used to a nursing student who was working with the second patient, and then collected data on the student–patient interaction.

Part III: Believability of Results

This study purported to describe a phenomenon of concern to nursing (i.e., mutual withdrawal) and to test the effect of nursing interventions on this pattern of staff–patient interaction. In that sense, it has both the elements of a case study, since qualitative descriptive data on two patients is described in detail, and of a single subject experimental design (Holm, 1983). Regarding the latter, Tudor used an ABAB design with both subjects to test the effectiveness of the nursing strategies in altering behavior. Baseline observations (A_1) were made followed by the introduction of the intervention (B_1). This phase was followed by ceasing the intervention (A_2) and then reintroducing the same or similar strategies a week later (B_2). In both cases, Tudor observed positive changes in the patient's behavior during the intervention phases in contrast to the baseline phases.

Tudor selected a convenience sample of two female patients with schizophrenia that exemplified the pattern under investigation. However, she provided insufficient information other than diagnosis for one to judge whether the subjects were representative of other women admitted to the 80-bed private psychiatric hospital. The setting suggests that the subjects were white, middle or upper class women and, hence, dissimilar from many women admitted to public mental hospitals in the 1950s. Tudor also makes no mention of obtaining informed consent, although not obtaining consent of subjects was common practice in observational studies at that time.

Unfortunately, Tudor did not elaborate on extraneous variables that may have influenced her results. However, she did identify changes in ward management that may have contributed to the ability to introduce alternative interventions and that may have affected the nature of data obtained in the earlier and later phases of the study. Since only one person collected data, there is no way to assess the consistency and accuracy of the data collected through examining interrater reliability. As previously noted, the use of the sociologist as an expert consultant external to the study was a method used to mitigate against Tudor's subjective biases during data collection and analysis.

Tudor reported her data and analysis procedure in considerable detail, enabling the reader in part to judge the adequacy of the conclusions she drew. The study does not reflect more sophisticated methods of qualitative analysis for identifying phenomena discussed in current literature. But the methods of analysis were similar to those used in sociological field studies of that time.

Part IV: Generalizability of Results

Tudor essentially used a single case design in her study. Only recently has nursing returned to a position of valuing this approach for studying clinical problems. Holm (1983) makes a strong case for the use of this approach by nurses practicing in clinical settings who wish to engage in research. Holm also argues that results obtained from systematic observations of a single subject can be generalized to similar individuals if a process or effect has been carefully established.

In fact, Tudor did replicate her study. She observed and identified the pattern of mutual withdrawal in the first subject, and then tested the effect of interpersonal contact as an intervention. After she established that the pattern occurred with the second subject, she taught a nursing student to successfully implement the intervention she had previously tested. Hence, she demonstrated that the strategies could be easily taught to, and carried out by, nursing personnel through the use of clinical instruction and supervision. Although the study lay dormant for 20 years, Hall (1976) documented that the pattern of mutual withdrawal still described the interpersonal behavior of nursing staff and psychiatric patients who were nonparticipants in the milieu of an inpatient setting in the mid 1970s.

The conclusions Tudor drew about the effect of the social structure of the ward and the interpersonal relations between nursing personnel and patients on patients' progress are still relevant today even though theories about mental illness, treatment approaches, and length of hospitalization have changed. For example, current nursing research on difficult young adult chronic patients (Gallop & Wynn, 1986) may assist staff in understanding what factors contribute to staff avoidance of such patients and how the milieu can be used effectively in managing their behavior. Moreover, Tudor's vision of the psychiatric nurse as one who incorporates conceptual and research approaches with clinical skills is congruent with primary nursing and clinical nurse specialist roles as described today in the current literature.

Part V: Other Factors to Consider in Utilization

Because of the single case design and the nature of the intervention (i.e., one that is clearly within the domain of nursing practice), systematic evaluation of the interventions Tudor introduced is clearly feasible in current inpatient settings. The benefits of using the research are that nursing staff may gain a better understanding of how both staff and patients contribute to the patterns of interaction that develop on inpatient units. Patients may benefit from more skillful interactions of staff aimed at altering problematic patterns of participation. The risk of not trying the practice suggested by the research is that nursing staff may underestimate and devalue the therapeutic use of self and that patients may be deprived of a major benefit of being in a protected milieu. Given that the benefits outweigh the risks, the relevant question seems to be: what system factors mitigate against the incorporation of both the process and the outcomes of the study in the daily practice of a psychiatric nurse in all inpatient settings?

In general, Tudor's study has stood the test of time. The therapeutic use of self and social milieu to change behavior patterns and the use of a systematic nursing process in providing patient care are part of the current standards for psychiatric nursing. We are indebted to her for demonstrating to us 35 years ago that theory and research are an integral and enriching aspect of nursing practice.

REFERENCES

American Nurses' Association. (1982). *Standards of psychiatric and mental health nursing practice*. Kansas City, MO: Author.

Gallop, R., & Wynn, F. (1986). Difficult young adult chronic patients: Re-evaluating short-term clinical management. *Journal of Psychosocial Nursing and Mental Health Services*, *24*(3), 29–32.

Hall, B. (1976). Mutual withdrawal: The non-participant in a therapeutic community. *Perspectives in Psychiatric Care*, *9*(2), 75–79.

Holm, K. (1983). Single subject research. *Nursing Research*, *32*(4), 253–255.

Attitudes of Patients with Schizophrenia toward Taking Medication

Ruth E. Davidhizar
Logansport State Hospital
Logansport, IN

Joan K. Austin
School of Nursing
Indiana University
Indianapolis, IN

Angela B. McBride
School of Nursing
Indiana University
Indianapolis, IN

The attitude of 50 hospitalized persons with schizophrenia toward taking their medication was examined. Both open-ended and fixed-response estimates of attitude were made. Insight also was measured, and the relationships between insight and attitude and between hallucinations and insight were analyzed. Patients were able to provide information about beliefs and feelings about taking medication and about insight toward illness and treatment. Attitudes varied, and both strongly positive and strongly negative beliefs about taking medication were held simultaneously. Some of the implications for nursing are explained.

In both medicine and nursing there is awareness that the patient's beliefs and feelings toward medication and the patient's insight about illness and treatment are significant information for the health care professional. These issues were addressed in the present study by three research questions:

1. What is the attitude of patients toward taking medication?
2. How much insight do patients with schizophrenia have about psychiatric illness?
3. What is the relationship between attitude about medication and insight about illness?

Among the variables found to affect medication behavior (Battle, Halliburton, & Wallston, 1982; Durel & Munjas, 1982; Whiteside, 1983; Witt, 1981) are patient beliefs and feelings. Investigators have studied attitude toward ambulatory treatment (Serban & Thomas, 1974), outcome (McGlashan & Carpenter, 1981), changes in medication (Lesser & Friedmann, 1981), and placement in seclusion (Binder & McCoy, 1983). In some reports the operationalization of attitude is unclear. In only one (Binder & McCoy, 1983) was attitude considered a phenomenon composed of both beliefs and feelings. The term attitude has been used in a variety of ways: to describe feelings about illness, beliefs about illness and/or understanding of illness. The studies suggest that it is possible to obtain information on attitude from patients with schizophrenia, however, and that some relationship exists between attitude and future behavior.

There is interest in patient insights about illness and treatment (Del Campo, Carr, & Correa, 1983; Greenfeld, Strauss, & Bowers, 1983; Kane, Quitkin, Rifkin, Wegner, Rosenberg, & Borenstein, 1983; Lin, Spiga, & Fortsch, 1979; McEvoy, Aland, Wilson, Guy, & Hawkins, 1981; Nelson, Gold, Hutchinson, & Benezra, 1975; Van Putten, Crompton, & Yale, 1976). These studies indicate a beginning and an evolving understanding of insight as experienced by the patient with schizophrenia. While each researcher operationalized insight differently, the definition has progressed from an initial recognition of illness to the broader view of insight as encompassing a variety of facets (McEvoy et al., 1981; Greenfeld et al., 1983). Insight probably is a multidimensional phenomenon involving assessment of the possible sources of the disorder, the impact of symptoms on others, perception of the presence of symptoms, perception of the need for treatment, perception of treatment benefit, and perception of vulnerability to recurrence of illness in the future. In most reports a clear operational definition of insight was not presented making it difficult to compare data across studies. A further problem has been the interchangeable use of the terms attitude and insight.

Fishbein's Expectancy-Value Model (Ajzen & Fishbein, 1980) provided the theoretical base for this study of attitude. In this model, "A person's attitude toward any object is a function of beliefs about the object and the implicit evaluation responses associated with those beliefs" (Fishbein & Ajzen, 1975, p. 29). An attitude was defined as having two components. The first was the individual's perceived probability (i.e., subjective probability) that the object is associated with the attribute or issue under scrutiny. The second component was the individual's evaluation of the attribute that is associated with the attitude object. This typically is estimated on a bipolar scale ranging from very positive to very negative. The midpoint (0) may be chosen when feelings are neutral.

The Fishbein Expectancy-Value Model has been used extensively in studies of attitude over the past 20 years. Attitudes toward personal characteristics, for example, Negroes (Fishbein, 1963), health related behavior, having another child (Vinokur-Kaplan, 1978), donating blood (Bagozzi, 1981b), adolescent alcohol use (Schlegel, Crawford, & Sanborn, 1977), and religious behavior (Fishbein & Ajzen, 1974) have been measured. Some studies have been reported by nurses using the model in clinical settings. Austin, McBride, & Davis (1984) studied attitudes of parents of children with epilepsy; Millican (1982) studied characteristics of parents who physically abuse their children; and Schmidt (1980) studied attitudes of nurses toward charting behavior.

Among the studies reporting on validity of the model are studies that reported positive correlations between expectancy-value and semantic differential measures (Fishbein, 1963; Fishbein & Coombs, 1974; Jaccard & Davidson, 1972). The Guttman, Likert, Thurstone, and Guilford Self-Rating Scales have been used in validity studies (Fishbein & Ajzen, 1974). The correlations obtained in these studies provided measures of concurrent or criterion-related validity. In addition to concurrent and criterion validity, construct validity was studied by Bagozzi (1981a, 1981b) and Ajzen and Fishbein (1980).

METHOD

Subjects

The subjects were 50 patients who were consecutively admitted to an acute-care psychiatric unit with schizophrenia, and who met the criteria. The criteria in the *Diagnostic and Statistical Manual of Mental Disorders* (SPS, 1980) determined the operationalization of schizophrenia for this study. Patients were all on a voluntary status and on a psychotropic medication regimen. The conceptual definition of schizophrenia used was an illness in which patients experience splitting off of portions of the psyche. These portions may then dominate the psychic life of the patient for a time and lead to an independent existence even though these may be contrary and contradictory to the personality as a whole (Hinsie & Campbell, 1973).

Patients ranged in age from 18 to 75 with a median age of 33. The group included 22 men and 28 women; 27 were never married, 14 were married, and 9 were either separated, divorced, or widowed. High school had been completed by 54% of the patients but only 20% had regular employment; 4 patients were 65 or older, and therefore in the retirement years. The number of previous psychiatric hospitalizations for the patients in the study ranged from 0 to 10 with an average of 3.85 for 49 patients. While patients were interviewed within the first month of being hospitalized, more were interviewed in their third or fourth day of hospitalization than any other. According to hospital records, 64% of the subjects were complying with their medication regimens before admission. No medication regimen had been previously prescribed for six patients. Of the 50 patients, 23 hallucinated during the hospitalization.

Measures

Each patient responded to questions on three instruments: an open-ended attitude instrument, a fixed-response attitude instrument, and an insight instrument. The open-ended instrument was administered first so that patients would not be prompted by the beliefs in the fixed-response instrument, but would volunteer their individual beliefs. The fixed-response instrument, with 26 belief statements, was constructed from a review of the compliance literature (Davidhizar, 1982) and was modified after a pilot study. An insight instrument was administered last.

Open-Ended Instrument. In the open-ended attitude assessment, patients were asked to state beliefs in response to four questions: What do you think about taking your medication in the hospital? Why do you take your medication in the hospital? What are the advantages of taking your medication in the hospital? and What are the disadvantages of taking your medication in the hospital? Each belief stated was rated by the subject on: (a) strength of the beliefs on a scale of +2 to −0, and (b) feeling about the belief on a scale of +2 to −2. Although Fishbein and Ajzen (1975) suggested that the strength of beliefs can be estimated on a scale of −3 to +3, special modifications were made in this study because of the cognitive difficulties of patients with schizophrenia. Since patients responding to the open-ended instrument only volunteered beliefs important to them, patients only had to distinguish between +1 (being slightly sure) and +2 (being very sure). Examples of items volunteered included "It causes sleepiness", "It tastes bad", "It causes my mouth to be dry", and "It won't help me."

Fixed Response Instrument. On the fixed-response instrument, patients rated their belief strength on a 5-point scale ranging from +2 (strongly agree) to −2 (strongly disagree). As on the open-ended instrument, a 5-point scale ranging from +2 (strongly positive to −2 (strongly negative) was used for feeling evaluation. Items included taking it is a way the doctor can help you, taking it pleases your doctor, and taking it will help you get better. The belief statements were varied so that in some cases agreeing affirmed a belief likely to be positive and in some cases agreeing affirmed a belief likely to be negative.

Insight Instrument. In the absence of an instrument for assessing insight, a 10-item tool was developed incorporating the five dimensions identified by Greenfeld et al. (1983) and the factors identified by McEvoy et al. (1981) (see Table 1). Each statement was rated on a 5-point scale: strongly agree (5), slightly agree, not sure, slightly disagree, and strongly disagree (1).

The 10 items were arranged randomly in the instrument. Items varied so that in some cases strongly disagree showed insight, while at other times it was necessary to check strongly agree to indicate insight. The range of possible scores was 10-50 with 10 showing the least insight and 50 showing the most insight. A pilot study with the insight instrument indicated patients could vary their responses to demonstrate no insight, questionable insight, and insight. No modifications were made after the pilot study. A .903 reliability

Table 1
Measurement of Insight into Illness and Treatment

1. My hospitalization was caused by symptoms of psychiatric problems.
2. I do not need psychiatric treatment.
3. I am psychiatrically ill.
4. I am getting psychiatric treatment.
5. I should be at home instead of in the hospital.
6. I will always have to be careful about getting a psychiatric problem in the future.
7. I should not be hospitalized in a psychiatric unit.
8. I have symptoms that need psychiatric treatment.
9. I should have care by psychiatric professionals.
10. I am psychologically healthy.

coefficient indicated strong internal consistency on the insight instrument when Cronbach's Alpha was computed on the data obtained in this study.

Procedures

A memorized verbal presentation was used in explaining the procedure and obtaining consent. The presentation emphasized the voluntary nature of participation, that failure to participate would not affect subsequent care. The verbal consent was witnessed by a staff member not directly involved in patient care who did not remain for the interview. Only one patient who was asked to participate declined.

RESULTS

Attitude toward Medication

Open-Ended Instrument. On the open-ended instrument a total of 198 beliefs were volunteered by the 50 patients. The open-ended attitude for each of the 50 patients toward taking medication was determined by summing the product of the strength and feeling for each volunteered. The mean of these 50 scores was −.420. The scores ranged from -24 to +24 with a median score of .357 and a mode of 0. These scores indicate that the average patient attitude was essentially neutral, though this overall neutrality was achieved most of the time because positive perceptions and negative perceptions canceled each other out.

The largest number of beliefs (53.5%) were negative. Patients tended to have more negative beliefs about medication than positive. Of the negative beliefs, the largest number (33%) concerned physiological effects or side effects related to medication. Another category of negative beliefs (11.5%) fell in a subgrouping called cognitive effects. A further grouping were beliefs involving control and power issues. Control and power beliefs were defined as those involving a feeling of being directed or restrained by something or someone else, such as a feeling of dependency or force. Statements such as, "I don't need it" also were included since they carried the implication of "I don't need this control, I can take care of myself." Power and control beliefs appeared to be an issue of emerging significance with this patient group. A third category of negative beliefs concerned perception of medication effects. The largest group of positive beliefs (17%) involved psychological effects. Other positive beliefs concerned cognitive effects and feelings of well-being.

Fixed-Response Instrument. Attitude about taking medication was determined on the fixed-response instrument by summing the product of the belief strength and feeling for each of the 24 beliefs. The mean attitude score for the 50 patients was 20.3 with a range from -32 to 76 and a standard deviation of 23.8. The median score was 16.5, while the attitude score obtained by the most respondents was 0. Again, as in the open-ended instrument, these scores indicated an essentially neutral attitude about taking medication. The attitude score did not vary significantly when compared with age and sex of the patients.

The strength of beliefs on the fixed-belief instrument was computed and the beliefs were ranked from those with which patients most agreed to those with which they least agreed (see Table 2). Only two beliefs received a mean rating of greater than 1, slightly agree: "Taking it is a way the doctor can help you" ($M = 1.76$) and "Taking it pleases your doctor" ($M = 1.46$). Both of these beliefs involve the doctor and indicate that patients made an association between medication and the doctor. These beliefs were the ones with the smallest standard deviation, indicating that there was consistency among the patients that these beliefs were true.

The salience of the individual belief items is an important subject deserving consideration. Salient beliefs are those that determine attitude at any given moment. It is easier to evaluate salience in an open-ended situation in which the volunteered beliefs usually are salient. In the fixed-response instrument, salience can be considered by taking those beliefs with a rating of at least .5, halfway between not sure and slightly against or disagree. Using this criterion, only the eight beliefs between .5 and 2 were salient.

The 24 items on the fixed-response instrument were internally consistent (r = .738) when Cronbach's Alpha was performed. A Pearson correlation coefficient was computed on the two attitude instruments. A correlation of .71 ($p < .001$) was obtained which accounted for 54% of the variance. This is noteworthy considering the very different elicitation procedures used and indicates that the instruments measured similar content.

Table 2
Beliefs of Schizophrenic Patients Toward Taking Medication [Fixed-Response Instrument]

Belief	Belief Strength[a] M	SD	Evaluation[b] M	SD
Taking it is a way the doctor can help you.	1.76	.74	1.46	1.03
Taking it pleases your doctor.	1.46	1.11	0.78	1.33
It will help you get better.	0.86	1.55	1.38	.95
It makes you feel calm and/or relaxed.	0.78	1.42	1.26	1.19
It can be changed by your doctor if you request it.	0.78	1.60	1.34	1.08
It is expensive for you.	0.76	1.36	-.38	1.03
Taking it pleases your family.	0.64	1.42	0.72	1.05
It causes you to have dry mouth.	0.52	1.69	-1.02	1.25
Taking it will help you feel like yourself again.	0.28	1.79	1.08	1.14
It controls your confusion.	0.16	1.49	0.96	1.09
It makes you sleepy during the day.	0.16	1.79	-0.80	1.58
It alters your sexual drive.	0.16	1.25	-0.24	1.19
Taking it is something you are forced to do.	0.14	1.86	-0.48	1.54
It requires the nurses to watch you closer to make sure you take it.	0.02	1.64	-0.16	1.18
It reduces your hallucinations.	-0.10	1.47	0.68	1.13
It makes you dizzy.	-0.14	1.62	-1.08	1.14
Taking it results in the nurses spending more time with you explaining the medication.	-0.18	1.34	0.38	.88
Taking it results in your doctor spending more time with you explaining the medication.	-0.24	1.42	0.58	1.01
It makes you feel restless and/or makes your feet move back and forth.	-0.38	1.58	-0.86	1.39
It helps you feel like getting along with others.	-0.40	1.96	0.44	1.23
It makes your legs ache and your joints stiff.	-0.48	1.74	-1.06	1.43
It tastes bad and/or leaves a bad taste in your mouth.	-0.56	1.63	-0.98	1.15
It causes you to feel shaky or have tremors.	-0.72	1.53	-1.02	1.52
It prevents you from sleeping at night.	-0.80	1.59	-1.08	1.28

[a] Scale ranged from +2 (strongly agree) to −2 (strongly disagree).
[b] Scale ranged from +2 (strongly positive) to −2 (strongly negative).

Since patients with schizophrenia may experience loosening of associations, patients may be inconsistent in their responses at different times. Two questions were repeated in the fixed-response instrument, one positive and one negative, to test for consistency.

A strong negative correlation was obtained for the belief strengths of "It is expensive for you" and "It is inexpensive for you" ($r = -.863$, $p < .001$), as well as for the evaluation rating on these two items ($r = -.917$, $p < .001$) Relatively strong negative correlations also were obtained for the belief strength of "It has no effect on your getting better" and "It will help you get better" ($r = -.789$, $p < .001$), as well as for the evaluation rating ($r = -.540$, $p < .001$) on these two items. These negative correlations support the notion that patients with schizophrenia were consistent in their responses on the fixed response instrument. In addition, when the products of the belief and evaluation score for the net regarding expense were analyzed, a positive correlation ($r = .917$, $p < .001$) was found. A positive correlation coefficient of .712 ($p < .001$) also was found for the product scores of the other set. "It has no effect on your getting better" and "It will help you get better." There was a stronger positive correlation for the belief concerning expense than for the belief concerning a more abstract phenomenon, evaluation of well-being. These relatively strong positive correlations indicate that patients were generally able to be consistent in their judgments.

Insight into Psychiatric Illness. The possible range of scores on insight about illness and treatment was 10-50. Arbitrarily, scores ranging from 10 to 20 indicated no insight and from 40 to 50 indicated insight; scores between 21 and 39 indicated questionable insight. The scores obtained by the 50 patients ranged from 10 to 50. Only 14% of the patients met the criterion for no insight, 38% of the patients met the criterion for questionable insight, and 48% met the criterion for insight. Most patients had insight for some statements yet lacked insight for others. The item on the insight instrument receiving least agreement was: "My hospitalization caused by symptoms of psychiatric problems."

Insight and Attitude. The correlation between insight and attitude on the open-ended instrument was $r = .371$, $p = .004$, and the correlation between insight and attitude on the fixed-response instrument was $r = .368$, $p = .005$. While there was a relationship between the scores on the insight instrument and the scores on both attitude instruments, the correlation was modest, accounting for only 13.7% and 13.5%, respectively, of the total variances. A point biserial correlation between insight and the presence of hallucinations was $r = .276$, $p = .026$, indicating that patients who had hallucinated during the hospitalization had less insight. The researchers had thought that hallucinations were related to a positive attitude toward treatment; this was not supported.

DISCUSSION

Patients demonstrated a range of attitudes toward medication. An assortment of widely varying beliefs composed individual attitude. Patients were able to both generate a variety of beliefs about medication and to respond to a set of beliefs. Beliefs were rated with varying belief strengths and feelings. For most patients both positive and negative feelings about medication contributed to attitudes toward medication. Some individuals had a positive attitude and others had a negative attitude.

Common negative beliefs concerned side effects. This is in keeping with other reports of patient reaction to side effects. Van Putten (1974) reported that a significant number of patients discontinued and altered doses of medication due to side effects. Supporting this finding, Slater, Linn, and Harris (1981) also found reports of side effects higher among relapsers than the general population of an outpatient clinic. In a study comparing patients who refused neuroleptic treatment with those who consented, it was not the history of side effects, but patient perception of "adequate explanations of side effects" which varied significantly in the two groups (Marder, Mebane, Chien, Winslade, Swann, & Van Putten, 1983).

Beliefs about power and control also contributed to negative attitudes. Some patients felt forced by others to take medication, for example, "I'm forced to take it." Amarasingham (1980) explained that medication may be associated with a feeling of being pressured and may be resisted by a patient who wishes "to make a direct statement of autonomy." Feelings of control by the medication, for example, "They are trying to control me with medication," and feelings of dependency, "Being on medication is a dependency," and "I don't want to be on any medication," were other aspects of feeling controlled mentioned by patients.

On the open-ended instrument, patients commonly related positive feelings to therapeutic effects of the medication, such as physiological effects, cognitive effects, and feelings of well-being. The beliefs about the doctor, "Taking it is a way the doctor can help you," and "It pleases your doctor," received the strongest belief strength and positive evaluation in the fixed-response interview. In a study by Marder et al. (1983), the patient view that the physician had the patient's best interest in mind was found to be a significant variable between refusers and acceptors of neuroleptic treatment.

Patients ranged from having no insight about illness and treatment to having insight. Only 48% of the patients in this study met the criterion for having insight. This corresponds with deficits in insight by patients with schizophrenia which have been identified by many authors including McEvoy et al. (1981), Havens (1963), and Applebaum, Mirkin, and Batemen (1981).

Insight and attitude were found in this study to be related. Since previous studies have not operationalized insight and attitude in the manner used in this study, it is not possible to compare the correlation obtained in this study with others. A relationship has been alluded to by many authors (Marder et al., 1983; McEvoy et al., 1981), but the nature of the relationship is unclear.

Attitude scores on the two instruments were significantly and positively correlated. This correlation occurred in spite of very different elicitation procedures. Both attitude instruments demonstrated that attitude was commonly composed of a variety of positive and negative beliefs. The positive relationship indicated that both procedures provided similar information about attitude.

A number of implications for practice emerged from this study. Since patients with schizophrenia are willing and able to give their attitude about medications, professionals should request this information. Since patient beliefs were found to be very individual, education for patients should include specific beliefs of individual patients rather than a group approach without individual consideration. A teaching technique such as that used by Comon (1979) and Sclafani (1977), combining both individual and group teaching, would seem more appropriate than the most common educational program implemented which involves only group teaching. Intervention strategy of professionals cannot assume a set attitude by the patient but must determine the attitude of the individual being taught. Some patients in this study explained their beliefs were not based on their own present experience, but on the experience of others or their experience in the past. Exploration of the origin of beliefs can enhance the understanding of patients and discussion may change their evaluation of the beliefs and consequently their attitude.

The prevalence of beliefs about side effects and the large contribution of these beliefs to negative attitude about medications implies that it is important to carefully monitor patients for side effects and to discuss both the possibility that they may occur and that the patient can be treated if they occur. It is necessary to deal with beliefs about side effects if attitude is to be improved.

Many aspects of the attitude of patients with schizophrenia toward medication have not been thoroughly investigated. There are little data available about the reaction of patients to individual psychotropic medication or when medication is monitored by one therapist versus several therapists. No studies have been reported on patients who have only been on medication a short time in contrast to those who have had extensive experience with the medication. There has been little study on the effect of dysphoric reactions on attitude of patients. Information is needed on the relationship of individual and group teaching on attitude and on the relationship of attitude to compliance. The Reasoned Action model (Ajzen & Fishbein, 1980) provides a method to investigate both intention and actions and would appear appropriate to use in an investigation of the intention and actions of adherence to a treatment regimen.

The need for further study about insight toward illness and treatment is evident since studies have related insight to increased compliance (Nelson et al., 1975). While McEvoy et al. (1981) found that lack of insight continues in spite of education, more research is needed to study the effect of individual versus group educational programs on patient insight. Investigation is needed on the nature of the relationship of insight and attitude.

REFERENCES

Ajzen, I., & Fishbein, M. (1980). *Understanding attitudes and predicting social behavior.* Englewood Cliffs, NJ: Prentice-Hall.

Amarasingham, L.R. (1980, March). Social and cultural perspectives on medication refusal. *American Journal of Psychiatry, 137,* 353–357.

American Psychiatric Association, Committee on Nomenclature and Statistics. (1980). *Diagnostic and statistical manual of mental disorders (3rd ed.).* Washington, DC: The American Psychiatric Association.

Appelbaum, P., Mirkin, S., & Bateman, A. (1981). Empirical assessment of competency to consent to psychiatric hospitalization. *American Journal of Psychiatry, 138,* 1170–1176.

Austin, J., McBride, A., & Davis, H. (1984). Parental attitude and adjustment to childhood epilepsy. *Nursing Research, 33(4),* 92–96.

Bagozzi, R.P. (1981a). Attitudes, intentions, and behavior: A test of some key hypotheses. *Journal of Personality and Social Psychology, 41,* 607–627.

Bagozzi, R.P. (1981b). An examination of the validity of two models of attitude. *Multivariate Behavioral Research, 16,* 323–359.

Battle, E, Halliburton, A., & Wallston, K. (1982). Self medication among psychiatric patients and adherence after discharge. *Journal of Psychosocial Nursing and Mental Health Services, 20(5),* 21–28.

Cohen, M., & Amdur, M. A. (1981, February). Medication group for psychiatric patients. *American Journal of Nursing, 81,* 343–345.

Comon, A. (1979, Summer), Released patients get medication education. *Innovations, 37.*

Davidhizar, R. (1982). Tool development for profiling the attitude of clients with schizophrenia toward their medication using Fishbein's expectancy-value model. *Issues in Mental Health Nursing, 4,* 343–354.

Del Campo, E., Carr, C., & Correa, E. (1983). Rehospitalized schizophrenics: What they report about illness, treatment and compliance. *Journal of Psychosocial Nursing and Mental Health Services, 21(6),* 29–33.

Durel, S., & Munjas, B. (1982). Client perception of role in psychotropic drug management. *Issues in Mental Health Nursing, 4,* 65–76.

Fishbein, M. (1963). An investigation of the relationships between beliefs about an object and the attitude toward that object. *Human Relations, 16,* 233–240.

Fishbein, M., & Ajzen, I. (1974). Attitudes towards objects as predictors of single and multiple behavioral criteria. *Psychological Review, 81,* 59–74.

Fishbein, M., & Ajzen, I. (1975). *Belief, attitude, intention and behavior: An introduction to theory and research.* Reading, MS: Addison-Wesley Publication.

Fishbein, M., & Coombs, F. (1974). Basis for decision: An attitudinal analysis of rating behavior. *Journal of Applied Social Psychology, 4,* 95–124.

Greenfeld, D., Strauss, J., & Bowers, M. (1983). *The nature of insight in recovery for psychosis: An exploratory study.* Unpublished manuscript, 1–8.

Hinsie, L., & Campbell, R. (1973). *Psychiatric dictionary.* New York: Oxford University Press.

Havens, L. (1963). Problems with the use of drugs in the psychotherapy of psychotic patients. *Psychiatry, 26,* 289–296.

Jaccard, J., & Davidson, A. (1972). Toward an understanding of family planning behaviors: An initial investigation. *Journal of Applied Social Psychology, 2,* 228–235.

Kane, J., Quitkin, F., Rifkin, A., Wegner, J., Rosenberg, G., & Borenstein, M. (1983). Attitudinal changes of involuntarily committed patients following Rx. *Archives of General Psychiatry, 40,* 374–377.

Lesser, I., & Friedmann, C. (1981). Attitudes toward medication change among chronically impaired psychiatric patients. *American Journal of Psychiatry, 131,* 801–803.

Lin, I. F., Spiga, R., & Fortsch, W. (1979). Insight and adherence to medication in chronic schizophrenia. *Journal of Clinical Psychiatry, 38,* 430–432.

Marder, S., Mebane, A., Chien, C., Winslade, W., Swann, E., & Van Putten, T. (1983). A comparison of patients who refuse and consent to neuroleptic treatment. *American Journal of Psychiatry, 140,* 4.

McEvoy, J., Aland, J., Wilson, W., Guy, W., & Hawkins, L. (1981). Measuring chronic schizophrenic patients' attitudes toward their illness and treatment. *Hospital and Community Psychiatry, 32,* 856–858.

McGlashan, T., & Carpenter, W. (1981). Does attitude toward psychosis relate to outcome? *American Journal of Psychiatry, 138,* 797–801.

This article is printed with permission of *Research in Nursing and Health.*
Copyright © 1986 John Wiley & Sons.

Original article:
Davidhizar, R. E., Austin, J. K., & McBride, A. B. (1986). Attitudes of patients with schizophrenia toward taking medication. *Research in Nursing and Health, 9*(2), 139–146.

CRITIQUE BY: VALERIE GOWDY, BSN, RN

Part I: Clinical Relevance

This study examined three questions relating to the attitude and insights of hospitalized schizophrenic patients toward taking medication. In the first question, the investigators addressed the attitude of patients towards taking their medication. In the second question, they asked about the insight that patients have toward their illness. In the third question, they looked at "the relationship between attitude about medication and insight about illness." From a nursing perspective, it is essential that professionals become aware of the feelings, beliefs, and insights that our patients employ in order to facilitate appropriate care. In light of the importance of the research questions, I feel that this study has the potential to further nursing knowledge and provide additional assessment tools, as well as providing possible teaching and learning concepts which could be utilized in patient education.

This study has the potential to aid in identifying patients who are at risk for possible medication noncompliance. By observing negative and positive attitudes about medication and illness, the nurse may be able to intervene and identify those patients at risk for medication noncompliance. Completing an assessment of patients' attitudes and insights would give the nurse a better understanding of the patients' feelings and beliefs toward their medication regimen. This information then could prove valuable in planning care for the psychiatric patient and providing the nurse with a way to identify possible blocks in the treatment plan.

While the investigators provided a specific theoretical framework for studying attitudes and beliefs, they failed to provide any theoretical framework for studying insight. They cite numerous other studies of insight amoung psychiatric clients which indicate a beginning and evolving understanding of this condition. However, the investigators of the present study go on to state that there remains no clear operatonal definition of insight, which makes it difficult to compare data across studies. They mention that there has been a problem with the terms (*attitude* and *insight*) being used interchangeably, which makes me wonder if the investigators can adequately separate out and measure the two terms sufficiently. However, they did not test an intervention in this study but rather interviewed each participant and measured the dependent variables of attitude and insight.

Since the research problems were clearly identified, the study has the potential to help identify and possibly solve a problem which practitioners currently face. It also makes available two assessment tools which have the potential to add much information to the patient's data base. Hence, I believe that this study deserves futher consideration and has potential for use in practice.

Part II: Conceptualization and Internal Consistency

This study is written clearly and is logically developed. The investigators also cited numerous additional studies to aid the reader in understanding the concepts involved. They provided clear operational definitions for their dependent variables, as well.

The investigators find justification for their study by assuming that knowledge about a patient's attitudes toward taking medication (which is comprised of his or her beliefs and feelings about medications) and a patient's insight about illness and treatment are significant information for the health care professional. Unfortunately, this assumption is not sufficiently supported.

For example, the investigators stated that there is interest in patient insights about illness and treatment, but they failed to document the need for health care providers to become knowledgeable about a patient's beliefs and feelings. On the other hand, the investigators did provide documentation to explain that both beliefs and feelings are aspects of attitudes which support the underlying conceptualization. In this regard, the three study questions proposed relate to the aforementioned justification.

The subjects, setting, and sampling procedures were congruent with the study conceptualization and questions. The investigators used a convenience sample: they asked subjects to participate in the study if they met the criteria and were assigned to an acute-care psychiatric unit. The various instruments employed were congruent with the underlying conceptualization and study questions. They included two instruments for measuring attitude, a fixed-response and an open-ended tool. Insight was measured using a fixed-response instrument only. The open-ended instrument was given first so that patients would not be sensitized by the beliefs in the fixed-response instrument and, therefore, bias the results. The insight tool was given last. The analysis also fits the conceptualization and study questions in that the investigators answer all three study questions individually.

Part III: Believability of Results

This study purported to describe a phenomenon of concern to nursing by way of quantitative data. The investigators chose a relatively small sample of schizophrenic patients as defined by the "Diagnostic and Statistical Manual of Mental Disorders" (APA, 1980). The sample contained nearly equal numbers of male and female subjects and incorporated a wide range of ages and number of hospitalizations. The investigators selected subjects by using a convenience sampling method of patients consecutively admitted to the unit. Unfortunately, the investigators made no mention of controlling for extraneous variables or potential biases which might lead to a skewed sample.

The investigators discuss the reliability of the insight tool but they do not mention its validity: since this is a new tool constructed for this study, such information would be important. However, the open-ended and the fixed-response attitude instruments appeared to be valid measures of attitude ($r = .71$) in that they measured similar content. The reliability coefficient ($r = .738$) indicates that items in the fixed-response instrument are internally consistent.

The investigators drew conclusions that appear to be congruent with the measures, subjects, and procedures of this study. There was a positive correlation between the two attitude instruments in spite of the two different approaches used to obtain information. Both of the instruments displayed patients' attitudes composed of both positive and negative feelings toward medication. Another possible explanation for the positive correlation is that there may have been some interviewer bias which could have positively skewed the results. Unfortunately, the investigators provided no information concerning how they administered the instruments to the subjects. Did one person administer all three instruments? If so, were all subjects exposed to the same person administering the instruments? These data would have provided a better understanding of the research protocol and may have possibly allayed some doubt concerning the positive correlation obtained between the two attitude instruments.

The investigators concluded that insight and attitude were positively related; however, this modest correlation, although statistically significant, still makes me wary. The investigators had anticipated that hallucinations were related to a positive attitude toward treatment. However, when they performed a correlation between insight and the presence of hallucinations, this was not supported. In fact, the correlation showed that patients who had hallucinated had less insight. Additionally, the investigators did mention that it would be hard to compare their findings with other studies since previous studies have not operationalized insight and attitude in the same manner.

Given these considerations, I propose that the study results have adequate believability. Even though the investigators utilized a relatively small convenience sample, their sampling appeared adequate to tap all viewpoints on the nursing phenomenon under study. In most cases, they provided reliability and validity for their tools, proving them appropriate for this study. However, the investigators should have provided information concerning the validity of the insight tool since it was newly constructed. In general, the believability of results are such that I would consider using them in future practice.

Part IV: Generalizability of Results

The sample and setting were similar to many facilities that focus on acute care for the psychiatric client. The study does not indicate, however, who administered the tools, so one questions whether they were typical of practicing nurses or whether they were specially trained. If other clinicians were to use these tools as an addition to patient assessment, such validity would be important to know. In addition, I know of no replication studies that support the theory or evaluate the consistency of findings presented with other samples. However, the investigators discussed and built on other studies in which similar results were found.

In conclusion, the ability to generalize these findings to similar subjects and settings appears high.

Part V: Other Factors to Consider in Utilization

Before deciding to use this research in practice, there are several practical aspects one must consider. First, one must examine the feasibility of doing systemic evaluation of the research-based practice.

According to Polit and Hungler (1985), there are several issues relating to the question of feasibility: time, availability of subjects, needing special facilities or equipment, and ethical considerations. However, I believe that this study poses no problems in their regard.

The risk of changing practice based on this study would be the possibility of practitioners labeling their prospective patients. Practitioners may assume that certain attitudes are inherent in certain psychiatric illnesses and that all patients with schizophrenia may have difficulty following medication regimes. Although this risk is a possibility, I doubt it would happen with members of the professional psychiatric field.

However, a risk would be involved if the practitioner decided to maintain current practice and not assess attitudes toward medication in the schizophrenic population. The practitioner would not be able to identify positive and negative attitudes of patients toward medication, an identification that might prove helpful if the patient is noncompliant. Also, this information might prove helpful when planning teaching sessions regarding medications.

Increased knowledge about the patient characterizes the benefits of changing practice based on this study. Such knowledge also might provide a richer therapeutic relationship if the practitioner can help the patient explore the origin of his or her beliefs toward medication. Indeed, this exploration may change the patient's evaluation of his or her beliefs and consequently his or her attitude.

Financially, there may be some cost in implementing study findings. At the present, most hospitals teach in a group setting because it is cost effective for the hospital. If the staff were to do individual and group teaching for each of their schizophrenic patients, it would be more time consuming and more costly. Also, there would be an expense to the hospital to construct the attitude and insight tools and have them incorporated into the assessment procedure for schizophrenic patients.

In summary, there are both risks and benefits to implementing these study findings. However, I feel that the benefits of increased depth of knowledge about the patient outweigh the primarily financial risks.

REFERENCES

American Psychiatric Association. (1980). *Diagnostic and statistical manual of mental disorders* (3rd ed.). Washington, DC: Author.

Polit, D. F., & Hungler, B. P. (1985). *Essentials of nursing research: Methods and applications.* Philadelphia: Lippincott.

Original article:
Davidhizar, R. E., Austin, J. K., & McBride, A. B. (1986). Attitudes of patients with schizophrenia toward taking medication. Research in Nursing and Health, 9(2), 139–146.

CRITIQUE BY: BEVERLY HOEFFER, DNSc, RN

Part I: Clinical Relevance

Compliance with or adherence to a prescribed regimen of psychotropic medications is documented in the literature as enhancing recovery from acute psychotic episodes, remission of troublesome symptoms, and prevention of relapse for patients with schizophrenia. Yet, noncompliance occurs at a high rate among these patients, ranging from 24–66 percent in studies of outpatients (Davidhizar, 1987). Although patients' attitudes toward treatment and insight into their illness is believed to affect their adherence to medication regimens, only a few studies address these factors. In part, patients with schizophrenia have been viewed as unable to provide reliable information because of the nature of their mental illness.

Davidhizar, Austin, and McBride questioned this latter assumption. They believed that patients with schizophrenia could provide information to psychiatric nurses about their attitudes toward medication, insight into their illness, and need for treatment. Such information has clinical relevance for psychiatric nurses because they are directly involved in monitoring patients' adherence to medication regimens and educating patients about their medications. Hence, knowledge about patients' attitudes toward medication and insight into their illness could assist psychiatric nurses in making clinical decisions about which patients might be at risk for noncompliance. Furthermore, such information could be used by psychiatric nurses to determine what issues to address when teaching patients how to manage their medications.

Three research questions were posed by the investigators to address the clinical problem they identified.

1. What is the attitude of patients [with schizophrenia] toward taking medication?
2. How much insight do patients with schizophrenia have about psychiatric illness?
3. What is the relationship between attitude about medication and insight about illness?

The investigators inferred from previous research that a relationship exists between attitudes, insight, and future behavior. Consequently, assessing patients' attitudes toward taking medications and their insight into their illness would seem to be a logical step in determining what factors contributed to patients being at risk for noncompliance. Moreover, the research questions suggest that understanding patients' illness experiences from *their* perspective is important, and that even acutely ill psychiatric patients can share meaningful observations and feelings about aspects of their treatment.

The investigators used Fishbein's Expectance-Value Model as a theoretical model for the study. According to this model, a person's attitude toward anything is comprised of two components:

beliefs about the object and an evaluative response (i.e., feelings about the object) that can range from very negative to very positive. This model and a review of the compliance literature guided the development of a four-item open-ended assessment instrument and a 24-item fixed-response assessment instrument to measure attitudes toward medications. The investigators also developed a 10-item Likert scale to measure insight into illness and treatment based on factors identified in the literature. Although developed for research purposes, each of the three instruments could potentially be used by psychiatric nurses in assessing patients. Unfortunately, no information was provided on how long it took to administer each instrument. A detailed, quantified assessment of both the strength of beliefs about medications and the intensity of feelings attached to the beliefs might be a tedious undertaking during a clinical interview. However, the theory (i.e., Fishbein's model) used to construct the instruments is of clinical value. For example, a patient who slightly agrees with the beliefs that a medication tastes bad, causes sleepiness, and won't help and feels slightly negative or neutral about those beliefs may be more likely to adhere to a medication regimen than a patient who strongly agrees with those beliefs and feels very negative about them.

Part II: Conceptualization and Internal Consistency

The investigators developed and presented their study in a logical and readable manner. They justified the importance of studying attitudes toward taking medication with a review of the research literature on attitudes of patients with schizophrenia toward various aspects of treatment. They operationally defined attitudes to correct a deficit they noted in previous studies. They supported their selection of Fishbein's model for studying attitudes by reviewing the use of the model in nursing and non-nursing studies of attitudes over 20 years. In contrast, their justification for studying insight was more tentative. In their brief literature review on insight of patients with schizophrenia, they failed to elucidate the relationship between insight about illness and attitudes toward taking medication. As a result, the investigators did not adequately address the link between attitudes and insight in their conceptualization of the study.

Because all subjects were patients with schizophrenia who were receiving psychotropic medications, subject selection was consistent with the population of interest. The methods employed in the study also were appropriate for the nature of the research questions. The first two questions asked for a description of two phenomena involved in the illness experience of patients with schizophrenia: attitudes toward medications and insight into psychiatric illness and treatment, respectively. The third question asked what relationship existed between these phenomena. The instruments developed and administered to subjects provided a means of quantifying the variables representing the phenomena.

The investigators drew conclusions that were consistent with the findings as reported for each question. For example, the investigators made no attempt to infer a cause and effect relationship between attitudes and insight: however, they did infer that a modest association existed between them. Similarly, the investigators made no attempt to imply that the study answered questions about the relationship between attitudes and behavior or between insight and behavior. Their discussion focused on implications for clinical practice, specifically for patient teaching about medications.

Part III: Believability of Results

This study purported to describe phenomena of concern to nursing through quantitative methods. The investigators used a convenience sample of 50 patients with schizophrenia who were consecutively admitted to an acute-care inpatient psychiatric unit. All subjects were involved in the phenomenon of concern in that they met the DSM III diagnostic criteria for schizophrenia and were currently receiving psychotropic medications. The investigators also presented information on demographic characteristics (e.g., age and marital status) so that the reader could judge whether the convenience sample was typical of persons with schizophrenia. One limitation concerns the type of subjects studied: only hospitalized patients. Hospitalized patients' attitudes toward taking medications may differ from their attitude after discharge when they believe they are "well" and no longer need treatment (Davidhizar, 1987). Additionally, persons with schizophrenia residing in the community who adhere to ongoing treatment and do not require hospitalization may have more positive attitudes toward medications and insight into their illnesses.

The investigators descibed the procedure for obtaining informed consent. However, they did not discuss how the interview procedure for the open-ended assessment of attitudes may have affected subjects' responses. For example, did one investigator conduct all interviews or were multiple interviewers used? Did the patients openly share their attitudes toward taking medication in the face-to-face interview? We are somewhat assured that the latter concern was not an issue because of the strong positive correlation ($r = .71$) obtained between patients' scores on the open-ended and fixed-response instruments. This suggests that patients were consistent in the beliefs and feeling that they shared regardless of which method was used (i.e., that similar perceptions were elicited with the two different approaches).

The investigators also were concerned that disturbances in thought processes which occur during exacerbations of the illness may have affected how subjects answered the questions since the majority completed the instruments during the first week of hospitalization when they were acutely ill. Hence, the investigators repeated two questions each in a positive and negative manner on the fixed-response attitude instrument. As a result, they found strong negative correlations between subjects' responses to negative and positive versions of the questions, suggesting that patients were generally consistent in their responses and could provide reliable information.

The investigators reported the internal consistency of the 24-item fixed-response attitude instrument and the 10-item insight into illness and treatment Likert scale. High alpha coefficients (.74 and .90, respectively) suggest that the items "hang together" in measuring the respective concepts of the scales and attest to the instruments' reliability. The investigators reported on previous studies that supported the validity of the Fishbein expectancy-value model used in constructing both attitudinal instruments. They did not discuss the validity per se of any of the instruments except to indicate that items were developed based on the literature review. However, since the two different methods (open-ended interview and fixed-response questionnaire) used to collect data about patients' attitudes toward medication elicited consistent information, some evidence of concurrent validity for these two instruments is provided by the findings.

Study results were reported in sufficient detail. Summary and descriptive statistics were used appropriately to answer the first two questions; correlational procedures were used appropriately to answer the third question. Regarding research question one, scores on both open-ended and fixed response attitude instruments indicated that patients held a wide range of attitudes toward taking medications. Most patients had both negative and positive attitudes, although some patients held predominantly either positive or negative attitudes. Findings from the open-ended instrument indicated that the majority (54 percent) of the beliefs were negative. Of these, concerns about medication side effects accounted for the largest percent. Findings from the fixed-belief instrument indicated that patients associated taking medications with physicians' efforts to help them. Regarding research question two, scores obtained on the insight scale indicated a considerable range in the amount of insight subjects had about their illness and treatment. Over half had questionable insight (38 percent) or no insight (14 percent). Regarding research question three, significant but modest positive correlations between insight and attitudes toward taking medication were found as measured by the open-ended ($r = .37$) and fixed-response ($r = .37$) instruments. Contrary to the investigators' expectations, hallucinating during hospitalization showed only a weak though significant positive correlation with insight ($r = .28$).

The investigators clearly stayed within the boundaries of their analysis in drawing conclusions about the findings. For example, they concluded that patients with schizophrenia are able and willing to give reliable information about their beliefs and feelings toward taking medications even when acutely ill. Hence, psychiatric nurses can have confidence in what patients say about their medication regimens. Because side effects accounted for the largest percentage of negative attitudes, the investigators advocated that nurses pay particular attention to monitoring and discussing side effects with individual patients in an attempt to change negative attitudes.

The investigators were cautious in drawing conclusions about the relationship between attitudes and insight because only a modest correlation was found. In other words, the investigators did not strongly relate insight into illness to attitudes toward taking medication. Nor did they offer explanation for this finding. However, a plausible explanation suggested by the data is that patients who are acutely ill (e.g., have hallucinations) may be less insightful in general about their immediate illness and treatment even though they hold very specific negative and positive attitudes toward taking medication based on past and present experiences.

Part IV: Generalizability of Results

The study results may be generalized to patients with schizophrenia admitted voluntarily to inpatient psychiatric units because the sample, as described, is fairly typical of this population. Less is known about the setting since it was only briefly described as an acute-care psychiatric unit. One limitation of the study that appears at this point concerns the findings themselves: they cannot be generalized to persons with schizophrenia residing in the community or involuntarily admitted inpatients. Attitudes toward medications and insight into psychiatric illness and treatment may differ during an exacerbation of the illness that requires hospitalization in contrast to periods of remission and for patients who do not wish treatment.

The four questions asked of patients in the open-ended interview to elicit their beliefs and feelings ("What do you think about taking your medication in the hospital? Why do you take your medication? What are the advantages of taking your medication? What are the disadvantages of taking your medication?") are clear and could be asked by practicing nurses. A salient question, however, is whether patients would respond as openly to these questions if the interviewer were a staff member whom patients perceived as responsible for their care or having some control over treatment outcomes.

Our confidence in the implications of the findings for practice is strengthened because Davidhizar (1987) replicated the study a year later with another 50 patients with schizophrenia consecutively admitted to the same facility. The findings were very similar. For example, patients demonstrated a wide range of individual attitudes toward taking medication that included both positive and negative beliefs. Concerns about side effects accounted for the largest proportion of negative beliefs. Davidhizar noted that a greater number of beliefs were elicited from the second group of patients, suggesting that experience in asking patients for information about their beliefs and feelings may result in obtaining more complete data.

Part V: Other Factors to Consider in Utilization

Although not explicitly stated, the investigators' ultimate goal seemed to be to identify strategies that psychiatric nurses could use to enhance patients' compliance with psychotropic medications. Hence, a logical step would be to determine the relationship between patients' attitudes toward medications and their adherence to medication regimens in future research. A nursing intervention study could be developed to test if individualizing patient education by incorporating specific beliefs and feelings of individual patients toward medication was more effective than group teaching in changing patients' attitudes and compliance (Davidhizar, 1987). Because the nursing staff time involved in individualized teaching approaches would increase costs to a psychiatric facility, findings from such a study would be helpful in determining if the benefits outweigh the costs of changing practice to an institution.

Nonetheless, the current descriptive study can be used to improve nursing practice even though the relationship between attitudes and compliance was not addressed. Taking patients' beliefs and feelings about aspects of their treatment seriously is very congruent with nursing's philosophy of treating patients as individuals and trying to understand illness experiences from the patient's perspective. The findings from this study could be used to reinforce this philosophy on inpatient psychiatric units. It may "cost" a psychiatric nurse additonal time to explore with patients their beliefs and feelings about taking medication, but the information gained could enhance the effectiveness of nursing interventions. For example, if specific side effects (e.g., shakiness) were identified as troublesome to a patient, the nurse could focus monitoring and explanations on these side effects. Then the nurse and the patient could evaluate together whether the information had a positive effect on the patient's attitude using items from either the open-ended or fixed response questionnaire. In this way, a nurse could assess the benefit of changing practice (i.e., individualizing medication teaching) for individual patients as an intergral aspect of nursing care.

REFERENCES

Davidhizar, R. E. (1987). Beliefs, feelings and insight of patients with schizophrenia about taking medication. *Journal of Advanced Nursing*, *12*, 177–182.

Recovery From Rape and Prior Life Stress

Ann W. Burgess, PhD
Professor and Chairperson
Department of Nursing
Boston College
Chestnut Hill, MA

Lynda L. Holmstrom, PhD
Associate Professor and Chairperson
Department of Sociology
Boston College
Chestnut Hill, MA

This longitudinal study on rape victims looks at four life stress events and their association with recovery from rape. Data from 88% of the original sample of 92 adult victims 4 to 6 years after rape suggest that life stress before rape may act to hasten or to inhibit the recovery process. Stress is not uniform in its effect. Different types of stress have different effects. Earlier victimization and chronic life stressors such as economic hardship, lack of social support, and pre-existing biopsychosocial problems tend to delay recovery. In contrast, family grief stress may act as an energizing factor in that coping skills may have been developed through experiencing the grief process and are available to the victim for settlement of rape trauma. Recent life changes have a lack of association with recovery although they may be important in some individual cases.

The subject of rape has received marked attention from clinicians, researchers, feminists, activists, and the media over the past 5 years (Brodsky, Klemmack, Skinner, Bender, & Polyson, 1978). However, while studies of victims have become increasingly common, studies dealing with the long-term effects are much less common, especially those in which the victim is interviewed both at the time of the attack and also later.

Clinically, victim recovery from rape is an important concern. Thus, a follow-up study of rape victims focusing on their progress over the years was undertaken. In keeping with one of the assumptions of the original project—the value of the client's perspective of the situation—this follow-up report analyzes and interprets what the victims themselves report to be relevant to recovery from rape trauma.

There are many factors that could influence recovery: prerape factors, rape-related factors, and postrape factors. One factor that has a major impact on health is stress. Stress is a multifaceted concept that is also a popular area of interdisciplinary research. Stress can be a strengthening or a hindering force. It can contribute, disrupt, energize, or inhibit. It can affect a person's recovery to health by helping or hindering the process.

Certain external variables have been documented as being capable of producing stress in a person's life (Levine & Scotch, 1970). Some of these may be related to the physical environment, the social environment, population characteristics, or a crisis problem. In addition, internal psychological variables are known to be stress producing (Appley & Trumbull, 1967).

In a conference proceedings text titled *Stressful*

Life Events: Their Nature and Effects, the Dohrenwends (1974) pulled into focus two sets of concerns shared by stress researchers: (a) the stressful situations to which everyone is exposed to a greater or lesser extent in the natural course of life, or "life events" and (b) the role of stressful life events in the etiology of various somatic and psychiatric disorders.

An important question specific to rape trauma is: What is the relationship between prior stress in a victim's life and the pattern of recovery following rape? One way to study this problem is to see if there is a correlation between certain stressors experienced by victims before rape and the length of time they report that it takes for recovery. For example, are there some chronic or current stressors that delay or hasten recovery for a victim, and are there some life history stressors that weaken or strengthen the coping capacity of a person to help her deal subsequently with other life stressors? This paper looks specifically at stress factors before rape that might influence the adult victim's recovery: (a) prior victimization, (b) chronic life stressors, (c) family grief stressors, and (d) recent life change stressors.

Prior Victimization

A major clinical observation is that rape creates a crisis and/or a highly stressful situation in the life of the victim (Burgess & Holmstrom, 1974b). This basic finding has become a cornerstone in rape counseling. The amount of life style disruption and of physical and psychological symptoms caused by rape is striking. Being raped also stirs up memories and feelings from previous attacks. This suggests that repeated victimization may have a different impact than one-time victimization. It would be important to see if there is a correlation between previous victimization and length of recovery from rape.

Chronic Life Stressors

Stressors may be short-term or chronic. The concern in this paper is with chronic stressors; that is, with stressors that have persisted over time, from which there is no relief, and over which the person has relatively little control. In interviews with rape victims, three types of chronic stressors emerged: economic stress, lack of social support, and pre-existing biological, psychological, and/or social problems.

The question is whether the existence of chronic stressors before rape is related to the length of recovery from rape. Chronic life stressors would continually call for coping behavior by the person. After rape, the victim would have the combined stress of dealing with the existing chronic stressor and the situational crisis of rape. Existing crisis theory would predict that the two together would be more difficult to handle because there would be a cumulative impact. However, it is possible that the opposite effect might occur. It is possible that rape would have less effect on victims under chronic stress, either because they gain experience in coping with chronic stress or because the rape is less salient when embedded in a series of serious problems.

Family Grief Stress

The crisis that can develop after rape results from an encounter with a life-threatening situation. The resulting trauma reaction is in the service of self-preservation (Burgess & Holmstrom, 1974a). In reviewing coping behavior of people dealing with highly stressful or crisis situations, the work on grief and loss is clinically relevant. Lindemann's work on acute grief reactions (1944) and Kübler-Ross' work on death and dying (1972) are excellent examples of the process of coping with major life stress. Analogies can be made between the psychological work in grief resolution and in rape trauma resolution. Grief, as a psychological process that occurs after loss, allows a person to cope in a gradual way with an overwhelming situation so that it can be accepted as a reality. The psychological work required by rape victims includes freeing oneself from the fears caused by the rape, acknowledging and bearing the pain caused by the rape, redefining the feelings of vulnerability and helplessness, and gaining control of one's life again.

Because coping behavior is necessary to deal with major human crises, it seemed relevant to analyze past family grief stress to see whether it is associated with length of recovery. Family grief stress is defined as the loss, separation or death of a family member within 2 years before the rape. Two predictions about such a relationship could be made drawing on stress literature. First, one might reason that stress is cumulative, and thus, one might predict that family grief stress would be related to longer recovery. Second, one might reason that stress allows one to learn coping skills, and thus, one might predict that family grief stress would be related to more rapid recovery.

Recent Life Change Stressors

The importance of everyday life events to the processes of health and illness was the focus of Adolph Meyer's research (Lief, 1948). Life events that have the potential to cause stress include such changes as entering school, graduations, employment, relocating a residence, illness, births, and deaths. Recent life change stressors are defined as events occurring within 6 months before the rape. Because life changes can cause stress, it seemed important to see if there was an association between recent events and length of recovery. The reasoning was, again, that the stress might be cumulative and that life changes would hinder recovery. Or, stress might provide learning, and life changes would facilitate recovery.

METHOD

Sample

This paper reports part of a three-phased longitudinal study consisting of (a) an initial interview at the time the victim was admitted to the hospital; (b) short-term follow-up by telephone and/or home visit, weekly for the first 3 months and then at 6-, 9-, and 12-month intervals: and (c) long-term follow-up by telephone and/or home visit 4 to 6 years after the rape.

The original research project on rape victims was started in July 1972. Over a 1-year period, the authors were notified by the Emergency Department of the Boston City Hospital each time a rape victim was admitted, and went immediately to the hospital to gather data. The rape victim sample included 92 adult victims (age 17 to 73) and 23 preadult victims (age 5 to 16). In 1976, the authors began to contact the rape victim sample again. The sample for this paper consisted of 81 victims, 88% of the original adult victim sample, who were reinterviewed (78 women) or for whom there were good indirect data (3 cases). Three victims from the original sample have since died and although there are considerable data on them, they are not included in the statistics for this paper. The adult rape victim group represents a heterogeneous sample in terms of ethnicity, race, religion, social class, employment, education, marital status, and age.

Procedure

Data for the initial and short-term follow-up project, in the majority of cases, were collected by both authors. Typically, one author interviewed while the other author took notes at the time of the victim's admission to the hospital. The initial interview was followed by weekly and then monthly follow-up telephone calls or home visits for 3 months. Both methods of data collection for the first two phases of the study are described in a prior publication (Burgess & Holmstrom, 1974b, pp. 163-196). Victims entering the criminal justice system were accompanied to court, also, and participant observation methods of data collection were used (Holmstrom & Burgess, 1978, pp. 5-29). The various methods of collecting information are important for this paper because considerable life history data regarding stress factors were recorded during these contact times. At the time of the first interview, victims were informed verbally and in writing that the project was an ongoing study about the problems women encounter as a result of being assaulted, and that they would be contacted periodically. They could consent or they could refuse to participate at any point during the project.

Instrument

For this long-term follow-up study, the authors used a standard schedule of questions that were flexible and open-ended. The following general categories of information were asked of each person: biographical data; recurring thoughts, feelings, and actions related to the rape; symptoms of the acute phase of rape trauma; symptoms of the reorganization phase of rape trauma; length of trauma reaction; coping behavior; legal outcome and memories; information on the assailant; need for additional professional help; partner and social network reaction and changes; reactions to police, hospital, and counseling services; life style changes; and recovery patterns. Some questions that were asked during the initial interview and during the short-term follow-up were repeated; in addition, new questions were added. The combined sources of data provided the information on the prerape stress.

Dependent Variable

The dependent variable in this paper is the time required for the victim to feel recovered. The classification of length of recovery was developed by looking at the answers to two major questions asked during the long-term follow-up: (a) Do you feel back to normal; that is, the way you felt prior to the rape? If yes, when did this occur, and if not, in what ways are you not back to normal? (b) Has the rape interfered in your life, and if so, in what areas? These data are subjective reports by victims of their own recovery and/or life events over the intervening years. One question, of course, is how to define normal. Rather than the authors assuming this task, the victims provided the definition. This approach allowed for a wide variance of what victims considered normal. The victims' reports of their recovery were categorized into three groups: victims who felt recovered in months, in years, or not by the time of long-term follow-up 4 to 6 years after the rape.

The statistical test used in the analysis of data was the Goodman-Kruskal gamma, which is an index of association between two ordered dimensions of a cross classification table. The statistical tests are not necessarily independent.

RESULTS

Patterns of Recovery

The majority of victims (74%) felt recovered by the time of the long-term follow-up study. Equal numbers of victims reported feeling recovered within months (N = 30 or 37%) as did within years (N = 30 or 37%). The smallest group of victims (N = 21 or 26%) did not feel recovered by the time of follow-up.

Prior Victimization

Victims were asked, as part of the initial interview, if they had ever been raped before. In addition, on follow-up, victims were asked if they had experienced any type of prior victimization. Victims were then categorized as having prior victimization if they reported having been subjected to either attempted or completed sexual assault, assault, mugging, or verbal or physical sexual harassment before the rape in 1972-73.

Prior victimization is related to a longer recovery time, as shown in Table 1. Without prior victimization 47% recovered within months, but

Table 1
Prior Victimization and Length of Recovery

Length of Recovery[a]	No Prior Victimization	Prior Victimization
Months	24 (47%)	6 (20%)
Years	20 (39%)	10 (33%)
Not yet recovered	7 (14%)	14 (47%)
Total	51 (100%)	30 (100%)

Note. Goodman-Kruskal two-tailed test γ = .57 (z = 3.15, p < .01).
[a] Reported in terms of victims' verbatim statements 4 to 6 years after the rape.

with prior victimization only 20% recovered this fast. Without prior victimization only 14% were not yet recovered 4 to 6 years later, but with prior victimization 47% were not yet recovered.

In reviewing the dynamics in the 14 cases with prior victimization where victims were not recovered, several clinical observations were noted.

1. *The time interval between victimizations.* Four victims were raped a second time within a 2-year period, and the second rape represented a setback. The victim might comment on this setback in terms of relating to people ("I was just beginning to trust people again.") or might talk in terms of the anticipated trauma affects of the new rape as in the following example.

I was just getting over the first time—not sitting up everytime I heard a strange noise or getting jittery being alone. What makes me mad is my life is disrupted: every part of it upset. I have to move and do all kinds of difficult things, and he just leaves...it is not right.

2. *Victim's point in the life cycle.* It has been previously reported that the sexual assault takes on specific meaning to victims according to their stage of development in the life cycle (Burgess & Holmstrom, 1974b). Thus, it was important to see if there was any specific age period in which victims who had not recovered reported a prior victimization. Six of the 14 victims reported that a prior rape or attempted rape had occurred during their adolescence. One 18-year-old victim stated that a prior gang rape was also her first sexual experience.

I was only 15. It was my first sex and three boys raped me. The police brought me here...but I wouldn't let them examine me.

3. *Similarity with prior victimization.* The current rape may remind the victim of similar characteristics of a prior victimization. One 33-year-old victim who was badly beaten during the current rape and who refused hospitalization for her injuries talked of a prior rape resulting in similar physical trauma, as well as a family member's response.

I was 20...The man grabbed me, beat me so badly my jaw was broken and my eye closed shut...had multiple injuries to my face...My mother came to visit me in the hospital and cried...I must have looked so bad.

The victimization does not necessarily have to be of the same type to prompt an association to a prior incident. In one case, a friend who accompanied a 28-year-old victim to the hospital made the association and said:

About 3 months ago, a guy hassled her at a bus stop. She got so upset she went into a store nearby to get away from him. I don't know if she even connected this with that incident. But I thought of it. I wonder if the two are connected.

4. *Comparison with prior victimization.* The victim may compare the current rape with a prior victimization. Sometimes the victim denies to herself that such a situation could ever happen again:

This all reminded me of the time when I was 12 years old and the same thing happened. It took me so long to get over that and here I am a grown woman...I never thought this would happen.

Or the victim might describe the rape as being even worse than the prior situation.

[Before] it wasn't like this. It was my own fault the other time...I should have been wiser. But this was something else...I was sleeping.

5. *Prior victimization is an unresolved issue for the victim.* It became clear that the disclosure of a victimizing situation to outsiders continues to be a conflict area for victims. A number of women in the original sample stated spontaneously that they had been raped or molested at a previous time, often when they were children or adolescents. Often, these women had not told anyone of the rape and had just kept the burden

within themselves. This behavior did not allow for the victimization to be discussed and settled as a major life event.

Chronic Life Stressors

The data on chronic stress support predictions from current crisis theory in terms of recovery from rape. Chronic stress is related to a longer recovery time. Table 2 shows that without chronic stress 51% recovered within months, but with chronic stress only 21% recovered this fast. Without chronic stress only 16% are not recovered 4 to 6 years after the rape, but with chronic stress 37% are not recovered.

Economic Stress Most adults in the study had, at best, modest financial resources. Over 60% were employed at the time of the rape. But not surprisingly for women, they tended to be concentrated in service jobs with modest incomes: secretary, clerk, waitress, teacher, research assistant.

Victims were categorized according to their economic resources. Victims were considered to be under economic stress if they (a) were on outside financial support, (b) had very low paying jobs making them and their children eligible for state medical benefits, (c) had transitory or modest paying jobs that required supplementation by families or partners, or (d) did not maintain any steady kind of job. Of the 35 victims under economic stress, 13 also were responsible for supporting their children as well as themselves. Of the 28 victims with outside financial support or with state medical benefits, hospital records indicated that 17 had earnings under $4,000 a year.

Economic stress is related to length of recovery, as shown in Table 3. Without economic stress 50% recovered within months, but with economic stress only 20% recovered this fast. Without economic stress only 15% had not recovered 4 to 6 years later, but with economic stress 40% had not yet recovered.

The dynamics of the relationship between economic stress and length of recovery are undoubtedly very complex. One focus of victims' comments is how lack of economic resources decreases their ability to make the changes they desire in their life style after rape occurs. In the following case of a 33-year-old rape victim who had not recovered, the difficulties this victim had in finding a suitable place to live, and the limits placed on the victim via her welfare check are described.

I moved...but it didn't work out...there was a mix up over my payment from welfare...confusion about getting my money back. I was so mad. I lost my temper...Then I got my money

Table 2
Chronic Life Stressors Prior to Rape and Length of Recovery

Length of Recovery[a]	Chronic Stress	
	Without Chronic Stress	With Chronic Stress
Months	22 (51%)	8 (21%)
Years	14 (33%)	16 (42%)
Not yet recovered	7 (16%)	14 (37%)
Total	43 (100%)	38 (100%)

Note. Goodman-Kruskal two-tailed test $\gamma = .51$ ($z = 2.80$, $p < .01$).
[a]Reported in terms of victims' verbatim statements 4 to 6 years after the rape.

Table 3
Economic Stress and Length of Recovery

Length of Recovery[a]	Economic Stress	
	Without	With
Months	23 (50%)	7 (20%)
Years	16 (35%)	14 (40%)
Not yet recovered	7 (15%)	14 (40%)
Total	46 (100%)	35 (100%)

Note. Goodman-Kruskal two-tailed test $\gamma = .54$ ($z = 2.99$, $p < .01$).
[a]Reported in terms of victims' verbatim statements 4 to 6 years after the rape.

back...Don't have a phone yet, but plan to as soon as I get my welfare check.

Lack of Social Support. Most victims in the study had social relationships for meeting many of their psychosocial needs. However, a minority (19%) did not. These victims, who were categorized as lacking social support, had no stable back-up group that was available when a crisis developed and to whom they could turn for emotional support. Thus, their needs were not met on a consistent basis. Usually, these victims were living alone, unemployed, and either not in regular communication with family members or geographically distant from them. They lacked access to people who could offer support.

Table 4 shows that social support is related to length of recovery. The data are striking. With social support 45% recovered in months, but without support not a single victim recovered in months. With social support only 20% were not recovered, but without support 53% were not recovered.

The dynamics of this relationship are revealed in comments from victims. One victim who lacked social support lived in a state-financed halfway house for alcoholics after the rape. She described her feelings:

I am so lonely and I can't seem to talk to people. I need money and I have to get a job, and I feel everyone is against me because I am in here. I go to get a job and they hear where I live, and I don't think they want me. There are some nights when I feel so terrible; so lonely inside. I want someone to care about me. I am so alone and I really am the only one who cares what happens to me. I should have someone to care about me. I know that is what is important but how do I go about getting someone?

Another victim who lacked social network support at the time of the rape and who took years to recover commented:

Right after I left the hospital, I was walking through the park and saw an old man I knew. I went to sit with him. He said, "My god, what happened to you—your face is a mess." He was scared to have me sit with him and said, "You better not sit here. Whoever did that to you, I don't want them coming after me." I felt dirty and worthless. No one even wanted to talk to me. I wasn't getting along with my parents. Men were abusing me sexually. I felt like a rag. There was nowhere else I could turn.

The tragic outcome that may occur when a person faced with a crisis lacks social support and is also reluctant to seek professional support is dramatically illustrated in one case. The woman, a 21-year-old college student when attacked, was the victim of an attempted rape. She was extremely upset by the attack. She explained to us that in her culture loss of virginity was especially significant, no matter how it occurred. "In my culture this is serious—it's 'a big deal.' It's very important to be a virgin when you marry." She was extremely worried about anyone finding out what had happened. She was, therefore, reluctant to contact anyone for help. Her ethnic background restricted her from freely expressing her feelings about the victimization. Despite this, she was able to resume her previous life style with the help of crisis counseling. We learned on follow-up that she soon had become romantically involved with a young man. Unfortunately, he was killed in an accident. His death triggered a severe depression, and she hung herself. Her

Table 4
Social Support and Length of Recovery

Length of Recovery[a]	Support	
	With Support	Lack of Support
Months	30 (45%)	0 (0%)
Years	23 (35%)	7 (47%)
Not yet recovered	13 (20%)	8 (53%)
Total	66 (100%)	15 (100%)

Note. Goodman-Kruskal two-tailed test γ = .75 (z = 3.39, $p < .01$).
[a] Reported in terms of victims' verbatim statements 4 to 6 years after the rape.

suicide occurred within months after his death and 18 months after the attempted rape. It is speculated that her suicide was related to a sense of isolation from others. She was geographically distant from her parental family, from a culture that discouraged discussing an issue such as rape, and lacked a group of from which she could receive support and comfort. She then lost her boyfriend, apparently one of the few people with whom she was close. Her ties with others were tenuous at best. Presumably, this heightened her sense of loneliness and her feelings of loss. These feelings then were acted on with a lethal result.

Prior Biological, Psychological, and Social Problems. Some rape victims have a pre-existing biopsychosocial problem such as psychosis, alcoholism, drug use, mental retardation, or homosexuality. All these patterns of behavior and of relating to others cause difficulty for persons living in our society. Such people often seek professional services through an institutional system and thus have the added stress of dealing with these institutions. Victims with such difficulties were identified as having a pre-existing chronic problem (Burgess & Holmstrom, 1974a).

Since these victims had a greater number of problems and range of physical and psychological symptoms at the time of crisis, it was predicted that they would take longer to recover. The data in Table 5 show this to be the case. Without prior problems 44% recovered in months, but with problems only 16% recovered this fast. Without prior problems only 19% were not recovered, but with prior problems 47% were not recovered.

The dynamics of the relationship between prior biopsychosocial problems and length of recovery are revealed in the comments made by victims. Alcohol and drug abuse were the most common prior problems, and they caused difficulties for recovery. One victim who took years to recover described her drinking problem before the rape and the problem after the rape.

I was in such bad shape [at the time of the rape.] I was drinking very heavy at the time and into anything that would keep me high...I stayed constantly drunk after that. I just hit rock bottom.

Table 5
Biopsychosocial Problems Prior to Rape[a] and Length or Recovery

Length of Recovery[b]	Prior Problems	
	Without	With
Months	27 (44%)	3 (16%)
Years	23 (37%)	7 (37%)
Not Yet recovered	12 (19%)	9 (47%)
Total	62 (100%)	19 (100%)

Note. Goodman-Kruskal two-tailed test $\gamma = .54$ ($z = 2.55$, $p < .01$).
[a]18 victims were diagnosed as having compounded rape trauma at time of initial interview. On follow-up, of the 18 victims, 2 had died and 1 could not be located. Follow-up data also revealed that an additional 4 victims should be regarded as having compounded rape trauma.
[b]Reported in terms of victims' verbatim statements 4 to 6 years after rape.

I drank to pass out—not to have to think of how bad things had gotten.

Of the victims with an alcohol and/or drug problem, 58% were not recovered at the time of the long-term follow-up.

Psychiatric difficulties were the next most common prior problem. These victims also had difficulty recovering—43% were not yet recovered at the time of the 4 to 6-year follow-up. One 29-year-old victim with a prior psychiatric history said, "The rape made me manic for 4 months. Then I was depressed for 5 months. Then I attempted suicide."

Victims may have combinations of problems. One victim who had not recovered describes her difficulties with depression and drug dependence.

At the time of the rape I was addicted to Darvon, and I was very depressed...I spent the next few years in and out of state hospitals trying to get off Darvon. Coping with my drug and depression problem took up most of my time in the past few years.

Family Grief Stress

Victims were categorized as having family grief stress if they had lost a family member prior to the rape. None of the victims had lost a family member within 2 years before the rape, but 64 had lost family members over 2 years before the rape. The experience of losing a family member either through death, divorce, or separation is related to whether victims recover more rapidly. The data in Table 6 support the reasoning that undergoing major crisis can be a learning experience. With family grief stress 56% recovered in months, but without family grief stress only 24% recovered this fast. With family grief stress only 16% had not recovered, but without family grief stress 33% had not recovered 4 to 6 years later.

Clues to the dynamics of this relationship are provided in the comments made by victims. One victim, for example, explained how she was accustomed to being on her own and to dealing with problems:

I'm here alone in Boston...my mother and grandmother live in New York, and a sister lives in Tennessee...I've been pretty much on my own since my father died when I was 10...I've had many problems, and this tonight is just one more...but I think the worst is over...I got through it.

Table 6
Family Grief Stress[a] and Length of Recovery

Length of Recovery[b]	Family Grief Stress	
	Without	With
Months	12 (24%)	18 (56%)
Years	21 (43%)	9 (28%)
Not yet recovered	16 (33%)	5 (16%)
Total	49 (100%)	32 (100%)

Note. Goodman-Kruskal two-tailed test $\gamma = -.50$ ($z = 2.66$, $p < .01$).
[a]Defined as loss of family member through death, separation, or divorce more than 2 years before rape.
[b]Reported in terms of victims' verbatim statements 4 to 6 years after the rape.

Another victim, who felt recovered in years, indicated that her mother's death provided a basis for comparison:

My mother's death [in 1966] was worse. This rape reaction didn't last as long...it was not as intense a reaction.

Recent Life Change Stressors

Life changes can cause stress. The data in Table 7, however, show that there is little connection between life changes occurring within 6 months before the rape and length of recovery. For example, without recent life changes 36% recovered in months, and with recent life changes 38% recovered in months. It should be emphasized that in most cases the type of life change that occurred was one leading to a modest amount of upheaval. The most common life changes were changes in residence or social living status. Different results might occur with more serious recent life changes.

The majority of victims with recent life change stress had only one such event. Although the findings show a lack of association with length of recovery, it is clinically interesting to note two different responses by victims who experienced more than one recent life change stress in addition to the rape. When several events coincide, we noted that recent life changes affected different victims in two different ways. The victim might describe such changes as facilitating her recovery from rape, as in the following case of one victim who recovered in months.

The rape happened at a time in my life when lots of heavy things happened. I had the court record, and then I had that serious car accident...I had to have plastic surgery. Those three things happened in a 6 week period.

This victim felt that the court indictments and her car accident were more serious than the rape, and she turned her attention more toward them. She felt recovered within months. She was able to continue in her work, married her boy friend, and ranked herself as being in good emotional health on long-term follow-up.

In contrast, the victim who experienced several recent life stresses might describe these changes as hindering recovery from the rape, as in the following case:

The rape scared me...it was just another thing in a series of situations in which I had been trusting and then it backfired—one situation with my boss and then with a friend. The rape was the straw that broke the camel's back. My head said to get out of town.

This victim, who felt it took her years to recover, made two short transition moves before settling into a counterculture group in an isolated resort area in the state. She remained there for 2 years before moving back into a more traditional life style, returning to college and beginning to work again.

DISCUSSION

The data on recovery from rape, collected from victims after their rape, have clinical implications. Clinicians may find it useful when obtaining the victim's life history to assess prior victimizations, chronic stressors, family grief stressors, and recent life change stressors. Clinicians can evaluate these prior life stressors in terms of the type, number, intensity, and similarity of stressors, and the client's perception of them. This type of clinical information may help (a) to plan crisis counseling or (b) to determine if the victim needs more than crisis counseling. The client may fall into a high-risk category and need interventions beyond rape counseling.

Important factors for assessment of prior victimization include the following: (a) the type of prior victimization in comparison with the current victimization, (b) whether the prior victimization was attempted or completed, (c) whether the victim disclosed the prior victimization to others, and (d) whether the prior victimization has been psychologically settled. A victimization may be unresolved at the time of a subsequent victimization if the issue had not been discussed or if sufficient time had not passed for the psychological work to be completed. This latter point may be one reason why a brief time interval between victimizations may result in a longer length of time for recovery.

Some victims are already under chronic stress and may need additional interventions. Low income can cause chronic stress in our cash-based economy. In addition, economic resources may be especially important during an emergency. Financial resources are an advantage to someone experiencing a crisis because they can act as a buffer. Persons seeking professional services, for example, have a greater choice if they are able to pay. If a person has savings or an income not based on hourly wages, a day of work lost due to an emergency may have less monetary impact. If the stressful situation would be eased by making a costly change such as moving, adequate finances can facilitate it.

The stress literature emphasizes the importance of social structural factors in successful adaptive behavior. The ability of persons to maintain psychological comfort is believed to depend not only on intrapsychic resources but also on the social supports available in the environment. Few persons can survive without support from some segment of their group network (Mechanic, 1970). Lack of support can lead to self-destructive behavior. This insight was made in the last century by Durkheim, who reported that rates of suicide vary inversely with the degree of cohesiveness of

Table 7
Life Change Stress Six Months Before Rape and Length of Recovery

Length of Recovery[a]	Recent Life Change Stress	
	Without	With
Months	14 (36%)	16 (38%)
Years	17 (44%)	13 (31%)
Not yet recovered	8 (20%)	13 (31%)
Total	39 (100%)	42 (100%)

Note. Goodman-Kruskal two-tailed test $\gamma = .07$ ($z = .31$, $p < .01$).
[a] Reported in terms of victims' verbatim statements 4 to 6 years after the rape.

the group in which the individual is embedded (Durkheim, 1951).

People under stress need access to people who understand and who will provide emotional comfort and support. This is so whether or not the nature of the stress is revealed. A variety of social groups may provide the support, including family members, friends, colleagues, employers, and school officials. People who lack access to supportive people have to rely more exclusively on their own psychological resources to cope with the stress. This action may be difficult and, thus, contribute to the cumulative effect of the stress.

Victims who had a prior problem and who typically had extended association with an institution (hospital, mental health facility, or court) were diagnosed as having compounded rape trauma reaction at the time of crisis counseling. This group was found to be at high risk for developing not only symptoms associated with rape trauma syndrome but also additional symptoms related to their prior problem. These additional symptoms included depression, psychotic behavior, psychosomatic disorder, suicidal behavior, and acting out behavior associated with sexual activity, alcoholism, or drug use.

The data suggest that having to cope with the loss of a parent, spouse, or child through death, separation, or divorce more than 2 years before the rape may facilitate recovery from rape. There are two possible reasons why this may occur. First, coping skills learned and mastered when a person is confronted with family grief stress may be useful in other situations. Thus, if raped, one is able to use the psychological coping skills used in a previous crisis. Second, the successful resolution of previous family grief may strengthen a person psychologically. Caplan (1959), in discussing the positive aspects of crisis recovery, said that a crisis is a time in one's life when one can either gain strength psychologically or regress to a lower level of mental health.

Recent life change stressors, although not associated with length of recovery, need to be identified for two reasons. First, the recent life stressor assumes some degree of magnitude of impact to the victim, and this needs to be assessed. Construction of rating scales for life events is a specific area of research through which the magnitude of the event is cited (Holmes & Rahe, 1967). Second, the recent life event may have special meaning to the victim, and this is important information for the clinician in working with the client.

In summary, the data on prerape stress suggest that the stress may either facilitate or delay the recovery process for the victim. Stress is not uniform in its effect; different types of stress have various consequences for an individual. Stressors delaying recovery were found to be prior victimization and chronic life stressors of economic hardship, lack of social support, and pre-existing biopsychosocial problems. In contrast, family grief stress may act as an energizing factor for the victim. Recent life change stressors were not found to have an association with recovery although in individual situations they are clinically important.

REFERENCES

Appley, M. H., & Trumball, R. (Eds.). (1967). *Psychological stress*. New York: Appleton-Century-Crofts.

Brodsky, S. L., Klemmack, S. H., Skinner, L. J., Bender, L. Z., & Polyson, A. M. K. (1978). *Sexual assault: A literature analysis*. Center for Correctional Psychology: Report No. 33, Department of Psychology, University of Alabama, Tuskaloosa, Alabama.

Burgess, A. W., & Holmstrom, L. L. (1974a). Rape trauma syndrome. *American Journal of Psychiatry, 131*, 981–986.

Burgess, A. W., & Holmstrom, L. L. (1974b). *Rape: Victims of crisis*. Bowie, MD.: Robert J. Brady.

Caplan, G. (1959). *Concepts of mental health and consultation*. Washington, D. C.: U.S. Government Printing Office.

Dohrenwend, B. S., & Dohrenwend, B. P. (Eds.) (1974). *Stressful life events: Their nature and effects*. New York: Wiley.

Durkheim, E. (1951). [*Suicide*] (J. A. Spaulding & G. Simpson, Trans.) Glencoe, IL: Free Press, 1951. (Originally published 1897; translated from 1930 edition.)

Holmes, T. H., & Rahe, R. H. (1967). The social readjustment rating scale. *Journal of Psychosomatic Research, 11,* 213–218.

Holmstrom, L. L., & Burgess, A. W. (1978). *The victim of rape: Institutional reactions.* New York: Wiley.

Kübler-Ross, E. (1972). On death and dying. *Journal of the American Medical Association, 221,* 174–79.

Lief, A. (Ed.). (1948). *The commonsense psychiatry of Dr. Adolf Meyer.* New York: McGraw-Hill.

Levine, S., & Scotch, N. A. (Eds.). (1970). *Social stress.* Chicago: Aldine Press.

Lindemann, E. (1944). Symptomology and management of acute grief. *American Journal of Orthopsychiatry, 45,* 813–24.

Mechanic, D. (1970). Some problems in developing a social psychology of adaptation to stress. In J. McGrath (Ed.), *Social and psychological factors in stress.* New York: Holt, Rinehart & Winston.

This article is printed with permission of *Research in Nursing and Health*

Copyright © 1978 John Wiley & Sons.

10

Community Health Nursing

Caroline McCoy White, DrPH, RN
Jean Regier, BSN, RN
Dianne Wheeling, BSN, RN

INTRODUCTION BY: CAROLINE McCOY WHITE DrPH, RN

Selected because their content is central to the practice of community health nursing, the three studies in this chapter are relevant to other areas of nursing practice as well. In addition to describing nursing interventions, the studies illustrate ways in which methods of research might be incorporated into practice.

The research reported in the studies was conceived and conducted by nurses. As might be expected, the impetus for each study was different. Also characteristic of the research of nurses and research relevant to nursing, the reports of the studies were published in two different types of journals. One journal focuses on the development of nursing knowledge through research. The other journal, through its editorials, emphasizes the research and practice implications of the studies published: it is an interdisciplinary journal wherein the knowledge and practice of nursing overlap with that of other disciplines.

The first study in the chapter is frequently cited in nursing and community health textbooks. Long, Whitman, Johansson, Williams, and Tuthill collaborated in the design of a program of nursing interventions to a population of school children with records of high absence. One prescription strongly associated with community health nursing is reflected here: interdisciplinary collaboration to solve problems through pooling of expertise and access to resources. The study also illustrates the collaboration between health professionals in what might be called a service setting and health professionals in an academic institution. Such collaboration is often prescribed in hope that the interventions of practitioners might be systematically derived and examined and so that the research and teaching of academicians might have greater real-world relevance. A second prescription, one that nursing shares with many other disciplines and practices, also is reflected: build the design and plan for evaluation concurrently, then plan for the intervention.

The second study in the chapter is a report of the investigation of two frequently asked questions in nursing: what factors are associated with certain behaviors and what is the most effective way to assist patients to incorporate new behaviors into their life styles. Brailey, working with nurses in an occupational health program, sought to determine whether individual or group teaching was more effective in increasing: (1) the frequency of breast self-examination, (2) the extent of knowledge of participants with respect to techniques for thorough exam, and (3) the perception of susceptibility to breast cancer and benefits of breast self-examination. The selection of variables for study was guided by an explicit framework derived from existing literature. Measurement of the dependent variables was done with instruments developed by other researchers and modified for use in the study. The study could be described as theory testing research, since aspects of the framework are often presented as a theory. Teaching, the independent variable, is a strategy widely used in nursing. Preventive health behaviors, such as breast self-examination, are a major focus in community health nursing where the emphasis is on the developent and implementation of measures, both for individuals and groups, that are conducive to the prevention and early recognition of disease.

The third study in this chapter, in contrast to the first two that report evaluations of nursing interventions, is particularly relevant to the assessment phase of the nursing process. Also in contrast to the first two articles, the research methods used are more qualitative than quantitative. For her doctoral dissertation, Duffy sought to discover the way in which women heading single-parent families thought about their family life styles in relation to conscious decisions to engage in behaviors thought to be conducive to health. In research and practice the qualitative methodology of asking open-ended questions is necessary in order to approach accurate understanding of the client's perspective. This understanding is considered important in nursing. It is critical in community health where the achievement of positive health outcomes is the result of active working together of nurse and client.

The three studies in this chapter were selected from many in nursing journals and community/public health journals. Because the practice of the community health nurse is guided by research in many disciplines, the nurse seeking to discover justification for current practice or for practice innovations must search widely. The studies presented here reflect the fragile and tentative nature of our understandings. Each was selected so that the group would cover a range of practices, populations, and research strategies that would be within the scope of expertise of the baccalaureate prepared nurse; each is not necessarily more meritorious than others in the literature.

Evaluation of a School Health Program Directed to Children with History of High Absence: A Focus for Nursing Intervention

Gene V. Long, MN, RN
Assistant Director of Nursing
Palm Beach County Health Department
Palm Beach, FL

Caroline Whitman, MEd, RN
Director
Indian River County Health Department
Vero Beach, FL

Mabel S. Johansson, MPH, RN
Director
Palm Beach County Health Department
Palm Beach, FL

Carolyn A. Williams, PhD, RN
Assistant Professor
Department of Epidemiology
University of North Carolina
Chapel Hill, NC

Robert W. Tuthill, PhD
Assistant Professor
Department of Public Health
Amherst, MA

INTRODUCTION

In recent years nursing personnel associated with the Palm Beach County Health Department have become involved in efforts to assess the effectiveness of their services with particular emphasis on determining the benefits to the populations they serve. The present study was developed in response to questions concerning whether the skills of professional nurses were being utilized to best advantage within the school system.

In Palm Beach County public health nurses are responsible for providing generalized nursing services to the community as well as services to children in the schools. Thus, except for vision and hearing programs, services provided as part of their school-related responsibilities are frequently limited to one-time or episodic encounters with individual children who are referred by teachers, principals, and occasionally themselves. Although response to such service demands may be necessary, confining the school program to these activities results in episodic problem solution rather than a balanced program with an appropriate concentration on preventive services. A major implication of such an approach is that children with unidentified problems, particularly problems at an early stage of development, may never come to the attention of the nurse. Awareness of the possible existence of these difficulties within the school health program in Palm Beach County led to a decision to continue the usual services to the school while also testing the feasibility of a pilot program, preventive in spirit and directed to a defined group of children.

Industrial studies have shown that a small proportion of persons are responsible for the majority of illnesses in work groups.[1] Likewise, a recent school health study[2] indicated that a good predictor of a pupil's future absence record is his past year's absence record. Other national studies[3,4] have found that at least 80 per cent of the school absences are for health reasons. In addition, the nursing staff of the Palm Beach County Health Department conducted a small preliminary pilot study of 40 high absence pupils randomly selected from the high absence group in two schools which indicated that these children had a high prevalence of health problems.

On the basis of the data cited above it was decided that identification of children with a past record of high absence would be a reasonable way of defining a group of children with a high risk of future episodes of illness and possibly a high prevalence of basic health problems. Since it was anticipated that children so defined—and their families—could benefit from nursing service, it was concluded that high absence children constituted an appropriate risk group to which nursing services could be profitably directed. This group was therefore selected for the pilot program. The major objectives of the study were (1) to consider the utility of directing nursing services to a defined risk group and (2) to document the results of the experience in terms of patient outcomes, specifically, change in absence experience. The basic working hypothesis was that focused nursing attention would be positively associated with a reduction in days absent.

METHODOLOGY

Research Design

Since the research design was detailed in an earlier paper[5] only highlights will be presented here. The basic strategy was to: (1) select two groups of high absence children comparable in factors thought to be associated with absence experience; (2) direct professional nursing services to one of the two groups (intervention group); and (3) document the results of the program in terms of change in absence.

The total group of 68 elementary schools in Palm Beach County was stratified into three socioeconomic levels (high, middle, low). From each socioeconomic level two schools were randomly selected as intervention schools (for a total of six schools) and two schools matched on socioeconomic level were selected as controls for each intervention school (a total of 12 schools). Within each intervention and control school, pupils in grades 2 through 5 with 14 or more absence days in the previous school year (1969-70) were identified. Each high absence pupil from an intervention school was matched with a pupil from a control school on number of days absent, grade level, sex, and race. In September, 1970, the new program was begun in the intervention schools.

Pilot Intervention Program

During the study year a public health nurse was assigned to each of the six intervention schools, with no nurse being responsible for both an intervention and a control school. All schools, intervention and control, continued to receive the usual nursing services: nurse participation in "staffing" (an interdisciplinary team approach to assessment and planning for children with complex problems), routine vision and hearing screening and follow-up, teacher-nurse conferences, and referral by school personnel for home visits regarding identified or suspected problems. In addition, the high absence pupils in the intervention schools received focused attention from the nurse assigned to that school which was initiated at the start of the 1970-1971 school year and continued throughout the academic year.

At the beginning of the school year, each nurse assigned to an intervention school was given a list of high absence pupils in her school and asked to make a family-centered assessment of each pupil as early in the year as possible. In the process the nurse was expected to utilize her assessment skills to identify possible explanations for the previous year's absences, to determine the child's current health status, and to assist the family in recognizing and coping with any problems or situations which might result in future difficulties. The plan for the intervention program was systematic in that nursing services were to be directed to each high absence child and his family; yet nurses were to exercise their professional judgment in the intervention program within the overall guidelines provided.

Two major aspects of the intervention program were the activities of the nurse and the record of her activity. A uniform record of contact was designed to record the nurse's activities and to increase the possibility of describing the relationship between input (activities of the nurse) and patient progress. For each contact made the nurse was asked to record on the contact record identifying information, the reason for contact, findings, and the plan of action. For each child in the experimental group brief continuous accounts of the contacts and results were also recorded on a summary sheet. It was anticipated that such a record would be helpful to the nurses by providing a means of quickly noting problems identified, problem solving efforts, and the presence or absence of progress toward solutions.

Activities involved in carrying out the program included: (1) examinations of all available school and health records of the child, (2) home visits, and (3) conferences with the classroom teacher. Other types of contacts utilized for assessment and management purposes were: (1) nurse-pupil conferences, (2) nurse-principal conferences, (3) participation in "staffing" (the interdisciplinary case review), (4) phone calls, and (5) written communications. Close communication was maintained between the nurses and the study supervisory staff. In addition to participating in initial in-service sessions designed to prepare the nurses for involvement in the program, the project coordinator met monthly with the nurses serving in the intervention schools during the study year to discuss any problems they were having. Individual conferences were arranged as needed.

The nurses in the control schools were not given the names of the high absence children matched with the intervention group but were asked to provide services in the school as usual. When a child was seen, information was recorded on the child's cumulative health record at the school, in the school folder maintained for each school, and on the contact record which was adopted systemwide. Thus, a mechanism for recording contacts with control children was provided.

The Study Sample

At the beginning of the 1970-1971 school year there were 349 children in the intervention schools who met the criteria for high absence, that is, who had absences of 14 or more days during the previous (1969-1970) school year. Of these pupils, 47 withdrew from school during 1970-1971 and were dropped from the study.

The 47 intervention pupils lost to the study during the school year had more days of absence in 1969-1970 than the rest of the intervention group (mean of 25.8 versus 21.6 days of absence); this difference was found to be statistically significant

Table 1
Percentage Distribution of Intervention Children and Controls by Socioeconomic Level of School and Matching Status

Socioeconomic Level of School	Pairs Matched on Socioeconomic Level of School		Children Not Matched on Socioeconomic Level of School			
			Intervention		Control	
	No.	%	No.	%	No.	%
High	93	38.1	19	32.8	10	17.2
Middle	87	35.7	33	56.9	8	13.8
Low	64	26.2	6	10.3	40	69.0
Total	244	100.0	58	100.0	58	100.0

($t = 2.30$ with p less than 0.05 for a two-tailed test). Loss rates differed little between schools of different socioeconomic levels and between grade levels (nonsignificant by chi-square analysis). Although the differences were not statistically significant, the dropout rates for white females (16.8 percent) and white males (12.8 percent) were higher than for nonwhite females (8.1 percent) and nonwhite males (7.1 percent). It is possible that these differences may have been related to the integration experience which took place during the study year. As compared to the original sample the final study sample was, due to losses, somewhat underrepresentative of the higher absence pupils and of whites, although not to any great extent.

The original design of individual matching had to be modified somewhat because of the implementation of integration in the schools and the resulting transfers of large numbers of children. Of the 302 pairs of children remaining at the end of the study period, the majority of the intervention children (N = 199) were matched with a child from one of the two matched control schools as called for in the original design. In a second group (N = 45) the matches for the intervention children were selected from either of two control schools matched with the other intervention school within the same socioeconomic level. In the remaining group (N = 58) the matches for the intervention children were drawn from the eight control schools outside the socioeconomic level of the intervention school (Table 1).

The accuracy of the matching procedure in regard to days of absence can be assessed from Table 2, which shows that the difference in days of absence between the children in the intervention group and their matched controls was quite small.

RESULTS

As previously mentioned, it was anticipated that by directing professional nursing service to children who experienced high absence levels during the 1969-1970 school year, it would be possible to decrease their health problems and thus their

Table 2
Means, Standard Deviations, Medians, and Modes for Days of Absence, 1969-1970* School Year, by Intervention Group and Matched Controls

Days Absent 1969-1970	Intervention Group (N = 302)	Control Group (N = 302)
Mean	21.65	21.34
Standard deviation	8.14	7.53
Median	19.28	19.17
Mode	14.00	14.00

*This was the school year immediately prior to the initiation of the study.

absences during the study year. The data in Table 3 indicate that between 1969-1970 and 1970-1971 the intervention group experienced a mean decline in absence of 7.08 days. The control group's mean decline was 5.10, resulting in a statistically significant mean difference of 1.98 between the intervention and control groups. In other words, pupils in the intervention group showed a decline in absences which averaged 2 days more than the reduction experienced by those in the control group, and this difference can be viewed as a nonchance occurrence. The decline in mean absence for the intervention group was 32.7 per cent while the decline was only 23.9 per cent for the matched controls, the difference between the groups being 8.8 per cent. When the decline is expressed in actual days there were 597 less days of absence among the 302 intervention children during the study year than among their matched controls.

The difference in absence decline between the intervention and control groups exceeded the minimum level specified as worthwhile from a programmatic point of view. In the original estimate the control group was expected to have a natural decline of 30 percent in days absent without intervention from one year to the next. It was decided before the study began that if the program effort and expense were to be worthwhile the intervention should bring about a 10 percent greater relative reduction in absences among the

Table 3
Change in Mean Days of Absence for Intervention Children and Matched Controls, 1969-1970 to 1970-1971

Days of Absence	Intervention Group (N = 302)	Matched Controls (N = 302)	Mean Difference: Intervention and Control Groups
1969-1970			
Mean	21.65	21.34	0.31
Standard deviation	8.14	7.53	
1970-1971			
Mean	14.57	16.24	-1.67
Standard deviation	10.57	11.18	
Change in days absent (1970-1971) to (1969-1970)*			
Mean	-7.08	-5.10	-1.98*
Standard deviation	9.93	10.87	
% change	32.70	23.90	8.80

*t for difference of means, matched pairs = 2.53 with 301 df. p is less than 0.01, one-tailed test.

experimental group than the control group or an absolute difference of 3 percent (0.03 X 0.10 = 3 percent). The actual difference which occurred was 8.8 percent or almost 3 times that expected. The results can therefore be considered meaningful from a practical point of view.

In an attempt to discover whether the intervention program was more successful for certain types of students, a series of individual t-tests (matched pairs) were done for each race/sex and each grade level. The null hypothesis tested was that within each subgroup no difference in absence decline

Table 4
Means and Standard Deviations for Differences between Intervention and Control Group in Change in Days Absent, 1969-1970 to 1970-1971 by Race/Sex Group and Grade Level

	Race/Sex Group				
	White Male	White Female	Nonwhite Male	Nonwhite Female	Total
Mean*	-0.813	-2.706	-0.385	-4.882	-1.980
Standard deviation	14.629	12.521	16.130	10.688	13.575
No. of observations	123	119	26	34	302

	Grade				
	2	3	4	5	Total
Mean†	-1.867	-2.773	0.467	-3.913	-1.980
Standard deviation	15.482	13.709	12.929	11.362	13.575
No. of observations	83	75	75	69	302

*t values for difference of means, matched pairs: WF $p < 0.025$; NWF $p < 0.01$; total $p < 0.01$. Analysis of variance = F with 3,298 df = 1.055, nonsignificant.
† t values for difference of means, matched pairs: Grade 3 $p < 0.05$; Grade 5 $p < 0.005$; total $p < 0.01$. Analysis of variance = F with 3,298 df = 1.371, nonsignificant.

would be found between the intervention and the control groups. The data in Table 4 show that statistically significant differences ($p < 0.05$) in decline of days of absence between the intervention and control groups were found in females and in third and fifth grade pupils (both sexes combined), indicating that these groups contributed most to the overall difference between the two groups. The next step in the analysis was to determine whether there were significant differences in the magnitude of the mean change scores (determined by subtracting the mean decline in absence for the control group from the mean decline for the intervention group). A series of one-way analyses of variance was done to assess differences by race/sex and grade level; no statistically significant differences were found (Table 4).

To summarize, it is clear that the absence decline experienced by the intervention group differed significantly from that experienced by the control group. And, although the females and the third and fifth graders seemed to contribute most to the overall differences between the intervention and control groups, analyses of variance showed that the relative differentials in absence decline experienced by these groups were not sufficient to conclude that nonchance differences existed between them and the other subgroups. The data thus indicate that a real difference cannot be attributed to the effect of sex/race group or grade level.

DISCUSSION AND IMPLICATIONS

Data generated by the study indicate that the intervention group showed a difference in absence decline from that of the control group which was statistically significant and of some practical consequence. However, the question still remains whether the differences observed between the intervention and the control groups can be attributed to nursing service. Information available on nursing activities showed that there was a considerable difference in the amount of service effort expended on behalf of the intervention group as compared to the controls. For 99.7 percent of the children in the intervention group (all but one) the nurse reported an attempt to make some type of assessment. These assessments led to additional interventions on behalf of about 32 percent of the children. In contrast, only 3.9 percent or 12 of the 302 children in the control group were even mentioned by name in any of the records associated with them.

Despite the clear difference between the nursing service provided to the two groups, associations between nursing service and the change in absence can only be viewed as suggestive, for two basic reasons. First, it is possible that the differential in absence decline experienced by the intervention group can be partially attributed to a Hawthorne effect. In other words, perhaps during the assessment of the child and his family the nurse called undue attention to the child's absence history and this and/or the nurse's interest in the child—rather than the resolution of any underlying health problem—was responsible for the absence reduction. Second, it is difficult to relate absence decline to actual nursing intervention because of: (1) inability to obtain systematic assessment data on each child and family, and (2) difficulty in determining the nature of the nursing service actually rendered.

A special record for reporting every contact made on behalf of a child was developed for use throughout the school system. However, because of a decision not to develop and use a common approach to family and child assessment, and because of a general lack of uniformity among the nurses in recording patterns, an audit of the records did not provide adequate reliable information on problems identified and strategies utilized by the nurses in problem resolution.

Despite inability to be certain about the role which provision of nursing service might have had in the absence reduction experienced by the intervention group, the study validated that with careful planning it is possible to incorporate a prevention-oriented service directed to a defined risk group into an on-going school health program. Further, the data suggest the need for additional study of the contribution which nursing service might make by focusing on vulnerable groups of children such as those defined as high risk due to past absence experience.

Recent data suggest that through the identification of high absence children within the schools it is not only possible to offer preventive services to these children but it may also be possible to locate families in the community who are in particular need of health service. In a cross-sectional survey Boardman[6] identified two pools of elementary school children: one group who had experienced 10 or more episodes of absence in two successive school years and one who had had three or fewer episodes in the same time period. From these groups 100 randomly selected families of children defined as high absence were matched (according to race, sex, grade, and school of the index child) with 100 families of low absence children. The data indicated that family members of the high absence children were reported to have almost twice as much chronic disease as family members of the low absence children.

The present study points up the need (1) to develop systematic and reliable approaches to assessing children and their families and (2) to document nursing action. Clearly, before it will be possible to understand the contribution which nursing may be able to make to children with a history of high absence, or to study the processes involved, it will be necessary to describe in a systematic way the child and his family in terms of health status and other characteristics, such as family and child attitudes toward school attendance, which may affect absence experience. Further, it will be necessary to conceptualize and specify the nature of the services provided by the nurse. And finally, in order to understand the processes involved it is essential that attempts be made to study the interaction between child and family characteristics, nursing actions, and change in absences which may be due to change in health status or behavior of the child and/or his family. It is encouraging to note that such work is proceeding[7].

In Palm Beach County, following analysis of the data in 1971-1972, plans were made to reorganize the school health services in order to further explore the processes and interactions between the nursing services and the target populations. In 1973-1974, a public health nurse coordinator position was established to assist in planning, assessing, and evaluating nursing intervention activities, with implementation in 1974-1975.

From the perspective of the service agency some of the concomitant benefits from the study are: (1) the methodology, using absence as an indicator, suggests a practical approach to identification of a high risk population; (2) the school health program can be planned to further explore emphasis on prevention through selected priorities rather than continuing to be crisis-oriented; and (3) efforts can be directed toward development of improved documentation of nursing intervention not only to provide an improved data base for evaluation but also to meet the current demand for accountability.

In addition to providing a meaningful experience in program evaluation for nursing staff within the health department, participation in the study has promoted more effective communication between the school system and the health department which share joint responsibility for the school health program.

ACKNOWLEDGMENTS

Appreciation is gratefully extended to Dr. Cecil Slome, Dr. Steve Zyzanski, Dr. John Cassel, and other members of the training faculty; Dr. Doris E. Roberts, Division of Nursing, National Institutes of Health; and Dr. John A. Demming, Director, Pupil Personnel Services, Palm Beach County Public Schools.

REFERENCES

1. Hinkle, L. E., Jr., Plummer, N., & Whitney, L. H. (1961). Continuity of patterns of illness and prediction of future health. *Journal of Occupational Medicine, 3*, 417–423.
2. Roberts, D. E., Basco, D., Slome, C., Glasser, J. H., & Handy, G. (1969). Epidemiological analysis in school populations as a basis for change in school nursing practice. *American Journal of Public Health, 59*, 2144–2156.
3. Rogers, K. D., & Reese, G. (1965). Health studies—Presumably normal high school stu-

dents. *American Journal of Diseases of Children, 109,* 9–27.
4. Metropolitan Life Insurance Company. (1950). School absenteeism. In statistical bulletin, No. 31. New York: The Author.
5. Tuthill, R. W., Williams, C. A., Long, G. V., & Whitman, C. (1972) Evaluating a school health program focused on high absence pupils: A research design. *American Journal of Public Health, 62,* 240.
6. Boardman, V. (1972). School absences, illness, and family competence. Unpublished doctoral dissertation, University of North Carolina, Chapel Hill.
7. Basco, D., Eyres, S., Glasser, J. H., & Roberts, D. E. (1972). Epidemiological analysis in school nursing practice—Report of the second phase of a longitudinal study. *American Journal of Public Health, 62,* 491–497.

This article is printed with permission of *American Journal of Public Health.*

Original article:
Long, G. V., Whitman, C., Johansson, M. S., Williams, C. A., & Tuthill, R. W. (1975). Evaluation of a school health program directed to children with history of high absence. *American Journal of Public Health*, 65, 388–393.

CRITIQUE BY: DIANNE WHEELING, BSN, RN

Introduction

People are always looking for new and better ways to accomplish tasks and solve problems in their community. Community health nurses often search for the right answer to clinical issues or problems that surface daily in their practice. Nursing research is one source of information, but it is often difficult to know whether a particular research study can answer questions raised in specific situations. The purpose of this paper is to systematically evaluate the study entitled "Evaluation of a School Health Program Directed to Children with History of High Absence" to determine clinical relevance for a community health nurse practicing in a school setting.

Part I: Clinical Relevance

This study addresses two nursing issues. First, are professional nurses using all their available skills and resources in the school health program? Second, would school children benefit if nurses focused their interventions on high-risk groups in a preventive manner rather than continuing the current standard practice of treating referred individuals?

The study is particularly relevant in today's changing health care environment where emphasis is placed increasingly on cost-effective health care. As health services fall under scrutiny, the nursing profession must be able to verify the need for nursing services and provide data that indicate the cost effectiveness of interventions. The study may provide valuable data regarding the effectiveness of health promoting programs over a more traditional screening-referral approach.

The investigators selected children with high absence records for their high-risk groups and measured intervention effectiveness in terms of decreasing absence rates. Attendance records can be used as a basis for judging the effectiveness of many community nursing programs. A decrease in absences is an indicator that both school officials and business management can appreciate. Occupational health nurses, for example, watch for trends of high absenteeism among employees and may establish preventive programs aimed at the high-absentee employee. A reduction in sick days through preventive health care reduces costs for the employer as well as possible cost to the employee for secondary care for an illness that may have been prevented. Nurses in a hospital or clinic setting are in a position to assess days absent from school or work and may identify high-risk patients, thus cueing the health team to investigate further the extent of a client's health needs.

The investigators do not use any single theory as a basis for designing the intervention. They propose that primary preventive nursing may decrease the need for later nursing intervention or other medical expenses. Working under this assumption, a community health nurse would want to identify high-risk groups within the community being served and focus on health promoting nursing care.

The investigators do not test any particular nursing intervention in the study. The fact that nurses are intervening in a more preventive manner is more the focus. Nurses in the experimental group identified high-risk pupils and intervened before a referral was made. In the control group, the high-risk children received standard care in the school system and were only seen if referred to the school nurse. In either case, the nurse was to document any time spent with a child through charting.

If a more independent, preventive nursing approach is undertaken and successful, professional nurses would be well advised to consider such an assertive approach. Preventive nursing assessment and intervention is an area in the health care field in which a nurse can make an independent nursing decision and intervene appropriately. Also, gathering data on groups within a population provides information on the community system and can be critical in terms of assessing the community as client.

The investigators measured the dependent variable or outcome by an increase or decrease in the number of days absent during a school year for each high-risk child. This is a concrete measurement which can be utilized in other research studies or by nurses in practice.

In general, one can begin to see the possibility of using the study in practice; not only in terms of community health nurses wishing to experiment with preventive program development, but also in terms of nursing as a profession wishing to document effective nursing care as an economic necessity.

Part II: Conceptualization and Internal Consistency

The investigators have written a clear and readable study, which develops section by section and from topic to topic. In addition, they provide answers and explanations to the questions they pose at the beginning of their work.

The investigators are attempting to justify nursing in the public sector. They question the current utility of professional nurses working with the school population and want to examine the relevance of nursing interventions with a preventive focus. The investigators set out to answer this question by focusing on school absences and preventive services. They label those children who have high absence records as high-risk for future health problems and cite several studies supporting their selection of absenteeism as a health indicator and viable tool for research use. Thus, the investigators logically link their research question to their study justification.

In addition, the investigators link the independent variables of regular school nursing services or "focused attention" nursing care to the dependent variable, number of days absent, in a logical manner. They define "focused attention" as the completion of a family-centered assessment followed by a health care plan, interventions, and follow-up evaluation to the defined high-risk population.

The investigators also define their population of interest and select the sample accordingly. From 68 elementary schools in the county district, they randomly selected 12 after stratifying them into three socioeconomic categories. Then they selected 359 children from grades two through five as high-risk; that is, as having 14 or more day absences from the previous school year. The investigators matched each experimental school to a control school in terms of socioeconomic level; then they matched each child from an experimental school to each child from a control school in terms of sex, race, and grade level. In addition, to further reduce possible study bias, they assigned nurses to work either with the experimental schools or the control schools.

In theory, although a reduction of days absent is appropriate to measure effective nursing care, there may be several other reasons for a decline in absences. Appropriately mentioned by the investigators is the problem of Hawthorne effect, where just increasing the attention given to the child decreases his or her absence from school. Other reasons could include better teaching staff, a chicken pox epidemic one year and not the next, or a more organized PTA group this year. Changing an established pattern of behavior is difficult, and reduction of absences may be a very temporary change.

In general, then, the investigators have designed their study to reduce bias and provide information on the effectiveness of preventive nursing care. However, they did not provide a systematic method for nurses to record their assessment data or interventions with the experimental group. Charting methods varied and it was difficult to determine what nursing interventions actually took place. Although this is a disappointing gap in the study and does prevent the investigators from drawing concrete conclusions, they examine this shortcoming in detail and provide a clear discussion of the subsequent implications for their study and future research.

Part III: Believability of Results

This study purported to test the effects of two types of nursing intervention styles—health promoting nursing or a more passive referral approach—by way of quantitative data gathered by recording the change in number of days absent in two consecutive school years for a group of high-risk children.

The investigators selected a convenience sample of elementary school children if they had absences of 14 or more days during the previous school year. Cause of absence, illness or otherwise, is unknown to the reader. While the investigators assume that absence is due to illness, this may be invalid. After using their convenience sample, they took steps to reduce factors within the sample that might bias results. As mentioned previously, they matched children in both groups for several biosocial variables. Through statistical analysis, they measured the commonality and differences between the two groups. They also discussed the 47 children who moved or withdrew and were lost to the study. These students who had higher absence rates than the other children may have changed the outcome of the study. Thus, the investigators examined research validity in terms of subject attrition and group equivalency.

Although the investigators utilized a contact record sheet for every child in the school system, they failed to implement a common assessment tool or method of charting for the intervening nurses. This resulted in an inconsistent record of nursing data which is not reliably or uniformly documented. As a result, the validity of study results is decreased considerably.

The investigators stratified schools into three socioeconomic levels then randomly labeled them as either control or experimental. Therefore, high-risk children had an equal chance of being in a control or an experimental environment. In addition, nurses assigned to experimental schools could not also have a control school and nurses working in the control schools did not receive a list of high-risk students. All schools received standard nursing services.

The investigators reported results, measured in change of days absent, in terms of mean, standard deviation, and percent change between the two groups. Also, they used further statistical analysis, t-tests, and analyses of variance to determine whether particular kinds of students were influenced to a greater degree than others by focused nursing. Although I would need assistance in interpreting the more complicated statistics, I believe the investigators described their analysis clearly and with concision. On the other hand, the use of simpler statistics would have facilitated the interpretation of data and provided an easier understanding of results.

The investigators report a significant drop in absence for their experimental group (8 percent) and consider this drop large enough to warrant initiating a preventive nursing program on a county-wide basis. They concede that the significant drop may not be totally related to nursing intervention and further state that they cannot positively identify the nature of nursing service performed on the experimental group. In addition, they believe the difference is large enough to warrant further study and the activation of preventive health care programs. These opinions seem realistic. An eight percent reduction does not, at first, appear impressive; however, this is only a first-year figure. Perhaps the rate of absences would be further reduced if the program continued and was initiated from grade one. The eight percent figure corresponds to 597 less days of absence among the intervention children than their matched controls, which is a more impressive number to quote.

The investigators do not allow the statistical results to cloud their awareness of the study's limitations. Rather, the statistics provide incentive for exploring preventive nursing care as an economically sound alternative in the health care system.

Part IV: Generalizability of Results

The investigators drew subjects from Palm Beach County public schools in Florida and selected nurses from Palm Beach County Health Department. Although the investigators do not state how similar their sample is to the population of American school children, generalizability of results is probable. Perhaps private or rural school students would be excluded from generalizability, however.

The investigators did not specially train the nurses practicing in the school system for the experiment. Those working with the control group provided services as usual without knowledge of the high-risk pupils. Nurses working in the intervention schools met monthly with the research team but were allowed to intervene with the subjects at their discretion. No special assessment tool was used nor were there special care plans or intervention protocols for clarification or direction.

Since other variables can interfere with the experimental process and results are not easily quantifiable, the problem of testing the efficacy of a preventive nursing program presents difficulties. I am not aware of other studies addressing the issue of preventive nursing versus a more traditional approach. However, studies showing the importance of preventive prenatal care in reducing intrapartal and postpartum complications are well documented. The investigators also do not cite replication studies or those which utilize the number of day absences as a dependent variable.

In general, average public health nurses worked with average public school children trying a new approach within the framework of a well-established system. Although the investigators do not attempt to generalize, one can assume that similar results can be obtained under similar circumstances.

Part V: Other Factors to Consider in Utilization

Since absence records are easily obtainable, the feasibility of repeating a similar study is high. A practicing nurse could utilize records to identify high-risk groups, make some assessments, intervene, and calculate some yearly comparisons with simple statistics. However, before another study of this kind is undertaken, further clarification is needed on the description and documentation procedures of actual nursing interventions. With the support of the employer and accurate documentation, a nurse could provide data which supports preventive health care as economically appropriate.

There is little risk involved in implementing a preventive school health program. Such a program may be more costly and require more staff; however, more children could be seen sooner for their concerns and perhaps costly illness could be avoided. Maintaining the status quo school health program means shutting the door on promoting wellness in school age children and limiting lifetime health maintenance values. Also, current practice tends to curb responsibility and initiative in nursing at a time when professional nurses should push forward and assume a leadership role in the changing health care arena. In addition to increasing wellness opportunities for their clients, nursing as a profession would benefit greatly from a preventive health care approach.

I consider the present study as appropriate for utilization in practice based on the discussion and criteria reviewed in this critique. Such research is an important addition to the body of nursing knowledge. If appropriate and relevant, nursing research can be a valuable resource for community health nurses trying to provide the best possible care for their community.

Original article:
Long, G. V., Whitman, C., Johansson, M. S., Williams, C. A., & Tuthill, R. W. (1975). Evaluation of a school health program directed to children with history of high absence. *American Journal of Public Health*, 65, 388–393.

CRITIQUE BY: CAROLINE McCOY WHITE, DrPH, RN

This study describes an innovative program for the delivery of school nursing services and the evaluation of its effectiveness. Components of the innovative program included the identification of children with a history of high absence and the delivery of focused nursing attention to these children and their families. The impetus for the study included questions about whether a new way for delivering service that emphasized those most in need could achieve results more effectively while not compromising ongoing service programs.

Part I: Clinical Relevance

As presented by the investigators, their theory purported that nursing attention focused on individual children in a high-risk group would result in a decrease in overall absence in that group. The nursing attention included: (1) a family-centered assessment of each high-absence child that was completed as early in the year as possible and (2) interventions directed toward assisting the family to recognize and cope with problems or situations that might result in future difficulties. The investigators implemented the program as an experiment by which to compare the absence experience of the group receiving the innovative program to that of a matched control group. They derived the theory and assumptions underlying the innovative program from previous studies. It was assumed that children with history of high absence were at risk for future high absence and that they were likely to have a high prevalence of health problems.

This study is useful to the nurse seeking to decide about the most efficient and effective use of time and program effort where responsibilities are for groups of essentially well individuals. It is particularly relevant to nurses in school health programs. Although elementary school children constituted the study population, I would consider targeting effort to absentees in programs for other groups as well—children in pre-school and kindergarten, and junior and senior high school students and workers, because absence is costly in terms of lost opportunities for learning and decreased productivity. In addition, the nurse seeking to evaluate change in attendance behavior or other behavior where some variation in frequency could be expected to be due to chance would find the model for measuring meaningful change useful.

The innovation described in this study is clearly within the realm of nursing practice. However, a nurse seeking to implement nursing care on the basis of this study needs to consider whether the new model for care could be accomplished within the constraints of other responsibilities. While approval might not be essential, concurrence from school and health program supervisors might be desirable. Possible supporting evidence for making the change is that the processes described in this study have become part of "routine practice" in many school health programs.

The main measure used in the study, school absence, is accessible to the nurse. It is usually considered necessary by school officials that the nurse have access to such data in order to fill position responsibilities. History of absence, indicator for intervention and outcome, is based on routinely collected data to which school systems attach great significance. Data regarding absence also is routinely collected information in work places.

Part II: Conceptualization and Internal Consistency

The study describes the absence experience of two groups of elementary school children enrolled in a large public school system. Children in both groups had a history of high absence. Pairs of children were individually matched on the basis of factors thought to be associated with absence experience. Children in the experimental group received the usual nursing services *plus* focused nursing attention. Children in the control group received the usual nursing services at the usually provided intensity.

The study report begins with a description of the basic concern: how can the skills of professional nurses be used to best advantage within the school system? After brief reference to relevant literature, the investigators describe their study methodology: the intervention, its documentation, and the sample. They present results in narrative and tabular forms. Their discussion covers implications for practice, limiting factors to the study, and possible reasons for findings other than the effects of the intervention (i.e., competing hypotheses or explanations). Throughout, investigators use terms consistently and with a minimum of jargon. Their presentation is clear, one section of the report building on and consistent with preceding sections.

In addition, the investigators state the underlying conception for the study with concision. The intervention and the evaluation measure are congruent with the conception and logically related to one another. The subjects of the study, children with history of high absence, are the population of interest and their absence experience during the study year is the dependent variable.

The key variables of the study make sense. The logical relationship of the dependent variable (change in school absence) to the independent variable (focused nursing attention) rests on the assumptions that: (1) factors that cause children to be absent from school might be altered and (2) that nursing attention to the health and social situation of individual children and their families might influence those factors in a way to decrease absence.

The investigators obtained the dependent variable (change in school absence) from records routinely kept by the schools. They measured the phenomenon of interest (change in school absence) by direct comparison of days absent in the study year to those in the previous year for each subject. Bias in regard to study results, potentially due to the way this measure was obtained, is difficult to envision. It would seem that school officials in both intervention and control schools have the same overriding interests with respect to recording absences accurately and that these transcend the possible gain from any fabrication of study results.

The independent variable consists of the existence of the innovative program in particular schools and the delivery of "focused nursing attention" to the children identified as having a history of high absence the previous year. Documentation of whether or not the targeted children received "focused nursing attention" came via a uniform record of activity designed for the study. Such a record does seem likely to measure one component of the independent variable (the service to individual children and their families) and allow verification of the other component (that all those on the list of high absence children received service). However, the investigators do state that the records were insufficient to allow them to understand exactly what aspect(s) of focused attention were most strongly associated with change in absence. Maintained by the nurse assigned to the school, and thus the one delivering the intervention, there was to be a record for each child who had been on the list of high-absence children. The forms for the intervention were designed to promote efficiency and effectiveness on the part of nurses, and, as such, contribute to the intervention. Since the nurse also was the recorder, it is possible, though not likely, that a particular child could have been identified as receiving service but who in fact did not. Services to children in the control schools (the individual children matched to individual children in the intervention schools) were documented by the nurse on the student's cumulative health record at the school, in the school folder maintained for each school, and the contact record that was adopted system-wide.

Part III: Believability of Results

The investigators used quantitative methods to test the effect on school attendance of an innovative program of focused nursing attention to school children with history of high absence. This supplemented the program that all children, as school enrollees, received. All children were either present or absent on particular school days.

The investigators randomly selected schools in which to implement the innovative program. They included, within each of these schools, all members of the eligible population: the intervention group. Subjects for the innovative intervention became eligible: (1) if they were enrolled at one of two schools randomly selected from the three socioeconomic strata into which the 68 elementary schools in one county had been classified; (2) if they were in grades two through five; and (3) if they had 14 or more absences during the previous school year. The investigators included these eligible subjects in the analysis if they continued to be enrolled in the innovative program school for the entire school year. Since 47 of the 349 eligible children in the innovative program schools withdrew from school during the study year, the investigators based their final sample on the remaining 302 enrollees. They selected control group subjects on the basis of their "match" to an intervention group subject. Two-thirds of the "control" subjects became eligible for the study because: (1) they attended a school matched to an innovative program school and (2) they were matchable to an experimental group child from that school on the basis of number of days absent during the previous school year, grade level, sex, and race. This procedure matched 199 control children with intervention group children. Forty-five children came from the other control school at the same socioeconomic level and 58 came from a control school outside the socioeconomic level of the intervention school; in both instances, these subjects were matched by number of days absent during the previous year, grade level, sex, and race.

The investigators, having identified potential intervening variables prior to the study, incorporated them into the study design via matching procedures: socioeconomic level of the school; sex, race, and grade level of the child; and number of days absent during the previous year. Possible intervening variables not accounted for (but mentioned by the investigators) are attitude of the student's family toward school attendance and actual child and family health. Possible intervening variables not accounted for (and not mentioned by the investigators) include variables associated with the schools that might motivate attendance, such as the effects the integration instituted that year, the general morale of faculty and children, the general quality of the school program, and differential experience with contagious diseases.

It appears that the investigators stayed within usual bounds for practice research. They were implementing a study in a school system inviting the study and were using, for the most part, data collected as part of normal system operations. Unfortunately, the investigators do not discuss reliability of measures. In addition, they present no operational definitions for the variable absence;

presumably the school system had guidelines for that. Nor do they address validity issues, as such, in the report. The extent to which recorded absence is a measure of absence depends upon the criteria by which time in classroom was defined as absence. For example, a problem could exist if a child missed three hours but was counted as absent that day. The measure for focused nursing attention is self-reported and refers to a variety of possible activities whose common elements were initiation by the nurse and attention to family context. Therefore, at best, face validity can be applied to the measure. However, while the investigators discuss the interests of persons recording data that might affect reliability, they assume them as unimportant to the study results.

The investigators report their results in narrative form and via tables that provide additional detail about the quantitative measures used. For example, the investigators compared decline in days absent in the intervention groups to the decline for the control group. The difference (1.98 days) was statistically significant ($p < .01$) on the basis of a test for differences of means for matched pairs. Thus, the investigators rightly attribute the difference to the program with reasonable assurance that results were not due to chance. Criteria for determining "real world" or clinical significance were identified in advance. These took into account possible decline in absence that could be attributed to expected yearly variation in attendance. Thus, in order for findings to be "considered meaningful from a practical point of view," 10 percent or greater decline would have to occur for the intervention group. The actual difference was greater than that.

Both the form of t-test used and the test for difference greater than might be expected minimized the likelihood that differences between groups would be exaggerated. The investigators used their professional judgment to further analyze data to see if "the intervention program was more successful for certain types of children." Their conclusion was that "a real difference cannot be attributed to the effect of sex/race group or grade level."

Part IV: Generalizability of Results

Several features of this study can be cited as justification for considering the study results as generalizable, including: (1) the investigators randomly selected six schools for the intervention from all schools (68) in a large school system with a racially mixed population; (2) the intervention group subjects were all those eligible; (3) the investigators developed the control group through a process of matching individual subjects; (4) the nurses who delivered the innovative program were the nurses already employed in the school system—they were selected because their schools were selected for the project; and (5) their training and orientation most likely did not include principles and practices for nursing different from those they had learned in school and from their practice experiences.

To my knowledge, this study has not been replicated. However, its results are cited as rationale for programs directed to high absence persons in both school and work settings.

In my view, the risk of changing practice is minimal if provision can be made to ensure continuity of essential routine services. This may require anticipatory development of alternative ways of doing things (including use of non-nurses for some activities). A current concern is that, in general, school nursing programs have been stripped of personnel such that one nurse per one to two schools no longer prevails. Nurse coverage of schools is thin or nonexistent. Thus, the decision to implement the new program may be quite difficult if it means, for example, that screening activities might not occur or that resources for communicable disease control become depleted beyond acceptable risk.

Part V: Other Factors to Consider in Utilization

My impression is that there are no particular dollar costs directly associated with implementation of the innovative program beyond those of mileage for home visits and, perhaps, increased telephone charges.

A direct replication of evaluation may not be practical because the matched pair design would need to be carefully planned. However, the measure of program effectiveness is easily obtained. In addition, the variables on which matching should occur are routinely collected data. Since age, sex, and grade were not important in this study, it is possible that one or all of these factors could be disregarded. A stronger evaluation would give attention to more extensive documentation of the independent variable and to health-related child and family characteristics.

Given the increased scarcity of nurses in school health programs, the risk of maintaining current practice may be greater now than ever before. Thus, serious attention should be given to targeting interventions to those whose history of school absence puts them at academic risk, and perhaps is a sign of health risk as well.

Effects of Health Teaching in the Workplace on Women's Knowledge, Beliefs, and Practices Regarding Breast Self-Examination

L. Joan Brailey, PhD
Associate Professor
University of Toronto
Toronto, Ontario, Canada

This study had two primary purposes: to examine the effects of group and individual teaching by nurses in the workplace on 140 female office employees' health knowledge, beliefs, and practices regarding breast self-examination and to identify factors associated with frequency of practice. Skill in technique, confidence in the skill, and frequency of breast self-examination increased significantly with both teaching formats, but there were areas of technique that needed further improvement. Perceived susceptibility to breast cancer and perceived benefits of breast self-examination increased significantly only with individual teaching; knowledge was not increased with either teaching format.

Cancer of the breast is the foremost cause of cancer deaths in North American women (American Cancer Society, 1984). One out of eleven American women, about 9%, will develop breast cancer at some time in their lives (American Cancer Society, 1984). No means have been found to prevent breast cancer, but the earlier diagnosis and treatment occur the better the long-term prognosis. There is a 5-year survival rate of 87% when breast cancer is discovered in a localized stage within breast tissue, whereas when axillary nodes are involved at the time of discovery, survival rate is reduced to 47% (American Cancer Society, 1984). Thus the best means of breast cancer control are early diagnosis and early treatment.

Regular and competent breast self-examination, when carried out as an adjuvant to annual professional examination and/or mammography, is an economical, safe, and effective means for early detection of breast abnormalities (Cole & Austin, 1981). A relationship between the self-examination and the discovery of breast cancer at a favorable clinical stage has been demonstrated (Foster et al., 1978; Greenwald et al., 1978; Huguley & Brown, 1981). Yet most women do not practice this simple routine. Percentages of women reporting regular monthly self-examinations vary from 12% (Parkinson et al., 1982) to 36% of the population (Phillips & Brennan, 1976).

Occupational health nurses are searching for effective teaching strategies to promote breast self-examination. They often have the opportunity to do either group or individual teaching. This study was conducted to compare the effectiveness of a group teaching-discussion session with individual instruction by the same nurse in the same setting.

Educational interventions to promote self-examination have included films, pamphlets, lectures, discussion groups, personal demonstration, and guided practice. Few evaluations of the effectiveness of these interventions have been done.

Use of an educational film (Hall, Goldstein, & Stein, 1977) and filmstrip (Hobbs, 1971) were effective in increasing the frequency of practice. Bond (1956), however, found that film demonstrations alone did not provide sufficient training for competent practice. Adding demonstration and guided over-the-clothing practice to group sessions resulted in more women practicing more frequently and in the prescribed fashion than a standard group teaching program with a film (Lieberman Research Inc., 1977). The guided practice was particularly effective in convincing women that breast self-examination is an easy and nonembarrassing procedure (Lieberman Research Inc., 1977).

Edwards (1980) presented instruction to 130 women at a cancer screening clinic in small groups through a short lecture and a demonstration of technique, both with the investigator serving as a model and by using a silicone breast model with implanted abnormalities. Analysis of variance of preclinic and 6-month postclinic reports of self-examination behavior revealed significant effects in frequency of self-examination, knowledge of self-examination, and confidence in ability to detect breast abnormalities.

In a study of 871 women, Bond (1956) found that the group discussion-decision method was more effective than lecture in promoting attitude change, individual commitment to action, and increased frequency of practice. Parkinson and associates (1982) found that participating in large groups of 60 or small groups of 15 or fewer did not influence breast cancer knowledge, attitudes, or behavioral change. The instructors, however, judged the small groups as more conducive to discussion of personal concerns than the larger groups.

Individual instruction by a doctor or a nurse has been demonstrated to be particularly effective in promoting competence in self-examination techniques. Phillips and Brennan (1976) compared self-examination techniques after education by film and pamphlet only with education by film, pamphlet, and individual instruction. More thorough examination was performed by those who had the additional individual instruction.

No study was found which compared the effectiveness of a group teaching-discussion session and individual instruction by the same professional in the same setting in promoting knowledge, beliefs, and practices regarding breast self-examination.

CONCEPTUAL FRAMEWORK

Many theories have been developed to explain and predict health behaviors, yet no single theoretical model has been universally accepted. The PRECEDE (predisposing, reinforcing, and enabling causes in educational diagnosis and evaluation) model for health education planning (Green et al., 1980) was chosen as the conceptual framework for this study. Figure 1 illustrates the conceptual framework, focusing attention on assumptions about relationships among factors that affect the practice of breast self-examination. The factors included in the model were those found to influence breast self-examination in previous research.

Predisposing factors arise prior to breast self-examination and provide the rationale or contribute to the motivation for the behavior. Enabling factors also arise prior to self-examination and include the skills and resources necessary to perform this health behavior. Reinforcing factors are factors subsequent to the health behavior that provide the continuing reward, incentive, or punishment of a behavior and contribute to its persistence or extinction. The predisposing, enabling, and reinforcing factors are the processes through which health education should be expected to influence health behavior.

All the predisposing, enabling, and reinforcing factors shown in Figure 1 have a collective influence on the desired behavioral outcome, the monthly practice of breast self-examination. However, the specific factors on which health education interventions might be expected to have an effect were: the predisposing factors of health knowledge and health beliefs (perceived susceptibility to breast cancer and perceived benefits of breast self-examination), and the enabling factors of skill in self-examination technique and confidence in technique skill. Therefore, in evaluating the health education interventions, these factors are measured as intermediate variables leading to frequency of breast self-examination. Although the ultimate health outcome, early detection of breast cancer is included in Figure 1, it was not measured in this study.

The two purposes of this quasiexperimental study were: (a) to examine the effects of two health education interventions by occupational health nurses on women employees' health knowledge, beliefs, skill, and confidence in practicing breast self-examination, and (b) to identify factors that influence the frequency of this practice. The two educational interventions were a group teaching/discussion session and individual instruction.

The specific questions were: What are the changes in the frequency of breast self-examination and the identified predisposing and enabling factors from the pretest to the posttest 4 months after the teaching? What is the association between each predisposing, enabling, and reinforcing factor and the frequency of breast self-examination?

METHOD

Sample

The study was carried out in one large business firm in south central Canada. The sample of women employees was selected by convenience over a 2-month period from 7000 female office staff. The women employees were included in the study if they had not received breast self-examination teaching at this workplace for at least 2 years.

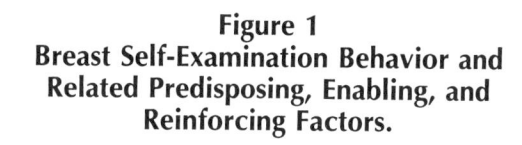

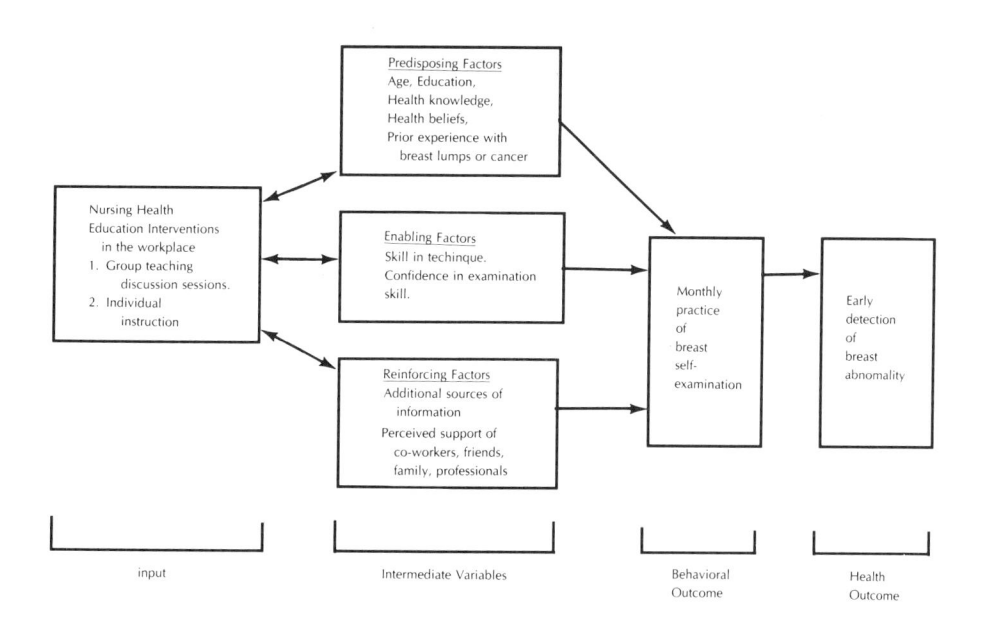

Figure 1
Breast Self-Examination Behavior and Related Predisposing, Enabling, and Reinforcing Factors.

The five nurses who conducted the teaching sessions were chosen randomly from the staff of 11 nurses employed by the firm. Each of the five nurses obtained approximately 30 women from her geographic area of the company, 10 for each of two teaching groups and 10 for a no teaching group. The refusal rate was 10%. The overall sample size was: group teaching 55; individual teaching 50; and no-teaching 49, a total of 154 women.

Instrument

A 34-item questionnaire modified from the studies of Stillman (1977) and Trotta (1980) was designed to measure the predisposing, enabling, and reinforcing factors as well as frequency of self-examination practice. In spite of the limitations of self-reported behavior, a self-administered questionnaire was the most appropriate measure for this study in the work setting, since it was inappropriate to ask the women to demonstrate their breast-examination technique. The content validity of this instrument was based on studies by Stillman (1977) and Trotta (1980). In addition, content validity of the questionnaire was assessed by four of the occupational health nurses teaching breast self-examination. No reliability can be claimed for the tool because it has not had adequate use. The questionnaire was pilot tested with 10 employees representative of the potential sample and only minor word changes for clarity were made. The questionnaire was divided into four sections.

Section I measured frequency of self-examination and posed questions covering the two enabling factors, skill in breast self-examination technique and confidence in examination skill, and the two reinforcing factors, additional sources of information and perceived support of co-workers, friends, family, and professionals. Skill in technique was scored on the basis of the woman's self-report of the steps she took the last time she examined herself. Skillful self-examination was expected to include the use of two positions (supine plus standing or sitting); inspection of breasts in a mirror; placing the hand of the examined side up behind the head; moving fingers in a regular circular direction; taking between 5 and 10 minutes for the examination; and giving a specific and appropriate time for the examination (American Cancer Society, 1975). Possible score range was 0 to 8. Confidence in examination skill was measured with two questions: How confident are you that you know the right way to do breast self-examination? How sure are you that, if you had a lump, you would find it in your self-examination? Each question was scored 0–3, giving a total range for confidence of 0–6.

In Section II, the predisposing factor, health knowledge, was measured by four questions regarding prevalence of breast cancer, incidence of malignant and benign tumours, and age of greater susceptibility to breast cancer. Each correct answer received a score of 2, partially correct 1, and incorrect 0. Possible scores were 0–8.

In Section III, another predisposing factor, health beliefs, was measured by scores obtained on the Perceived Susceptibility to Breast Cancer and the Perceived Benefits of Breast Self-examination Scales developed by Stillman (1977). Each answer received a score of 1–4 depending on the respondent's degree of agreement or disagreement. A total score was assigned to the five perceived benefit questions with a score range of 5–19. A total score was assigned to the five perceived susceptibility questions with a score range of 5–20. These ranges were divided to indicate low, moderate, or high beliefs. Section IV covered additional predisposing factors: prior experience with breast lumps or breast cancer in self or significant others, age, and education.

Procedure

The five nurses explained the study to all potential subjects and asked for their written consent to participate in the study. For group teaching, each nurse asked company supervisors to allow her to meet with 10 women for approximately 1 hour during work time. The nurse made introductory comments about breast cancer and breast self-examination; showed the 25-minute film, *It's your decision* (Canadian Cancer Society, 1979); led a discussion regarding the women's beliefs about breast cancer and self-examination; reviewed the technique shown in the film by modeling over her own clothing; and encouraged the participants to mimic the demonstration over their clothing. The Canadian Cancer Society (1980) flip-chart, *Breast self-examination*, was used as an aid in the introductory remarks and review of technique. The nurses attempted to help the women think about and understand breast cancer and breast self-examination and encouraged them to make a decision to carry out this health practice on a regular monthly basis. The Canadian Cancer Society pamphlet, *Breast self-examination: It could save your life* was given to each woman.

For individual teaching, the next 10 women who were scheduled for a routine nursing health evaluation were asked by each nurse to take part in the study and were taught individually by the nurse at the time of the health evaluation. The content and order of the teaching was the same as for group teaching except for omission of the film and inclusion of its content in the dialogue. The complete nursing health evaluation lasted approximately 1 hour. For the no-teaching group, each nurse asked the next 10 women who visited the health center for whatever reason to participate in the study by completing the questionnaires only. These women were taught breast self-examination after the study was completed.

The five nurses administered the pretest to all subjects before any teaching took place and sent the posttest questionnaire to the subjects in the company mail system 4 months after the teaching was completed. Changes in each group in the identified predisposing and enabling factors, and frequency of self-examination between the two measurements, were analyzed using Wilcoxon matched-pair signed rank tests. If more than one group showed significant change on any variable, the chi-square statistic was used to test for difference between groups. Relationships between predisposing, enabling, and reinforcing factors and frequency of practice at each measurement time were assessed using Spearman's rank correlation coefficient. All statistical tests used .05 as the preset alpha level.

RESULTS

By the time of the posttest, 4 months after the teaching interventions, 140 subjects (91% of the original sample) remained in the study; 49 from group teaching; 48 from individual teaching; 43 from the no teaching groups. The 14 subjects for whom followup data were unobtainable were demographically similar to the responding subjects. The women in the study ranged in age from 20 to 63 years with an average age of 31.1 years; the majority had completed high school.

Frequency of Practice

The women in both teaching groups and in the no teaching group showed significant increase in the frequency of practice. This result is displayed in Table 1. Of the total group, the percentage of women reporting self-examination three or more times in a 4-month period increased from 12% in the preteaching measurement to 38.5% in the postteaching measurement. Of the 97 women in the two teaching groups this percentage rose to 43%. Since subject reports of their practice of breast self-examination were classified as "never," "at least once but not in the last 4 months," "one or two times in the last 4 months," and "three or four times in the last 4 months" the following two categories were used in analyzing changes in practice: (a) positive change in frequency or maintained high practice and (b) no change, low practice or negative change in frequency. Subjects who reported their pretest practice as "three or four times in the last 4 months" and in the posttest maintained their practice at this level were placed in the maintained high practice category. Subjects who reported their pretest practice as "never," "at least once but not in the last 4 months," or "one or two times in the last 4 months," and who subsequently gave the identical response in the posttest, were placed in the category no change low practice.

Eighty-three percent of women in group teaching, 76% in individual teaching, 58% in the no-teaching group were in the positive change in frequency or maintained high practice category. A significantly greater proportion of women from

Table 1
Practice of Breast Self-Examination before and 4 Months after Teaching

Times Examined in Last 4 Months	Group Teaching Before	Group Teaching After*	Individual Teaching Before	Individual Teaching After*	No Teaching Before	No Teaching After*
0	34	11	30	3	20	10
1-2	9	19	14	22	15	19
3-4	6	19	4	23	8	14
Total	49	49	48	48	43	43

*$p < .01$.

the two teaching groups made a positive change in frequency of practice or maintained a high level of practice than from the no-teaching group, $x^2 (1.140) = 5.9, p < .05$. However there was no significant difference between the two experimental groups in the proportion of women who were in this change category, $x^2 (1,97) = .91, p > .05$. Thus it can be concluded that the teaching was effective in increasing the frequency of practice, but that there was no difference in the effectiveness of the two teaching formats.

Predisposing Factors

Pretest health knowledge scores ranged from 1 to 8, with a median of 4, and indicated lack of knowledge regarding the prevalence of breast cancer. For example, less than 25% of the women knew that only 15% of breast lumps "turn out to be breast cancer." Only 22% of the sample chose correctly the statement that 1 in 11 women will develop breast cancer. Health knowledge scores showed no significant change after teaching in any of the three groups.

Of the possible scores 5 (low)–19 (high) on perceived susceptibility to breast cancer, the sample's pretest median score was 16 with a range of 6–19. The statement, "The older I get, the more I think about the possibility of getting breast cancer someday" provoked the greatest variation along the agree-disagree continuum, with 24.4% disagreeing with this statement to some extent. The sample's pretest median score on perceived benefits of breast self-examination was 17.9 with a range of 10–20. Thirty-five women (23%) agreed with the statement: "Even though it's a good idea, I find examining/having to examine my breasts an embarrassing thing to do," while 102 women (66%) disagreed with this statement. Twenty-eight percent of the women agreed that "Examining my breast often makes/would make me worry unnecessarily about breast cancer," while 72% disagreed with this statement. Table 2 shows that, in the posttest, the women taught individually increased their scores in both of the health beliefs; perceived susceptibility to breast cancer, $T (48) = 147, p < .05$, and perceived benefits of breast self-examination, $T (48) = 54, p < .01$. Those women taught in groups and the no-teaching subjects made no changes in these beliefs.

Prior experience with breast lumps or breast cancer in themselves was low at the pretest time. Only 14 women (9.1%) previously had a lump in their breasts; none had had a mastectomy. Experience was much greater with breast lumps or breast cancer among significant others; 96 women (62%) had a family member or close friend who had either a breast lump or breast cancer. Three women discovered a breast lump between the pretest and the posttest.

Enabling Factors

Possible scores in technique skill were 0-8, with a low score indicating low skill. Scores achieved on the pretest were 0-7 with a median of 4.3. Serious deficiencies were revealed in technique, especially in timing with the menstrual period,

Table 2
Scores in Health Beliefs before and 4 Months after Teaching

Score	Group Teaching Before	Group Teaching After	Individual Teaching Before	Individual Teaching After	No Teaching Before	No Teaching After
	Perceived susceptibility to breast cancer					
6-13	11	8	9	2*	11	4
14-16	19	20	14	15	13	18
17-19	19	21	25	31	19	21
Total	49	49	48	48	43	43
	Perceived benefits of breast self-examination					
10-16	19	12	13	5**	5	6
17-18	16	21	16	17	12	17
19-20	14	16	19	26	26	20
Total	49	49	48	48	43	43

*$p < .05$. **$p < .01$.

length of time for the examination, body positions used, and inspection of the breasts in a mirror. After teaching, the members of both group teaching, $T(28) = 10.5, p < .01$, and individual teaching, $T(27) = 23.5, p < .01$, groups made significant improvements in their skill (see Table 3), but there was no significant difference between the two groups. The no teaching group's skill remained unchanged.

Although both types of teaching interventions were effective in increasing the women's skill in technique, there were still areas in their practice that needed improvement. Of the 91 women in the teaching groups reporting on their practice in the postteaching questionnaire, 37 (41%) were still examining their breasts "whenever I think of it" rather than at a regular appropriate time. More than 33% of the women were still taking less than 5 minutes for the procedure. Seventy women (77%) were now incorporating an inspection of their breasts in a mirror into their practice, but only 26 (29%) were using two positions (including the supine) for palpation of their breasts. The supine position is especially recommended to ensure that the breast tissue is spread evenly over the chest wall for easier examination. Sixty-four women (70%) were now putting one hand up behind their head while examining the breast on that side.

Subjects in both teaching, $T(30) = 17, p < .01$, and the individual teaching, $T(32) = 4.5, p < .01$, groups made gains in confidence in their skill in breast self-examination technique between the two measurement times. This result is displayed in Table 4. There was no significant difference between the two teaching groups. The no teaching group showed no improvement in confidence.

Association of Factors with Breast Self-examination

Looking at the total sample and using Spearman's rank correlation coefficient (2-tailed test), significant correlations were found between the following four factors and the frequency of breast self-examination in the pretest: three predisposing factors, perceived susceptibility to breast cancer ($r_s = .19, p < .05$); perceived benefits of breast self-examination ($r_s = .20, p < .05$); prior experience with breast lumps or breast cancer in self or significant others ($r_s = .28, p < .01$); and one enabling factor, confidence in skill in breast self-examination technique ($r_s = .29, p < .01$).

Thirty-one women had high pretest scores in both perceived susceptibility to breast cancer and perceived benefits of breast self-examination. A

Table 3
Skill in Breast Self-Examination before and 4 Months after Teaching

Score	Group Teaching Before	Group Teaching After*	Individual Teaching Before	Individual Teaching After*	No Teaching Before	No Teaching After
0-3	11	8	8	3	11	10
4-5	12	16	14	16	12	16
6-8	5	21	5	27	11	12
Not applicable°	21	4	21	2	9	5
Total	49	49	48	48	43	43

°These women had never examined their breasts.
*$p < .01$.

Table 4
Confidence in Skill in Breast Self-Examination before and 4 Months after Teaching

Score	Group Teaching Before	Group Teaching After*	Individual Teaching Before	Individual Teaching After*	No Teaching Before	No Teaching After
0-1	4	0	10	0	6	5
2-3	16	22	14	12	13	9
4-6	10	23	8	34	16	24
Not applicable°	19	4	16	2	8	5
Total	49	49	48	48	43	43

°These women had examined their breasts.
*$p < .01$.

significantly higher proportion of those women who had high scores in both beliefs had carried out breast self-examination at least once in the previous 4 months than of those women who had a high score in perceived susceptibility only, $x^2 (1.69) = 7.14$, $p < .05$. There was no significant difference in the proportion of those with high scores in both beliefs and those with a high score in perceived benefits of breast self-examination only who had carried out self-examination in the previous 4 months. In the postteaching data, the correlations of factors with the frequency of breast self-examination practice remained almost identical to preteaching correlations, except that now skill in breast self-examination technique replaced prior experience with breast lumps or breast cancer as a factor relating to frequency of practice ($r_s = .26$, $p < .01$).

Differences between Groups before Teaching

Since the subjects were not randomly assigned to groups, Kruskal-Wallis ANOVA by ranks tests were performed on the pretest data to test the hypothesis that the subjects in the three groups came from the same population. Significant differences among the three groups were found in: perceived benefits of breast self-examination, confidence in skill in technique, and frequency of breast self-examination. With each of these three variables the no teaching group showed the highest variable and group teaching showed the lowest. The two teaching groups did not differ significantly. No differences among the three groups were found in age, education, health knowledge, perceived susceptibility to breast cancer, prior experience with breast lumps or breast cancer, skill in technique, number of additional sources of learning, or number of sources of perceived support.

DISCUSSION

Both group and individual health teaching interventions led to significant increases in women's frequency of breast self-examination, skill in the technique, and confidence in their skill. Individual health teaching also was effective in increasing women's perceived susceptibility to breast cancer and perceived benefits of breast self-examination. It was unexpected that those taught individually would show greater gains in these health beliefs than those taught in a group. Green and Roberts (1974), in a review of health education methods, concluded that group discussion has the potential for imparting a sense of realism about susceptibility, severity, and efficacy, because these beliefs are easier to internalize in the company of others and easier to rationalize away when one is faced with them alone. Bond (1956) also found group discussion effective in attitude change toward examining one's breasts. Nurses should continue with teaching breast self-examination both in groups and on an individual basis until further research indicates that one method is more effective than the other in promoting competent monthly practice of self-examination.

The importance of health beliefs in the promotion of health behaviors requires further investigation. The pretest scores indicate that the women already had quite realistic beliefs before teaching took place. The association between perceived susceptibility to breast cancer and frequency of self-examination before teaching was statistically significant, yet it is notable that 41 subjects (28%) with high scores (17-19) on perceived susceptibility to breast cancer had not examined their breasts once in the previous 4 months. Similarly, although the correlation between the scores on the perceived benefits of breast self-examination and the frequency of practice reached statistical significance, there were 32 women (21%) who had very high scores (19-20) on perceived benefits of breast self-examination who had not examined their breasts in the previous 4 months. These are almost identical findings to those of Stillman (1977) and Schleuter (1982).

Previous research has revealed that perceptions of susceptibility to a disease and benefits of a health action interact to exert a joint influence on health-related behaviors (Kirscht, Becker, & Eveland, 1976; Rosenstock, 1974). This study demonstrated that as many women with a high score on perceived benefits of breast self-examination alone as with high scores on both beliefs examined their breasts. Perhaps if one perceives the benefit of breast self-examination, one does not need to feel personally susceptible to breast cancer to make self-examination a regular health practice. This finding was supported by Hallal's (1982) study. Nurses should stress the benefits of breast self-examination as a lifelong health habit in their teaching.

Since level of health knowledge did not show a significant correlation with frequency of practice, one could conclude that it is not important to try to raise the level of knowledge related to the incidence of breast cancer. Yet research has shown that unwarranted fear and anxiety due to lack of knowledge may cause a delay in seeking medical attention for breast symptoms (Magarey, Todd, & Blizard, 1977). Thus improving knowledge is important even if the knowledge level does not influence the practice of breast self-examination.

Other researchers also reported concern about the lack of skill demonstrated by subjects after teaching (Celentano & Holtzman, 1983; Feldman, Carter, & Nicostri, 1981; Hall, 1981; Zapka & Mamon, 1982). Hall (1981) concluded that competent technique is not easily adopted even with a class and practice session. She recommended follow-up teaching, redemonstration of technique, and reinforcement of both technique and practice. The present study would support these recommendations. Assessments of women's skills should be carried out after teaching sessions and follow-up teaching instituted as necessary.

Confidence in technique, an enabling factor, had a low but significant relationship to frequency of practice in the posttest. Edwards (1980) also found confidence level related to the frequency of practice. Mahoney (1977) concluded that a woman's confidence in her skill in breast self-examination was the "only significant criterion" in the success of breast self-examination promotion. Bandura (1977) emphasized the importance of confidence in one's skill or "efficacy expectations" in determining whether an individual will adopt and persist with any health behavior. Thus a woman will not likely persist with regular monthly practice unless she is confident that she is carrying out the technique correctly, and is confident she would discover an abnormality if present. Nurses, therefore, should question women regarding confidence in their skill after teaching has taken place and give reinforcement when necessary.

In general, the study results support the conceptual framework selected for the study. It would be premature to delete any predisposing, enabling, or reinforcing factors which did not correlate with the frequency of self-examination. Further research with other samples of women may support retention of all the factors in the framework.

It is clear that the findings of this study are limited by the purposive sample selection, use of self-report as a measure of behavior, lack of assessed reliability of the instrument, and the brief 4-month measurement period. However, the study has contributed to nursing knowledge regarding the effects of two teaching interventions by occupational health nurses in one work setting, on the frequency of breast self-examination, and the predisposing, enabling, and reinforcing factors associated with this health practice. Findings suggest that nurses explore other teaching strategies that might further increase the frequency of and competency in this health behavior.

REFERENCES

American Cancer Society. (1975). *How to examine your breasts*. New York: The Author.

American Cancer Society. (1984). *Cancer facts and figures*. New York: The Author.

Bandura, A. (1977). Self-efficacy: Toward a unifying theory of behavioral change. *Psychological Review, 84*, 191–215.

Bond, B. W. (1956). *Group discussion-decision*. Minneapolis: MN: Department of Health.

Canadian Cancer Society (Producer). (1979). *It's your decision* (Film). Toronto: Canadian Cancer Society.

Canadian Cancer Society. (1980). *Breast self-examination* (Flip-chart). Toronto: Canadian Cancer Society.

Celentano, D. D., & Holtzman, D. (1983). Breast self-examination competency: An analysis of self-reported practice and associated characteristics. *American Journal of Public Health, 73*, 1321–1326.

Cole, P., & Austin, H. (1981). Breast self-examination: An adjuvant to early cancer detection. *American Journal of Public Health, 71*, 572–574.

Edwards, V. (1980). Changing breast self-examination behavior. *Nursing Research, 29*, 301–306.

Feldman, J. G., Carter, A. C., & Nicostri, A. D. (1981). Breast self-examination, relationship to stage of breast cancer at diagnosis. *Cancer, 47*, 2740–2745.

Foster, R. S., Lang, S. P., Costanza, M. C., Worden, J. K., Haines, C. R., & Yates, J. W. (1978). Breast self-examination practices and breast cancer stage. *The New England Journal of Medicine, 299*, 265–270.

Green, L. W., Kreuter, M. W., Deeds, S. G., & Partridge, K. B. (1980). *Health education planning. A diagnostic approach*. Palo Alto, CA: Mayfield Publishing.

Green, L. W., & Roberts, B. J. (1974). The research literature on why women delay in seeking medical care for breast symptoms. *Health Education Monographs, 2*, 129–177.

Greenwald, P., Nasca, P. C., Lawrence, C. E., Horton, J., McGarrah, R. P., Gabriele, T., & Carlton, K. (1978). Estimated effect of breast self-examination and routine physician examinations on breast cancer mortality. *The New England Journal of Medicine, 299*, 271–273.

Hall, J. A. (1981). Technique of breast self-examination. In American Cancer Society, *Proceedings of Second Conference on Cancer Nursing Research* (p. 14–16). Seattle: University of Washington.

Hall, D. C., Goldstein, M. K., & Stein, G. H. (1977). Progress in manual breast examination. *Cancer, 40,* 364–370.

Hallal, J. C. (1982). The relationship of health beliefs, health locus of control, and self concept to the practice of breast self-examination in adult women. *Nursing Research, 31,* 137–142.

Hobbs, P. (1971). Evaluation of a teaching programme of breast self-examination. *International Journal of Health Education, 14,* 189–195.

Huguley, C. M., & Brown, R. L. (1981). The value of breast self-examination, *Cancer, 47,* 989–995.

Kirscht, J. P., Becker, M. H., & Eveland, J. P. (1976). Psychological and social factors as predictors of medical behavior. *Medical Care, 14,* 422–431.

Lieberman Research, Inc. (1977). A study of the effectiveness of alternative breast cancer public education programs. Summary report. Prepared for the American Cancer Society, New York.

Magarey, C. J., Todd, P. B., & Blizard, P. J. (1977). Psychosocial factors influencing delay and breast self-examination in women with symptoms of breast cancer. *Social Science & Medicine, 11,* 229–232.

Mahoney, L. J. (1977). Early diagnosis of breast cancer. The breast self-examination problem. *Canadian Family Physician, 23,* 481–483.

Parkinson, R. S., Denniston, R. W., Baugh, T., Dunn, J. P., & Schwartz, T. L. (1982). Breast cancer: Health education in the workplace. *Health Education Quarterly, 9,* 61–72.

Phillips, A. J., & Brennan, M. E. (1976). Reactions of Canadian women to Pap tests and breast self-examination. *Canadian Family Physician, 22,* 1261–1264.

Rosenstock, I. M. (1974). The health belief model and preventive health behavior. *Health Education Monographs, 2,* 354–386.

Schleuter, L. A. (1982). Knowledge and beliefs about breast cancer and breast self-examination among athletic and nonathletic women. *Nursing Research, 31,* 348–353.

Stillman, M. J. (1977). Women's health beliefs about breast cancer and cancer self-examination. *Nursing Research, 26,* 121–127.

Trotta, P. (1980). Breast self-examination: Factors influencing compliance. *Oncology Nursing Forum, 7*(3), 12–17.

Zapka, J. G., & Mamon, J. A. (1982). Integration of theory, practitioner standards, literature findings and baseline data: A case study in planning breast self-examination education. *Health Education Quarterly, 9,* 330–356.

This article is printed with permission of *Research in Nursing and Health*. Copyright © 1986 John Wiley & Sons.

Original article:
Brailey, L. J. (1986). Effects of health teaching in the workplace on women's knowledge, beliefs, and practices regarding breast self-examination. *Research in Nursing & Health*, 9, 223–231.

CRITIQUE BY: JEAN REGIER, BSN, RN

Part I: Clinical Relevance

In this quasiexperimental study, the investigator addressed two research questions. First, what is the change in frequency of breast self-examination from the pretest to the posttest, a period of four months. This question included changes in the identified predisposing and enabling factors during the same period. Second, what is the association between each predisposing, enabling, and reinforcing factor and the frequency of breast self-examination? Of special concern to the investigator are the specific issues relevant to nursing practice: the multiplicity of factors that influence people's behavior and, therefore, the practice of primary prevention behaviors.

This study tests the PRECEDE (predisposing, reinforcing, and enabling causes in educational diagnosis and evaluation) model for health education planning. The investigator describes the conceptual framework in the text and illustrates it in a figure. The predisposing, reinforcing, and enabling factors included in the model were those found to influence breast self-examination (BSE) in previous research. The investigator assumed this prior research as thorough, reliable, and valid. Health education strategies could potentially be guided by this model in nursing practice.

The two educational interventions implemented were group and individual instruction on BSE. For both groups, the teaching sessions lasted approximately one hour and included the same content in a discussion and demonstration format. Because these interventions fall within the scope of nursing practice, immediate potential exists for their use. In addition, an individual nurse may decide to try these interventions without permission or approval from a physician or other health care professional.

The investigator measured the questionnaire outcomes by scoring the pretest and posttest responses. The 34-item self-administered questionnaire was modified from previous research. The questions required a rank order response. The use of this questionnaire would be beneficial because it measures factors associated with the frequency of practicing BSE. Again, since a nurse can make an independent decision for its use, this measure could easily be used in practice.

This reviewer appreciated the investigator's study of multiple factors and her attempt to understand and explain the practice of positive health behaviors. This research study dealt with health teaching strategies that potentially increase the frequency of breast self-examination. Regular and competent BSE increases the likelihood of early detection of breast abnormalities, which lead to earlier detection and treatment of cancer. Specifically, it would seem that the findings could potentially be applied to testicular self-examination, and generally, to other preventive health practices.

In general, potential exists for both the community health nurse as well as nurses in other clinical settings to make the independent decision to use these health education techniques and to measure the outcomes by using the questionnaire.

Part II: Conceptualization and Internal Consistency

Brailey states that the two purposes of this quasiexperimental study were: "to examine the effects of two health education interventions by occupational health nurses on women employees' health knowledge, beliefs, skill, and confidence in practicing breast self-examination, and to identify factors that influence the frequency of this practice." The specific study questions arise directly from these two stated purposes. In general, from the introductory paragraphs through the results/discussion sections, the report has a logical flow. The conceptualization has surface plausibility but an awkward writing style makes it difficult to develop a true understanding of the model.

Because early diagnosis and treatment are empirically determined to be the best means of breast cancer control, justification exists for initiation of this type of study. BSE is an effective adjuvant to annual physical examination or mammography to detect breast abnormalities. The investigator relates the study questions to this justification by way of this rationale: they attempt to explore what influence the intermediate variables have on the frequency of BSE. The investigator also describes the conceptual framework in the introductory paragraphs. However, the illustration she provides, rather than her description, presents the clearest understanding of the process.

The investigator's study answered the questions that were initially presented. Her conclusions were consistent with the type of research questions and methods of the study. The questionnaire she developed was a suitable vehicle to answer questions of frequency and associated factors related to BSE. Data collection procedures are such that they should not interfere with the usual practice of nursing. The independent variables (health education interventions) and dependent variable (monthly practice of BSE) are logically related. The sample subjects are consistent with the population of interest, working women. The testing tool is likely to measure the phenomenon of interest because it directs questions to the intermediate variables.

Part III: Believability of Results

This study purported to test the effects of two independent variables (group and individual teaching) on the dependent variable (monthly practice of BSE). The type of data collected is primarily quantitative; that is, the manipulation of numerical data through statistical procedures for the purpose of describing phenomena of interest or assessing the magnitude and reliability of relationships among them (Polit & Hungler, 1985).

The investigator selected a convenience sample of 154 women from a total of 7000 female office staff, all employees at one large business firm in south central Canada. To further limit her study sample, she included subjects only if they had not received self-breast examination teaching during the past two years at this particular work place. The investigator made an assessment of sample characteristics but offered no analysis of their potential influence. She chose nurses randomly out of all the nurses employed by the company. Unfortunately, she did not discuss potential biases or intervening variables.

The investigator claimed that the 34-item questionnaire designed to measure BSE had content validity based on use in previous studies, but she provided no description or evaluation of that research. Therefore, one would have to determine content validity from the references provided. In addition, the investigator claimed content validity by having four of the five occupational health nurses, who participated in teaching the self-breast exam, evaluate the tool. The study also provides an adequate description of how the tool was put together, the type of questions it contained, and the rank order scaling of the responses.

On the other hand, the investigator states, "no reliability can be claimed for the tool because it has not had adequate use," which points to a seeming contradiction between content and tool validity. In addition, she fails to provide description of the procedures used for achieving consistency of content and format between the five nurses. In general, however, the investigator stays within the parameters of her stated objectives and proposed study, but the reliability of her tool remains unknown.

Brailey did not apply randomization to the three experimental groups, only to the selection of the five nurses involved in the teaching. Her interchangeable use of convenience sample and purpose sample confused this reviewer according to definitions provided by Polit and Hungler (1985). Brailey analyzed differences between groups before they received teaching by using a Kruskal-Wallis ANOVA by ranks test, but did not control for possible initial differences in the groups in the sampling procedure. The control group received no treatment but this reviewer was pleased they received teaching after the study was completed. It seems ethically sound to provide health information that could potentially save a woman's life, rather than not providing it just because of the boundaries of a particular research study.

The statistics used appear to be appropriate for the type of data collected and the kind of research questions asked. Spearman's rank correlation coefficient (designed for two sets of ranks) is appropriate. However, since I am not familiar with a Kruskal-Wallis by ranks test, I would need to seek further consultation on the appropriateness of its use.

Brailey produced several statistically significant findings but offered no precise explanation of them. Both group and individual health teaching interventions led to significant increases in women's frequency of breast self-examination, skill in the technique, and confidence in their skill. Individual health teaching also was effective in increasing women's perceived susceptibility to breast cancer and perceived benefits of breast self-examination. However, due to the study design, Brailey could have produced results just by instituting it, which is known as the Hawthorne effect. Since Brailey also based her data on self-report, the significant increase in frequency of breast self-examination could be a result of other factors she did not account for, such as wanting to please the investigator or reporting what is thought to be wanted and not what is necessarily true.

An unexpected finding appeared in the study: those taught individually showed more significant positive changes in their scores related to health beliefs (perceived susceptibility and perceived benefits) than those taught in a group. In addition, the investigator cited studies which both supported and disagreed with her findings, which remain inconclusive. Therefore, this reviewer would tend to agree with Brailey's conclusion that "the importance of health beliefs in the promotion of health behaviors requires further investigation." To conclude from the study design, other explanations for these results are possible. The pretest/posttest tool cannot be claimed as reliable, the sample was not selected by a random procedure, nor does its use of self-report of behavior necessarily measure true behavior.

Part IV: Generalizability of Results

Health teaching, the procedure employed in this study, is an intervention typically implemented in current nursing practice. The sample population were women who worked in a large business in Canada. Considerable similarity exists between the study's sample population and the target population of working women in general. The nurses actually administering the teaching and testing were practicing nurses of that particular setting. They were performing functions that were basically the same as what they typically did in that setting and they were not specially trained for this study.

Numerous studies that relate to this topic have been done but I am unaware of research that has replicated this particular study. I am also unfamiliar with comparable studies that address this particular problem.

Part V: Other Factors to Consider in Utilization

It would be feasible to repeat, evaluate, and implement these health education interventions into nursing practice. Because teaching increased reported BSE, I would feel free to use either teaching or BSE without compromising effectiveness regarding behavioral outcome. However, Brailey's findings are limited by the flaws in her study design: the nonrandomized sample selection procedure, the use of self-report, and the lack of reliability of the assessment tool. Nonetheless, the study has provided nursing information related to two health education interventions in the work setting and the intermediate variables associated with the frequency of practice of BSE.

Only minimal risk is involved in the implementation of this teaching intervention. Because current nursing practice already employs these teaching techniques, little change is required in practice routines. Two components of feasibility are cost and benefit. Here, the only cost involved would be the expenditure of time by the instructor. The study findings indicate that one method of teaching is not more effective than the other. However, this raises a further question: is it more efficient to teach ten people in one hour or one person in the same amount of time?

Increased frequency of BSE potentially leads to earlier detection of breast abnormalities. Earlier detection of breast abnormalities leads to earlier detection and treatment of breast cancer. As this study indicates, more research needs to be done to examine teaching strategies which would be effective in increasing behavioral outcomes regarding positive health behaviors.

REFERENCES

Polit, D. F., & Hungler, B. P. (1985). *Essentials of nursing research: Methods and applications.* Philadelphia: Lippincott.

Original article:
Brailey, L. J. (1986). Effects of health teaching in the workplace on women's knowledge, beliefs, and practices regarding breast self-examination. *Practice in Nursing & Health, 9*, 223–231.

CRITIQUE BY: CAROLINE McCOY WHITE, DrPH, RN

This study compares the effects of a group method for health teaching to those from a program of individual teaching. Breast self-examination, the focus of the teaching, can assist in early detection of breast cancer, which may lead to better survival for affected women. Since one in eleven women can be expected to develop breast cancer, the topic is clearly relevant. As employers develop more interest in health promotion programs, there is need for the type of research reported here for it provides the basis for decisions about teaching strategy in the workplace.

Part I: Clinical Relevance

This study addresses a common practice problem: What method will effectively and efficiently convey health information to clients? Nurses are often expected to teach about breast self-examination. They are expected to teach about other practices that would lead to early detection of disease or change in health-related behaviors. This study could help the nurse decide whether to use what is often considered a more costly individual approach or to use a possibly less costly (at least in terms of the nurse's time) group approach. Moreover, this study alerts the nurse to (1) possibly relevant factors to include in a program of teaching about breast self-examination and (2) an instrument that could be the basis for evaluation of a similar program.

The nurse has clear authority—and, in fact, is generally expected—to assist well persons by providing health information that will enable them to initiate lifestyle changes and other behaviors that have as their likely outcome better health. In many settings, including occupational health settings, nurses are responsible to others (nurses and non-nurses) for the way in which they allocate themselves as resources to specific programs and activities that comprise their contribution to the health effort of the organization. From the perspective of resource allocation, the individual nurse seeking to implement a practice change on the basis of Brailey's study probably needs to consult others. This is necessary because shifts in resource allocation created by one practice change are likely to impact resource allocations for other nursing activities. Moreover, nurses in workplaces must consider work schedules (involving both on and off the job time) and, possibly, the nature of the workers' union contract specifications with regard to on-the-job health programs.

In her study, Brailey included two treatment groups and one control group. She compared two nursing interventions, which she also compared to what she described as no intervention. Both interventions are within the scope of usual nursing practice and the competence of recent baccalaureate graduates. Both interventions involve focused teaching. The investigator highlighted the difference between the two interventions by way of group size: one method used an individual approach (nurse to subject) and the other used a group approach (nurse to 10 subjects). However, the investigator did not highlight an additional difference in method: women in the group session saw a film; for those in the individual teaching intervention "the content and order of the teaching was the same as for the group teaching except for omission of the film and inclusion of its content in the dialogue." The pretest received by the control group would be considered an intervention, as well (the awareness of individuals can be changed by the content of questionnaires); however, the investigator did not consider this possible influence in her discussion of the posttest scores of women in the control group.

Brailey used the same 34-item measure for the pretest and posttest. The use of this measure, or one similar, is within the scope of nursing practice. The nurse could make an independent decision regarding its use, though it would be necessary to contact the investigator for a copy since the instrument is not presented in the report.

In the absence of evidence to the contrary, I would consider the interventions explored in this study about breast self-examination relevant to other areas of health teaching. Three factors interrelate to support this view. First, all health-related behaviors have personal meanings that may make individual teaching more appropriate than group teaching. Second, individuals are often influenced by the experience of others and their common culture. Third, I am willing to assume that most other topics are less "threatening" than the topic of concern for this study: the potentially very significant concerns of touching one's breasts and fear of cancer.

Part II: Conceptualization and Internal Consistency

As the practical reason for conducting her study, Brailey cites the lack of clear evidence on which to plan health teaching programs. My reading of the literature supports Brailey's contention. In addition, Brailey presents a literature review that highlights the results of several studies.

Programs of health teaching are based on the assumption that the attitudes, knowledge, and behavior of individuals can change as a consequence of exposure to information that is conveyed by the educator and educational package. It is likely that the specific trigger for changes varies according to individual and environmental factors, the subject matter, the change required, and the nature of the teaching situation. With regard to the teaching situation, the individual being taught may respond to the factual information or to whatever else he or she may experience during the teaching session (e.g., the expression of interest by a significant other).

The conceptual framework for this study is widely used in health education. Specifically, I refer to the PRECEDE model (predisposing, reinforcing, and enabling causes in education diagnosis and evaluation). Also part of the framework, but not of the health belief model, is the subject's ability to perform the necessary actions. In this way, Brailey derives study variables directly from the framework and logically relates both independent and dependent variables. Since the subject of concern is breast self-examination, the subjects are all women.

In this study, mode of teaching comprises the independent variable. The practice of breast self-examination comprises the major dependent variable. Also incorporated into the study are variables relating to elements of the health belief model (e.g., perceived susceptibility) that might be expected to change as a consequence of a health teaching program. In addition, these same variables could influence the variable of major interest (practice of breast self-examination) at both pretest and posttest.

There are two major conceptual and methodological dilemmas that confront the investigator designing studies evaluating the effects of health teaching, however. The first dilemma concerns time: what is the appropriate time(s) to assess outcomes, considering both the nature of the intervention and its purpose; right after exposure to the intervention or sometime later? Brailey administers the posttest to subjects in all three groups four months after the teaching occurred but does not explain her rationale. The second dilemma concerns behavior: how does one measure the actual change in behavior. In many studies, only knowledge change is assessed, or only attitudinal change with regard to possible motivating factors, or only self-report of behavioral change. In contrast, Brailey measures all three categories of change. However, all are proxy measures, substituting for the variable of most concern, the actual behavior of subjects. We cannot know for certain their behavior, let alone its ultimate impact on their health, on the basis of pen and pencil test, or verbal report.

Numerous studies of the impact of educational programs use pen and pencil tests. In terms of usual practice in occupational health nursing, the instrument Brailey used collected more information relevant to BSE practices in a more standardized way than would occur in a clinic visit. In itself, this probably does not bias results. However, a variety of factors could lead subjects to misrepresent their attitudes and behaviors.

The large number of variables measured, the language of the frameworks used in health education, and the investigator's extensive presentation of results make the report slow reading. However, Brailey does follow the standard format for presentation of research, uses terms consistently, and inserts quotations from informants as examples of responses. In general, Brailey also relates all components of the report to one another.

Part III: Believability of Results

This study purported to test the effects of a nursing intervention on the attitudes and beliefs of women relevant to breast self-examination (BSE) and their reported practice of BSE. The investigator selected 140 of 7000 female office staff employed by a large company as subjects for the study. Their age range was 20–63 years (mean 31.1 years). The majority were high school graduates.

To identify which 5 of 11 nurses employed in the workplace would implement the program with employees for whom they were responsible, Brailey used a random procedure. To assign subjects to treatment and control groups, Brailey used a convenience procedure based on the order in which women came to seek services for various health matters: the first 10 were assigned to the group teaching; the next 10 to individual teaching; and the next 10 to the control group. Women were not eligible for the study if they had received BSE teaching at that workplace in the last two years. The control group received individual teaching at the end of the data collection period. It is not clear why a random procedure was not used here.

It is difficult to identify what factor(s) were operating to influence the characteristics of subjects in the three groups. Nonetheless, Brailey's comparison of pretest scores for the groups on all variables produced statistically significant differences between the control group and the treatment groups, but not between the treatment groups.

Initial differences in the three groups, for those variables where there were differences (perceived benefits of BSE, confidence in technique, and frequency of BSE), are presented as a relation between posttest and pretest scores. The relative (not absolute) change was used to establish teaching impact.

In her study, Brailey used an instrument modified from those used by two other researchers in studies of BSE. However, because it has not had adequate use, Brailey claims no reliability for the tool. Nor does Brailey report any reliability tests that she might have made. Nonetheless, Brailey attributes content validity to the instrument on the basis of its development by two other researchers and a review by four of the five nurses doing the teaching. In addition, she mentions that the American Cancer Society was the source of the skill questions.

There were no statistically significant differences in the practice of BSE when the reports of women exposed to the two teaching methods were compared. Given ordinal data and the nonrandom sampling procedure, the chi square statistic was appropriate. The differences therein did not appear clinically significant either, and Brailey made no claim for such. However, those women who experienced the teaching did have statistically significant increases in frequency in practice of BSE and skill from those in the control group. These differences lend support to the idea that teaching can influence beliefs and practices with regard to breast self-examination.

Brailey extensively analyzed the study findings in terms of before and after measures and relationships between the predisposing and reinforcing variables taken two at a time. However, if Brailey had used a larger sample, she would have been able to make a more extensive statistical analysis. This would have allowed one to know if more complex relationships among the variables existed. It also would have given one greater confidence in the conclusions. For example, it would have been possible to know if initial differences on variables different from those compared on a pretest posttest basis influenced the posttest scores. In the absence of such knowledge, Brailey's analysis leaves me curious whether factors associated with the nurses' teaching effectiveness (in each of the modes of teaching) had any impact on results. (This seems relevant given that Brailey indicates that a unique feature of this study is that the same nurse did both group and individual teaching.)

Such problems notwithstanding, Brailey did assess some potentially important intervening variables (e.g., womens' prior experience with breast lumps; which nurse did the teaching). However, these were not incorporated into the statistical analysis to see if they influenced results. Brailey also failed to assess several potentially important intervening variables (e.g., experience of BSE teaching at other than the workplace within the last two years; participant satisfaction with the teaching session).

Brailey's conclusions—that teaching makes a difference, but that there is no evidence that supports selecting either group or individual teaching—are reasonable given the data and methods. Further, Brailey uses the data to justify continued inclusion of all health belief model content in teaching programs. This is reasonable in light of what is known from this and other studies. However, it may not be reasonable if time for teaching is limited. In that case, it may be more important to ensure that more emphasis is given to ensuring that technique is taught and confidence building is attended to. Discussing perceived susceptibility to breast cancer and perceived benefit from engaging in BSE may not be important since, even when these predisposing factors are present, the enabling factors may not be.

Part IV: Generalizability of Results

The sample and interventions of this study are generally similar to those in most workplaces. That the study was done in Canada probably is not significant since I assume the population studied was in the English-speaking part of the country. That the population is working and of wide age range, although weighted toward the younger ages, and not college educated, would make it similar to many working populations in the United States. It is possible that the women coming to the nurse were different from those in the workplace, perhaps being more motivated regarding health or more illness prone. Nothing is said about any special preparation undertaken by the nurses conducting the intervention. My sense is that if nurses were to incorporate this intervention into their practice, they would require some review regarding breast cancer and breast self-examination.

The cumulated findings from studies of other health education programs are as inconclusive as the present study. In addition, this study has not been replicated to the best of my knowledge.

Part V: Other Factors to Consider in Utilization

The practices evaluated by this study are discrete health teaching "packages." Nurses and all teachers are exhorted to evaluate outcomes. The measures used in this study are straight-forward and require no special resources, once the instrument is obtained. However, even these tests require paper and are more easily scored and analyzed— especially for large groups—if there is an automated score reader or a microcomputer to develop frequency distributions and cross-tabulations. What must be appreciated is the limitation of pen and pencil testing as indication of actual behavior.

An important factor to consider when deciding to implement a teaching program is the comparative cost and effectiveness of the various modes of teaching suitable for the purpose. If there are no differences, as this study leads one to believe, then comparative costs of the modes should be assessed and strategies implemented on the basis of least cost. Among the costs to be weighed are (1) nurse time in preparation, delivery of content, and organizing attendance, and (2) worker time in attendance and disruption to schedules and work processes. In other words, the findings of the study allow the nurse to implement either group or individual teaching regarding breast self-examination without worry that one method or the other is more likely to have less good outcomes for the learners. Thus, method of teaching could be selected on the basis of what additional "goods" might be realized through use of one method rather than another.

Primary Prevention Behaviors: The Female-headed, One-parent Family

Mary E. Duffy, PhD
Assistant Professor
College of Nursing
Brigham Young University
Salt Lake City, UT

The purpose of this study was to describe the primary prevention behaviors of 59 female-headed, one-parent families and the barriers which deter their practice. Two interviews, a health diary, and a card sort were used for data collection. Descriptive statistics and content analysis were used to analyze the qualitative data. Nutrition was the behavior the families felt was most important for maintaining health. Time was the major barrier to primary prevention practices. A relationship was found between the family's ability to change and grow and their practice of primary prevention behaviors. Families that consciously risked lifestyle changes also were willing to try to incorporate primary prevention behaviors. On the contrary, families with stagnant lifestyles expressed the desire to change their primary prevention behaviors but made no visible attempt to do so.

The one-parent family headed by a woman culturally is perceived as "less than" the family ideal (Norbeck & Sheiner, 1982; Richardson & Pfeiffenberger, 1983). Many innuendos evolve from that perception which affect the woman and her children. Two such myths are relevant to the health of the one-parent family members: (a) The one-parent family generally is neglectful of their health and responds only to acute care needs (Patton, Harvill, & Michal, 1981). (b) A woman is not worthy without a man. This latter perception degrades a woman's feelings about herself and influences the formal and informal societal responses to the one-parent family headed by a woman (Worrell & Garret-Fulks, 1983).

The practice of primary prevention behaviors in the female-headed, one-parent family is an uninvestigated phenomenon. The literature on female-headed, one-parent families suggests that stressors in these families differ qualitatively and quantitatively from those in other family types (Berman & Turk, 1981; Herman, 1977; Horowitz & Purdue, 1977; Smith, 1980). The interaction between stressors and primary prevention practices in these families is unknown. The purpose of this study was to investigate the practice of primary prevention behaviors within the context of the one-parent family headed by a woman.

Women are neither prepared nor expected to assume the role of head of the household (Duffy, 1982). Gender gaps in salaries, career commitments, and occupational choices thwart women's inherent abilities to succeed in this role. The stressors from decreased economic resources, increased parental responsibilities, and isolation place the one-parent family at a greater psychological risk than the two-parent family experiencing the same stressors (Pearlin & Johnson, 1977). These stressors, coupled with the significance in this society of being unmarried, place the female head of a one-parent family at the greatest risk of depression (Herman, 1977; Jacobsen, 1980; Pearlin & Johnson, 1977).

Although the female-headed, one-parent family is experiencing greater acceptance by society (Norbeck & Sheiner, 1982), the emphasis of health care has been on existing problems rather than on preventive care and normalcy (Schorr & Moen, 1980). Until recently, there have been two major limitations to research into the one-parent family. According to Norbeck and Sheiner (1982), the research focus has been on the needs or satisfaction of the one-parent family rather than functioning patterns. The patterns of coping and adaptation were described as passive processes, ignoring the family's active self-help behaviors (Berman & Turk, 1981). The samples for these studies usually were drawn from a clinical population, however. Such samples lend credence to the perception that the one-parent family is pathological. More recently studied samples were drawn from a nonclinical population and the one-parent family was found to be a functional structure (Brandwein, Brown, & Fox, 1974; Burgess, 1970; Cherlin & Furstenberg, 1982; Le Masters, 1971; Malouf, 1979; McCord, McCord, & Thurber, 1962). Variables such as socioeconomic status, parenting skills, and family size were more potent influences in child development than the absence of a father.

The female-headed, one-parent family represents a major family form. The most recent predictions indicate that by the year 2000, 50% of all children will spend some time in a one-parent family before the age of 18 (Cherlin & Furstenberg, 1982). Therefore, it is necessary to understand the potential relationship between the contextual or environmental factors of the female-headed, one-parent family and the family's practice of primary prevention behaviors.

Health transcends all aspects of family functioning. Patton, Harvill, and Michal (1981) surveyed a sample of Parents Without Partners as to their attitudes toward health issues. Time, finances, and lack of information were problems confronting the one-parent family. First, the cost of health care contributed to a decrease in the use of health care services, particularly for prevention or routine care. Second, the need for health information increased with decreased service use. Third, other responsibilities—work or school—complicated the single parent's ability to care for an ill child or to make health care appointments.

Family research on primary prevention behaviors has focused on medically sanctioned activities: immunizations, physical examinations, medication regimens, dental care, diet plans, and so forth. These behaviors are disease specific and prescribed by a professional member of the health care team. Harris and Guten (1979) assumed that everyone engages in self-perceived, health-protective, behaviors whether medically approved or not. When they asked 842 individuals, "What are the three most important things you do to protect your health?", only 2.5% reported that they did not take any health-protective actions. Nutrition, sleep, and exercise were cited with the highest frequencies.

This study was based on three factors: the paucity of research on the practice of health behaviors in female-headed one-parent families, the intensity of reported stress in these families, and the need to examine the relationships between the family structure, functions, health practices, and lifestyles (Friedman, 1981). Two research questions that emerged were addressed:

1. What primary prevention behaviors are practiced by the members of female-headed, one-parent families?
2. What barriers prevent the family from practicing primary prevention behaviors regularly?

The following definitions guided the investigation:

1. Primary prevention behaviors: Those health practices to promote health or prevent illness identified by the woman for her family (Leavell & Clark, 1965; Pender, 1982).

2. Barriers influencing primary prevention practices: Those factors identified by the woman as deterrents to the family's practice of primary prevention behaviors.

METHOD

Sample

Families who met the following criteria were invited to participate in the study: A unit consisting of a woman and her children in which the woman stated she was the head of the household and there was no male residing in the home; the family was created by separation, divorce, death, or no legal marriage; and the female parent was at least 18 years old and English speaking. Community social service agencies and the participants themselves were sources of families for this study. The staff at the community agencies read a letter of explanation to each potential participant. Women interested in participating in the study were referred to the researcher for further information. Also, in conjunction with a presentation by the researcher at the agencies, a verbal explanation of the study was given and volunteers signed a form indicating willingness to be contacted by the researcher. A similar procedure was followed when participants were asked to suggest women for the study. Of the women the researcher contacted, 86% agreed to participate in the study.

Instruments

There were four instruments used for data collection: two interview guides, a health diary, and a card sort. Interview Guide 1 had three areas. The demographic data collected in section one included religion, length of time as a one-parent family, and income source and amount. The second area of the interview used open-ended questions to understand the meaning, for the family, of living in a one-parent family headed by a woman. The questions focused on how the woman felt heading a one-parent family, what her experiences had been in this role, how she felt about herself, and what effect the experience had on the children. The third and last area on family health status and behaviors included questions on the family's health, their health practices, their source for health information, the barriers to desired health practices, and so forth. Interview Guide 2 built on the first interview guide and focused on the last two areas of Interview Guide 1. Each woman was asked to identify the three most important things her family did to maintain health, what her major concerns were for her family, and what changes needed to be made in the health care delivery system to better accommodate the female-headed, one-parent family.

The health diary was completed by the participants over a 2-week period using questions and a notebook supplied by the investigator. The women were asked to answer the following five open-ended questions on a daily basis.

1. What kinds of things did you do today that were good for your health?
2. What did you do today that might hurt your health?
3. Keep track of any thoughts you have about health: questions, concerns, etc.
4. What encouraged you to do something for your health today?
5. What stopped you from doing something for your health today?

The purposes of the diary were twofold: to sample the family's health and health practices and to compensate for memory decay which could affect the interview responses. This instrument was suggested by the women who participated in the pilot study when they realized important data on primary prevention practices was omitted because they had not thought of it during the interviews.

Last, a card sort of primary prevention behaviors and barriers to their practice was completed by each woman. The list of 53 primary prevention behaviors and nine barriers was developed from the pilot study interviews and the literature. The cards were sorted into one of three categories: not applicable or not practiced, sometimes practiced, or regularly practiced (Harris & Guten, 1979). The definitions of sometimes and regularly were from the participant's perspective. The cards sorted into the sometimes category were resorted by the woman to determine which behaviors she would like to see her family practice regularly and which she was content with practicing sometimes. A card sort of nine barriers to primary prevention practices was then given to the woman and she matched those behaviors that she would like to practice regularly with one or more barriers deterring the desired behavior.

Procedure

All data collection occurred in the home of each participant after a signed informed consent was obtained. The interviews of the female household head, responding for family members, were tape recorded and later transcribed. The health diary was completed by the woman for her family during the 2-week period between the first and second interviews. The card sort was administered at the second interview.

A pilot study was conducted with 18 female-headed, one-parent families to pretest the interview guide and to develop the card sort. As a result of the pilot study, the second interview was added, the card sort was compiled, and the health diary was developed.

The data analysis consisted of two segments. First, the primary prevention behaviors and barriers to practice were analyzed by descriptive statistics. Second, the behaviors and barriers were categorized to describe the family's health practices. For example, the behaviors were divided according to whether the woman considered it a conscious health practice or an unconscious part of the daily routine. During the interview each woman was asked to classify into one of the two categories the health behaviors the family regularly practiced. Conscious health practices were identified by the woman as health behaviors the family purposefully engaged in regularly to promote health or prevent disease. Unconscious daily routines were behaviors the family practiced regularly but considered part of their lifestyle rather than for the purpose of health promotion or disease prevention. Next, the families were divided into those who practiced only unconscious routine behaviors and those who identified conscious health practices in addition to the unconscious routines. The family data were analyzed to understand the differences between the family's lifestyle and their practice of primary prevention behaviors (Duffy, 1984). The content analysis primarily was completed by the researcher. The completed analysis was shared with the study participants and a group of health professionals who worked with female-headed, one-parent families. This panel was asked to judge the face validity of the conclusions of the content analysis.

RESULTS

Fifty-nine, female-headed, one parent families participated in this study. These families consisted of 228 individuals. The mean number of children per family was 2.4 with a range of 1 to 6. The majority of women (26 or 44%) were in the 30 to 39–year–old age category; ages ranged from 18 to 51–years–old. The women had become single parents through divorce, death, separation, or never having been married; two-thirds of the families had been through a divorce. Nineteen of the 59 families had lived as a one-parent family for less than 2 years. The majority of families (28 or 48%) had consisted of one-parent for 2 to 5 years.

Fifty-two percent of the families were receiving Aid to Dependent Families. Sixty-eight percent of the families had an income of less than $10,000 per year. Incomes between $10,000 and $20,000 per year were reported by 24% of the families, and the remaining families, 8.5%, earned more than $20,000 per year. These incomes are reflected in the employment status of the women. Thirteen (22%) were full-time homemakers, 19 (32.2%) were employed, 22 (37.2%) were students, and 5 (8.5%) were temporarily unemployed and actively seeking employment. The employed women were concentrated in traditionally female job categories: secretaries, clerks, waitresses, aides, and so forth. On the other hand, slightly more than half of the students, 12 women, were

Table 1
Primary Prevention Behaviors Reported by Female-Headed, One-Parent Families

Behavior	Practiced Regularly (N = 59) Number	Percent	Designed for Regular Practice (N = 48) Number	Percent
Exercise	47			
Walking	38	65.5	10	21.8
Dancing	25	43.1	12	25.0
Calisthenics	22	37.9	8	16.6
Biking	19	32.7	17	35.4
Swimming	18	31.0	16	33.3
Gardening	16	27.5	10	20.8
Hiking	16	27.5	15	31.2
Jogging	10	17.2	12	25.0
Skiing	4	6.8	5	10.4
Nutrition	55			
Balanced meals	46	79.3	9	18.7
Take vitamins	35	60.3	9	18.7
Eat low sugar diet	28	48.3	5	10.4
Eat low salt diet	20	34.5	2	4.1
Eat low fat diet	20	34.5	6	12.5
Take nutrition supplements	19	32.7	3	6.2
Eat high fiber diet	11	19.0		
Make special dietary alterations	9	15.5		
Substance use decline	15			
Stopped or decreased alcohol	9	15.5	1	2.0
Stopped or decreased smoking	8	13.8	4	8.3
Stopped or decreased illegal drug use	6	10.3		
Stopped or decreased medication use	4	6.8		
Health care system	56			
Immunizations	50	86.2	2	4.1
Dental examinations	47	81.0	6	12.5
Medical care as needed	37	63.8	6	12.5
Eye examinations	37	63.8	5	10.4
Physical examinations	34	58.6	8	16.6
Follow physicians' orders	33	56.9	2	4.1
Pap smear	27	46.6	5	10.4
Use mental health counseling	15	25.9	8	16.6
Use prescribed medications	12	20.7		
Use naturopath or chiropractor	3	5.2		
Personal health—physical	56			
Dress for weather	56	96.6	2	4.1
Hygiene	54	93.1		
Adequate sleep	38	65.5	14	29.1
Clean, uncluttered house	36	62.1	14	29.1
Breast self-examination	20	34.5	12	25.0
Birth control	19	32.7		
Lose weight	15	25.9	18	37.5
Wear seat belts	13	22.4	2	4.1

Table 1
Primary Prevention Behaviors Reported by Female-Headed, One-Parent Families

Behavior	Practiced Regularly (N = 59) Number	Percent	Designed for Regular Practice (N = 48) Number	Percent
Personal health—emotional	53			
Close friends	42	72.4	4	8.3
Someone supportive to talk to	41	70.7	8	16.6
Relaxation	30	51.7	16	33.3
Do something for myself	28	48.3	19	39.5
Pray for health	19	32.7	3	6.2
Safety	37			
Check house for safety	24	41.4	11	22.9
Home fire extinguisher and smoke detector	21	36.2	4	8.3
Learn first aid	13	22.4	13	27.0
Learn CPR	12	20.7	6	12.5
Health knowledge	27			
Read about health	25	43.1	10	20.8
Talk with someone about my family's health	17	29.3	10	20.8
Work on community health program	5	8.6	3	6.2
Other				
Symptom identification and early treatment	5	8.6		
Keep thermostat down	4	6.8		
Clorox in water	1	1.7		
Good bed	1	1.7		

pursuing career pathways nontraditionally female.

Primary Prevention Behaviors

In Table 1 is a list of the number of families who regularly practiced each primary prevention behavior. The responses were dominated by two categories: health care system related behaviors and behaviors routinely learned during childhood (such as the basic four food groups, hygiene, rest, and proper clothing).

Other primary prevention behaviors such as eating a low salt or low fat diet, examining the breasts, using seat belts, checking the home for safety, and so forth, were less frequently practiced. These behaviors usually were not carried over from the woman's family of origin and had to be learned by the woman in order to teach her children. For six of the nine category headings in Table 1 over half of the families indicated that they engaged in one or more of the health behaviors in that category.

When asked to respond to the following question: "What are the three most important things your family does to maintain health?", a balanced diet was the overwhelming response. The responses to the questions are listed in Table 2. In addition to a balanced diet, the nutrition practices included taking vitamins, eating balanced meals, decreasing junk foods, and increasing the amounts of fruits and vegetables. Rest was identified as the second most important behavior by 49% of the families, exercise third (46%), and personal hygiene fourth (24%). The four most important behaviors could be practiced with minimal, if any, intervention by members of the health care delivery system.

The families in this study participated in two categories of primary prevention behaviors: unconscious or long-standing and new or conscious. Long-standing behaviors either originated in the woman's childhood or prior to the family becoming a one-parent unit. These behaviors were integrated into the lifestyle of the family members and instead of labeling them as primary prevention behaviors, the women called these practices "common sense" behaviors. Long-standing behaviors were practiced regularly without conscious thought of their health effect. Most of the primary prevention behaviors practiced by the families were long-standing. One participant summarized this category by saying: "I cannot think of anything I set out to do. I do not set out to do something healthy that day."

The second category of primary prevention behaviors were relatively new and undertaken specifically for promoting health and preventing disease. These behaviors either were attempted intermittently but not adopted, or eventually became integrated into the family's life-style. Either way, the woman identified these behaviors as prevention practices consciously undertaken. Primary prevention behaviors were categorized as new behaviors if the woman reported that the behavior began during the time the family had been a one-parent unit. The following excerpt is an example of a successful change in a primary prevention practice and its integration into the family's lifestyle:

> Along with the weight is trying to establish good eating habits and not have a lot of junk around the house. We do not use sugar as much as we used to. I used to let the kids munch a lot like after supper on cookies. We hardly ever have cookies and stuff like that in the house anymore. I like to keep fruit and fresh vegetables and stuff if they want to munch on that.

Barriers to Practice

Overall the women cited 61% of the behaviors that they practiced sometimes as behaviors they would like to practice regularly. In Table 1 the distribution of the desired behavior is shown. A woman may have cited more than one behavior

Table 2
Most Important Primary Prevention Behaviors Identified by 59 Female-Headed One-Parent Families

Behavior	Number	Percent
Nutrition	56	95.0
Rest	29	49.0
Exercise	27	45.8
Personal hygiene	14	23.7
Physical examinations	9	15.2
Dress for weather	7	12.0
Emotional support	7	12.0
Symptom identification and early treatment	5	8.5
Keep active	2	3.4
Pray for health	2	3.4
No alcohol	1	1.7
Safety	1	1.7

per category. The specific behaviors most frequently cited were: do something for myself, 19 or 40%; lose weight, 18 or 38%; and biking, 17 or 35%.

The women were asked to identify barriers to the desired primary prevention practices with the card sort. The women's responses are presented in Table 3. Time was the most frequently stated barrier, appearing 153 times. Feeling lazy was second, followed by money. Needing someone's

Table 3
Barriers to Primary Prevention Behaviors of Female-Headed, One-Parent Families (N = 48)

Barrier	Number of Times Cited
Time	153
"Lazy"	83
Money	71
Need someone's support	64
Don't feel good about doing	39
Never thought about it	35
Need more information	32
Wasn't allowed to by someone else	10
Other	2

support was cited 64 times. Support, if present, was frequently identified as a motivation to primary prevention practices.

Additionally, the women described factors which occurred in their life circumstances and influenced their primary prevention practices. These concerns were economics, day care, parenting, inadequate support systems, and low self-esteem. These stressors were perceived as negative influences on the family's ability to practice primary prevention behaviors; habitual prevention practices were maintained, but the energy resources were insufficient for establishing new behaviors. The continuum of transcending options (Duffy, 1984) relates these stressors of life circumstances and the barriers to primary prevention practices.

DISCUSSION

When working with families, it is imperative that the nurse understand primary prevention practices from the families' perspectives. Equally imperative is the nurse's understanding of the contextual milieu or environment of the family. The physical and emotional demands of one parent, combined with a typically low income, contribute to the single female parent being "overworked, overstressed, often so depressed" (Weltner, 1982, p. 205).

Health professionals can complicate the situation and nurses are not immune from contributing to the problem. One woman's comments about health professionals summarizes the comments of many of the women.

I think a lot of them are kind of insensitive to where you are coming from. Maybe that is just because they do not understand. I do not think they understand the frustration of a single parent trying to raise kids.

The findings of this study indicate that families perceive themselves as practicing primary prevention behaviors. These results suggest that certain environmental factors limit the practice of additional primary prevention behaviors. For example, time and money are major contributors to role strain. Previous research was consistent in identifying role overload and poverty as two major stressors in the one-parent family (Pearlin & Johnson, 1977). Regardless of socioeconomic level, Pratt (1976) found that families could practice effective health behaviors if other characteristics of the family were altered: family interaction, power, and coping. The management of role overload may be critical in impeding the one-parent family's practice of primary prevention behaviors. Further study is needed to understand time demands on one-parent, the family's priority-setting patterns, and the woman's use of available resources, i.e., social support systems. Woods (1985) suggested that the number of roles a married woman performed was a less critical influence on her mental health than the context for role performance, including social support. The effects of social support on the role performance of women heads of one-parent families needs study.

The lack of social support systems was another barrier to the practice of primary prevention practices. Social support systems, when available, were identified as motivators in trying out new behaviors and then sustaining those behaviors. Research is needed to investigate the types and amounts of social support which contribute to the practice of primary prevention behaviors in the one-parent family. A future study could test the differences in primary prevention practices between women with support systems and those without. The duration, intensity, and types of social support are critical questions.

Longitudinal studies also are needed to observe changes in primary prevention practices as families adjust to their one-parent status. This type of study should contribute to an understanding of the factors which influence the family's practice of primary prevention behaviors.

In addition, various socio-demographic variables must be isolated and studied in relation to the practice of primary prevention behaviors. Money was frequently cited as a barrier. Are there differences in primary prevention practices based on income?

This study identified variables related to the families' practices of primary prevention behaviors. The major limitations of this study were the use of a convenience sample and the identification, through qualitative analysis, of potentially influencing contextual variables. Further investigations are needed which identify and measure the relationships between these specific contextual variables and the families' practices of primary prevention behaviors.

Nursing practice, especially community health nursing, often involves the female-headed, one-parent family client. First, the nurse must assess those primary prevention behaviors the family perceives themselves as practicing. These behaviors are a family strength to acknowledge and enhance. Second, the nurse, with the family, can identify both the motivators and barriers to desired primary prevention practices. The female-headed, one-parent family experiences role overload, stereotyping, and poverty, which can deter the practice of primary prevention behaviors.

REFERENCES

Berman, W. H., & Turk, D. C. (1981). Adaptation to divorce: Problems and coping strategies. *Journal of Marriage and the Family, 43*(1), 179–189.

Brandwein, R. A., Brown, C. A., & Fox, E. M. (1974). Women and children last: The social situation of divorced mothers and their families. *Journal of Marriage and the Family, 36*(3), 498–514.

Burgess, J. K. (1970). The single-parent family: A social and sociological problem. *The Family Coordinator, 19*(4), 137–144.

Cherlin, A., & Furstenberg, F. F. (1982). *The shape of the American family in the year 2000.* Washington: American Council of Life Insurance.

Duffy, M. E. (1982). When a woman heads a household. *Nursing Outlook, 30*(8), 468–473.

Duffy, M. E. (1984). Transcending options: Creating a milieu for practicing high level wellness. *Health Care for Women International, 5*(1–3), 145–161.

Friedman, M. M. (1981). *Family nursing theory and assessment.* New York: Appleton-Century-Crofts.

Harris, D. M. & Guten, S. (1979). Health-protective behavior: An exploratory study. *Journal of Health and Social Behavior, 20,* 17–29.

Herman, S. J. (1977). Women, divorce, and suicide. *Journal of Divorce, 1*(2), 107–117.

Horowitz, J. A., & Purdue, B. J. (1977). Single-parent families. *Nursing Clinics of North America, 12*(3), 503–511.

Jacobsen, A. (1980). Melancholy in the 20th century: Causes and prevention. *Journal of Psychiatric Nursing and Mental Health Services, 18*(7), 11–21.

Leavell, H. R., & Clark, E. G. (1965). *Preventive medicine for the doctor in his community: An epidemiologic approach* (3rd ed.). New York: McGraw-Hill.

LeMasters, E. E. (1971). Parents without partners. In A. S. Skolnick & J. H. Skolnick (Eds.), *Family in transition.* Boston: Little, Brown and Company.

Malouf, R. E. (1979). *Social bases of power in single and two-parent families.* Unpublished doctoral dissertation, University of Utah, Salt Lake City.

McCord, J., McCord, W., & Thurber, E. (1962). Some effects of paternal absence on male children. *Journal of Abnormal and Social Psychology, 61,* 361–369.

Norbeck, J., & Sheiner, M. (1982). Sources of social support related to single-parent functioning. *Research in Nursing and Health, 5,* 3–12.

Patton, R. D., Harvill, L. M., & Michal, M. L. (1981). Attitudes of single parents toward health issues. *Journal of the American Medical Women's Association, 36*(11), 340–348.

Pearlin, L. I., & Johnson, J. S. (1977). Marital status, life strains and depression. *American Sociological Review, 42*(5), 704–715.

Pender, N. J. (1982). *Health promotion in nursing practice.* Norwalk, CT: Appleton-Century-Crofts.

Pratt, L. (1976). *Family structure and effective health behavior: The energized family*. Boston: Houghton-Mifflin.

Richardson, R., & Pfeiffenberg, C. (1983). Social support networks for divorced and stepfamilies. In J. K. Whittaker & J. Garbarino (Eds.), *Social support networks: Informal helping in the human services*. (pp. 219–247). New York: Aldine Publishing Company.

Schorr, A. L., & Moen, P. (1980). The single parent and public policy. In A. Skolnic & J. H. Skolnic (Eds.), *Family in transition* (3rd ed.). Boston: Little, Brown and Company.

Smith, M. J. (1980). The social consequences of single parenthood: A longitudinal perspective. *Family Relations, 29*, 75–81.

Weltner, J. S. (1982). A structural approach to the single-parent family. *Family Process, 21*, 203–210.

Woods, N. F. (1985). Employment, family roles, and mental ill health in young married women. *Nursing Research, 34*(1), 4–10.

Worrell, J. & Garret-Fulks, N. (1983). The resocialization of single-again women. In V. Franks & E. D. Rothblum (Eds.), *The sterotyping of women* (pp. 201–229). New York: Springer.

This article is printed with permission of *Research in Nursing and Health*.
Copyright © 1986 John Wiley & Sons.

11

Health Promotion and Primary Care Nursing

Pamela Hellings, PhD, RN
Grace A. Lin, BSN, RN
Karen S. Davis, BSN, RN

INTRODUCTION BY: PAMELA HELLINGS, PhD, RN

One of the reasons that nurses have conducted research in the area of health promotion is to study the impact of lifestyle changes on health. There is increasingly compelling data which suggest a relationship between certain health behaviors and maintenance of health. The growing recognition that encouraging certain behaviors (e.g., weight loss, exercise, smoking cessation, and avoiding stress) may prevent major catastrophic illness or at least alter the degree of impairment has added urgency to finding solutions to the question of how to support lifestyle changes both before and after a health problem is recognized. What is not known, however, is how to promote these lifestyle changes.

The three studies selected each offer a different perspective on the issue of promoting health behaviors. Alexy examines the effectiveness of client participation in selecting goals for reducing risk factors. Laffrey and Isenberg study participation in one health promoting behavior—exercise—and its relationship to locus of control, value placed on health, and perceived importance of health. Finally, Pender and Pender examine the relationships among attitudes, subjective norms, and the intention to engage in the health behaviors of exercising, maintaining weight, and avoiding stressful situations.

These particular studies were selected for inclusion because of their currency, their potential for utilization in nursing practice in a variety of settings, and the differing perspectives that they offer within the framework of promotion of health behaviors. The variation in methods and the contrast in the conceptualization of the questions also offer the practitioner an opportunity to examine the issue of health promotion from several frameworks.

Goal Setting and Health Risk Reduction

Betty Alexy, DNSc, RN
Associate Professor
College of Allied Health Sciences
Thomas Jefferson University
Philadelphia, PA

The effectiveness of client participation in goal selection aimed at health risk reduction was compared with the effectiveness of provider-selected goals and of no goal setting. No difference in goal attainment was found between the two groups with goals. However, analyses of covariance for selected subsamples of individuals at risk revealed a significant difference between goal-setting groups for weight reduction, with the collaborative goal-setting group being more effective. Covariance analyses for other subsamples at risk showed significant differences between the goal-setting groups for current health age and potential for life expectancy increase; the provider goal-setting group proved to be more effective. Paired t tests within groups revealed that the provider goal-setting group made significant change in alcohol intake, seat belt use, and exercise as well as in global measures of current health age, estimated life expectancy, and potential for life expectancy increase. For the collaborative goal-setting group, significant change was found in weight reduction, exercise levels, and the global measures of estimated life expectancy and potential for life expectancy increase. The control group made a significant change in exercise, but not in any of the global measures of risk reduction.

Although chronic disease is a problem of immense proportion in this country, its incidence can be influenced to some degree by individual behavior. Even with information regarding the effect of personal behavior on health, however, some persons choose not to change their life-styles. In other words, after considering the alternatives, some individuals decide that the costs outweigh the benefits.

To date, health care providers have given little consideration to personal choice behavior. For the most part, health management plans are determined by the provider. Input from the client is seldom solicited even though the client has primary responsibility for carrying out the plan. Because nurses traditionally play a prominent role in health teaching and counseling, knowledge about effectiveness of client participation in health planning is important.

This study investigated (a) if collaboration between the health care provider and the client in developing a plan for risk reduction resulted in greater reduction in risk behaviors than a plan formulated entirely by the provider and (b) if health risk reduction would occur independently of the goal-setting interventions.

Edwards' (1954) value expectancy model served as the theoretical framework for this study.

Edwards (1954, p. 411) demonstrated that in situations of risk choices an individual is able to consider probabilities, set priorities related to alternatives, and make a choice that is likely to lead to the most favorable outcome. This study predicted that collaboration in goal setting would result in a greater reduction of health risk than when risk-reduction goals were set by health care providers.

REVIEW OF THE LITERATURE

Client participation in health planning and management for health prevention or health promotion and maintenance has seldom been studied. Traditionally, the physician has been the dominant force in designating the therapeutic plan. With the recent interest in consumer involvement, the time seems right to extend this notion to the health care field.

Increased consumer involvement has been investigated in several studies. In some instances, individuals have been provided with information and encouraged to assume more responsibility for their own care. Green (1974), using health education related to asthma, demonstrated significantly fewer visits to the emergency room for patients in the experimental group. Rosenberg (1971) showed that group discussion and individual counseling with patients with congestive heart failure significantly increased the experimental group's knowledge of their health problem, diet and drug therapy, and reduced the number of subsequent hospital admissions for patients with cardiac failure. Both of the preceding studies indicate that individuals can profit from health information and can learn behaviors that may contribute to a decreased frequency of episodes of illness.

Behavioral contracts have been used to increase client participation and influence management outcomes. Steckel (1976) investigated the influence of knowledge and contingency contracting on adherence to hypertensive treatment regimens. She concluded that a great deal of interaction between client and researcher was needed to identify behaviors that had a high probability of being achieved and rewards that were sufficiently valued to reinforce the selected behavior. She found that clients became more active in negotiating a behavioral goal as they became more comfortable in the role.

Setting goals has been investigated as a means of motivating change. Locke, Cardledge, and Koeppel, (1968) found that setting goals facilitated self-regulation in studies of mathematical computation and performance in driving tests. After analyzing several goal-setting studies they concluded that knowledge of results such as a test score was not sufficient to motivate change, but knowledge of results plus goal setting produced significant changes in performance. It should be noted that the investigations took place over short, discrete time intervals, generally with a single goal requirement.

Hefferin (1979) explored health goal setting in Veterans Administration facilities. A group of patients that received nurse assistance in developing their own health goal was compared with another group with nurse-developed health goal plans. Goal statements were based on identified needs from medical and nursing assessments and patient comments and were related to direct management of a health problem or adaptive or preventive activities. Specific goals included such factors as finding living arrangements, obtaining eye glasses, controlling a rash, learning signs of infection, and stopping smoking. Hefferin found that the group that had input into the goal plan achieved more goals within a shorter period of time. Although a content analysis of the goal statements revealed little difference between groups in the proportion of management care concerns, patients from the input group were more likely to identify problems of an immediate practical nature. The immediacy of the patient-identified goals may have contributed to the greater success with this strategy.

Risk-reduction programs have been shown to be effective in stimulating life-style change. The Stanford Heart Disease Prevention Program (Maccoby, Farquhar, Wood, & Alexander, 1977) found that a mass media-intensive instruction was most effective in increasing knowledge of cardiovascular disease and changing dietary and smoking behavior. Meyer, Nash, McAlister, Maccoby, and

Farquhar (1980) continued the study of subsamples of higher risk and concluded that mass media, plus intensive instruction, induced immediate and reasonably stable change, whereas mass media alone took longer to achieve an effect that was partially maintained after maximal treatment.

Morisky et al. (1983) examined the effects of a 5- to 10-minute counseling session, family instruction, and group sessions on blood pressure control and mortality over a 5-year period. A continuing positive effect on weight control, appointment keeping, and blood pressure control was found with all intervention groups, demonstrating a reduction in mortality over the 5-year period.

From the preceding studies it appears that behavioral change can be maintained over time and can result in decreased mortality. Moreover, the Morisky et al. (1983) study suggests that modest interventions may stimulate the change.

METHOD

Sample: Participation in this study was solicited in three industrial or corporate settings. Participants represented a convenience sample obtained from individuals who were eligible for periodic health examinations at their place of employment and who agreed to participate. To be eligible for the study, individuals had to have at least one risk factor identified by the Personal Risk Profile (PRP) (General Health, 1981) which could be lowered by changing behavior.

One hundred four males and 48 females participated in the study. This ratio reflected the composition of the work force at the study locations. Four participants were lost from the control group over the 3-month study period, leaving 52 subjects in the provider group, 54 in the collaborative group, and 46 in the control group. Ages of the participants ranged from 27 to 66, with a mean age of 45.6 years. Educational background ranged from completion of 10th grade to completion of graduate study. The majority of the participants (58.9%) had completed baccalaureate or graduate college programs. Subjects reported a family income of from less than $20,000 (1.7%) to more than $40,000. The average salary was higher than $40,000 per year (51.77%).

Instrument: The instrument used to identify health risks and as the reference point for goal setting was the PRP (General Health, 1981). This instrument was developed using morbidity and mortality data from the 20-year Framingham Study of Cardiovascular Disease, the Third National Cancer Survey, the US Bureau of Vital Statistics, and a variety of other reputable sources. The PRP is one of a number of health-risk instruments based on age, sex, and race factors.

Information contained in the PRP was organized into categories of risk for heart disease, cancer, stroke, and motor vehicle accidents. In addition to risk categories, an individual's health risk age (which may be higher or lower than the individual's chronological age), life expectancy, and potential for life increase were indicated. The latter three factors were considered global measures of overall risk reduction.

The test-retest reliability of the instrument was estimated by repeating the questionnaire 3 to 5 days after the first administration to a sample of 28 individuals. Test-retest reliabilities of the questions relating to weight, exercise, smoking behavior, alcohol intake, and wearing seat belts were calculated using Pearson product moment correlation coefficients. Test-retest reliability coefficients ranged from .83 to 1.00. Reliability for the question on breast self-examination was not estimated because there were only two females in the reliability sample.

Procedure: Individuals at the three sites were asked by the investigators to participate in a study of health risk reduction that involved completing a questionnaire containing questions about their personal and family health history and personal habits. They were assured that confidentiality would be maintained and that they might withdraw from the study at any time. After the study was explained, persons from each site who agreed to participate were randomly assigned to one of three groups: provider goal setting, collaborative goal setting, or control.

All three groups completed the PRP and returned for a review of the initial profile results. Risk areas in order of priority for each individual were discussed, and any questions regarding risk factors or resources were answered for all individuals in all groups.

Two graduate nursing students assisted the investigator in data collection. The assistants followed established protocols for goal setting whereby goals were designated for the provider group and selected by the collaborative group. Review of the pre- and posttest profile by investigators and clients systematically followed each risk category, highlighting significant areas for each individual in each group. Risk factors selected for goal-setting interventions included weight management, cigarette smoking, alcohol intake, exercise, seat belt usage, and breast self-examination for women. These specific factors were chosen because behavioral change seemed possible within the 3-month study period.

In the provider goal-setting group, goals were structured according to the following protocol: cessation of smoking; weight reduction of 1 pound a week or achievement of ideal body weight; exercise three times a week for at least 30 minutes each; reduce alcohol to 1 or 2 ounces of liquor, or two beers, or two glasses of wine a week; and wear seat belts at least 76% of the time. Monthly performance of breast self-examination was advised for women. After reviewing the priority risk areas, the collaborative group selected the goals they wished to achieve from the six investigated categories. Some individuals selected only one or two goals; others chose more. Control group members completed the questionnaire and received feedback from the profile, but were not involved in goal setting. The control group was included to determine if health risks would be reduced independently of the goal-setting intervention. Each individual in the goal-setting groups received a copy of the profile results and a goal sheet indicating identified risks and goals selected or recommended. Individuals in the control group were given only a copy of the profile results.

Three months after the goal-setting intervention, members of the three groups again completed the PRP, and the performance of the two intervention groups in relation to goal setting was determined. The second PRP results provided updated calculations of current health risk age, estimated life expectancies, and potential life expectancy gains as well as calculations for the various risk factors.

Potential changes in current health risk age, life expectancy increase, or potential life expectancy gain were assumed to result, in most part, from factors investigated, because changes in the health history itself were likely to be minimal.

Data Analysis: A method was needed to adjust for the initial differences in goal-setting between individuals in the collaborative goal-setting group, who were able to select a number of goals from the identified risks, and members of the provider goal-setting group, who had goals set for them if a risk was identified. Thus, each risk category was weighted according to the total group difficulty of achieving it. This computation was performed in the following manner: The number of identified health risks for all individuals was summed for each risk category. This sum was divided into the number of unachieved goals in each risk category. The resulting weight was considered a difficulty of achievement (D/A) measure for the specific risk category.

The weights for the six risk categories investigated were as follows: D/A smoking = .75; D/A weight = .65; D/A seat belts = .54; D/A exercise = .43; D/A breast examination = .43; D/A alcohol = .36.

A goal-met ratio for each subject was obtained by dividing the sum of the D/A weights of the recommended or selected goals into the sum of the D/A weights of the achieved goals. A t test was then done on the difference in means between the provider and collaborative goal-setting groups, with the goal-met ratio as the dependent variable and the type of goal-setting group as the independent variable.

Significant differences were found to exist between groups prior to the intervention in spite of randomization. Therefore, analyses of covariance were performed on overall measures of risk reduction (current health age, estimated life expectancy, and life expectancy increase) as well as on each of the investigated risk factors with the pretest score as the covariate, type of goal-setting group the independent variable, and posttest scores the dependent variable.

As individuals did not have identified risks in all six investigated risk categories, analyses of covariance were performed on selected subsamples of individuals who reported fewer than 4,000 calories a week in exercise, smoked cigarettes, drank more than 2 ounces of alcohol a week, were at least 10% overweight, wore seat belts less than 76% of the time, and women who did not perform monthly breast examinations.

To determine success in risk reduction, paired t tests were done on all participants in each of the three groups, with the subject's performance on the first PRP matched with the subject's performance on the second PRP. Paired t tests were also performed on selected subsamples as identified previously. The level of statistical significance for all tests was .05.

RESULTS

No significant difference was obtained between the means of the provider group's goal-met ratio and that obtained by the collaborative group, $t = .18$, $df = 104$, $p = .86$. Thus, achievement of health goals, as measured by the goal-met ratio composite score, was not differentially influenced by the type of client participation in goal setting.

The analyses of covariance for subjects who had potential for improvement in the risk categories revealed a significant difference between goal-setting groups for weight reduction; the collaborative goal-setting group was more effective. Covariance analyses for selected subsamples further revealed significant differences between the goal-setting groups for current health age and potential for life expectancy increase; here the provider goal-setting group proved to be most effective. These findings are shown in Tables 1 and 2.

Associated Findings: Given the general lack of significant findings based on the previous analyses, the data were subjected to paired t tests.

After selecting subjects with identified risks and potential for change in the various risk categories, the greatest amount of change was found in the provider goal-setting group (alcohol, seat belts, and exercise). Less change was observed in the collaborative goal-setting group (exercise and weight) and change only in exercise levels was found in the control group (see Table 3).

The paired t tests for each group further indicated significant overall gains from pretest to posttest in estimated life expectancy and potential life expectancy increase for both goal-setting groups. Significant change in current health age was also found in the provider goal-setting group. Changes in current health age, life expectancy, or potential life expectancy increase were not found to be statistically significant in the control group (Table 4).

DISCUSSION

Although findings from this study suggest that setting goals for risk reduction can be effective in changing behavior, results provided no indication that client participation in setting goals was superior to a directive approach. In fact, using paired t tests, the provider goal-setting group made statistically significant changes in three of the six investigated risk categories.

These results may be explained in part by studies of goal setting relative to listing objects and mathematical computation (Locke, 1966; Locke & Bryan, 1966, 1968), which revealed that higher levels of expectation resulted in higher levels of performance.

In general, the provider goal-setting group had greater total numbers of goals to achieve, as well as specifically defined goals. This may have been viewed by the participants as a more difficult task to achieve and thus may have been more challenging, resulting in a higher degree of success. The provider group made significant changes in exercise levels, alcohol intake, and seat belt usage.

Table 1
ANCOVA of Risk Categories for Selected Subsamples with Baseline Data and Covariates

Risk Categories	Provider n	Provider X̄ Pretest	Provider X̄ Posttest	Collaborative n	Collaborative X̄ Pretest	Collaborative X̄ Posttest	Control n	Control X̄ Pretest	Control X̄ Posttest	F	p
Exercise (calories per week)	37	1513.30	2726.00	42	1482.83	2939.29	35	1847.23	2950.37	0.15	.86
Weight (10% above average)	19	22.47	19.42	20	27.55	22.00	15	33.87	28.93	27.11	<.001
Alcohol (ounces a week)	35	2.61	2.45	26	2.50	2.43	23	2.65	2.46	0.52	.60
Smoking 1 = <10 2 = 10-19 3 = 20-39 4 = 40 or more	15	2.60	2.47	6	2.00	2.50	12	2.50	3.08	1.03	.37
Seat belt use 1 = <10% 2 = 11-50% 3 = 51-75% 4 = >75%	39	1.45	1.95	31	1.45	1.58	36	1.44	1.59	2.24	.11

Table 2
Analyses of Covariance of Global Measures of Risk Reduction for the Selected Subsamples with Baseline Data Covariates

Global Measures	Provider n	Provider X̄ Pretest	Provider X̄ Posttest	Collaborative n	Collaborative X̄ Pretest	Collaborative X̄ Posttest	Control n	Control X̄ Pretest	Control X̄ Posttest	F	p
Current health age	44[a]	47.64	46.77	49[a]	43.18	42.88	45[a]	-43.44	43.36	32.89	<.001
Estimated life expectancy	52	76.42	77.94	54	77.41	78.30	46	77.15	-77.65	2.67	.07
Life expectancy increase	52	5.58	4.37	54	4.54	3.80	46	5.01	4.54	-3.92	.02

[a]Entire sample is not included because some second profile results did not contain a calculated current health age. (In these instances, the profile noted that the participant was exceptionally healthy.)

The control group, which had knowledge of the results of the questionnaire and received the same feedback as the treatment groups, made significant changes in exercise and achieved marginal significance in weight reduction. These changes in behavior, however, were not sufficient to make significant overall changes in current health age, life expectancy, or potential life expectancy increase.

The collaborative goal-setting group also changed significantly in exercise and weight reduction. Overall changes in this group were sufficient to make significant differences in life expectancy and potential life-expectancy increase.

Although significant change occurred in exercise levels and weight reduction in the collaborative group, and change occurred in exercise levels in the provider goal-setting and control groups, such change may be related to the current emphasis on these factors in modern culture. Exercise and weight-reduction facilities are readily accessible to urban and suburban dwellers and have been the subject of intensive membership marketing campaigns. Their current popularity can be demonstrated by looking at the numbers of individuals in the collaborative group who selected these goals. Exercise ($n = 39$) and weight reduction ($n = 30$) were the two most frequently chosen goals of all the risk areas, even though for some subjects cessation of smoking would have made more potential difference in their life expectancy.

A study by Meyer, Kay, and French (1965) relative to performance appraisal in a business setting may help to explain the above results. The authors concluded that although employee participation in goal setting did affect performance in a positive manner, a more important factor was the presence or absence of goals. The fact that no significant change occurred in smoking behavior needs to be explained. Bernstein and Glascow (1981), in a comprehensive discussion of smoking cessation programs, noted that multicomponent programs combining such techniques as rapid smoking, self-monitoring, nonsmoking skill training, stimulus control, and social and material reenforcement of nonsmoking behavior were no more successful than single treatment components. Bandura (1969, 1971), a well-known social learning theorist, indicated that psychological treatment procedures involve several stages and must address the induction of behavior change, individual incorporation of that change, and maintenance of change over time. This observation implies that the process is complex and that a multifaceted approach at definite intervals may be necessary to achieve long-term cessation, which may explain the lack of significant change in smoking behavior in this study.

For breast self-examination, consistent results were obtained across both goal-setting groups and the control group. There are several possible explanations for this result. Breast self-examinations were recommended on a monthly basis at specific times. However, an event that is planned at sporadic intervals may be more difficult to incorporate into one's routine than an event that occurs on a daily or weekly basis. Other factors such as fear and attitudes may inhibit performance of breast examination. Two women told the investigators that they were reluctant to carry out this procedure because they were afraid they would discover some abnormality. This type of expressed concern must be managed effectively if health promotion programs are to succeed. Results from this portion of the study need to be viewed in relation to the sample size for the groups at risk (total $n = 25$ for all three groups).

Weight losses, when compared by paired t tests for subjects who were at least 10% overweight, were statistically significant for both the provider and the collaborative goal-setting groups. The control group was marginally significant. Weight loss in pounds for all three groups was relatively modest (provider goal setting = 4.79 pounds; collaborative goal setting = 6.70 pounds; and control = 3.80 pounds). However, individuals in the study were, for the most part, mildly overweight, so great changes in weight would not be expected. Also, since one pound a week of weight loss was recommended for those who were overweight, the 6.7 pound loss for the collaborative goal-setting group over the 12-week study period represents modest success.

The structure of the interventions is another factor potentially affecting the outcome of the investigation. In many instances, the goals formulated

Table 3
Paired *t* test Comparisons for Selected Subsamples Within the Three Groups for All Risk Factors

Risk Categories	n	X̄ Pretest	X̄ Posttest	SD Pretest	SD Posttest	t	p
PROVIDER GOAL-SETTING							
Alcohol (ounces a week)	37	11.85	9.12	8.83	6.90	2.50	.017
Seat belt use	52	19.48	15.34	11.26	12.53	3.22	.011
Weight (10% above average)	27	18.04	15.85	11.74	11.45	1.82	.08
Exercise (calories per week)	37	1513.29	2726.00	1094.74	1845.15	-3.49	.001
Breast examination for women	9	2.00	1.66	0.00	0.50	2.00	.08
Smoking	15	2.60	2.47	0.91	1.06	0.62	.55
COLLABORATIVE GOAL-SETTING							
Alcohol (ounces a week)	28	8.98	9.41	5.02	6.35	-0.65	.518
Seat belt use	54	14.46	13.70	12.86	13.06	0.91	.369
Weight (10% above average)	29	21.17	17.10	17.69	15.03	4.11	<.001
Exercise (calories per week)	42	1482.83	2939.28	1010.71	2023.73	-4.76	<.001
Breast examination for women	7	2.00	1.57	0.00	0.535	2.12	0.78
Smoking	6	2.00	2.50	0.89	1.38	0.75	.400
CONTROL GROUP							
Alcohol (ounces a week)	23	11.45	10.53	6.02	5.93	1.39	.178
Seat belt use	46	20.89	19.32	11.20	11.51	1.32	.193
Weight (10% above average)	21	26.09	22.14	17.29	16.26	2.07	.059
Exercise (calories per week)	35	1846.23	2950.37	1132.14	2192.68	-3.23	.003
Breast examination for women	9	2.00	1.66	0.00	0.50	2.00	.081
Smoking	12	2.50	3.08	1.00	1.16	-1.63	.131

in this study focused on outcome criteria rather than specific intermediate behaviors. An example of this was the recommendation for over-weight individuals that weight loss should be one pound a week during the course of the study or until ideal weight was achieved.

Mahoney (1974) found that goals specifying behavior change, such as eating habits, rather than outcome criteria, such as body weight, were more effective in weight reduction. In addition, Bandura and Simon (1977) found that proximal (daily) goals were more effective than distally, it is possible that individuals in choice situations (i.e., the collaborative goal-setting group) have difficulty setting goals that they can realistically achieve. Steckel (1976) noted in her research on contracting that it took time for participants to learn to negotiate achievable behaviors. Much of the work related to goal setting has been conducted in a laboratory setting (Locke, 1966; Locke & Bryan,

1966, 1968) in studies performed over short time spans, generally with one stated goal. Intervening variables such as social support systems or environmental factors would not likely influence the results. Since the present investigation took place over a 3-month period, there is more chance for either of the above to influence the outcome.

The basic underlying issue is to determine if behavioral change can be stimulated regardless of risk and then to determine how to maintain change over time. In the current investigation, no contact was made with the participants during the 3-month study interval. It may be necessary to provide periodic psychological support to encourage behavioral change. In addition, the higher level of success with the provider goal-setting group may indicate that individuals prefer specified programs. Interventions focusing on intermediate behavior change (daily or weekly goals) rather than outcome criteria might represent a more successful strategy. Successful techniques over short periods could then be investigated over longer time frames to determine what is necessary to maintain behavior change.

REFERENCES

Bandura, A. (1969). *Principles of behavior modification*. New York: Holt-Rinehart-Winston.

Bandura, A. (1971). Psychotherapy based upon modeling principles. In A. E. Bergin and S. L. Garfield (Eds.), *Handbook of psychotherapy and behavior change: An empirical analysis*. (pp. 653–672). New York: John Wiley & Sons.

Bandura, A., & Simon, K. M. (1977). The role of proximal intentions in self-regulation of refractory behavior. *Cognitive Therapy Research*, *1*, 177–194.

Table 4
Paired t test Comparisons for Selected Subsamples on Global Measures of Risk Reduction

Global Measure	n	X̄ PRETEST	X̄ POSTTEST	SD PRETEST	SD POSTTEST	t	p
PROVIDER							
Current health age (years)	44	47.64	46.77	10.34	9.93	2.18	.03
Estimated life expectancy (years)	52	76.42	77.83	4.54	3.53	-4.53	<.001
Potential life expectancy increase (years)	52	5.68	4.47	2.97	2.35	4.25	<.001
COLLABORATIVE							
Current health age (years)	49	43.18	42.88	10.27	10.10	1.31	.196
Estimated life expectancy (years)	54	77.41	78.30	3.24	3.22	-3.47	<.001
Potential life expectancy increase (years)	54	4.54	3.81	2.44	2.31	3.08	.003
CONTROL							
Current health age (years)	45	43.44	43.35	11.25	10.96	.24	.811
Estimated life expectancy (years)	46	77.15	77.65	4.55	4.63	-1.38	.174
Potential life expectancy increase (years)	46	5.01	4.54	3.03	3.21	1.69	.099

Bernstein, D. A., & Glascow, R. E. (1981). The modification of smoking behavior. In O. F. Pomerleau & J. P. Brady (Eds.), *Behavioral medicine: Theory and practice*. (pp. 233–253). Baltimore: Williams and Wilkins, Inc.

Green, L. W. (1974). Toward cost-benefit evaluations of health education: Some concepts, methods, and examples. *Health Education Monographs, 2* (Supplement): 34–60.

Hefferin, E. A. (1979). Health goal-setting: Patient-nurse collaboration at Veterans Administration facilities. *Military Medicine, 144*(12), 814–822.

Locke, E. A. (1966). The relationship of intentions to level of performance. *Journal of Applied Psychology, 50*, 60–66.

Locke, E. A., & Bryan, J. R. (1966). Effects of goal-setting, rule-learning, and knowledge of score on performance. *American Journal of Psychology, 79*, 451–457.

Locke, E. A., & Bryan, J. R. (1968). Goal-setting as a determinant of the effect of knowledge of score on performance. *American Journal of Psychology, 81*(3), 398–406.

Locke, E. A., Cardledge, N., & Koeppel, J. (1968). Motivational effects of knowledge of results: A goal-setting phenomenon? *Psychological Bulletin, 70*(6), 474–485.

Maccoby, N., Farquhar, J. W., Wood, P. D., & Alexander, J. (1977). Reducing the risk of cardiovascular disease. *Journal of Community Health, 3*(2), 100–114.

Mahoney, M. J. (1974). Self-reward and self-monitoring techniques for weight control. *Behavior Therapy, 5*, 48–57.

Meyer, A. J., Nash, J. D., McAlister, A. L., Maccoby, N., & Farquhar, J. W. (1980). Skills training in cardiovascular health education campaign. *Journal of Consulting and Clinical Psychology, 48*(2), 129–142.

Meyer, H. H., Kay, E., & French, J. R. P. (1965). Split roles in performance appraisal. *Harvard Business Review, 43*, 123–129.

Morisky, D. E., Levine, D. M., Green, L. W., Shapiro, S., Russell, R. P., & Smith, C. R. (1983). Five-year blood pressure control and mortality following health education for hypertensive patients. *American Journal of Public Health, 73*(2), 153–162.

Rosenberg, S. G. (1971). Patient education leads to better care for heart patients. *HSMHA Health Reports, 86*, 793–802.

Steckel, S. B. (1976). Influence of knowledge and of contingency contracting on adherence to hypertensive treatment regimens. Doctoral dissertation, University of Michigan. *Dissertation Abstracts International*, 1979 (University Microfilms No. 76–19, 249).

This article is printed with permission of *Nursing Research*. Copyright 1985 American Journal of Nursing Company.

Orginal article:
Alexy, B. (1985). Goal setting and health risk reduction. *Nursing Research, 34,* 283–288.

CRITIQUE BY: GRACE A. LIN, BSN, RN

Part I: Clinical Relevance

The clinical problem of concern was to measure the effectiveness of goal setting on health risk reduction. When goal setting is implemented, health care providers usually take a major role in planning. Little input from clients is taken into consideration. In my clinical practice, we have begun to emphasize more mutual goal setting which allows the nurse and the patient to work together in selecting and achieving goals. This study has the potential to show us whether collaborative goal setting has impact on a client's health behaviors.

The investigator used a value expectancy model as the theoretical framework for this study. From the model, she generated a proposition predicting that collaboration in goal setting would result in a greater reduction of health risk when compared with provider-only or no goal setting. This proposition can guide nurses in deciding the usefulness of client participation in planning care.

The investigator tested two specific interventions in her study: collaborative and provider goal settings. She stated that both have potential to be used in practice because of their positive influence on health behaviors. These interventions also are based on independent nursing decisions, which can be carried out without doctor's order.

The investigator measured the study outcome by having participants complete the Personal Risk Profile (PRP) before and after the three-month study period. She then compared and analyzed results from both tests to determine whether improvement in specific health behaviors and whether changes in current health age, life expectancy, or potential life expectancy increase occurred. The potential for using this measure in nursing is great if the PRP were readily available. Since nurses can make the independent decision to use this assessment form, PRP can be beneficial in identifying patients at risk and in evaluating the effectiveness of interventions.

This study is enlightening not only because it may provide a way of modifying health behaviors, but also because we can expand its concept to support a major emphasis in nursing: client-centered care. In collaborative goal setting, nurses give clients more personal choice and independence. This sense of control may then become a motivator for better performance.

Part II: Conceptualization and Internal Consistency

In general, the investigator presented her study in a consistent manner concisely identifying research questions in the introductory paragraph. She followed this with a detailed explanation of methods, results, and reasons for discrepancies. As previously noted, the investigator derived the underlying conceptualization of her study from Edwards' (1954) value expectancy model. She further justified this conceptualization by referring to a number of similar studies in the literature review. Based on this conceptual framework, the investigator formulated her study questions to determine factors of health behaviors.

Provider and collaborative goal setting constitute the independent variables for this study. Health risk reduction constitutes the dependent variable. The investigator presumes variability in the dependent variable to depend on variability in the independent variables. In other words, she presumes that the level of health risk reduction is in some ways influenced by the intervention, goal setting.

The population of interest for this study includes individuals who have at least one identified health risk factor that could be lowered by changing behavior. The subjects selected for this study all met this criterion and were, therefore, consistent with the population of interest.

For her measuring instrument, the investigator used the Personal Risk Profile, which is based on demographic and health data provided by participants to identify health risk factors for each individual. Unfortunately, the investigator provided only a brief description of this instrument. In general, PRP seems an appropriate tool for this study. However, more examples of the data contained in PRP are needed to determine whether it is likely to measure the phenomenon of interest.

Data collection for this study proceeds systematically. The investigator collected data by questionnaire only; her data collectors analyzed the data by established protocols, not by observation or self-interpretation, thus limiting the possibility of introducing personal biases.

Part III: Believability of Results

This study purported to measure the effects of two nursing interventions in health risk reduction by way of quantitative (statistical) data procedures.

The investigator selected her subjects by way of a convenience sample from three industrial or corporate settings. As she selected subjects, however, she did not consider sample characteristics. Demographic data indicated that more males were involved in the study and the majority of participants had completed higher education or had higher family income. Therefore, while this convenience sample may not be representative of the general population, it is in the phenomenon of interest since each subject was identified to have at least one health risk factor.

The investigator estimated reliability of the measuring instrument (PRP) by test–retest, a procedure testing the stability of the tool over time. The resulting coefficient, ranging from .83 to 1.00, indicated that the tool is reliable. However, with a sample of 28 individuals taking the test and retest, and with a short period of three to five days between the two tests, the scores may not be accurate because (1) the sample size is too small and (2) the result of the second test may be influenced by the memory of the first. To achieve consistency between the three data collectors (investigator and two graduate nursing students), they have all followed established protocols for goal setting whereby goals were designated for the provider group and selected by the collaborative group.

Unfortunately, the investigator did not discuss tool validity. She mentioned only the sources from which she developed the tool. Nor does she supply examples of kinds of material contained in PRP or criteria used for measuring the phenomenon of interest. Such limited information about the tool makes it difficult to determine validity.

There were two experimental groups and one control group in this study. The investigator assigned a total of 152 subjects randomly to each group. To control the initial differences, the investigator performed analyses of covariance on overall measures of risk reduction and on each risk category with the pretest score as the covariant. The control group received no goal setting intervention while the other two groups did.

The investigator reported study results in Tables 1–4. However, she could have elaborated more on each finding based on the numerical values written in the tables. Due to my limited understanding of statistical procedures, I cannot determine whether the statistics used here are appropriate for the collected data or whether there is a better procedure to analyze the data in this study.

Findings from this study indicated a positive correlation between the independent and dependent variables. But, unexpectedly, the clients participating in goal setting did not yield a more effective change of behaviors than clients in provider goal setting. The investigator presented a thorough explanation of how these findings might have resulted and why they deviated from the theoretical expectation of this study. She used her professional judgment to evaluate some of the intervening factors that could have influenced the study, but she did not refute the statistical findings. Other influencing factors not discussed by the investigator may be invalid or insensitive measuring tool, mistakes in data collection and calculation, and weak or inconsistent interventions. The above intervening variables may result in inaccurate findings.

Part IV: Generalizability of Results

The target population for this study should be people in any setting and who have at least one identified health risk which can be reduced by behavioral change. However, because the investigator drew her sample from industrial and corporate settings, she did not use true random measures. This sample of convenience then cannot be representative of the target population. While its homogeneity might have exerted more control over extraneous variables, its limitations prohibit generalizability of the study.

The individuals doing the testing and implementing the intervention were all at graduate school level and above. Since they may have had more training in conducting a research study, it is hard to determine whether the study would yield similar results if practicing nurses with no special training in doing research had implemented interventions.

Besides the studies mentioned in the literature review, I am not aware of other studies that address the same problem, test the same intervention, evaluate the same measure or test the same theory. There might be studies that are related or similar to this one, but I will need to look for them in order to compare results.

Part V: Factors to Consider in Utilization

A scientific study is a controlled, systematic investigation that aims to develop generalizable knowledge about natural phenomena (Polit & Hungler, 1985). The findings from a nursing research activity help nurses to make more informed decisions, to improve, modify or eliminate certain interventions, and to identify factors that prevent persons from achieving their optimal level of health. But a research-based practice needs to be evaluated systematically in order to establish its validity and applicability. After evaluating this particular research, regardless of some of the flaws discussed, I can conclude that goal setting is a better intervention than no goal setting when intending to reduce health risk. I am still uncertain of what kind of goal setting is more effective since the study findings at hand do not indicate significant differences between the two. Therefore, before I can decide on an intervention that will promote optimal health for clients, more studies are needed.

In current practice, there are nurses who do not do goal setting as part of their intervention. This may be due to their lack of knowledge, lack of interacting time with clients, or lack of interest and motivation. In order to promote utilization of this research in practice, nurses must have awareness of its importance. Also, they need to spend more time with clients to identify their health risk and to help in setting goals. Educational programs will be necessary to improve nurses' knowledge levels and sharpen their assessment skills. A lighter patient load may allow nurses more time to interact with patients and carry out goal setting. Finally, nurses will need ongoing positive reinforcement to keep them interested and motivated in using this intervention. If we were to maintain the current no goal-setting practice, clients may develop more chronic illnesses and require more extensive nursing care. If we were to change the practice based on this research, cost for educational programs and other changes could be high, however. To decide whether the potential benefits outweigh the cost, we still need to conduct more studies on this issue.

REFERENCES

Polit, D., & Hungler, B. (1985). *Essentials of nursing research: Methods and applications*. Philadelphia: Lippincott.

Original article:
Alexy, B. (1985). Goal setting and health risk reduction. *Nursing Research, 34*, 283–288.

CRITIQUE BY: PAMELA HELLINGS, PhD, RN

Part I: Clinical Relevance

This study focuses on the effectiveness of client participation in determining a plan for reduction of risk for certain health problems. Using the Personal Risk Profile (PRP) to measure risk categories for heart disease, cancer, stroke, and motor vehicle accidents as well as health risk age, life expectancy, and potential for life increase, the investigator tests the theory that client participation in goal setting may increase the effectiveness of interventions aimed at risk reduction. She compares the attainment of goals for the client participation group with the result of groups in which goals are provider determined or in which goals are not formulated.

An understanding of factors which contribute to patient compliance with a plan of risk reduction offers the nurse an opportunity to develop intervention strategies which are more likely to produce the desired outcome. This question is a relevant one for nurses practicing in a variety of settings as an increase in our understanding of the factors which contribute to client participation in health promoting activities may be applied in many areas of nursing practice. The nurse who practices in an outpatient setting or inpatient facility must be able to work with the client to develop appropriate goals. The client's role in the development of the plan is an important aspect to be considered and studied.

An independent decision by a clinician experienced in the administration of an instrument, such as the PRP, to individual clients is certainly within the realm of nursing practice. The PRP also has the potential to improve the assessment of client health status as well as to measure change in health status over time. Both of these potential benefits to practice make the study worth reviewing for relevance for implementation in practice.

Part II: Conceptualization and Internal Consistency

The focus on personal choice behavior that this study offers provides an interesting area for investigation. The need to provide support for change in health behaviors serves as justification for the effort. The study questions flow naturally from a conceptual framework based on the notion that a favorable outcome is more likely in situations of risk when an individual is allowed to make choices. The links between the conceptual framework, the justification, and the study questions are clearly made. The instrument selected to measure health risk factors (PRP) appears to measure the factors of interest. However, because the investigator does not explicate the nature and number of questions related to each risk factor, the ability of the instrument to measure change over the three-month period of the study is questionable.

The convenience sample that participated in the study were well educated (over 50 percent had a baccalaureate degree) and largely male (104 as compared to 48 females). The risk factors selected for goal setting include weight management, cigarette smoking, exercise, seat belt usage, alcohol intake, and breast self-examination. These appear to be consistent with the focus on risk assessment and the design of the PRP. It would seem, however, that a sample which represents a population more consistent with the general nature of the risk factors under investigation, at least from the standpoint of sex of the participant, might have proven more illuminating.

In summary, the study does provide a justification related to the study questions and does have a conceptual basis related to theory and to nursing practice. The report is understandable and deserves further consideration for evaluation of use in practice.

Part III: Believability of Results

In this study, the investigator tests the effects of an intervention, client participation in goal setting, by way of quantitative data gathered preintervention and postintervention; the investigator calculated a risk status score using the Personal Risk Profile at both time periods. From employees who were eligible for periodic health examinations in three industrial/corporate settings, the investigator obtained a sample of convenience. Each participant had to have at least one risk factor identified by the PRP that could be lowered by a change in behavior. In the first group, the clients selected the goals they wished to achieve. In the second group, the investigator, using a protocol, determined the goals. In the control group, participants did not set any goals but were given the results of the health risk analysis. Despite random assignment into one of these three groups, the investigator found significant differences in risk scores between groups. Analyses of covariance were calculated to account for initial differences. However, since not all subjects had identified risks in all categories, the ANCOVA could only be calculated on a selected subsample. Therefore, although the investigator tried to take the initial differences in risk into account in the presentation of her results, she failed to mention other differences in the groups, such as mean age, sex of members of the group, and educational differences. It is possible that these differences may be a factor in the differences in baseline scores and exert a lingering effect on the effectiveness of the intervention—a possibility which must be considered in future research efforts. In addition, the investigator subjected each risk category to a rather complicated calculation in order to weight the total group difficulty in achieving that goal. These weightings help adjust for differences in goal setting between the collaborative goal setting group and the provider goal setting group. The resultant goal-met ratio for each subject did help address the issue of whether the achievement of goals was significantly influenced by the type of behavior risk selected for change. In addition, the calculated results supported no evidence of differences. As a consequence of all of these manipulations, the results became difficult to interpret—a definite drawback to the utilization of this research in practice.

Although the investigator discussed test–retest reliability characteristics of the tool, she made no mention of validity. Because so little is revealed about the nature of the tool, the question of its validity is an important one and needs to be clarified before consideration is given to further use of the tool.

The investigator presented results in four tables detailing the ANCOVAs for risk categories and global measures of risk reduction. In addition, she detailed results of the paired t-tests for within group comparisons. Despite the use of tables, however, this reviewer found the results difficult to interpret. Ultimately, there were very few significant findings. The provider goal-setting group was more effective in increasing current health age and in the potential for life expectancy increase. Because the scores were subject to so many weightings and division into subsamples, it is difficult to consider repeating this study, at least using the same instruments and methods.

Ultimately, the findings of the study support the notion that setting goals may be effective in changing client behavior. However, the investigator failed to substantiate the importance of client participation in the effort. In this respect, the investigator did provide potential explanations for the lack of significant findings in the use of collaborative goal setting, including the sensitivity of one aspect of the tool's results to other changes. For instance, changes in exercise and consequent weight reduction had the potential to alter scores significantly in the life expectancy and potential life expectancy increase scores. Thus, a change in one risk factor could make a significant alteration in another score. The lack of tool validity, which the investigator does not consider as a source of the lack of significant findings, should be considered here as well.

In general, the investigator goes to great lengths to make adjustments for differences in the nature of the groups and the behaviors selected for change. Yet a basic question regarding validity of the tool remains. Due to the lack of significant findings, it would be hard to justify utilization of the findings in practice, but the questions asked and the approach to answering them makes this study worthy of consideration as one attempts to plan for health promotion practice.

Part IV: Generalizability of Results

The subjects used in this sample are relatively healthy, highly educated, and predominantly male. Therefore, generalizability is limited. However, they may be representative of the typical individual who seeks health promotion counseling. They are potentially more motivated as a result of their likelihood to seek intervention in an early stage of health risk. One must question the advisability of applying the results, although minimal, to a higher risk or more diverse group.

The graduate nurses who assisted in the study followed a protocol for data collection and goal setting. Their training is not highlighted, but it is likely that practicing nurses with proper orientation to the methodology could assist in the conduct of the study. Because the investigator does not discuss interrater reliability, it is not clear if she attempted to ensure that data collective methods were similar. If they were not similar, their effect on results remains unknown.

In summary, although there are limits to generalizability, further consideration of this study for utilization in practice is justified by the relevance of an evaluation of methods of goal setting in clinical practice.

Part V: Other Factors to Consider in Utilization

In light of the limited significance of findings of this study, any recommendation to change activities in the practice setting must be made with great caution. However, this study provides a preliminary look into a relevant practice question and may serve as a first step to identifying important factors in the effort to change health behaviors in clients. The need for additional study goes without saying. The practice arena offers an ideal setting for further study. The risk is minimal and the possibilities great.

The Relationship of Internal Locus of Control, Value Placed on Health, Perceived Importance of Exercise, and Participation in Physical Activity during Leisure

Shirley Cloutier Laffrey
Department of Mental Health and
Community Nursing
University of California
San Francisco, CA

Marjorie Isenberg
College of Nursing
Wayne State University
Detroit, MI

Health promotion has traditionally been a basic function of nursing and the study of health promoting behavior is appropriate for the development of nursing science (Donaldson and Crowley, 1978). One health promoting behavior that is receiving increasing attention is physical exercise. Beyond the controversy about the relative benefits and dangers of specific exercises, the beneficial effects of regular physical activity on the quality of life are generally accepted. People enrolled in physical activity programs are said to experience feelings of well-being, increased work capacity and ability to relax, an improved self-image, and decreased anxiety and depression (Pollack, 1979; Joesting, 1981). But even widespread acceptance of these benefits has not induced many people to engage in regular physical exercise. There is, therefore, a need to identify the factors that distinguish active from sedentary people.

Dotson and Stanley (1972) and Kenyon (1968) state that the decision to engage in a physical activity is based upon the instrumental value of the activity for the individual. Instrumental value of leisure activity, chosen freely by the individual, can differ from instrumental value of work related activity, mandated by one's job. However, these two are not mutually exclusive. Many job related activities are chosen freely by individuals for their inherent value. An example would be walking up and down stairs rather than using the elevator in one's place of employment. On the other hand, many leisure activities are chosen for job related purposes. For example, an individual might engage in a sport because this leads to valuable contacts with persons who can further the individual's career. In general, however, one is more likely to find voluntary, freely chosen activities as part of leisure rather than work. For this reason, the present research focused on leisure activities in an attempt to study some of the factors associated with an individual's decision to engage in physical activity.

This study examined three factors postulated to be associated with participation in physical activity during leisure, namely the internal locus of control, the value placed on health, and the perceived importance of physical exercise.

Theoretical framework

Rotter's Social Learning Theory (1954, 1966) postulates that a particular behavior is more likely to occur if it is associated with high reinforcement value and expectancy. Reinforcement value is the degree of preference for a particular reinforcement if various alternative reinforcements are available. Expectancy is the probability that the particular reinforcement will occur as a result of an individual's behavior (Rotter et al., 1972). The potential for a particular behavior to occur, therefore, is a function of the expected occurrence of reinforcement following the behavior (Rotter, 1954).

The term "locus of control" describes the degree to which the reinforcement is contingent on one's own behavior (internal locus of control) rather than on control by other persons, chance, fate, or luck (external locus of control). Rotter measures locus of control by the Internal/External scale (I/E) on which high scores reflect external locus of control and low scores reflect internal locus of control.

Wallston et al. (1978) have developed the Multidimensional Health Locus of Control (MHLC) scales as a specific health related measure of locus of control. These scales measure locus of control as a multidimensional construct instead of internality and externality as polar opposites. The MHLC consists of three scales; one for internal health locus of control (IHLC); one for chance health locus of control (CHLC); and one for health locus of control by powerful others (PHLC). Each scale ranges from low to high score.

Locus of control has been examined in many health related studies, usually with the assumption that internally controlled individuals will engage in health promoting behavior to a greater extent than externally controlled ones. The assumption has only partially been supported. Studying single and married women's use of family planning methods, Macdonald (1970) found that single women who were internally controlled were more likely to use family planning methods. Lee and Mancini (1981) found that internally controlled single women were more likely to use effective contraceptives than were externally controlled women. Manno and Marston (1972) found a positive relationship between weight loss and internal control in a group of overweight persons. Although reinforcement was not a variable in the latter two studies, one can infer that subjects associated their behavior (family planning practices and measures to reduce weight) with at least moderate reinforcement value. This is not so clear in other studies. Dabbs and Kirscht (1971) measured locus of control in two groups; one had received influenza vaccine and the other had not. They found no relationship of locus of control and the taking of influenza shots. Because reinforcement value is not discussed in their article, one could assume that the internally controlled persons who did not receive the vaccine simply did not associate any reinforcement value with this behavior. There is no theoretical reason to expect locus of control to be predictive of a health promoting behavior unless it is combined with a measure of the reinforcement of that behavior. Rotter (1975, p. 54) notes, "without doubt, the most frequent conceptual problem of a number of investigators is the failure to treat reinforcement as a separate variable."

Lowery and DuCette (1976) examined the relationship between patients' locus of control and their knowledge and control of diabetes in a group of newly diagnosed diabetics and a group of longer term diabetics. A positive relationship between internality and knowledge and control of disease was found in the newly diagnosed diabetics but not in the long term group. The authors offered as possible explanation that control mechanisms used by the internals did not lead to disease control and were, therefore, given up. This would support the notion that an important condition of an individual's taking an action is that the individual perceives that action to be worthwhile; that there be at least a moderate amount of expectancy that an action will produce a positive reinforcement value.

In a 1980 review of health locus of control research, Wallston and Wallston note that the samples showing the most internal control tend to be those exhibiting health behaviors (birth control use, smoking reduction), college students, and middle to upper-middle class samples, and that there is little indication that locus of control varies by age or sex. Although reinforcement value is not explicitly mentioned in many locus of control studies they reviewed, social learning theory postulates its importance as a variable associated with locus of control. We would suggest that the results of locus of control research might be more consistent if both reinforcement value and expectancy were explicitly measured.

In studies in which reinforcement value is considered, value of health is often the measure of reinforcement (Wallston and Wallston, 1980). Internally controlled persons who value health are hypothesized to seek more health information and engage in health behaviors to a greater extent than persons who are less internally controlled and value health less. In a study of participants in a smoking cessation program, Kaplan and Cowles (1978) found that high health value together with high internal locus of control was characteristic of persons who reduced the number of cigarettes smoked and maintained this reduction over a three month period. Saltzer (1981) studied weight loss behavior of persons who intended to lose weight. The internally controlled persons who placed a high value on physical appearance or health lost more weight than internally controlled persons with a low value on physical appearance or health. The relative influences of reinforcement value and locus of control are not clear however. Phares (1971) notes that the value of a situation declines following failure to successfully control that situation. Wallston and Wallston (1980) have suggested that internal locus and reinforcement value are more likely to be related to a given behavior if they are close to the behavior. That is, health specific internal locus of control would be more closely related to health behavior than general internal locus of control. Therefore, it is important that the measure of attitude toward a behavior be specific to the behavior in question.

We measured four variables: (1) internality of health locus of control, (2) value of health, (3) perceived importance of physical exercise, and (4) amount of physical activity engaged in during leisure. Internality of health locus of control is a measure of expectancy; value of health is a general measure of reinforcement value; perceived importance of physical exercise is a specific measure of reinforcement value; and amount of physical activity during leisure is a measure of health behavior.

The four hypotheses we tested were:
(1). The greater the internal locus of control, the greater the amount of physical activity during leisure.
(2). The greater the value placed on health, the greater the amount of physical activity during leisure.
(3). The greater the perceived importance of physical exercise, the greater the amount of physical activity during leisure.
(4). Internal locus of control, value of health, and perceived importance of physical exercise, taken together, are more predictive of amount of physical exercise during leisure than is each variable separately.

METHOD

Sample

Seventy women, aged 24-65 years (mean age: 43 years), comprised the sample. The women in this convenience sample were recruited from adult education classes that were not health related in three Midwest cities of the United States. All but one woman had completed high school. The reported mean number of years of education was 14. The mean yearly family income was in the $25,000 to $50,000 range; 38% reported incomes over $50,000, and 14% below $25,000.

Procedure

Adult education classes were contacted with permission of the school administration. The study purpose was explained to teachers and, if they consented, to their classes. Persons who indicated a willingness to participate in the study were given a questionnaire to be completed and returned during class the following week. Confidentiality was assured, and persons who wished an abstract upon completion of the study were asked to write their names and addresses on a separate sheet of paper. Questions about the study were answered at the time the questionnaires were distributed to the participants and at the time they were collected. Of 98 distributed questionnaires, 70 were completed and returned; a completion rate of 72%.

Questionnaire

The questionnaire took 10-15 minutes to complete. In addition to asking demographic data, the following variables were measured:

(1) *Physical activity during leisure*. The measure was adapted from the Physical Activity Recall

Record (Reiff et al., 1967) and the Minnesota Leisure Time Activity Questionnaire [LTA] (Taylor et al., 1978).

Subjects were asked to check each activity performed during the past month and indicate the usual number of minutes per activity session and the number of times per week they engaged in the activity. The score consisted of the summed products of the intensity code for the activities, number of minutes per activity session, and number of times per week.

Validity and reliability findings have been reported for the instrument (Reiff et al., 1967; Taylor et al., 1978). The rank order correlation between objectively scored questionnaires (the scoring method used in this study) and subjectively ranked subjects from "most active" to "least active" was 0.91. The LTA was found to discriminate effectively between swimmers and non-athletes (Taylor et al., 1978).

(2) *Internal health locus of control*. The IHLC, developed by Wallston et al. (1978), uses a 6-point Likert-like format for responses ranging from "strongly agree" (6) to "strongly disagree" (1). A subject's score is obtained by summing the scores for the six items on that dimension. Equivalent forms of the instrument have been developed. Form A was used in this study (Wallston et al., 1978).

Alpha reliabilities of 0.67−0.77 for individual forms and 0.83−0.86 for the combined forms have been reported (Wallston et al., 1978). The IHLC is negatively correlated ($r = 0.30$; $P < 0.01$) with the PHLC and positively correlated with perceived health status ($r = 0.40$; $P < 0.001$) and with its counterpart in Levenson's Internal, Powerful Others, and Chance Scales ($r = 0.57$; $P < 0.001$). The IHLC has been used in a large number of studies (Wallston and Wallston, 1980).

(3) *Health value*. Health value was measured by a scale of 10 values adapted from Rokeach's scale of 18 terminal values which force a subject to order a value at the expense of another (Wallston et al., 1978). Subjects were asked to rank the values from "most important" (scored "1") to "least important" (scored "10") as guiding principles in their lives. The rank position assigned to "health" was the score for the item. To be consistent with the other measures in this study health value was reverse scored for data analysis. No validity or reliability data are available for the adapted scale, but the original Rokeach scale shows satisfactory test-retest reliability ($r = 0.70$) and predictive validity (Robinson and Shaver, 1973).

(4) *Perceived importance of physical exercise*. A 9-point Likert-like scale ranging from "most important" (scaled "9") to "least important" (scaled "1") was used to measure this variable. The measure developed for this study, asked persons to mark the importance of physical exercise in their lives at this time.

The hypotheses were tested by means of zero-order correlations and stepwise multiple regression analyses. Although the data for the independent and dependent variables are considered ordinal to quasi-interval, multiple regression techniques were used based on the arguments of Kerlinger (1973) and Labovitz (1970) that the error is negligible when interval statistics are used for these data. The 0.05 level of significance was accepted. The Pearson Correlation and Multiple Regression Programs of the Statistical Package for the Social Sciences were used in all data analyses.

RESULTS

Ranges and means for the four major study variables are shown in Table 1. Inter-correlations of variables are shown in Table 2.

Table 1
Ranges, Means, and Standard Deviations for Major Variables ($n = 70$)

Variables	Range	Mean
Leisure time physical activity	0–5100	1342
Perceived importance of physical exercise	1–9	5.6
Value of health	1–9	7.7
Internal health locus of control	14–35	26

Table 2
Matrix of Pearson Correlations among Variables

of exercise	Perceived importance of exercise	Health value	IHLC	Education	Income	Age
Physical activity during leisure	0.53‡	0.07	0.10	0.34†	0.11	-0.24*
Perceived importance of exercise		0.17	0.19	0.36†	0.06	-0.24*
Health value			-0.16	-0.16	0.05	0.15
IHLC				0.14	-0.02	-0.05
Education					0.35†	-0.33†
Income						-0.38†

*$P < 0.05$.
†$P < 0.01$.
‡$P < 0.001$.

The correlation coefficients for the relationships between amount of physical activity during leisure and IHLC ($r = 0.10$) and health value ($r = 0.07$) were not significant at the 0.05 level. Hypotheses 1 and 2, which predicted that amount of physical activity during leisure would be positively associated with internal health locus of control and value placed on health, were therefore not supported.

The relationship between amount of physical activity during leisure and perceived importance of physical exercise was significant ($r = 0.53$; $P < 0.001$). Twenty-eight percent of the variance in physical activity during leisure was explained by perceived importance of physical exercise. Hypothesis 3 was therefore supported.

In the stepwise multiple regression procedure used to test hypothesis 4, the order of entry of variables into the equation was perceived importance of exercise, health value, and IHLC. The multiple correlation of the independent variables on physical activity during leisure was moderate, with a Multiple R of 0.46 (see Table 3).

Virtually all of the variance in physical activity during leisure was explained by perceived importance of exercise. Additional variance from health value and IHLC was minimal, increasing the R^2 by only 0.01. Hypothesis 4 was therefore not supported.

Two other variables most likely to predict amount of physical activity were age and education. The correlation coefficient for the relationship between physical activity during leisure and age was -0.24; $P < 0.05$, and the correlation coefficient between physical activity during leisure and education was 0.35; $P < 0.01$ (see Table 2).

Table 3
Multiple Regression of Perceived Importance of Exercise, Health Value, and IHLC on Amount of Physical Activity during Leisure Time

Independent variables	Multiple R	R^2	R^2 change	Beta	F
Perceived importance of exercise	0.46	0.21	0.21	0.44	12.3*
Health value	0.46	0.21	0.00	0.02	0.03
IHLC	0.47	0.22	0.01	0.08	0.37

*$P < 0.01$

Additionally, age and education were each significantly correlated with perceived importance of exercise (see Table 2). To detect whether these variables were confounding the relationship between perceived importance of exercise and physical activity during leisure, an additional stepwise multiple regression analysis was computed for perceived importance of exercise, age, and education on amount of physical activity during leisure.

As before, perceived importance of exercise account for virtually all of the variance in physical activity during leisure (Multiple $R = -0.47$) with age and education increasing the R^2 by only 0.03. Age and education therefore were not confounding the relationship between perceived importance of exercise and amount of physical activity during leisure.

DISCUSSION

Although literature suggests that such variables as health value and internality play a role in an individual's undertaking a health promoting activity, these variables proved to have little effect in the present study. It is likely that the women did not relate physical activity during leisure to health, *per se*. For example, leisure time physical activity might be associated with enjoyment, attractiveness, slimness; reasons not consciously associated with the notion of promoting health.

In 1968, Kenyon described physical activity as a multidimensional concept with six subsets based on the instrumental value of physical activity for the individual. Only one of these subsets was health. In the others, physical activity was seen as: (1) a social experience, meeting new people and perpetuating existing relationships; (2) pursuit of vertigo, perceiving risk and thrill through body movement and sudden changes in direction; (3) an aesthetic experience, perceiving body movement as possessing beauty or artistic qualities; (4) catharsis, providing release of tension and frustration; and (5) an ascetic experience, aspiring to high levels of achievement through strenuous physical training. If some of these nonhealth factors were operating in the present study, a nonhealth-related locus of control measure might have been more sensitive in correlating internality and leisure time physical activity. Sonstrom and Walker (1973), in a study similar to the present one, used a nonhealth measure, Rotter's I/E scale, to measure locus of control and found significantly higher amounts of physical activity for internal subjects with a concurrent positive attitude toward physical activity.

A possible explanation for the lack of relationship between IHLC and leisure time physical activity is a social desirability factor that was not measured here. If, in our sample, leisure time physical activity is considered a "socially accepted activity," then both high and low internals as well as externals might be likely to participate in high levels of exercise but for reasons that would warrant further study.

Another explanation would be the novelty versus publicity of a given behavior. Wallston and Wallston (1980) note that possibly health-related behavior that is much in the public domain is less tied to locus of control than less visible or less well publicized behavior. Rotter *et al.* (1972) note that generalized expectancies for locus of control are particularly predictive in novel situations but, as the person gains experience in these situations, the predictive power of generalized expectancies decreases and is supplanted by situation-specific expectancies.

Health clubs, spas, aerobic dancing, and physical education in various settings had been well publicized in the area in which the study was conducted. Our sample consisted of middle to upper-middle class women who had access to community resources for physical activities. They were already availing themselves of one community resource, namely, the adult education classes from which they were selected for the study. Although these classes were not physical exercise related, it is likely that women who attend adult education classes do not reflect the characteristics of the total female population. They, more than persons who must depend on their own surroundings for physical activities, may be more likely to engage in physical activities for purely social reasons. If this is so, a relationship between internality and physical activity might not be expected for this group. It would be important to study the relationships among internality, health value, and health behavior in persons who do not have ready access to community resources for health related behaviors.

Another factor that may account for the lack of relationship between internality and physical activity during leisure is the relationship between work and leisure activity. The amount of physical activity associated with one's work might very well affect the kinds of leisure activities that one chooses. Therefore, measurement of work related activities is warranted in future physical activity research.

The significant relationship between perceived importance of physical exercise and amount of physical activity during leisure is important for nursing. Many studies have examined the relationships of various health promoting behaviors and locus of control, but clients' perceptions of the importance of particular actions have generally been ignored in favor of the health professional's perception of importance. However, if the behavior is performed for nonhealth reasons, or if general health value is too remote from the behavior, then perceived importance on the part of the client becomes a more salient predictor of the behavior than the indicators generally seen in the health literature, such as locus of control. Ajzen and Fishbein (1980) argue the importance of a high degree of correspondence between attitude and behavior. If the attitude being measured is far removed from a given behavior, one wouldn't expect a relationship between the two. Value placed on health may have been far removed from engaging in physical activities during leisure, whereas the degree of importance of physical exercise was more specific to engaging in physical activities.

This is not to say that locus of control and value of health may not be factors with many behaviors, but simply that they may not be tapping into the perceptions of the client. Saltzer (1979) supports this idea with her finding that completers and drop-outs of a weight reduction program were not distinguished by the Multidimensional Health Locus of Control scale but were distinguished by a situation-specific Weight Locus of Control measure. High internals on the Weight Locus of Control scale who also held high values for personal appearance were more likely than others to complete the program. She concluded that the main motivation for women in the weight reduction program was a desire for improved physical appearance and not health, and therefore general health beliefs were less predictive than weight specific beliefs.

Wallston and Wallston (1980), in their study of dental maintenance behaviors, supported Saltzer's findings. They found a significant relationship between specific questions about perceived benefits and costs of carrying out the behaviors, but not with generalized health locus of control. Given these two studies, an exercise-specific locus of control measure might have been more closely related to physical exercise. This factor also helps to explain the relationship between perceived importance of physical exercise and amount of physical activity as contrasted to the lack of relationship between health value (a more remote measure of reinforcement) and amount of physical activity.

The relationship between perceived importance of physical exercise and amount of physical activity during leisure lends support to the traditional notion of assessing what is important to the patient/client and using client perceptions as the basis for nursing interventions. This is important for nursing practice in helping us understand how clients view physical activity. Further investigation of relationships between client perceived importance and other health related behaviors could elucidate the mechanisms of effective nursing interventions.

Probably more important would be the study of clients' views regarding benefits of health related behaviors. If benefits are seen in terms of broader reinforcements than we in the health professions customarily assume, then assisting clients by using these broader definitions may prove to be a more successful approach to encourage health promoting behaviors.

REFERENCES

Ajzen, I., & Fishbein, M. (1980). *Understanding attitudes and predicting social behavior*. Englewood Cliffs, NJ: Prentice-Hall.

Dabbs, J. M., & Kirsch, J. P. (1971). Internal control and the taking of influenza shots. *Psychological Reports, 28*, 959.

Donaldson, S. K., & Crowley, D. M. (1978). The discipline of nursing. *Nursing Outlook, 26*, 113–120.

Dotson, C. O., & Stanley, W. J. (1972). Values of physical activity perceived by male university students. *Research Quarterly, 43*, 148–156.

Joesting, J. (1981). Comparison of students who exercise with those who do not. *Perceptual and Motor Skills, 53*, 426.

Kaplan, G. D., & Cowles, A. (1978). Health locus of control and health value in the prediction of smoking reduction. *Health Education Monographs, 6*, 129–137.

Kenyon, G. S. (1968). A conceptual model for characterizing physical activity. *Research Quarterly, 39*, 96–105.

Kerlinger, F. N. (1973). *Foundations of behavior research, (2nd ed.)*. New York: Holt, Rinehart and Winston.

Labovitz, S. (1970). The assignment of numbers to rank order categories. *American Sociological Review, 35*, 515–524.

Lee, T. R., & Mancini, J. A. (1981). Locus of control and premarital sexual behaviors. *Psychological Reports, 49*, 882.

Lowery, B. J., & DuCette, J. P. (1976). Disease-related learning and disease control in diabetics as a function of locus of control. *Nursing Research, 25*, 358–362.

MacDonald, A. P. (1970). Internal-external locus of control and the practice of birth control. *Psychological Reports, 27*, 206.

Manno, B., & Marston, A. P. (1972). Weight reduction as a function of negative reinforcement (sensitization versus positive covert reinforcement). *Behavior Research and Therapy, 10*, 201.

Phares, E. J. (1971). Internal-external control and the reduction of reinforcement value after failure. *Journal of Consulting and Clinical Psychology, 37*, 386–390.

Pollack, M. L. (1979). Exercise—a preventive prescription. *Journal of School Health*, 215–219.

Reiff, G. G., Montoye, H. J., Remington, R. D., Napier, J. A., Metzner, H. L., & Epstein, F. H. (1967). Assessment of physical activity by questionnaire and interview. In M. J. Karvonen & A. J. Barry (Eds.), *Physical activity and the heart*, Springfield, IL: Charles C. Thomas, & J. P. Robinson, & P. R. Shaver. (1973). *Measures of social psychological attitudes*. Ann Arbor, MI: Institute for Social Research.

Rotter, J. B. (1966). Generalized expectancies for internal versus external control of reinforcement. *Psychological Monographs, 80*, 1–28.

Rotter, J. B. (1954). *Social learning theory and clinical psychology*. New York: Prentice-Hall.

Rotter, J. B. (1975). Some problems and misconceptions related to the construct of internal vs. external control of reinforcement. *Journal of Consulting and Clinical Psychology. 43*, 56–67.

Rotter, J. B., Chance, J. E., & Phares, E. J. (1972). *Applications of a social learning theory of personality*. New York: Holt, Rinehart and Winston.

Saltzer, E. B. (1979). *Causal beliefs and losing weight: A study of behavioral intention theory and locus of control in the prediction of health-related behavior*. Unpublished doctoral dissertation, University of California at Irvine.

Saltzer, E. B. (1981). Cognitive moderators of the relationship between behavioral intentions and behavior. *Journal of Personality and Social Psychology, 41*, 260–271.

Sonstrom, R. J., & Walker, M. I. (1973). Relationship of attitudes and locus of control to exercise and physical fitness. *Perceptual and Motor Skills, 36*, 1031–1034.

Taylor, H. L., Jacobs, D. R., Schucker, B., Knudsen, J., Leon, A. S., & Debacker, C. (1978). A questionnaire for the assessment of leisure time physical activities. *Journal of Chronic Diseases, 31*, 741–755.

This article is printed with permission of *International Journal of Nursing Studies*. Copyright 1983 Pergamon Press, Inc.

Original article:
Laffrey, S.C., & Isenberg, M. (1983). The relationship of internal locus of control, value placed on health, perceived importance of exercise, and participation in physical activity during leisure. *International Journal of Nursing Studies, 20*(3), 187–195.

CRITIQUE BY: KAREN S. DAVIS, BSN, RN

Part I: Clinical Relevance

The introduction to this study provides a succinct explanation of the importance of the topic to the nursing profession. The investigators indicate that by studying "factors that distinguish active from sedentary people" we might be able to generalize the results to the broad concept of health promotion, an important function of nursing.

Specifically, this study examines three factors that may influence physical activity level: internal locus of control, value placed on health, and perceived importance of exercise. Because I have interest in working on a cardiac step-down unit, this study could be of value to me. I believe exercise and physical activity to be of prime importance for patients recovering from open heart surgery, but often see a lack of motivation. In addition, if this study can help distinguish what internal or external factors motivate patients, then it is relevant to nursing practice in general.

Laffrey and Isenberg utilize Rotter's Social Learning Theory as a basis for their study. They define their variables as measures of "reinforcement value" and "expectancy." According to the theoretical framework, these are two basic concepts associated with the likelihood that a particular behavior will occur.

Through an understandable explanation of these concepts, I could appreciate that, in the clinical setting, by knowing the reinforcement value/expectancy of an activity for my client, I might better understand why he or she would choose or not choose to participate in an activity.

In this study, the investigators do not test a specific intervention. Rather they present a study that could provide information to help a nurse better understand underlying reasons for a client's health behavior. By integrating results from the four hypotheses tested I would hope to be able to use the information to analyze patient behavior toward activity. Instead of giving up on a patient who stubbornly refuses to get out of bed, I would be able to plan interventions based on my analysis of motivating factors.

At best, these interventions would be independent nursing actions subject to the level of activity determined best for the client by a multidisciplinary health care team and client input.

Laffrey and Isenberg use tools to measure the dependent variable (amount of physical activity) alone and also as related to each of the three independent variables: internal locus of control, value placed on health, and perceived importance of exercise.

They link these variables to the framework they use. To clarify the relationship for myself, I used the following diagram:

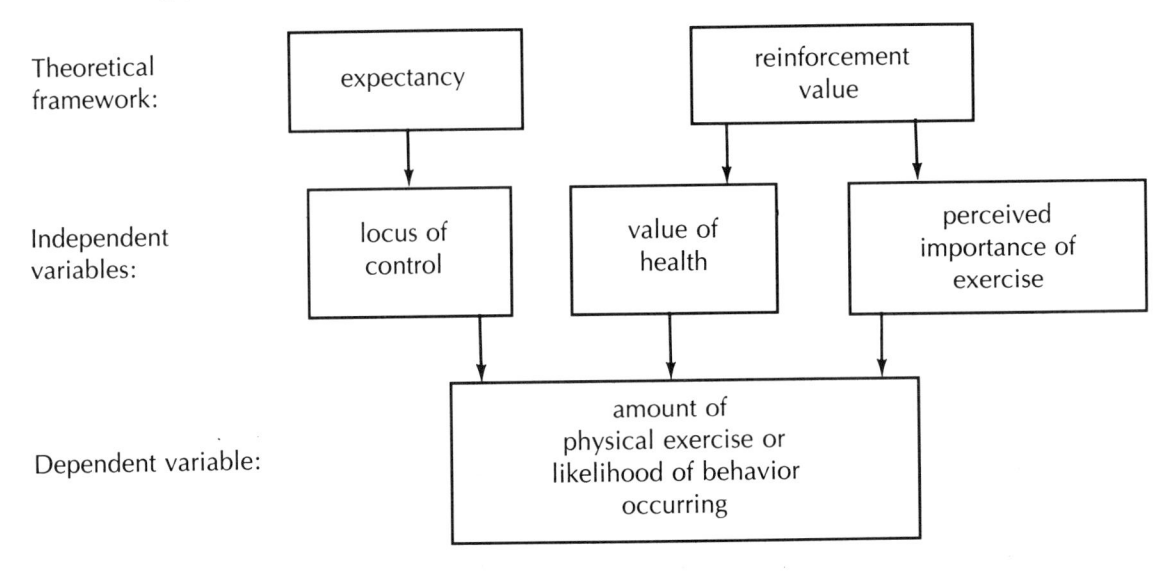

```
Theoretical          ┌───────────┐              ┌──────────────┐
framework:           │ expectancy│              │reinforcement │
                     │           │              │    value     │
                     └─────┬─────┘              └──────┬───────┘
                           │                ┌──────────┴──────────┐
                           ▼                ▼                     ▼
Independent          ┌───────────┐   ┌───────────┐         ┌──────────────┐
variables:           │  locus of │   │  value of │         │  perceived   │
                     │  control  │   │  health   │         │ importance of│
                     │           │   │           │         │   exercise   │
                     └─────┬─────┘   └─────┬─────┘         └──────┬───────┘
                           └───────────┐   │   ┌──────────────────┘
                                       ▼   ▼   ▼
                              ┌─────────────────────┐
                              │     amount of       │
Dependent variable:           │ physical exercise or│
                              │ likelihood of behavior│
                              │     occurring       │
                              └─────────────────────┘
```

The investigators used a demographic questionnaire and four tools to measure the dependent and independent variables. Beyond their use in the study, I did not investigate these tools further. In a hospital-based practice, however, their use would be difficult, as they would need to be given to each patient and analyzed separately, then together, for results. Therefore, instead of attempting to replicate the study, I plan to use its results to enhance my general understanding of behavior.

My initial reaction is that the study is well thought out and timely. There is one question the study left unanswered, however: what factors besides the three to be tested are associated with physical activity level, and how did the investigators choose these three over others?

Part II: Conceptualization and Internal Consistency

After reading the study, I found that the investigators did follow through on their research design by studying the concepts they outlined in their introductory comments. In addition, they have written their study with clarity and concision, systematically explained how they tested variables, and provided sufficient results.

For these reasons and because previous studies involving locus of control and reinforcement value have had conflicting results, I feel the study is justifiable. Actually, the majority of studies described in the literature review measured specific health behaviors rather than the more general concept of "physical activity" as measured in the present study.

In addition, this study tries to test individual factors that influence physical activity, and then combine those factors to see if their sum has a greater impact than each does alone. In this way, the investigators directly relate the four hypotheses to the theory their study is based on, and provide a way to test the concepts in question. The four hypotheses outlined in the study include: (1) the greater the internal locus of control, the greater the amount of physical activity during leisure; (2) the greater the value placed on health, the greater the amount of physical activity during leisure;

… (3) the greater the perceived importance of physical exercise, the greater the amount of physical activity during leisure; and (4) internal locus of control, value of health, and perceived importance of physical exercise, taken together, are more predictive of amount of physical exercise during leisure than is each variable separately.

The results and conclusions that Laffrey and Isenberg present relate directly to the hypotheses. In addition, they have designed their study so that independent and dependent variables relate logically.

Unfortunately, the sample they chose was very specific; it is not one that would be easily generalizable. For example, if the population I was working with was post-open heart surgery patients in a hospital, it would be mainly males age 50–80; the sample in the study was totally female with a mean age of 43 years.

This factor alone causes concern. I would want to find a research study with a more generalizable sample. However, I would still consider utilizing the results of this study if I felt they could broaden my general understanding of human behavior.

At first reading, the instruments used to collect data appear to accurately measure the variables. Then, too, I felt comfortable with the types of tools described. I will discuss them in greater detail in the following section.

Since study subjects took the questionnaires home, and post-surgical patients are confined to the hospital usually for seven to ten days, this data collection method could not be exactly replicated in the hospital. However, the tools conceivably could be given to patients at discharge if I wanted to replicate the study for my own specific population of interest. Patients then could return the tools via mail or at their first post-discharge doctor appointment. It would be important to note that the transition to home after heart surgery is often a traumatic time involving many lifestyle changes, and the home a very different setting than the one used in this study.

Despite several ways in which the study does not directly relate to my practice, it could still be of use. However, my understanding of the study would increase if I discussed it with someone more familiar with the tools or by investigating them more myself.

Part III: Believability of Results

This study purported to provide descriptive information about health promoting behavior, a topic important to nursing, since health promotion is one of nursing's main thrusts, and since many independent nursing interventions revolve around this concept. The data collected are primarily quantitative.

The subjects selected comprised a convenience sample of women aged 24–65 years. The investigators provide an explanation of the procedure used in selection. In the results section, the investigators described two variables of the population that could be confounding, and included these in the data analysis. However, they found that possibility to be negative and the variables *not* confounding.

In their conclusion, the investigators commented about their sample selection: "it is likely that women who attend adult education classes do not reflect the characteristics of the total female population." I agree with this statement as the age, health, income, and education level of the women are probably not representative of the total female population.

Laffrey and Isenberg do not comment on the threats that result from their sample selection procedure: those of selection, mortality, Hawthorne effect, novelty effect, and experimenter effect. For example, the sample is biased (threat of selection) because the investigators chose *only* women in an adult education class for convenience, and went through two additional groups (the school administrators and school teachers) to get consent to even approach the subjects and ask for participants.

In addition the investigators used a tool for each factor they tested by the hypothesis. For the "physical activity during leisure" factor, they used two instruments. They report validity and reliability, but it is not clear whether the figures are for *one* of the instruments or both combined. They include a sentence about the ability of these instruments to differentiate between "swimmers and non-athletes," which does not relate to the study at hand and makes me wonder if these tools are appropriate after all.

For the "internal locus of control" factor, the investigators reported on tool reliability but not validity. They described "alpha reliabilities" with which I am not familiar. To confirm the appropriateness of this test of reliability, I would have to seek consultation from one familiar with its use.

To measure the "health value" factor, the investigators adapted a scale with no reliability or validity reported. To measure "perceived importance of exercise," they developed a tool specifically for this study, again with no reliability or validity reported.

The investigators' description of the tools does not inspire confidence that any of the results would be reliable or valid. However, in a nonexperimental design utilizing psychologically oriented measures, it is difficult to establish the validity of an instrument (Polit & Hungler, 1985).

In their discussion, Laffrey and Isenberg provide several explanations of why they may have achieved the results they did. They also expand on how the study results could be used clinically in nursing, and this discussion remains within the boundary of the study.

An area included in the discussion that might better fit in the introductory material is the explanation of Kenyon's conceptual framework regarding physical activity. The investigators appear to have included it in the discussion section to provide an explanation for their results. If included earlier and in addition to Rotter's Social Learning Theory, it would have provided more depth in explaining other factors that impact physical activity.

This is a non-experimental design. The investigators did not test an intervention nor did they use a control group.

They reported results in both narrative and tabular form with descriptions of results for each hypothesis, including reasons for whether or not each hypothesis found support. In their methods section, the investigators state that they analyzed data using zero-order correlations and multiple regression methods. They indicate that these levels of measure may be inappropriate for the type of data collected (ordinal to quasiinterval) but defend using these levels based on arguments presented by other researchers.

Whether or not those arguments are valid is beyond my knowledge of statistics. Again, I would need to seek consultation with a nurse researcher fluent in such statistics. As a result, with the limited knowledge I have of methods of data analysis, I found the tables to be of no help at all in understanding the results.

The investigators offer explanations of why results were or were not statistically significant. The result that *was* statistically significant was the relationship between the perception of importance of physical exercise and actual amount of physical activity.

Laffrey and Isenberg contend that the two may be related because of the "high degree of correspondence often seen between attitude and behavior" as described by other researchers. Their discussion of this seems logical—basically, they say if something is perceived as important in one's life, one will attend to that activity. They expand this to clinical nursing by reminding us that it "lends support to the traditional notion of [the nurse] assessing what is important to the patient/client and using client perceptions as the basis for nursing interventions."

As far as the "locus of control" and "value of health" variables, the investigators use professional judgement to offer explanations as to why the results may not be statistically significant. They name the sample and instruments as playing a part in the fact that three of the hypotheses were not supported.

Questions regarding the applicability of this research to a hospital setting are raised in this section. Also, although the investigators continue to write in a clear and concise manner, to understand the tests of reliability, methods of data analysis, and tables would require consultation with other sources. The other option—to leave my questions unanswered—is not appropriate because it would diminish confidence in utilizing study results. The investigators should keep in mind when reporting their study results that the more roadblocks involved (i.e., needing to get experts to help interpret results) the less chance the results will be implemented in nursing practice. While it is appropriate for a practicing nurse to analyze research, including looking for help as necessary, often finding the time to do so is difficult.

The overall significant result of the study and recommendation—to assess what is important to the client—offers no risk and should be incorporated into any nursing assessment. This study reinforces that client behaviors are based on what is important to the client, not necessarily what is important to the other members of the health care team.

Part IV: Generalizability of Results

In several sections of this critique I have mentioned that the sample and setting of the study at hand are not similar to the population with which I would like to generalize results. Therefore, study results would be difficult to generalize to many settings.

Part V: Other Factors to Consider in Utilization

Based on using the information from this study with individual patients, I see no risks and numerous possible benefits in assessing with the patient what is important to him or her and whether the nurse and patient can relate these attitudes to physical activity in the hospital and at home after discharge.

A follow-up program would be helpful in the systematic evaluation of research-based practice, and would help us to discover if the client continues to be physically active at home based on his or her own motivations and attitudes.

The only cost I see for assessing what is important to the client (and relating this to physical activity) is time. If the assessment could not be done during the "official" nursing data base assessment, a creative nurse should be able to find other times to build up a knowledge base of what the client's interests are and what he or she perceives as important.

In conclusion, this study can provide motivation for nurses to include client input in their nursing care plans. It reminded me that nursing research can be used to point out and defend nursing interventions that have traditionally been paired with successful client outcomes.

Original article:
Laffrey, S.C., & Isenberg, M. (1983) The relationship of internal locus of control, value placed on health, perceived importance of exercise, and participation in physical activity during leisure. *International Journal of Nursing Studies*, 20(3), 187−195.

CRITIQUE BY: PAMELA HELLINGS, PhD, RN

Part I: Clinical Relevance

This study focuses on the importance of physical exercise as one type of health promoting activity. The investigators point out the need to identify characteristics that separate active from sedentary individuals. Therefore, they propose to study the relationship of internal locus of control, the value placed on health, and the perceived importance of physical exercise on participation in physical activity during leisure.

This study has the potential to impact on practice as one attempts to gain an increased understanding of the factors which may alter an individual's interest in or willingness to participate in health promoting behaviors. The ability to develop appropriate interventions is enhanced by an ability to understand the motivational factors which apply to the particular area of interest: participation in physical activity.

The investigators base their theoretical framework on Rotter's Social Learning Theory. This theory, which the investigators examined for utilization in practice, states that a behavior is more likely to occur if it is associated with a high degree of preference and expectation for reinforcement.

In their study, the investigators did not test a specific intervention; rather, they investigated the relationship between four variables, including: value of health, perceived importance of physical exercise, internality of health locus of control, and amount of physical activity engaged in during leisure time. From these four variables, they generated four hypotheses which predict the relationship between each of the first three and the fourth. The fourth hypothesis predicts that the three factors taken separately predict less than the three factors combined regarding amount of physical activity.

Three of the measures used in this study are readily available and may be used independently by clinicians in the practice setting. The fourth measure (perceived importance of physical exercise), which the investigators developed, would, I assume, be available with their permission. The measures, to be described in more detail in the following section, may be administered in a relatively short period of time and require little preparation to administer but more to interpret. The ability of the practitioner to assess an individual client's motivation to participate in physical activities would enhance the opportunity to develop appropriate intervention strategies. It also is noteworthy that the assessment may be completed in a relatively short period of time—an important consideration for busy nurses.

In general, an initial review of this study for relevance suggests that it is appropriate for further investigation for utilization in practice.

Part II: Conceptualization and Internal Consistency

The investigators move from a description of the theoretical bases to the development of the project in a logical fashion. As a result, the investigators make apparent the relationship between the theoretical framework and research hypotheses. Based on increasing understanding of the differences between those who engage in regular physical activity and those who do not, the investigators explicate and justify their study's relevance to nursing practice in health promotion.

They describe their research methodology with sufficient detail and logical concision. The instruments they selected to measure variables also appear to be appropriate.

In general, the conceptualization of the study is clear. In addition, the report of the study allows the reader to share in the conceptualization due to the clarity of the presentation. It is, therefore, appropriate to continue to evaluate this study for utilization in practice.

Part III: Believability of Results

The investigators recruited into their study 70 middle class women with a mean education of 14 years and who participated in adult education classes. Unfortunately, the investigators failed to justify or explain the reason for this selection of an all female sample. They did, however, take care to select classes which were not related to health topics.

To measure the variable of physical activity during leisure, the investigators adapted the Physical Activity Recall Record and the Minnesota Leisure Time Activity Questionnaire (LTA). Apparently, reliability and validity findings are available for the LTA, but are not reported. Likewise, no reliability and validity figures for the adapted version are given. This measure relies on recall of duration and frequency of certain activities for the previous month. However, accuracy of recall is open to question.

The investigators measured the variable—internal health locus of control—by the IHLC which uses a Likert-like format to gain responses ranging from "strongly disagree" to "strongly agree."

They report reliability figures of 0.67 to 0.77 for the individual forms. In addition, they report the correlation of the scale with other measures of similar concepts.

The investigators measured health value by a 10-item scale adapted from a longer version known as the Rokeach. Unfortunately, they report no reliability or validity data for this short version.

Using a Likert-like scale, the investigators designed the measure of the perceived importance of physical exercise. As with the above scale, they report no reliability or validity data.

The investigators tested hypotheses using zero-order correlations and stepwise multiple regression. They found no support for hypotheses regarding a positive relationship between amount of physical activity and internal health locus of control and between amount of physical activity and value placed on health. However, the correlation between amount of physical activity and perceived importance of physical exercise was significant, $r = 0.53$. When the investigators combined the three variables to examine total effect on amount of physical activity, they accounted for the variance by the perceived importance of exercise. Therefore, they rejected the hypothesis that the combination of factors would increase the predictability of amount of physical activity.

In a very logical discussion, the investigators attempt to examine reasons for their lack of significant findings. They recognize that the sample they used may not be reflective of the total female population; in addition, they note other considerations, such as social desirability and the need to measure work-related activities, not just leisure activities. They also highlight the potential importance of the significant relationship between perceived importance of physical exercise and amount of physical activity. In practice, the ability to assess the value of a particular intervention to a client may serve as an important step in designing interventions.

In general, although the study uses a female sample and some of the data regarding reliability and validity are missing, the investigators do provide a thorough presentation of the results and discussion of the findings. Therefore, it seems warranted to proceed with the evaluation of the study for use in practice.

Part IV: Generalizability of Results

The use of a questionnaire-type format would be useful in practice. The one used in this study requires only 10–15 minutes to complete. No additional training of staff to collect the data is needed.

Before the results of this study may be considered more seriously for utilization in practice, however, there is a need to replicate the study with a sample more representative of the population at large. A practitioner could include an assessment of the value of physical exercise to a particular client in the design of an intervention that may have physical exercise as one component. The ability to collect data in an actual practice setting and to systematically evaluate results would be an important addition to the present work.

Part V: Other Factors to Consider in Utilization

The research effort described in this study is one that could be attempted in an actual practice setting. The lack of significant findings in several of the hypotheses should not deter attempts to further evaluate the concepts explicated here. The ability to follow-up with each client and to make modifications in the intervention plan provides the practitioner with the ability to minimize risks. However, the risk inherent in not utilizing the study is one of stagnation in practice. There is an ongoing need to discover and describe strategies that work in the promotion of health. This study provides an avenue for assessment and evaluation of client attitudes that may prove useful in health promotion. The need to evaluate the results cannot be underestimated, however. The data that might be generated must be carefully analyzed for additional concepts as well as for support or criticism of the theory.

Attitudes, Subjective Norms, and Intentions to Engage in Health Behaviors

Nola J. Pender, PhD, FAAN
Program Director
Health Promotion Research
School of Nursing
Northern Illinois University
Dekalb, IL

Albert R. Pender, PhD
Associate Professor
Department of Business Education
and Administrative Services
Northern Illinois University
Dekalb, IL

The theory of reasoned action was used as the conceptual framework for analyzing the relationships among attitudes, subjective norms, and intentions to exercise regularly, maintain/attain recommended weight, and avoid highly stressful life situations. The sample (N = 377) consisted of adults between the ages of 18 and 66 living in two midwestern communities. Data were collected using a structured questionnaire designed according to guidelines developed by Ajzen and Fishbein (1980). The theory was supported in part by study results. Attitudes were useful in explaining intentions to engage in all three health behaviors studied. Subjective norms contributed only to the explanation of intentions to engage in regular exerise. Three factors, attitudes, subjective norms, and weight, affected intentions to engage in regular exercise, R = .364, p < .01. Attitudes, weight, and perceived health status were the principle determinants of intention to eat a diet consistent with weight control, R = .428, p < .001. Of the variables studied, only attitude was associated with intention to manage stress, R = .271, p < .01.

The quest to understand determinants of health behaviors has intensified as evidence accumulates concerning the impact of personal behavior on health. Investigations focusing on the phenomena of stress indicate that life-styles that reduce stress have a positive impact on health such as lowering blood pressure, increasing peripheral circulation, and lessening anxiety (Frumkin, Nathan, Prout, & Cohen, 1978; Rupert, Dobbins, & Mathew, 1981). In a series of studies, Belloc and Breslow (1972) found that specific health practices contributed significantly to longevity. A 9-year, follow-up study of the population originally surveyed indicated that significant relationships between five health behaviors and longevity had persisted over time: exercising regularly, maintaining normal weight, avoiding smoking, limiting alcohol consumption, and sleeping at least 7 hours a night (Wiley & Comacho, 1980). Widespread adoption of lifestyles that incorporate positive health behaviors could promote higher levels of health within the population, prevent or delay onset of chronic illness, and extend longevity.

THEORETICAL FRAMEWORK

The theory of reasoned action (Ajzen & Fishbein, 1980) offers one approach for explaining individuals' intentions to engage in health behaviors. According to the theory, overt behavior is a function of one's intention to perform the behavior. Behavioral intention is determined by two additive components: attitude toward the behavior and subjective norms. The model can be represented in terms of the following multiple regression equation:

$B ' BI = [w_1] A_B + [w_2] SN_B$ wherein B = overt behavior; BI = behavioral intention; A_B = attitude toward performing the behavior; SN_B = subjective norm regarding the behavior; w_1 and w_2 = empirically determined weights reflecting the relative importance of each component in determining BI.

Attitude toward a behavior reflects beliefs concerning the probability of specific consequences following the behavior and favorable or unfavorable evaluation of those consequences. Subjective norms represent perceived social pressure to engage in the behavior and motivation to comply with those norms or expectations. Thus, according to the theory of reasoned action, individuals are more likely to engage in health behaviors if such actions are seen as instrumental in achieving desired consequences and are considered worthwhile by persons or groups the individual wishes to please. Hecker and Ajzen (1983) proposed that all other variables that influence health behaviors are mediated through the attitudinal and normative components of the model.

REVIEW OF THE LITERATURE

The usefulness of the theory of reasoned action in explaining health promoting intentions such as family planning (Fishbein, Jaccard, Davidson, Ajzen, & Loken, 1980; Jaccard & Davidson, 1972, 1975) and weight loss (Saltzer, 1978, 1980; Sejwacz, Ajzen, & Fishbein, 1980) has been addressed in previous studies. In analyzing the determinants of family planning behavior, Jaccard and Davidson (1972) reported a correlation of .81 between attitude toward use of birth control pills and intention to use them. The correlation between subjective norms and intention to use birth control pills was lower, .68, but significant statistically.

Saltzer (1978) used the theory of reasoned action as a framework for investigating the determinants of intentions to lose weight in a college-age, obese population. Attitudes, subjective norms, value placed on health and physical appearance, and locus of control were measured. When regression analyses were computed on intention to lose weight for persons who highly valued their health, physical appearance, or both, the average variance explained by attitudes and subjective norms was 68%. Attitude (personal belief) was the most salient component of the equation for individuals with internal locus of control, and subjective norm (social pressure) was the most influential component of the regression equation for persons with external locus of control. However, at 6-week follow-up, extent of weight change did not correlate significantly with stated intentions to lose weight. In a later study of individuals actively involved in a weight-reduction program, Saltzer (1980) found a relationship between strength of intentions to lose weight and actual weight loss.

Sejwacz et al. (1980) investigated weight loss among 88 college women over a 2-month period. The measures of attitudes toward eating, dating, "me right now," "the fat me," and "the thin me" did not predict changes in weight. Thus, results of past studies have not consistently supported the validity of the model for explaining health behaviors.

The purpose of the present investigation was to determine the relative impact of attitudes and subjective norms on intentions of adults to exercise regularly, eat a diet to attain/maintain recommended weight for height and body build, and avoid highly stressful situations.

METHOD

Sample: The sample for this study consisted of 377 residents of households from two northern Illinois communities each with a population of approximately 30,000. The sample was predominantly white, consisting of 40% males and 60% females between the ages of 18 and 66 ($M = 38$, $SD = 12$). Of the respondents, 24% had completed high school only; 76% had attended college or were college graduates. Twenty-nine percent of the sample reported an income of less than $15,000; 71%, more than $15,000. Ninety-one percent reported being in good or excellent health; 9%, in fair or poor health. Thirty-nine percent were at least 15% above recommended weight, 56% were within recommended weight limits, and 5% were below recommended weight for height and body build, as determined from standardized tables.

Instrument: To obtain information essential for constructing the questionnaire, 100 residents from the two communities used for the study were interviewed to determine pertinent beliefs regarding each health behavior. Verbal consent was obtained prior to the interviews. Using a free-response format, individuals were requested to identify both positive and negative consequences of engaging in each of the three selected health behaviors. The three positive and the three negative consequences mentioned most frequently for each behavior by the 100 interviewees were incorporated into the questions measuring attitudes. Significant others whose opinions the interviewees valued were also identified. The six referents mentioned most frequently were the significant others included in the normative beliefs section of the questionnaire. These referents were: spouse/boyfriend/girlfriend, children, parents or closest older relative, friends, co-workers, and family physician.

The 75-item questionnaire developed from the interview data according to guidelines described by Ajzen and Fishbein (1980) was used to assess behavioral intentions, attitudes, and subjective norms for three health promoting actions. Each health behavior subscale consists of the following 25 items: measure of behavioral intention, 1 item; measure of attitude, 12 items (consequence beliefs, 6 items, consequence evaluations, 6 items); measure of subjective norms, 12 items (expectations of others' beliefs, 6 items, motivation to comply with expectations of others, 6 items). Examples of the measures are shown in Figure 1.

Consequence beliefs and expectations of others' beliefs were scored on a 7-point scale from -3 (unlikely) to $+3$ (likely). Consequence evaluation scores ranged from $+3$ (good) to -3 (bad). Motivation to comply was scored on a scale from 1 (not at all) to 7 (very much).

Attitude toward performing the behavior was calculated by multiplying each consequence belief score by the corresponding consequence evaluation score and then summing the six products for each behavior. The score for the subjective norm regarding the behavior was obtained by multiplying the expectation of others' belief score by the score on motivation to comply with the expectations of others and summing these six products for each health action. Multiplicative functions were used for combining the subcomponents of the attitude and subjective norm scores, as the theory of reasoned action is derived from the theory of subjective expected utility and, thus, must parallel the combinational rules of the parent theory.

In addition to measuring the theoretical constructs, the demographic variables of sex, age, education, and income were ascertained. Weight and perceived health status were also determined, as these have been associated with frequency of health behaviors (Dishman, 1981; Dishman & Gettman, 1980; Young & Ismail, 1977).

The instrument was evaluated for internal consistency reliability and test-retest reliability. Standardized coefficient alphas for the attitude components were: exercising regularly, .87; maintaining/attaining recommended weight, .75; and avoiding stressful situations, .78. Standardized coefficient alphas for the normative components were: exercising regularly, .90; maintaining/attaining recommended weight, .85; and avoiding stressful situations, .81. Test-retest reliability was conducted on a group of 30 graduate nursing students. The tool was administered twice to the same group of students at a two-week interval. Reliability was .93 for the measure of behavioral intention, .78 for the attitude component, and .82 for the normative component.

Data Collection: Using detailed maps, a random sample of blocks was drawn from each community. The interviewers stopped at every third

Figure 1
Examples of Measures Used in Health Behavior Scale

1. Behavioral intention
   During the next week, I intend to exercise regularly, that is, jog, run, brisk walk, or participate in active recreational sports at least three times during the week.

   unlikely ___/___/___/___/___/___/___ likely
   extremely quite slightly neither slightly quite extremely

2. Attitude
   a. Consequence belief
   Exercising regularly would improve my muscle tone.

   unlikely ___/___/___/___/___/___/___ likely
   extremely quite slightly neither slightly quite extremely

   b. Consequence evaluation
   For me, improving my muscle tone is:

   good ___/___/___/___/___/___/___ bad
   extremely quite slightly neither slightly quite extremely

3. Subjective norm
   a. Expectation of others belief
   My spouse/boyfriend/girlfriend thinks I should exercise regularly.

   unlikely ___/___/___/___/___/___/___ likely
   extremely quite slightly neither slightly quite extremely

   b. Motivation to comply with expectation of others
   Generally speaking, how much do you want to do what your spouse/boyfriend/girlfriend thinks you should do?

   not at all ___/___/___/___/___/___/___ very much

house on the selected blocks to request participation in the study by an adult resident over 18 years of age. The survey was explained and verbal consent for participation obtained. Interviewees were assured their responses would remain anonymous. If an individual was unable to answer the questionnaire at that time, the interviewer arranged to return at a later time or date. If no one was home, a second attempt to contact that household was made later the same week. Data were collected during late afternoon and evening hours to maximize response rate. Of 523 households selected, data were obtained from an individual in 377 households for a response rate of 72%.

Data Analysis: A stepwise multiple regression model was used to determine the extent to which attitudes, subjective norms, and other measured variables explained intentions to engage in the designated health behaviors. In addition, a series of two-tailed t tests were computed to identify differences in attitudes and subjective norms between individuals intending to engage in each health behavior during the next week and individuals without such intentions.

RESULTS

The multiple correlation between the two components of the model and intention to exercise was significant, $r = .233, p < .01$, but accounted for only 5.5% of the variance in intention. The correlation coefficient for the normative component with intention was higher, $r = .263, p < .01$, than for the attitudinal component and intention, $r = .177, p < .01$. When weight of the individual was considered in addition to attitude and subjective norm, the amount of variance explained in intention to exercise more than doubled, increasing to 13%, $R = .364, p < .01$. That is, individuals who were at or close to recommended weight (higher scores) as opposed to being overweight or underweight (lower scores) were more likely to have intentions to exercise during the following week. No other variables received significant regression coefficients.

Attitude, but not subjective norm, was associated weakly, $r = .127, p < .01$, with intention to eat a diet conducive to attaining/maintaining recommended weight. Other significant correlates of intention to control weight were present weight, $r = .382, p < .01$, and perceived health status, $r = .257, p < .01$. The multiple regression coefficient for attitude, weight, and perceived health status was .428, $p < .001$, with 18% of the variance in intention to control weight explained. These data indicated that having a positive attitude toward weight control, being at or near recommended weight, and perceiving health status as good or excellent increased reported intentions to eat a diet consistent with weight control.

When the effects of attitude, subjective norm, and other variables on intention to manage stress by avoiding highly stressful situations were examined, only attitude had a low but significant correlation, $r = .271, p < .001$, with intention. None of the other variables added significantly to the explained variance in intention to manage stress. Attitude explained only 7% of the variance in behavioral intention.

Table 1 presents the mean attitude scores and mean subjective norm scores of individuals intending and not intending to engage in the identified health behaviors during the following week. Individuals who stated they were neither likely nor unlikely to engage in the health behaviors were excluded from these analyses. The group intending to exercise regularly had significantly more positive attitudes toward exercise ($M = 21.01, SD = 4$) than those not intending to engage in physical fitness activities ($M = 15.26, SD = 6$), $t(356) = -3.82, p < .01$. Intenders also had stronger beliefs that significant others thought they should exercise ($M = 41.09, SD = 5$) than nonintenders ($M = 27.20, SD = 7$), $t(356) = -3.47, p < .01$. When each consequence belief was analyzed separately, intenders were more likely than nonintenders to believe that exercise improved mental outlook and less likely than nonintenders to believe that exercise could result in overexertion or a heart attack.

No significant differences were noted on either attitude or subjective norms between individuals intending and not intending to control weight. In examining intentions to avoid highly stressful situations, intenders were significantly more positive in their attitudes ($M = 8.76, SD = 3$) toward managing stress than nonintenders ($M = 0.09, SD = 2$), $t(331) = -4.74, p < .001$. Persons intending to avoid stressful situations also had a higher mean subjective norm score ($M = 41.34, SD = 4$) than those not intending to avoid stress ($M = 26.97, SD = 5$), $t(331) = -3.33, p < .01$. In examining specific behavioral beliefs, intenders were much less likely than nonintenders to be-

Table 1
Mean Scores on Attitudes and Subjective Norms for Those Who Intend and Do not Intend to Engage in Health Promoting Behavior

BEHAVIORS	MEAN ATTITUDE SCORES INTEND	MEAN ATTITUDE SCORES DO NOT INTEND	MEAN SUBJECTIVE NORM SCORES INTEND	MEAN SUBJECTIVE NORM SCORES DO NOT INTEND
Exercise regularly	21.01* ($n = 206$)	15.26 ($n = 152$)	41.09*	27.20
Maintain/attain recommended weight	21.56 ($n = 304$)	18.00 ($n = 58$)	42.80	39.12
Avoid stressful situations	8.76* ($n = 185$)	.09 ($n = 148$)	41.34*	26.97

*Difference between means for intenders and nonintenders is significant, $p < .001$.

lieve that stress avoidance would result in low achievement, withdrawal from the realities of life, and shirking of personal responsibilities.

DISCUSSION

The findings of this study provide limited support for the theory of reasoned action. Both the attitudinal and normative components of the model influenced intention to engage in physical fitness activities. Subjective norms exerted more influence than attitude on intention. Although the explanatory value of the model for exercise behavior was modest, the findings do suggest that social support expressed verbally or through family or group fitness activities may be more conducive to continued, regular exercise than unsupported individual attempts to sustain exercise adherence. Weight was not mediated by either component of the model, indicating that biologic variables may influence intention to exercise independent of attitudes and subjective norms. The finding that individuals who are overweight are less likely to intend to exercise than individuals near normal weight is consistent with previous studies (Dishman, 1981; Dishman & Gettman, 1980).

Intentions to eat a diet to control weight and to avoid highly stressful situations were associated with positive attitudes toward these behaviors. However, the normative component of the model did not influence intentions to engage in either behavior. Persons of normal weight and good or excellent perceived health status were more likely to intend to control weight than individuals who were overweight/underweight or in poor health. *Thus, persons at highest risk for health crises may be the least likely to engage in positive dietary behaviors.* Weight and perceived health status were not mediated by components of the model but exerted independent influence on weight control intentions.

Comparison of intenders and nonintenders indicated that persons who planned to exercise and control stress had more positive attitudes toward these activities. They also had stronger expectations that others expected them to engage in appropriate fitness and coping behaviors than persons without plans to engage in these behaviors.

Efforts to test the applicability of the theory of reasoned action to health-promoting behaviors should continue. In the present study, exercise, weight control, and stress management were viewed as indicators of the behavioral category, health-promoting behavior. Possibly these behaviors need to be further analyzed into component actions to increase precision of measurement. In future research, each of the health actions explored in this study could be considered as a separate behavioral category and an index consisting of multiple items constructed for each behavior. This specificity might increase the amount of variance explained in health behavior by components of the model. Another possible reason for the limited amount of variance in intentions to engage in health behaviors explained in this study by components of the theory of reasoned action may be lack of prior experience with health-promoting behaviors on the part of some respondents. Individuals who have never engaged in health-promoting behaviors may not have a well-defined belief structure concerning these behaviors. If further research yields inconsistent findings regarding the potential of the theory of reasoned action to explain various health behaviors, new behavioral models will need to be developed to provide more reliable explanation and prediction of health actions.

REFERENCES

Ajzen, I., & Fishbein, M. (1980). *Understanding attitudes and predicting social behavior.* Englewood Cliffs, NJ: Prentice-Hall.

Belloc, N. B., & Breslow, L. (1972). Relationship of physical health status and health practices. *Preventive Medicine, 1,* 409–421.

Dishman, R. K. (1981). Biologic influences on exercise adherence. *Research Quarterly for Exercise and Sport, 52,* 143,159.

Dishman, R. K., & Gettman, L. R. (1980). Psychobiologic influences on exercise adherence. *Journal of Sport Psychology, 2,* 295–310.

Fishbein, M., Jaccard, J. J., Davidson, A. B., Ajzen, I., & Loken, B. (1980). Predicting and understanding family planning behaviors: Beliefs, attitudes and intentions. In I. Ajzen, & M. Fishbein (Eds.), *Understanding attitudes and predicting social behaviors.* (pp. 131—147). Englewood Cliffs, NJ: Prentice-Hall.

Frumkin, K., Nathan, R. J., Prout, M. F., & Cohen, M. C. (1978). Non-pharmacologic control of essential hypertension in man: A critical review. *Psychosomatic Medicine, 40,* 294–320.

Hecker, B. I., & Ajzen, I. (1983). Improving the prediction of health behavior: An approach based on the theory of reasoned action. *Academic Psychology Bulletin, 5,* 11–19.

Jaccard, J. J., & Davidson, A. R. (1972). Toward an understanding of family planning behaviors: An initial investigation. *Journal of Applied Social Psychology, 2,* 228–235.

Jaccard, J. J., & Davidson, A. R. (1975). A comparison of two models of social behavior: Results of a survey sample. *Sociometry, 38,* 491–517.

Rupert, P. A., Dobbins, K., & Mathew, R. J. (1981). EMG biofeedback and relaxation instructions in the treatment of chronic anxiety. *American Journal of Clinical Biofeedback, 4,* 52–61.

Saltzer, E. B. (1978). Locus of control and the intention to lose weight. *Health Education Monographs, 6,* 118–128.

Saltzer, E. B. (1980). Social determinants of successful weight loss: An analysis of behavioral intentions and actual behavior. *Basic and Applied Social Psychology, 1,* 329–342.

Sejwacz, D., Ajzen, I., & Fishbein, M. (1980). Predicting and understanding weight loss: Intentions, behaviors and outcomes. In I. Ajzen & M. Fishbein (Eds.), *Understanding attitudes and predicting social behavior* (pp. 102–112). Englewood Cliffs, NJ: Prentice-Hall.

Wiley, J. A., & Comacho, T. C. (1980). Life style and future health: Evidence from the Alemeda County study. *Preventive Medicine, 9,* 1–21.

Young, R. J., & Ismail, A. H. (1977). Comparison of selected physiological and personality variables in regular and nonregular adult male exercisers. *The Research Quarterly for Exercise and Sport, 48,* 617–622.

This article is printed with permission of *Nursing Research.*
Copyright 1986 American Journal of Nursing Company.

12

Nursing Management

Marie S. Berger, PhD, RN
Colleen M. Engstrom, BSN, RN
Cynthia Lea Strunk, BSN, RN

INTRODUCTION BY: MARIE S. BERGER, PhD, RN

During the last decade, many changes have occurred in health care organizations. These changes have been brought about by a combination of factors including economic constraints and increased complexity of patient care. In addition, the rapid growth of the health care industry and skyrocketing costs have generated an unaparalleled interest in assessment of the efficiency and effectiveness of these organizations. To a large extent, nurses today find themselves caught between two cultures. On the one hand, we are trying to practice within the culture of nursing which values caring and compassion. On the other hand, we must contend with the culture of capitalistic economics which values efficiency and profit. We struggle to maintain the humanism that is fundamental to our practice, even as budgets are slashed, staffing is reduced, and workloads are increased. Nursing managers are particularly vulnerable to the pressures created by an industry forced to contain costs and maintain efficiency without sacrificing quality of care or the quality of nursing environment.

The first two studies included in this chapter address aspects of the quality of the nursing environment or the context of nursing practice. This can be defined as the interrelationship of factors in the external environment (i.e., the institution, state, and nation) and factors in the internal environment (i.e., the attitudes, perceptions, and behavior of the nurse that affect the practice of professional nursing).

The health care delivery system, and political, social, and economic factors have a significant influence on how nursing practice occurs. Learning to assess the impact of these factors on practice and to develop strategies for modifying those with negative impacts is a critical component of nursing administration. The study by McCloskey and McCain is a report of a study undertaken to assess changes in job satisfaction, commitment, and professionalism during the first year of newly employed nurses. All of these variables have been cited in nursing administration literature as important to the quality of the nursing environment. While job satisfaction can be expected to change over time, surveys can provide important information about the present state of affairs so that approximate interventions can be implemented. Commitment to the organization is considered a more stable attitude. The commitment tool has been used in business, industry, and less often in health care organizations to pinpoint an employee's readiness to leave the organization and predict turnover. Professionalism also is considered a more stable attitude. One could imply that a high level of commitment to professional values would lead to more innovative practice. On the other hand, the argument may also be made that commitment to the profession and commitment to the organization are mutually exclusive. The research reported here sheds some light on these notions.

The study by Duxbury, Henly, and Armstrong represents an attempt to measure organizational climate in an intensive care unit. Each work setting has its own unique characteristics, culture, traditions, and methods of action. An organization or work setting tends to attract and keep people who fit the climate, so that the culture, traditions, and methods of action can be perpetuated. Being able to describe the elements of climate important in an intensive care unit is the first step in enhancing staff morale by matching person and environment.

The final study reflects the continued efforts of nurses to adequately define the concept of quality of care, and to establish valued and reliable measurement tools. As a result, various conceptualizations of quality of care and methodologies to evaluate care have emerged. The relationship between two quality of care measures is examined in the study reported by Ventura, Hageman, Slakter, and Fox. The Quality Patient Care Scale (QualPacs) is frequently cited in nursing administration literature, while the Rush-Medius instrument is cited less often. Both instruments are designed to evaluate care as it is being given (concurrent) rather than through review of charts (retrospective).

The importance of this research for nurse administrators is the recognition that although both instruments measure quality of care, each is measuring different dimensions of that care. It is important that the conceptualization underlying measurement tools be understood and that tools are selected that can measure what one wants to measure.

In summary, each of the articles presented here represents an attempt to further our understanding about two important components of our practice, the quality of care and the quality of the environment in which we do this care. The research presented points out areas for further study and stimulates critical thinking about practice issues.

Satisfaction, Commitment and Professionalism of Newly Employed Nurses

Joanne C. McCloskey, PhD, RN, FAAN
Associate Professor and Chair
Organizations and Systems
College of Nursing
University of Iowa
Iowa City, IA

Bruce E. McCain, PhD
Assistant Professor
Department of Management Sciences
University of Iowa
Iowa City, IA

Over their first year of work all nurses employed in a large hospital reported decreased job satisfaction, decreased organizational commitment, and decreased professionalism. This happened with both new graduates and experienced nurses alike; only Master's prepared nurses did not report this decline. The results suggest that employers need to assess the initial expectations of new nurses and either meet more of those expectations or help new nurses form more realistic expectations about their jobs.

Job satisfaction represents the degree to which employees like or enjoy their jobs; organizational commitment represents employees' overall attachment to the organization; professionalism is attachment to a particular occupation or profession. These attitudes play an important role in employee performance, absenteeism and turnover.

While there is a good deal of research on job satisfaction of nurses, few studies have measured the satisfaction of newly employed nurses. Organizational commitment and professionalism are much discussed in the nursing literature, but little research has been done with nurses. Findings from other groups may not be relevant to nurses: moreover, few longitudinal studies have been undertaken, in nursing or elsewhere, to examine changes in these attitudes over time. This paper documents the changes in satisfaction, commitment and professionalism that occurred among nurses during their first year of work in a hospital.

METHOD

Sample and Data Collection

All of the 350 nurses who joined a large Midwestern hospital between June 1983 and September 1984 were asked to participate in this study; 320 (91%) agreed. During the first year on the job, 54 nurses (17%) resigned; of those who remained, 150 (59%) completed the study.

During the first year of work, each nurse was asked to complete six questionnaires, that is, the two-parts of a questionnaire exploring satisfaction, organizational commitment and professionalism were each administered three times: during the first month, at approximately six months and at the end of the year. The first administration was during the first week of hospital orientation with one of the researchers present. After that the questionnaire was mailed to the nurses' homes. A nonresponse was followed in two weeks by a reminder postcard; in another two weeks, by a second questionnaire; and in another two weeks, by a telephone call.

Instruments

The questionnaire was designed using four scales and a demographic section. The *McCloskey Reward/Satisfaction Scale*, revised from an earlier tool (McCloskey, 1974), has 33 Likert-type scaled items categorized as either safety rewards (to meet basic security needs, e.g., hours and benefits), social rewards (to meet needs to belong, e.g., contact with others or psychological rewards (to meet self-actualization needs, e.g., control over working conditions, responsibility and recognition). Internal consistency (Cronbach Alpha) coefficients on the overall scale for the responses to the three administrations of the questionnaire were .89, .89, and .90. A factor analysis confirmed the construction of the scale.

The *Organizational Commitment Questionnaire* developed by Porter and Smith (1970; Mowday, Steers, & Porter, 1979), has 15 items, each rated from 7 (Strongly agree) to 1 (Strongly disagree). The higher the score, the more committed to the organization an individual is judged to be. Organizational commitment, as defined by Porter and Smith, is characterized by acceptance of the organization's goals and values, readiness to exert effort on behalf of the organization and a strong desire to remain a member of the organization. The scale has shown good reliability and validity (Cook, Hepworth, Wall, & Warr, 1981; Mowday, Porter, & Steers, 1982). Cronbach Alpha coefficients for this sample were .86, .91, and .92.

The *Hall Professionalism Scale*, devised by Hall in 1968 and revised by Snizek in 1972, consists of 25 items representing 5 attitudes of professionalism: use of the professional organization as a major referent, belief in public service, belief in self-regulation, a sense of calling to the field and a feeling of autonomy. Overall scale reliabilities range from .84 (Hall's data, KR-20), .78 (Snizch's data, KR-20), to Cronbach Alpha coefficients of .69, .68, and .72 (our data for each of the three times the questionnaire was administered).

The *Kramer Professionalism Scale (Revised)*, measuring professional behaviors, was constructed for this study on the basis of a scale described by Kramer in 1974. The nurses reported the number of professional books purchased, subscriptions to professional journals, hours spent in professional reading and continuing education, participation in professional organizations, number of professional publications, speeches given, committee activity, and participation in research. Test-retest reliability with 11 subjects tested 3 weeks apart resulted in a correlation coefficient of .99. The Cronbach Alpha reliability coefficients for our sample were .62, .63, and .71. The factor analysis supported the notion of one overall scale.

A *demographic survey*, included in the originally administered questionnaire, obtained the usual demographic information (age, sex, marital status, job experience) as well as data on whether or not the nurse had been assigned a preceptor, whether or not the unit obtained was the nurse's first choice of area and what the job benefits were (e.g., salary, number of weekends off).

RESULTS

Sample Description

The sample consisted of 22 percent associate degree nurses, 16 percent diploma nurses, 59 percent baccalaureate nurses and 3 percent Master's degree nurses. At the end of the first year of employment the sample mix was approximately the same.

The majority of the sample (94%) were staff nurses, with the remainder hired for management or clinical specialty positions. This was the first job for 46 percent of the total sample and for 60 percent of the baccalaureate nurses. Most were young women (59% between 20 and 25 years of age). The baccalaureate nurses were the youngest: 90 percent were less than 30 years old. There were only 14 men in the sample. Approximately half the sample were single; 23 percent had children. Most (81%) were employed full time and

Table 1
Mean Scores of Four Educational Groups on Satisfaction, Commitment, and Professionalism

Group	Total Sample			Diploma			Associate Degree			Baccalaureate Degree			Master's Degree			Repeated Measures MANOVA	
Month	1	6	12	1	6	12	1	6	12	1	6	12	1	6	12	Time	Education
N*	293	210	159	48	34	27	63	40	77	174	129	98	8	7	7	p=	p=
Scale																	
McCloskey Satisfaction†																	
TOTAL	3.44	3.27	3.33	3.42	3.22	3.40	3.52	3.38	3.40	3.42	3.24	3.29	3.36	3.46	3.42	.008	.166
Safety	3.48	3.25	3.26	3.44	3.24	3.40	3.59	3.34	3.31	3.44	3.19	3.19	3.66	3.97	3.80	.040	.032
Social	3.44	3.43	3.62	3.41	3.36	3.64	3.50	3.52	3.67	3.45	3.43	3.60	3.22	3.18	3.57	.001	.587
Psychological	3.40	3.16	3.16	3.42	3.10	3.22	3.49	3.31	3.28	3.38	3.14	3.13	3.23	3.07	2.97	.000	.348
Porter & Smith Commitment†	5.08	4.04	4.41	5.18	4.03	4.46	5.18	4.12	4.59	5.06	4.02	4.38	5.20	3.92	4.12	.000	.342
Hall Professionalism†																	
TOTAL	3.30	3.21	3.20	3.21	3.09	3.13	3.30	3.22	3.20	3.30	3.24	3.24	3.50	3.28	3.14	.000	.165
Self-regulation	3.67	3.68	3.68	3.65	3.66	3.70	3.67	3.70	3.71	3.68	3.70	3.70	3.78	3.54	3.20	.099	.208
Public service	3.48	3.36	3.40	3.42	3.29	3.31	3.52	3.28	3.31	3.47	3.40	3.48	3.72	3.34	3.20	.000	.843
Professional organizations	3.25	3.05	2.97	3.01	2.79	2.73	3.08	2.94	2.84	3.37	3.09	3.02	3.82	3.87	3.74	.004	.000
Calling	3.16	3.00	3.00	3.14	2.89	3.06	3.32	3.20	3.19	3.11	2.99	2.99	2.90	2.77	2.63	.043	.005
Autonomy	2.91	2.99	2.97	2.80	2.83	2.83	2.94	3.00	2.95	2.92	3.04	3.03	3.28	2.89	2.91	.484	.098
Kramer Professionalism†	1.86	1.71	1.79	1.78	1.69	1.65	1.80	1.68	1.70	1.90	1.67	1.79	2.56	2.77	2.67	.064	.000

*N approximate sample size. Because of the reverse order of questionnaires during administration, sample sizes vary a little.
† Each item was rated on a 5 point scale except items from Porter and Smith which were rated on a 7 point scale.

the majority worked rotating shifts (51%) or 10-hour to 12-hour combinations (22%); 34 percent worked on intensive care units, 68 percent worked on the unit that had been their first choice; the majority (65%) were assigned to a preceptor who helped them learn the new job.

Satisfaction

The mean scores on the McCloskey Reward/Satisfaction Scale for the total sample (see Table 1) showed that satisfaction declined over the first six months and then remained steady over the second six months. Overall, the nurses were most satisfied with social rewards and least satisfied with psychological and safety rewards. Master's-prepared nurses, however, were the most satisfied with safety rewards.

The particular rewards with which the nurses were most satisfied were vacation time (5 weeks for all nurses at this hospital) and benefits (11 holidays, 18 sick days and an excellent insurance package). They were also satisfied with their nursing peers, their supervisor and their amount of responsibility (see Table 2).

The nurses were least satisfied with the lack of opportunity to work straight days (only 10 nurses or 3% worked straight days) and compensation for weekend work (there was a bonus only when a nurse worked more than every other weekend).

Table 2
Most Satisfied and Least Satisfied Rewards as Rated on McCloskey Scale

	1st Month (N = 298)		6th Month (N = 214)		12th Month (N = 150)	
Reward		$\bar{X}$ Reward		$\bar{X}$ Reward		$\bar{X}$
Rewards most satisfied with:						
Vacation	4.54	Vacation	4.40	Vacation		4.45
Benefits	4.23	Benefits	4.23	Child care		4.45
Peers	3.83	Peers	4.04	Benefits		4.26
Supervisor	3.81	Responsibility	3.95	Supervisor		4.26
Responsibility	3.78	Physicians	3.81	Care method		3.86
Rewards least satisfied with:						
Opportunity to work days	2.62	Weekend pay	2.34	Weekend pay		2.27
Child care	2.80	Opportunity to work days	2.46	Opportunity to work days		2.42
Weekend pay	2.88	Child care	2.68	Participation in decision making		2.85
Maternity leave	3.14	Recognition from superiors	2.87	Recognition from superiors		2.87
Participation in decision making	3.14	Flexibility in scheduling weekends off	2.92	Encouragement and feedback		2.93

They were also dissatisfied with participation in organizational decision making and recognition of work by superiors.

Satisfaction with opportunities to attend educational programs, compensation for working weekends, recognition of work from superiors, opportunities for career advancement and amount of encouragement and positive feedback dropped most over the year.

Commitment

Mean scores on the Organizational Commitment Scale (see Table 1) showed that the nurses' commitment to the organization declined over the first 6 months but recovered slightly by the end of 12 months. This was true for all nurses, regardless of educational preparation. In comparison to the employees studied by Mowday, Steers, and Porter (1979), nurses in this study did not show a high degree of commitment to the organization in their first year of work.

Professionalism

Mean scores for the total Hall Professionalism Scale (see Table 1) showed that newly employed nurses' professionalism declined slightly within six months and then held steady.

Scores on three of the subscales (belief in public service, use of the professional organization as a referent and a sense of calling to the field) also declined at six months. On average, belief in self-regulation was rated highest; the feeling of autonomy, lowest. Associate degree nurses reported a significantly greater sense of calling to the field ($p = .005$). This upscale reflects dedication to work and idealistic performance of work for psychological gratification even when few extrinsic rewards are available (Regoli & Poole, 1980). Master's-prepared nurses scored significantly higher ($p = 0$) on using the professional organization as a referent.

Only one other study has reported using the Hall scale (Regoli & Poole, 1980). In it, urban and rural police officers, 19 percent of whom had degrees beyond high school, scored very low on the professionalism measures. The nurses in the present sample did not score much higher despite the fact that 84 percent had either associate or baccalaureate degrees.

In a comparison of 11 occupational groups (nurses, physicians, accountants, teachers, lawyers, social workers, stockbrokers, librarians, engineers, personnel managers and advertising executives), Hall (1969) reported that nurses, librarians and social workers had the highest sense of calling in the field. Nurses, however, were the least autonomous of the 11 groups.

The mean scores on the Kramer Professionalism Scale, which measures professional behavior rather than attitudes, declined within 6 months. Master's—prepared nurses reported more professional behaviors than other groups and in fact showed significantly higher scores at 6 months than at 1 month. However, none of the groups scored high on professional involvement at any time. The Master's-prepared nurses subscribed to more professional journals, read more professional literature, were more active in the professional organization and participated more in nursing research than any other nurses. Only 50 of the 290 nurses (17%) who answered the question said that they belonged to the American Nurses' Association.

Experienced versus Inexperienced?

For a large number of nurses in this sample (46%), this was their first job as a Registered Nurse. It was the second job for 20 percent of the sample, while 34 percent had had three or more jobs. Nurses with different job tenures did not score differently on the satisfaction, commitment and professionalism scales—with a few exceptions: those in the second job scored lower on Hall's professionalism scale ($p = .04$) and on preceived autonomy ($p = .03$). This was most apparent at 12 months when the nurses were most satisfied with social rewards. Nurses in their second jobs can be characterized as being less idealistic than new graduates and not as independent as those who have worked longer.

Relationships Among Variables

The correlation matrix of the 4 scales at months 1 and 12 (see Table 3) demonstrates that the relationships between the scores on the same variable were strong. In addition, satisfaction and organizational commitment were correlated at 1 month and strongly correlated at 12 months. Professional attitudes (Hall) and commitments were modestly correlated at both 1 month and 12 months. Professional behavior (Kramer), however, did not correlate with either satisfaction or commitment, although attitudes about the profession and professional behavior were correlated with each other. Nurses who were most satisfied at 1 month tended to be less involved professionally at 12 months.

Several demographic variables were correlated with satisfaction. Nurses who were significantly ($p = <.05$) more satisfied at 1 month were younger, had less experience, had less family income, had more weekends off, were assigned to a preceptor and were more likely to be working on the unit of their choice. At 6 months the most satisfied had less family income, less years of education and more weekends off. At 12 months the most satisfied had less personal and family income, were less involved in the community and had more weekends off.

Very few of the demographic variables were related to organizational commitment. Nurses who were significantly ($p = <.05$) committed to the organization at 1 month were less involved in the community and more likely to be working on the unit of choice; at 6 and 12 months the most committed had less personal income.

Only two demographic variables were significantly ($p = <.05$) related to professional attitudes: at 12 months those who had the most professional attitude were less involved in the community, and at all three times those with the most professional attitude were more likely to be working on the unit of their choice.

All but two of the demographic variables (number of children and community involvement) were significantly ($p = <.05$) related to professional behavior, however. The relationships were strongest at six months, when those who demonstrated the most professional behavior tended to be older, male, married more years, with a larger personal and family income, more years of education and experience, more weekends off and a preceptor to help orient them to a unit of their choice.

Table 3
Satisfaction, Commitment, Professionalism Correlated with Each Other at Months 1 and 12

Scale	Month	McCloskey 1	McCloskey 12	Porter & Smith 1	Porter & Smith 12	Hall 1	Hall 12	Kramer 1	Kramer 12
McCloskey	1	1.000	r .527	.373	.382	.163	.190	.022	-.143
			N (143)	(158)	(265)	(158)	(267)	(152)	
			p .000	.000	.000	.004	.008	.362	.037
McCloskey	12		1.000	.264	.538	.078	.265	-.032	-.056
				(142)	(133)	(142)	(133)	(142)	(132)
				.001	.000	.179	.001	.352	.263
Porter & Smith	1			1.000	.467	.347	.242	.085	.083
					(156)	(287)	(156)	(289)	(155)
					.000	.000	.001	.075	.153
Porter & Smith	12				1.000	.051	.313	.007	−.110
						(155)	(159)	(156)	(158)
						.265	.000	.465	.085
Hall	1					1.000	.606	.263	.298
							(155)	(287)	(154)
							.000	.000	.000
Hall	12						1.000	.265	.301
								(156)	(158)
								.000	.000
Kramer	1							1.000	.651
									(155)
									.000
Kramer	12								1.000

McCloskey = Satisfaction.
Porter & Smith = Commitment.
Hall = Professionalism (Attitudes).
Kramer = Professionalism (Behavior).

There were few differences among units, with nurses on specialty medicine units (e.g., medical cardiology, psychiatry, neurology) tending to have more professional behavior and those on intensive care units tending to be more satisfied with safety and social rewards. Those who worked days were more satisfied but reported less self-regulation; those who worked nights reported more autonomy.

Discussion

In this longitudinal analysis of nurses in their first year on a new job, the most striking finding was the decline in satisfaction, commitment and professionalism during the first six months of work. This was true for all nurses no matter what their educational background or how many jobs they had held. The only exception was the small group with Master's degrees; they were more satisfied and had higher scores on professionalism at the end of six months.

According to Kramer (1974) and Schmalenberg and Kramer (1979), new graduates experience reality shock in their first job as they make the transition from the idealism of students to the realism of working nurses. Corwin, Taves, and Haas (1961) attributed this disillusionment of the new graduate to the conflict between professional and bureaucratic values. Our findings indicate that the disillusionment may also apply to experienced nurses. It appears that as nurses begin work they are relatively satisfied with most aspects of the job, have a modest commitment to the employing organization and hold the nursing profession in relatively high regard. But, when initial expectations are not met, the nurse becomes less attached to the job, the organization and the profession. Master's-prepared nurses, who in the present study were the least idealistic (sense of calling at one month was 2.90 compared with means of 3.16, 3.14, and 3.32 for other groups), appeared to cope with the realities of a new job somewhat better. Apparently, lesser prepared nurses see job rewards as they begin a new job, but they learn the job costs only with experience. Our findings are consistent with those of Rusbult and Farrell (1983), who found that, among both accountants and nurses, satisfaction and commitment declined over the first year of work.

Our results confirm those of Weisman, Dear, Alexander, and Chase (1981), who compared first-time employed and experienced nurses at two university hospitals. Both groups experienced the same acclimation process and displayed similar turnover, similar job-hunting behavior and similar job-satisfaction levels. The authors concluded that adjustment to the organization rather than to role transition was the salient process to study.

Our results also support McClure's (1984) suggestions to nurse managers. According to McClure, nurses enter an organization with expectations about career development, involvement in decision-making, amount of independence, responsiveness of others, job rewards and job stress. A manager, she says, must reduce the discrepancy between nurses' expectations and their actual experiences, and the best way to do this is to try to meet their expectations.

In our study, changes in satisfaction with particular rewards document the discrepancy between expectations and experience. Nurses in this sample experienced the largest decline in satisfaction with their opportunities to attend educational programs, compensation for working weekends, recognition of work from superiors, opportunities for career advancement and amount of encouragement and positive feedback. Employers either need to meet these expectations or better inform employees about these things before they take the job. (The fact that those who were most satisfied were younger and earned less is not an indication that organizations should hire only young nurses and pay them less, but it may demonstrate that young nurses have fewer expectations.) Realistic job previews, which have been promoted as a way to decrease turnover (RJPs, 1983; Wanous, 1975a & 1975b) may need to include more information than specific job duties and tangible benefits. The employee should be informed about leadership styles, informal relationships, employer expectations and career advancement opportunities.

Two large drops in satisfaction in this study— recognition of work from superiors and amount of encouragement and positive feedback—reflect on the leadership of immediate supervisors. Head nurses and other leaders in the institution apparently have a direct effect on the satisfaction of newly employed nurses. Institutions may be able to increase the satisfaction of their nurses by developing the leadership skills of first-line managers, specifically the skills of giving encouragement, feedback, and recognition.

A critical reader might point out that, while satisfaction, commitment, and professionalism all declined in the first 6 months, the turnover figure for the sample was only 17 percent for the year. Why should one worry about these attitudes if so many of the nurses stayed on the job? One must remember that these data were collected during a time when there were few nursing jobs available because of the high unemployment nationwide. Despite the fact that the nurses in this sample had little opportunity for alternative employment, 17 percent left in their first year of work and by the end of 18 months, 24 percent had left. Turnover rates were highest in the 7-to-15 month period, indicating that decreased satisfaction and job commitment at 6 months did affect turnover. Moreover, should dissatisfied or uncommitted nurses stay on the job, they might increase the problems of absenteeism, poor performance, and patient dissatisfaction.

The finding that attitudes about the profession and organizational commitment were correlated contradicts most of the literature on professionalism, which suggests that there is a conflict between professional and bureaucratic values (Gouldner, 1957; Miller & Wagner, 1971; Sorenson & Sorenson, 1974). From our study it appears that nurses experience no conflict between commitment to the nursing profession and commitment to the work organization. Rather, declining favorableness of the job and organization reflects on the nurse's image of nursing. Thus our findings confirm the evidence cited by Bartol (1979) that there is not an inherent conflict between professional attitudes and organizational commitment. As Bartol and others have suggested, compatibility between professional values and organizational values may depend on the organization's willingness to reward professional behaviors.

CONCLUSION

The decline of satisfaction, commitment, and professionalism during the first six months of employment for all nurses, new and experienced alike, suggests that beginning job expectations were not met. The correlation between organizational commitment and professionalism gives additional evidence that this reflects not a conflict between professional and bureaucratic values but rather an adjustment to a particular organization and job. Our results suggest that employers need to assess initial expectations of new employees and either meet more of these expectations or be clear before hiring that these expectations are unrealistic.

The assumption in nursing is that new graduates have higher and unrealistic expectations because of the professional socialization of their educational programs. Studies that support this assumption are largely based on cross-sectional analysis. In our longitudinal study of nurses in their first year of work, younger nurses were more satisfied than were older, more experienced nurses. Thus, while internship programs for students about to graduate and other role socialization programs for the new nurse should be continued, nurse employers and researchers need also to pay attention to experienced nurses employed in a new job. For all newly employed nurses, the first six months on the job are crucial for their satisfaction, commitment, and professionalism.

REFERENCES

Bartol, K. M. (1979). Professionalism as a predictor of organizational commitment, role stress, and turnover: A multidimensional approach. *Academy of Management Journal, 22*(4), 815–821.

Cook, J. D., Hepworth, S. J., Wall, T. D., & Warr, P. B. (1981). *The experience of work: A compendium and review of 249 measures and their use.* New York: Academic Press.

Corwin, R. G., Taves, M. J., & Haas, J. E. (1961). Professional disillusionment. *Nursing Research, 10*(3), 141–144.

Gouldner, A. W. (1975). Cosmos and locals: Toward an analysis of latent social roles. *Administrative Science Quarterly, 2,* 444–480.

Hall, R. H. (1968). Professionalism and bureaucratization. *American Sociological Review, 33,* 92–104.

Hall, R. H. (1969). *Occupations and the social structure.* Englewood Cliffs, NJ: Prentice Hall.

McCloskey, J. (1974). Influence of rewards and incentives on staff nurse turnover rate. *Nursing Research, 23,* 239–247.

McClure, M. L. (1984). Managing the professional nurse. Part II. Applying management theory to the challenges. *The Journal of Nursing Administration, 14*(3), 11–17.

Miller, G. A., & Wager, L. W. (1971). Adult socialization, organizational structure, and role orientations. *Administrative Science Quarterly, 16,* 151–163.

Mowday, R. T., Porter, L. W., & Steers, R. M. (1982). *Employee-organization linkages: The psychology of commitment, absenteeism and turnover.* New York: Academic Press.

Mowday, R. T., Steers, R. M., & Porter, L. W. (1979). The measurement of organizational commitment. *Journal of Vocational Behavior, 14*(2), 224–247.

Porter, L. W., & Smith, F. J. (1970). The etiology of organizational commitment. Unpublished paper, University of California at Irvine.

Regoli, R. M., & Poole, E. D. (1980). Police professionalism and role conflict: A comparison of rural and urban departments. *Human Relations*, *33*(4), 241–252.

RJPs: A cost effective way to reduce nursing turnover (1983). *The Journal of Nursing Administration*, *8*(9), 42.

Rusbult, C. E., & Farrell, D. (1983). A longitudinal test of the investment model: The impact on job satisfaction, job commitment, and turnover of variations in reward costs, alternatives, and investments. *Journal of Applied Psychology*, *68*(3), 429–438.

Schmalenberg, C., & Kramer, M. (1979). *Coping with reality shock*. Wakefield, MS Nursing Resources, Inc.

Snizek, W. E. (1972). Hall's professionalism scale: An empirical reassessment. *American Sociological Review*, *37*, 109–114.

Sorenson, J. E., & Sorenson, T. L. (1974). The conflict of professionals in bureaucratic organizations. *Administrative Science Quarterly*, *19*, 98–106.

Wanous, J. P. (1975a). A job preview makes recruiting more effective. *Harvard Business Review*, *53*, 166–168.

Wanous, J. P. (1975b). Tell it like it is at realistic job previews. *Personnel*, *52*, 50–60.

Weisman, C. S., Dear, M. R., Alexander, C. S., & Chase, G. A. (1981). Employment patterns among newly hired staff nurses: Comparison of nursing graduates and experienced nurses. *Nursing Research*, *30*(3), 188–191.

This article is printed with permission of *Image: Journal of Nursing Scholarship*.

Original article:
McCloskey, J. C., & McCain, B. E. (1987). Satisfaction, commitment and professionalism of newly employed nurses. *Image: Journal of Nursing Scholarship, 19*(1), 20–24.

CRITIQUE BY: COLLEEN M. ENGSTROM, BSN, RN

Part I: Clinical Relevance

McCloskey and McCain studied changes in job satisfaction, organizational commitment, and professionalism of newly employed nurses during the first year of employment. As a nursing student with plans for full-time employment after graduation, I believe that this study has valuable information for nurse recruiters. It also has valuable information for newly employed nurses as to their own expectations and how these might change over the first 12 months of employment.

Results of this study were not directly applicable for decision making regarding patient care. Rather, the investigators addressed attitudes regarding satisfaction, commitment, and professionalism of newly hired nurses during their first year of employment. One conclusion that might be drawn from results of this study is that newly employed nurses need assistance in developing realistic expectations about their jobs. Results also could be beneficial to hospital nurse recruiters in assessing the needs of newly employed nurses and assisting these nurses to identify potential problem areas. The problems could be addressed before nurses experience decreased job satisfaction. Nursing faculty could assist students in assuming a more realistic attitude about their expectations about employment and give them an idea of what to expect and how to avoid decreased job satisfaction and commitment.

Although the study has limited direct applicability to my own practice, it is sufficiently interesting to continue evaluation of other aspects included in the study.

Part II: Conceptualization and Internal Consistency

Even though McCloskey and McCain do not raise specific research questions, they do address issues related to job satisfaction, commitment, and professionalism briefly in their introduction. As mentioned, their focus is on attitudes of nurses newly hired in a large Midwest hospital during the first year of their employment. In general, their language makes sense and, to provide the reader with sufficient background for the study, they review previously completed studies of concern. However, at the end of the discussion section, where the investigators address findings about attitudes, their wording is somewhat confusing.

The investigators provide justification for their study in this way: They state that no longitudinal studies of nursing job satisfaction had been done prior to theirs, and more specifically, that none had been done on newly employed nurses.

The investigators designed the study to address the issues identified. Variables seemed logically related to one another. In general, the sample selection makes sense, given the purpose of the study, although it is not clear why nurses with master's degrees were included. It seems to me that nurses with advanced educational preparation may be different in terms of their expectations than other nurses. For example, they may have been dissatisfied with practice already or, on the other hand, greatly satisfied, leading them to return to school. Data collection was done in person at orientation, then by mail. If the questionnaires were not completed in the allotted time, a follow-up letter was sent, followed by a telephone call. Both the use of questionnaires and repeated measures are consistent with the purposes of the study.

Part III: Believability of Results

This study purported to describe a phenomenon of concern to nursing which has an impact on both the newly hired nurse and the hospital who employs him or her. The type of data collected was quantitative and the study design was descriptive. The investigators used four separate scales to categorize data and collected demographic information. For their study sample, the investigators seleted 320 nurses employed by a large Midwest hospital. There were no criteria used for sample selection other than newly hired. Although the investigators do not state what type of sample they used, I believe that this was a convenience sample.

Unfortunately, because the investigators obtained their study sample from one hospital in a Midwest city, generalizability may be problematic. To overcome this possibility, they could have chosen their subjects from several hospitals in the same city and then selected a random sample of newly hired nurses. Nonetheless, the sample used had varied education backgrounds ranging from associate to master's degree.

The investigators do not discuss potential biases in the sampling technique nor do they provide a rationale. One clear bias is that out of 320 nurses who started the study, only 150 completed it. What about those who did not respond? I cannot assume that nonrespondents are the same as respondents. The fact that all nurses worked at the same hospital also is cause for concern. There may have been something unique about this one hospital that led to changes in the major variables over time, rather than that the changes are a generalizable event regardless of the setting.

In describing each of the four scales used, the investigators comment on reliability and validity. The test–retest reliability on one instrument was .99, which is very close to perfect, and reliability coefficients for the sample were .62, .63, and .71, respectively. These indicate that reliability is satisfactory.

The investigators do not report any procedures for achieving consistency between two or more data collectors. The questionnaires were mailed twice, while the first questionnaire was done in person with a researcher present. The investigators described how the questionnaire was developed and administered. They report data collection strategies in some detail and provide information on how follow-ups were done with nonresponders.

From my clincial experience, I would have expected newly hired graduate nurses to experience a decrease in satisfaction, commitment, and professionalism far more profoundly than more experienced nurses who were newly hired. The study not only refuted this expectation, but found that the more experienced nurses had more expectations than the graduate nurses.

The investigators illustrated relationships among the concepts with appropriate statistical data. If there were areas in which direct application was more apparent to me, I would want to obtain advice from a statistician or nurse researcher about the appropriateness of the methods used, particularly the statistical analysis. However, with my limited knowledge of design and statistics, it seems appropriate.

Part IV: Generalizabiltiy of Results

As the investigators note, this study confirms the findings of other research (Weisman, Dear, Alexander, & Chase, 1981) that compared first-time employed and experienced nurses at two university hospitals. This 1981 study did not examine change over time. Again, because McCloskey and McCain conducted their study at only one hospital, their findings regarding change over time may not be generalizable to other settings.

Part V: Other Factors to Consider in Utilization

This study, as conducted, does not directly indicate a change in practice. One implication might point to development of educational programs which help people develop more realistic expectations. It also may be that newly hired nurses simply experience a change in expectations and no intervention is warranted—that is, that this is a naturally occurring cycle. However, further research is needed into ways in which these attitudes early in employment relate to dissatisfaction and turnover.

In general, this study provides food for thought regarding expectations of newly employed nurses. Beyond this, I would not use this research because: (1) the findings were inconsistent with my own expectations and I'm not sure that the results, given the potential sampling bias, are believable; (2) there have been no replication studies and generalizability is limited; and (3) there is limited direct applicability to my practice.

Original article:
McCloskey, J. C., & McCain, B. E. (1987). Satisfaction, commitment and professionalism of newly employed nurses. *Image: Journal of Nursing Scholarship,* 19(1), 20–24.

CRITIQUE BY: MARIE S. BERGER, PhD, RN

Part I: Clinical Relevance

This study researched change in nurses' job satisfaction, organizational commitment, and professionalism during the first year of employment. Organization commitment measures an employee's attachment or commitment to an organization and, in one sense, predicts turnover. Assessing the newly employed nurse could identify potential problems and remedial actions could be taken before the employee has made the decision to leave. Since turnover is such a major and costly problem in our health care organizations, it is important that research be conducted to explore its causes and cures. Recent reports have noted large numbers of nurses who are leaving the profession. Some of the reasons nurses give for leaving the profession involve traditional family commitments, but many are leaving because of dissatisfaction with the status, pay, and general working conditions of a nursing career. As with organizational commitment, it is important to assess nurses' level of commitment and job satisfaction so that realistic and research-based policies and programs can be planned and implemented. The research reported by McCloskey and McCain is important to nurse administrators who have responsibility for recruitment and retention of staff and development of a nursing practice environment conducive to professional practice.

The present study is a descriptive one with no interventions employed. Results of this study, while not directly applicable to patient care, do suggest policy decisions and actions the nurse administrator can employ to mitigate staff turnover.

Part II: Conceptualization and Internal Consistency

The investigators presented their study in a logical manner. However, in their introduction and discussion of concepts they used insufficient information. For example, they do not provide the reader with information about their conceptualization of the influence of organizational commitment, satisfaction, or professionalism on turnover and absenteeism, or on performance and quality of care. This same lack of adequate information also plagues their discussion of the instruments used. In addition, the investigators provide very little description of the underlying conceptualization and no range of possible scores for the instruments used.

Furthermore, the investigators do not pose specific research questions nor do they provide rationale to support the possible relationship between variables, organizational commitment, job satisfaction, and professionalism. Also, they present only minimal background data making it impossible to make judgments about how the sample in this study compares with that of women in other professional groups. This information would be useful in assessing the applicability of the instruments across settings.

Part III: Believability of Results

The investigators used a longitudinal study (12 month) design that enabled them to address the question regarding changes in scores over time along dimensions of interest. Unfortunately, they failed to note the threats to reliability and validity inherent in longitudinal studies.

The investigators asked 350 nurses in a single Midwestern hospital to complete several questionnaires three times during the first year of their employment: first, during orientation sessions in week one of their employment; second, at six months of employment; and, third, at 12 months of employment, with a mailed questionnaire. Out of the sample remaining after 17 percent (34) nurses resigned, only 59 percent (150) eventually completed the study. There is no description of the 43 percent (116) who did not complete the study. The majority of the sample (94 percent) were staff nurses, and 6 percent were mangers or clinical specialists. Forty-six percent of the total respondent group were in their first nursing position as were 60 percent of the 174 beccalaureate degree nurses. The investigators did not analyze for first job respondents and respondents with previous experience separately. This lack of analysis does have significance. It would have been interesting to see if there were any differences between these two groups. Another interesting analysis would have been of changes that occured in nurses working on different units.

An additional concern is in regard to the potential for an inflated organizational commitment score due to multiple factors. First, a person in the first week of employment in a face-to-face administration of a questionnaire may give a socially desired response rather than a "true" response because of fear, issues of confidentiality or general anxiety. New graduates in the sample also may respond in a more socially acceptable way. Thus, the timing of the procedure for administration of the first questionnaire may have led to biased scores in at least two of the measures: commitment and satisfaction.

In their study, the investigators used instruments appropriate for the research question posed. In addition, they reported acceptable levels of reliabiltiy and validity for these instruments. A Cronbach Alpha coefficients on the overall McCloskey Reward/Satisfaction Scale responses to the three administrations were .89, .89, and .90, respectively. It is not clear whether the factor analysis reported is that conducted for this sample or for a previous one.

The Organizational Commitment Questionnaire is designed to assess an individual's acceptance of the organization's goals and values, readiness to act on behalf of the organization, and a desire to remain with the organization. The investigators state that the instrument has good reliability and validity, but only report coefficients for the present study of .86, .91, and .92, respectively.

The Hall Professionalism Scale measures attitudes of professionalism, involving use of professional organization as a major referrent, belief in public service and self-regulation, autonomy, and a sense of calling. Previous reliabilities range from .78 to .84. The Cronbach Alpha coefficients for the present study are .69, .68, and .72, respectively.

The final instrument, the Kramer Professionalism Scale (revised), measures a different aspect of professionalism than Hall. The individual is asked to report the number of journal subscriptions and books purchased, membership in professional organizations, and such activities as number of hours in professional reading. Test–retest reliability with 11 subjects tested three weeks apart yielded a coefficient of .99. The Cronbach Alpha coefficients for the present study were .62, .63, and .71, respectively. Once again, it is not clear whether the factor analysis was for the present sample.

The investigators presented results in a clear and concise style with some comparisons to results of other research. There is little discussion about specific findings. However, there is a more general discussion about the decline in all scores during the first six months of employment and factors that seem to contribute to the decline. It is this discussion that provides nurse administrators with useful information. For example, at 12 months, three rewards for which the nurses expressed the least satisfaction included: participation in decision making, recognition from supervisors, and encouragement and feedback. Implementing actions that would promote greater satisfaction with these three rewards have little or no financial cost attached to them and great potential benefits.

The investigators correlated organizational commitment and satisfaction at one month and at 12 months. While they found correlation between professional attitudes (Hall) and commitment, they did not find correlation between professionalism (Kramer) and satisfaction or commitment.

Conclusions do not include acknowledgment of limitations or suggestions for further research. However, the conclusions presented offer suggestions to managers.

Part IV: Generalizability of Results

Generalization should be undertaken with caution. The decline in scores may be due to an inflated initial score from the first week of employment when the individual has high expectations and is generally excited. As this same individual gains experience in the organization, his or her expectations become more realistic. Results can be used, however, to suggest actions a nurse manager could take to reduce possibility of a decline in commitment, professionalism or satisfaction. In other words, one could be sensitive to the expectations newly employed nurses have and provide time for discussion. Nursing administrators can call attention to the importance of human relations skills in retaining satisfied staff and formal classwork or coaching can be provided for nurse managers who wish to improve.

Part V: Other Factors to Consider

The benefits of implementing actions suggested by results of this study outweigh any potential risk. A committed and satisfied staff with professional attitudes and behavior would provide quality patient care.

Measurement of the Nurse Organizational Climate of Neonatal Intensive Care Units

Mitzi L. Duxbury, PhD, FAAN
Professor
School of Nursing
University of Minnesota
Minneapolis, MN

George A. Henly, AB
Doctoral Candidate
School of Psychology
University of Minnesota
Minneapolis, MN

George D. Armstrong, PhD
Research Associate
School of Nursing
University of Minnesota
Minneapolis, MN

The concept of organizational climate is important for the study and understanding of work organizations. Researchers have not yet studied the organizational climate of hospital intensive care units, so it is not clear that the dimensions useful in description of other work settings will be appropriate for conceptualizing neonatal intensive care units (NICU's). This study investigated nurse perceptions of the organizational climate of NICU's in a sample of 18 hospitals. The Organizational Climate Description Questionnaire was modified for use in the NICU setting. A set of homogeneous climate scales was developed from the revised instrument. The six scales of the resulting instrument, the Nursing Organizational Climate Description Questionnaire, Form B (NOCDQ-B), demonstrated median internal-consistency reliability of .69 on cross-validation. Analysis of variance indicated that each of the six NOCDQ-B dimensions served to differentiate the NICU's in the study. Further, significant relationships were found at the unit mean level between three of the six NOCDQ-B scales and nurse satisfaction, as measured by the Minnesota Satisfaction Questionnaire.

Environments characterized by use of expensive and sophisticated life support systems for the critically ill pose pressing problems for care-givers (Frader, 1979). Intensive care unit (ICU) nurses report more depression, hostility, and anxiety than non-ICU nurses (Cassein and Hackett, 1975). NICU staffs experience high levels of burnout (Price, 1979) and are characterized by high turnover rates (Duxbury and Thiessen, 1979). Burnout and turnover may be related to poor patient outcome. Because of the high cost of orienting new staff, turnover adds to the already high cost of neonatal intensive care.

Previous studies of the critical care environment emphasize that the inherent nature of the work, caring for life-threatened patients, is the pervasive source of stress for care-givers (Oken and Hey, 1972); Lancaster, 1976; Jacobson, 1978). They suggest that characteristics of the work environment can exacerbate or allay the stress inherent in providing care to these patients. Organizational climate measures may be useful for describing intensive-care work environments.

The Concept of Organizational Climate. Organizational climate is a concept that has been of interest to organizational researchers and practitioners in business, health care, and other settings for several decades (Forehand and Gilmer, 1964; James and Jones, 1974). The term "organizational climate" refers to a set of organizational characteristics that are relatively stable, differentiate organizations, and influence the behaviors of organization members (Forehand and Gilmer, 1964). The organizational climate label has been applied to a broad set of situational variables— e.g., leadership, communication, equity—which function to differentiate organizations. These situational variables influence important organizational outcomes, such as job performance and employee satisfaction (Campbell et al., 1970; Hellriegel and Slocum, 1974; Pritchard and Karasick, 1973).

The relationship between such variables and outcomes point to the importance of organizational climate for nursing researchers and administrators. Thus far researchers have not studied the organizational climate of hospital IC units, and it is not clear that the same dimensions used to describe other work organizations would be useful in the organizational climate of IC units.

A wide range of definitions have been used to describe organizational climate. Many of the variables included under the organizational-climate umbrella bear little conceptual or operational relationship to each other. The term has been applied to objective organizational characteristics, such as size, as well as individual and group perceptions of the organization.

These varying approaches result in confusion (Guion, 1973; James and Jones, 1974). Consider organizational size as an attribute; it could be measured by counting the number of employees on the payroll. It could also be measured by asking employees to rate the size of their organization on a scale ranging from "very small" to "very large." The aggregate group response to this rating could be used as an index of organizational size.

Payne, Fineman, and Wall (1976) suggested that the term "climate" be reserved for perceptual measures that reflect group consensus, rather than individual perceptions. They argue that climate measures should be descriptive rather than evaluative. For the example of perceptual measurement of organizational size, collective group perceptions of the organization as "very large" would be considered a measure of organizational climate; individuals' evaluations of the organization as "too large" or "too small" would not.

The focus of organizational climate is on organizational attributes rather than individual attributes. Therefore, organizational climate measures should reflect a convergence of perceptions of individual members (Guion, 1973; James and Jones, 1974). In perceptual measurement of organizational size, if half the group rate an organization as very large and the remainder rate it very small, the average of these ratings, medium-size, scarcely represents a group consensus in describing the organization. It would not be appropriate to claim to be measuring an organizational attribute in this instance.

Measurement of Organizational Climate. Given the choice of a methodology for measuring organizational climate, the question of what situational variables to measure remains. A number of dimensions might be explored. Halpin and Croft (1962) have chosen to emphasize interpersonal relationships. That emphasis guided their development of the Organizational Climate Description Questionnaire (OCDQ) (Halpin and Croft, 1962). The OCDQ was designed to tap two classes of behaviors of the work group: those of the leader and those of the subordinate work group. The OCDQ was developed to measure the climate of elementary schools but has been adapted for use in other settings (Friedlander and Margulies, 1969; Lyon and Ivancevich, 1974). The eight scales that comprise the OCDQ are divided equally between leader and subordinate work group dimensions. Definitions of these dimensions are listed below:

SUBORDINATES' BEHAVIOR:

Disengagement—subordinates' tendency to be "not with it." This dimension describes a group that is "going through the motions," a group that is "not in gear" with respect to the task at hand.

Hindrance—subordinates' feeling that the leader burdens them with routine duties, committee demands, and other requirements which they construe as unnecessary "busywork."

Esprit—refers to morale. The subordinates feel their social needs are being satisfied, and that they are at the same time enjoying a sense of accomplishment in their job.

Intimacy—refers to the subordinates' enjoyment of friendly social relations with each other. This dimension describes a social-needs satisfaction not necessarily associated with task-accomplishment.

LEADER'S BEHAVIOR:

Aloofness—behavior by the leader that is characterized as formal and impersonal. The leader "goes by the book," is guided by rules and policies rather than deals with subordinates in an informal, face-to-face situation.

Production emphasis—behavior by the leader, which is characterized by close supervision of the staff. The leader is highly directive and plays the role of a "straw boss."

Thrust—behavior by the leader which is characterized by an evident effort to "move the organization." Thrust behavior is marked not by close supervision, but by the leader's attempt to motivate the subordinates through the example he or she personally sets.

Consideration—behavior by the leader which is characterized by an inclination to treat the subordinates "humanly" to try to do a little something extra for them in human terms.

Halpin and Croft (1962) viewed the climate of an organization as analogous to the personality of an individual. Their aim was the measurement of attributes of the organization through the collection of aggregate group perceptions. Their operationalization of this approach, the OCDQ, fits the definition of a perceptual measure of organizational climate. It purports to be a measure of the aggregate descriptive perceptions of the organization's members.

This study examined the use of a modified form of the OCDQ with registered nurses in neonatal intensive care units. It was part of a larger study designed to develop a causal model of staff nurse turnover in NICU's. The utility of the modified OCDQ as a measure of the organizational climate of NICU's was examined. The analysis had two purposes: to assess the validity of the revised OCDQ as a consensus measure of climate of NICU's and to investigate the relationship between organizational climate dimensions and an important outcome dimension, worker job satisfaction.

Method

Subjects were registered nurses employed in 18 NICU's distributed throughout the United States. A total of 901 staff nurses were employed in these NICU's; 682 (76 percent) participated in part or all of the research reported here.

The 18 NICU's were a subset of a random sample of NICU's reported elsewhere (Duxbury and Thiessen, 1979). The subset of 18 NICU's were non-randomly chosen to ensure the inclusion of units with a broad range of turnover rates (0 to 72 percent crude turnover). The deliberate inclusion of disproportionate numbers of low turnover units means that this sample is atypical of the general NICU population. In fact, the over-representation of low turnover units is not extensive. It ensures that the obtained findings are generalizable to units with a broad range of turnover rates.

Table 1
Items and Scales of the Nurse Organizational Climate Description Questionnaire

(FORM A)

Thrust
4. The head nurse sets an example by working hard her/himself.*
12. The head nurse is well prepared when she/he speaks at educational meetings.
24. The head nurse goes out of her/his way to help nurses.*
31. The head nurse used constructive criticism.

Consideration
7. The head nurse helps nurses solve their personal problems.
13. The nurse helps staff members settle minor differences.
20. The head nurse stays late to help nurses finish their work.
26. The head nurse does personal favors for nurses.

Production Emphasis
2. The head nurse orders work for the nurses according to her/his needs.
10. The head nurse makes all decisions regarding nursing care.
22. The head nurse checks the ability of nurses.
26. The head nurse corrects nurses' mistakes.

Aloofness
6. Staff meetings are mainly head nurse report meetings.
15. The head nurse runs staff meetings like a business conference.
17. Staff meetings are organized according to a tight agenda.
18. Nurses leave the unit during their assignments.

Disengagement
3. Nurses seek special favors from the head nurse.
11. The mannerisms of nurses at this unit are annoying.
19. There is a minority group of nurses who oppose the majority.
23. Nurses exert group pressure on nonconforming nurses.

Hindrance
1. Routine duties interfere with the job of practicing nursing.
5. Patient charting and reports require too much work.
25. Administrative paper work is burdensome at this hospital.
30. Nurses have too many committee requirements.

Intimacy
8. Nurses' closest friends are other nurses from this unit.
14. Nurses know the family background of other nurses.
21. Nurses talk about their personal life to other nurses in the unit.
29. Nurses invite other nurses to visit them at home.

Esprit
9. The morale of nurses is high.
16. Nurses at this hospital show much spirit.
27. Housekeeping service is available when needed.
32. The nurses accomplish their work with vim, vigor, and pleasure.

---

*In order to bring NOCDQ items into closer compliance with the guidelines for non-sexist language in the *Publication Manual* of the American Psychological Association (APA, 1977) the wording changes in several items have been adopted for future use of the NOCDQ.
  4. Head nurse sets an example by working hard.
12. Head nurse is well prepared when speaking at educational meetings.
24. Head nurse goes out of the way to help nurses.

The intent was not merely to assess high turnover situations—where something may be wrong—but to assess low turnover units, settings where things are going well.

Instruments

Organizational Climate—the Organizational Climate Description Questionnaire, Form IV (OCDQ) (Halpin and Croft, 1962) was modified for use in this study. Earlier research by Halpin and Croft (1962) and Lyon and Ivancevich (1974) suggests there is substantial overlap in the domains covered by the various OCDQ scales. It was felt that the number of items from the OCDQ could be reduced without serious loss of information. Four items were chosen from each of the original OCDQ scales; the number of items was cut in half, from 64 to 32. The objective was to create an instrument that would be more practical to use; administration time was markedly reduced.

A second modification involved item wording. References specific to a school setting were revised to reflect the NICU setting—for example, "principal," was changed to "head nurse"; "teachers" to "nurses" (Table 1). The revised version was referred to as the Nurse Organizational Climate Description Questionnaire, form A (NOCDQ-A).

Job Satisfaction—the Minnesota Satisfaction Questionnaire short form (MSQ) (Weiss, England, and Lofquist, 1967) was the second instrument in this study. This 20-item instrument provided a global measure of individuals' job satisfaction. The MSQ is a measure of individuals' evaluative perceptions of an outcome variable thought to be important as it related to organizational climate.

Procedure. As part of a larger study, all registered staff nurses in the 18 participating NICU's were asked to complete a series of questionnaires during the course of a 1 1/2-year period (1979 to 1980). An on-site study assistant at each NICU distributed the instruments and an explanation of informed consent. To assure anonymity, each participant was assigned a code number by the assistant. After completing the instrument, participants mailed it directly to the reseachers. The researchers remained blind to participant identity and hospital personnel remained ignorant to participant responses.

Not all nurses who completed the NOCDQ-A were still on-site when the MSQ was administered. Since relationships between NOCDQ-A and the MSQ are examined at the unit mean level, loss of some participants should not seriously bias the observed relationships. Any resulting bias should deflate the size of observed relationships between the two instruments. Since job satisfaction as measured by the MSQ is presumed to be a relatively stable trait (Anderson, 1969), it is believed that the intervention of several months between a nurse's completion of the MSQ and the NOCDQ-A is not a serious limitation of the analysis to be reported here. Separation of testing has an added benefit of minimizing any spurious linkage between the two instruments, due to their completion at a single sitting.

Item Dimensionality and Revised Scale Reliability. A total of 661 staff nurses completed and returned the NOCDQ-A. Initial analysis of the NOCDQ-A concerned the internal consistency reliability of the revised scales. Cronbach's alpha was computed for each of the eight NOCDQ-A scales (Table 2). Several of the scales, notably Production Emphasis and Aloofness, showed low reliabilities. The items were submitted to further

Table 2
Nurse Organizational Climate Description Questionnaire (Form A) Scale Reliabilities

Scale	(coefficient alpha)
Thrust	.78
Consideration	.51
Production Emphasis	.26
Aloofness	.34
Disengagement	.56
Hindrance	.54
Intimacy	.63
Esprit	.60

[2]Principal axes factoring was employed, with squared multiple correlations used as communality estimates. Using Kaiser criterion, nine factors were extracted and rotated to Varimax™ solution.

analysis to determine if a new set of more nearly homogeneous scales might be derived from the NOCDQ-A items. The goal was to better define the independent dimensions of climate being tapped by the items.

The responses of a subset of the 661 nurses—those of the first 545 respondents— were submitted to factor analysis[2]. The 32 NOCDQ-A items yielded nine factors, six of which had substantial loadings from three or more items and were readily interpretable. Six scales were constructed from the items to represent these factors (Table 3). Cronbach's alpha coefficients were computed for each of the new scales and ranged from .51 to .83, with a median of .61. These reliabilities were based on the 545 respondents whose item responses had been factored, or the "development" sample. Reliabilities were also computed for a "cross-validation" sample of 116 respondents whose questionnaires arrived later. Internal consistency reliabilities for the six new scales, based on the cross-validation sample, ranged from .45 to .78, with a median Cronbach's alpha of .69. This finding of substantial reliability upon cross-validation increases confidence in the generalizability of these new, revised NOCDQ scales across NICU settings. The instrument, scored on these six new scales, was referred to as the NOCDQ-B.

Six of the original eight NOCDQ-A scales were retained in modified form. Items from the original Production Emphasis scale were scattered across factors, so that scale was eliminated. Items from the Consideration scale loaded largely on the same factor as items from the Thrust scale, so these two scales were merged into a single scale.

NOCDQ-B scale 1 loads heavily on items from the NOCDQ-A Thrust and Consideration scales. Seymour (1978) reported a similar finding from his factor analysis of the OCDQ. His term for the dimension, "Humanistic Thrust," was applied to Scale 1 here. The items of Scale 1 are concerned with constructive leadership behaviors of the head nurse.

Scales 2 and 3 correspond closely to the original Esprit and Intimacy scales, respectively, and retain these labels. The new Esprit scale consists of three of the four items in the original NOCDQ-A Esprit scale. These items reflect nurse morale and spirit. The four items from the NOCDQ-A Intimacy scale were retained in the new Intimacy scale, and concern the social intimacy of the work group.

Scale 3 consists of three of the four items in the original Aloofness scale. All are concerned with the extent to which the head nurse structures staff meetings. The name "Aloofness" is retained for Scale 4. The four items from the NOCDQ-A Disengagement scale were augmented by an additional item (from the NOCDQ-A Aloofness scale) to form Scale 5. These items reflect disunity and conflict among nurses working on the unit; the "Disengagement" label was retained for this scale.

Items forming Scale 6 came from the Hindrance scale of the NOCDQ-A, with the exception of a single, negatively-weighted item from the NOCDQ-AEsprit scale. These items reflect hospital characteristics and requirements that interfere

Table 3
NOCDQ (Form B) Scales, Items, and Reliabilities

Scale	FACTOR Label	ITEMS[a]	RELIABILITY (Coefficient alpha) Development	Cross-validation
1	Humanistic Thrust	4,12,13,22,24,31	.83	.78
2	Esprit	9,16,32	.76	.71
3	Intimacy	8,14,21,29	.63	.73
4	Aloofness	6,15,17	.54	.67
5	Disengagement	3,11,18,19,23	.58	.65
6	Hindrance	1,5,25,27(−),30	.51	.45

[a]Item numbers are as they appear in Table 2.

with nursing practice. Scale 6 is referred to as "Hindrance." While items forming this scale have a common conceptual core, they have substantial variance independent of other items in the scale. As a result, the internal consistency reliability of this scale is low. This is the least satisfactory scale, psychometrically speaking, of the NOCDQ-B scales.

Consensus Measure of Climate. The ability of the NOCDQ-B to differentiate organizations was examined. Organizational climate is different from NICU to NICU. If the NOCDQ-B are valid climate measures, they should be able to detect such differences. Scores on the six NOCDQ-B scales were computed for each nurse respondent by summing item responses for the items defining each scale. One-way analyses of variance were run for each of the six NOCDQ-B scales, with NICU as the independent variable. Significant mean differences between NICU's were found for each of the six scales. In other words, the climate dimension scales of the NOCDQ-B differentiated hospital NICU's (Table 4).

Obtaining significant F-values in an analysis of variance gives an indication that sufficient convergence exists among nurses within each NICU regarding climate to differentiate the units. However, the F values do not reveal the extent to which consensus exists among nurses within the units. The eta-squared statistic, while related to the F ratio, gives a more sensitive reading of the extent of consensus within the NICU's. The eta-squared statistic tells how much of a reduction in error in predicting the climate rating of an individual results from knowledge of which NICU that individual is a member. An eta-squared value of 1.0 means that the individuals within each unit are in perfect agreement in their ratings of the climate of the unit on a dimension. If it is known to which unit an individual belongs, his or her perception of the unit is known. An eta-squared value of 0.0 tells us that no consensus exists within each unit; no mean differences exist between units.

Eta-squared values ranged from .08 to .24, with a median value of .12 (Table 5). This suggests that while sufficient consensus regarding organizational climate exists to differentiate units on these dimensions, substantial diversity remains in the perceptions of individuals within each NICU regarding the climate of their NICU. Put another way, the NOCDQ-B scales measure to a large extent attributes of individuals as well as attributes of organizations.

Organizational Climate and Job Satisfaction. The Minnesota Satisfaction Questionnaire (MSQ) (short form) was completed and returned by 304 staff nurses, 283 of whom had completed the NOCDQ-A. The MSQ provided a general satisfaction score for each respondent. Mean satisfaction

Table 4
Analysis of Variance for NOCDQ-B Scales and MSQ Across NICU's

	$\bar{X}$	SD	N[c]	F	p	eta-squared
NOCDQ-B						
1. Humanistic Thrust	14.55	4.12	553	9.90	<.001	.24
2. Esprit	6.43	2.03	595	7.21	<.001	.17
3. Intimacy	10.89	2.31	593	3.66	<.001	.10
4. Aloofness	6.17	2.05	554	2.64	<.001	.08
5. Disengagement	9.93	2.69	580	3.90	<.001	.11
6. Hindrance	5.70	2.46	564	5.25	<.001	.14
MSQ Satisfaction	67.30	9.52	288	2.79	<.001	.14

[a]N fluctuates from scale to scale due to missing responses and change in number of respondents in the interval from administration of NCDQ to administration of MSQ.

**Table 5
Correlation of Unit Mean Climate Scores
and Satisfaction Scores**

	MSQ	N[a]	p
1. Humanistic Thrust	.52	17	<.02
2. Esprit	.71	17	<.005
3. Intimacy	.35	17	n.s.
4. Aloofness	−.16	17	n.s.
5. Disengagement	−.47	17	<.05
6. Hindrance	.03	17	n.s.

[c]MSQ responses were unavailable from the eighteenth unit, which had withdrawn from the study subsequent to administration of the NOCDQ.

scores were computed for each NICU. Satisfaction is as an evaluative perceptual variable, an attribute of an individual; mean satisfaction of a group may be labeled "morale" (Payne et al., 1976). A one-way analysis of variance tested the hypothesis that there were no significant mean differences between NICU's on the MSQ. This hypothesis was rejected ($p<.001$), indicating that significant differences do exist between NICU's in terms of morale (mean satisfaction) (Table 4).

Satisfaction measures tap individual attributes, while climate measures tap attributes of organizations; therefore, climate measures should show greater consistency within an organization than satisfaction measures. This implies that the eta-squared statistic for climate measures should be larger than for satisfaction measures. Three of the six NOCDQ-B scales showed eta-squared values greater than or equal to the eta-squared value computed for the MSQ (Table 4).

Based on previous research in organizational climate, it was expected that important relationships between climate variables and satisfaction would emerge. Correlations between NICU mean scores on the MSQ and NOCDQ-B scales were computed. Statistically significant relationships were found between satisfaction and climate on three of the six scales of the NOCDQ-B (Table 5). Such relationships suggest that climate is related to satisfaction but to a large extent the climate scales measure something other than satisfaction.

DISCUSSION

Scale reliabilities for modified OCDQ items scored on the original OCDQ scales were not encouraging. Factor analysis of the sample responses resulted in construction of six revised scales. Those six factor scales reflected the original eight OCDQ scales except that Production Emphasis was dropped, and Consideration and Thrust merged into a single scale.

The internal consistency reliabilities of five of these six revised scales were satisfactory and remained stable when cross-validated on additional subjects. The Hindrance scale exhibited a marginal level of reliability, and may require lengthening or item revision.

The NOCDQ-B responses involve both a consensus and individual rating components, which should be kept in mind when using the NOCDQ-B in either applied or research application. While the goal was to measure the personality of the organization, a substantial amount of non-convergent individual perception was included in NOCDQ-B responses.

Support for the practical utility and construct validity of the NOCDQ-B comes from the correlations of its six scales with job satisfaction as measured by the MSQ. The content, measured by the NOCDQ-B, is related to but different from the important organization outcome of employee satisfaction.

The sizable ($r = .71$) relationship between Esprit and Satisfaction is not surprising. Both are measures of group morale, although they presume different perceptual sets (descriptive vs. evaluative) on the part of the raters. The relationship between a leadership dimension (Humanistic Thrust) and employee satisfaction was found in many other studies (Stogdill, 1974). The lack of substantial correlation between mean satisfaction and three of the NOCDQ-B scales does not diminish their importance. They may be related to other important outcomes, such as performance. It is possible that individual personality variables (needs or values) may mediate the relationship between these climate variables and satisfaction (Friedlander and Margulies, 1969).

The instrument used for measuring nurse organizational climate in NICU's appears satisfactory from a psychometric standpoint, with the reservations noted. Wider application is necessary before its generalizability is established.

The use of the NOCDQ-B involved nurses working in NICU's. Given the observed generalizability of the OCDQ items across differing organizations, it appears that our nursing version of the OCDQ may be useful in other hospital units in addition to NICU's. Insofar as NICU's represent unique organizational entities, the scale properties of the NOCDQ-B might not be optimal in other hospital settings. While NICU's do have unusual features, they still entail nurses working in hospitals under the supervision of a head nurse. We expect the NOCDQ-B scales to remain useful when applied to nurses in different units. Future use of the instrument in diverse hospital settings in conjunction with other measures will be needed to finally determine the utility and validity of the scales.

REFERENCES

Anderson, L. M. (1969). *Longitudinal changes in level of work adjustment*. Unpublished doctoral dissertation, University of Minnesota, Minneapolis.

Campbell, J. P., et al. (1970). *Managerial behavior, performance, and effectiveness*. New York: McGraw-Hill.

Cassein, N. H., & Hackett, T. P. (1975). Stress on the nurse and therapist in the intensive-care unit and the coronary care unit. *Heart Lung, 4*, 252–259.

Duxbury, M. L., & Thiessen, V. (1979). Staff nurse turnover in neonatal intensive care units. *Journal of Advanced Nursing, 4*, 591–602.

Forehand, G. A., & Gilmer, B. (1964). Environmental variation in studies of organizational behavior. *Psychological Bulletin, 62*, 361–382.

Frader, J. E. (1979). Difficulties in providing intensive care. *Pediatrics, 64*, 10–16.

Friedlander, F., & Margulies, N. (1969). Multiple impacts of organizational climate and individual value systems upon job satisfaction. *Personnel Psychology, 22*, 171–183.

Guion, R. M. (1973). A note on organizational climate. *Organizational Behavior and Human Performance, 9*, 120–145.

Halpin, A. W. (1966). *Theory and research in administration*. New York: Macmillan, pp. 150–151.

Halpin, A., & Croft, D. B. (1962). *The Organizational climate of schools*. Chicago: Midwest Administration Center, University of Chicago.

Hellriegel, D., & Slocum, J. W. (1974). Organizational climate: Measures, research, and contingencies. *Academic Management Journal, 17*, 255–280.

Jacobson, S. P. (1976). Stressful situations for neonatal intensive care nurses. *MCN, 3*, 144–150, May-June 1978.

James, L. R., & Jones, A. P. Organizational climate: A review of theory and research. *Psychological Bulletin, 81*, 1096–1112.

Lancaster, Jean. (1976). Stress factors for nurses. In *Iatrogenic problems in neonatal intensive care*. Report of the Sixty-Ninth Ross Conference On Pediatric Research, Columbus, Ohio, Ross Laboratories. pp. 90–97.

Lyon, H. L., & Ivancevich, J. M. (1974). An exploratory investigation of organizational climate and job satisfaction in a hospital. *Academic Management Journal, 17*, 635–648.

Oken, D., & Hey, D. The psychosocial stress of intensive care unit nursing. *Psychosomatic Medicine, 34*, 109–118.

Payne, R. L., et al. (1976). Organizational climate and job satisfaction: A conceptual synthesis. *Organizational Behavior and Human Performance, 16*, 45–62.

Price, M. E. (1979). Why NICU nurses burn out and how to prevent it. *Contemporary Ob-Gyn, 13*, 37–46.

Pritchard, R. D., & Karasick, B. W. (1973). The effects of organizational climate on managerial job performance and job satisfaction. *Organizational Behavior and Human Performance, 9*, 126–146.

Seymour, H. A. (1978). *The validity of the subscales of the organizational climate description questionnaire using selected Mississippi junior colleges*. Unpublished doctoral dissertation, State College, Mississippi State University.

Stogdill, R. M. (1974). *Handbook of leadership: A survey of theory and research*. New York: Free Press.

Weiss, D. J., et al. (1967). *Manual for the Minnesota satisfaction questionnaire*. (Minnesota Studies in Vocational Rehabilitation: No. 22) Minneapolis: Industrial Relations Center. University of Minnesota.

This article is printed with permission of *Nursing Research*. Copyright 1982 American Journal of Nursing Company.

Original article:
Duxbury, M. L., Henly, G. A., & Armstrong, G. D. (1982). Measurement of the nurse organizational climate of neonatal intensive care units. *Nursing Researh, 31*(2), 83–88.

CRITIQUE BY: CYNTHIA LEA STRUNK, BSN, RN

Part I: Clinical Relevance

In their study Duxbury, Henly, and Armstrong probed organizational climate and its relationship to worker job satisfaction. They tested a concept developed in school and business settings to assess its relevance and applicability to neonatal intensive care unit (NICU) settings. While they are unclear about whether the tool they developed is only for research or for practical application, this reported study does have potential for helping nurse managers, particularly in NICU or intensive care units, manipulate the environment to improve job performance and employee satisfaction.

In general, this study concerns the development of a research tool. If the investigators could provide evidence for the validity of the tool, it could have practical application in leading nurse managers to decisions which reduce risk for patients by improving staff nurses' job performance. The revised Nurse Organizational Climate Descriptive Questionnaire, form B (NOCDQ-B), developed by Duxbury, Henly, and Armstrong for their study, and the Minnesota Satisfaction Questionnaire (MSQ) they used, could help nurse managers identify problems in the organizational climate and reasons for dissatisfaction among nurses. Improving the work environment and decreasing stress on nurses should lead to improved patient care, and better patient outcomes.

Because the NOCDQ-B pinpoints specific areas of risk for nurses, it provides a guide for nurse managers to intervene to improve conditions which could lead to better job performance and increased employee satisfaction. For example, if most of the staff nurses feel that routine duties interfere with the job of praticing nursing, the nurse manager is directed to interventions which modify or decrease routine duties. If responses to the questionnaire indicate that morale is low, the head nurse can explore interventions aimed at improving employee morale.

This study is based on a well-developed concept — organizational climate — that has been supported by earlier investigators in other fields. The underlying theory embraces a set of characteristics of an organization which remain relatively stable, influence the behavior of its members, and distinguish it from other organizations. These characteristics include leadership, communication, and equity, which influence important outcomes, such as job performance and employee satisfaction. By modifying previous tools developed to measure organizational climate to apply to an NICU environment, the investigators may be generating a device which will give nurse managers keys to improving worker job satisfaction and thereby lead to decreased burnout and turnover rates in the nursing staff. This tool, the NOCDQ-B, can guide the nurse managers' decisions on staff nurse work load, personal involvement with staff, amount of paper work and committee service required, level of responsibility given to staff, and, most appropriate, leadership style to use with staff in particular situations.

In their study, the investigators do not test a specific intervention, but rather a measurement tool which could potentially help nurse managers improve the work environment for their staff nurses. They tested the NOCDQ-B and then used the data gathered to modify the tool to increase its reliabilitiy for possible application in practice. The decision to use this tool would rest on the nurse manager with approval by hospital management.

The hospital management evaluating this study would find it clinically relevant. It has the potential to identify nurses who are at risk for burnout and characteristics of the work environment which may be exacerbating nurses' stress. It also points to specific areas for intervention. It is relatively easy to put to use in practice and it may lead to improved patient outcomes. A final attractive advantage of the study is that by reducing employee turnover, costs associated with new employee orientation can be decreased. However, further studies on reliabilitiy and validity of the instrument must be conducted before widespread use is advised.

Part II: Conceptualization and Internal Consistency

In general, I do not feel that the study is well written. The investigators use language that is frequently opaque and unclear.

The investigators draw on previous research as justification for their study. They cite strong supporting evidence from these studies for the problems of concern. They draw study questions from relationships suggested by previous research, as well. This study is an attempt to expand and quantify those relationships. Because the concept they are studying —organizational climate— can be interpreted in a number of ways, the investigators carefully explain their operational definition of the term. Since job satisfaction is a perception of the nurse, it is consistent with the nurse practice questions that the investigators have chosen to test perceptual measures of organizational climate.

While the investigators provide clear justification for their study and consistent use of concepts, there are several areas of concern regarding the way they present their research. The wording of the first research question is unclear; the investigators do not specify what will be done to validate the instrument. Given the effort to sample units with a range of turnover, I would have expected the investigators to see if the tools could distinguish between units of high and low turnover. The reader also should have been given more information on the possible responses to the NOCDQ-B, and the questions and possible responses to the MSQ. Most importantly, the investigators continue to assert that the relationships they are testing exist when their statistical analysis shows that their tool does not have satisfactory reliability and, therefore, may be invalid.

Part III: Believability of Results

This study, which is part of a larger study, purports to describe relationships between organizational climate and worker job satisfaction, and to assess the validity of a measurement tool. Data is primarily quantitative.

The subjects of the study were nurses from 18 NICUs across the United States. Although not specified, the subjects appear to have volunteered—a group comprising 76 percent of staff nurses from those facilities. Unfortunately, this introduces possible selection bias. While the NICUs selected for the larger study were random, this subset was not randomly chosen to include units with a broad range of turnover rates. This makes it a stratified random sample. Since it is the subjects' perceptions which are being tested, they are directly involved with the phenomenon of interest. The investigators do provide rationale for using a stratified random sample, but they do not discuss the sources of ideas just mentioned. In addition, while the investigators comment on the possible bias introduced by having some different nurses complete the NOCDQ-B and the MSQ, they fail to control for potentially significant bias introduced by using a self-report instrument.

On the other hand, the investigators spend a significant amount of time reporting on the reliability of their measurement tool. The initial internal consistency reliability computed for each of the eight scales of the NOCDQ-B was quite low for several of the scales, which led to revision of the instrument. The revised six scales of the NOCDQ-B show higher reliabilities; however, one falls far below the standard accepted reliability of 0.70 at 0.45 and two additional scales fall just below at 0.65 and 0.67. In addition, even the revised scales show very little consensus amoung nurses on each unit regarding organizational climate. Eta-squared values of only 0.08 to 0.24 indicate there is very little consistency among respondents, a serious problem given the conceptualization of the tool. If one is truly measuring original climate rather than characteristics of the individual, there should be higher interrater agreements.

Without reliability, a tool cannot have validity. Since the investigators have not shown reliability, their instrument has questionable validity. Nonetheless, they assert that the validity of the NOCDQ-B comes from its correlations with the MSQ. Since only three of the six scales correlate with the MSQ, the investigators conclude that it is measuring related but different content. But, since the eta-squared values are so low, even partial validity cannot be accepted. In addition, the investigators do not discuss reliability or validity of the MSQ.

The investigators do a fairly good job of subject selection and sampling. They have a large sample size, which is good for collecting descriptive quantitative data. They give an adequate explanation of their data gathering and analysis techniques; however, they do not provide the reader with possible answers to the questionnaires completed by the subjects, or explain clearly how they translated these answers to quantitative statistics.

The investigators do not thoroughly or accurately report their results. They acknowledge that their statistics show that the NOCDQ-B "to a large extent" measures attributes of individuals rather than organizations. This provides strong evidence that the tool is not reliably measuring organizational climate, and yet the investigators still assert that the instrument is satisfactory. Also, there are problems with the method they used to correlate NICU mean scores on the MSQ and NOCDQ-B. Different nurses filled out the MSQ than the NOCDQ-B. Since both turn out to be measures of individual perceptions, having different samples complete them causes concern. This is important informaton because it establishes the relationship between organizational climate and worker job satisfaction, which is the second research question addressed in the study.

In addition, it is difficult to determine if the investigators used statistics appropriately because they do not describe how they derived scores. Assuming they did use appropriate statistical analysis, the statistics fail to show significant relationships. However, the investigators still claim the relationships exist. They maintain that organizational climate is being measured to a small extent, yet agreement among nurses within each unit of only 0.08 to 0.24 are not large enough to establish this.

At this point, the reviewer feels that the flaws pointed out in this study are significant grounds for nonutilization. Because the investigators have found no results that are supported as significant by their statistical analysis, questions of generalizability and replication cannot be addressed. In addition, assessment of the risks and benefits of using the NOCDQ-B in clinical practice cannot be accurately assessed because the instrument's reliability and validity were not adequately substantiated.

In general, this research addresses an important problem in the nursing field, but fails to validate the tools to address the problem. It does draw on a well-established research base, but fails to show that the concept of organizational climate applies in an NICU setting. The investigators do not adequately describe one of the instruments used (the MSQ) for all of their two research questions, so the meaning of the results is entirely unclear. This study fails to show with adequate significance that the instrument is indeed measuring organizational climate or that there is a significant relationship between worker job satisfaction and organizational climate. These deficits in the study are sufficient grounds for nonutilization at this time. Further research as indicated by the investigators is needed.

Original article:
Duxbury, M. L., Henly, G. A., & Armstrong, G. D. (1982). Measurement of the nurse organizational climate of neonatal intensive care units. *Nurse Research*, *31*(2), 83–88.

CRITIQUE BY: MARIE S. BERGER, PhD, RN

Part I: Clinical Relevance

This study investigated nurses' perceptions of the organizational climate of neonatal intensive care units (NICU) in 18 hospitals. Organizational climate is the human environment, the context, within which employees work. It can range on a continuum from favorable to neutral to unfavorable. The climate of an organization can influence employee motivation, job satisfaction, and performance. The investigators cited one element of climate, quality of leadership, as a powerful influence on recruitment and retention of staff. They also noted that nursing staff thought their work meaningful and that it was appreciated by their supervisors.

Assessment of the organizational climate is a necessary step to planning and implementing appropriate changes. Business and industry have been successful in improving employee productivity and morale by changing an unfavorable climate through training and education.

The research reported in this study could be helpful to nurse managers in describing the organizational climates in their units and in pinpointing specific elements of climate requiring attention. High turnover and burnout of intensive care nurses is well documented in the literature. The human and financial cost to nursing departments, in particular, and health care organizations, in general, gives a high priority to research that attempts to address these issues.

Because this was a descriptive study, the investigators tested no intervention. They conducted the study to assess the validity of an adaptation of the Organizational Climate Description Questionnaire for use in hospitals, where few such research studies have been conducted. The results of the reported study are not directly applicable to patient care, but have indirect implications for patient care. An initial assessment of organizational climate establishes baseline data on existing favorable and unfavorable conditions which affect staff performance. Periodic follow-up surveys can then be used to determine how the organizational climate has improved or deteriorated. Such information guides the nurse manager in planning strategies for change. It is well documented in management literature that an unfavorable climate can lead to performance problems, staff burnout, and eventually turnover. All of these conditions adversely affect patient care.

Part II: Conceptualization and Internal Consistency

Although the investigators presented their study in an organized and readable manner, they omitted much critical information regarding methods they used. Without this information, the reader must make a leap of faith to accept the results.

The sample was purposive in that NICUs representing low to high turnover rates were selected from a larger random sample of NICUs reported elsewhere. The crude turnover rate ranged from 0 to 72 percent. The subset sample for this study was disproportionately low turnover units. The investigators state that this was not an extensive over representation, but do not provide data that would allow the reader to make such a judgment. The discussion about high versus low turnover units in the sample is confusing and incomplete, as well. On the one hand, the deliberate over sampling of low turnover units is an appropriate strategy. Given the generally accepted conceptualization of organizational climate, however, one could assume that the climate on low turnover units would be more favorable and that staff would be more satisfied, thus introducing bias. Indeed, the investigators do state that on low turnover units "things were going well." However, they do not explore whether the instrument could predict low–high turnover units, which would seem to be one of the major reasons for ensuring representation from the extreme ends.

The instrument used to assess climate was adapted from the Organizational Climate Description Questionnaire, Form IV (OCDQ), typically used in schools. The original OCDQ is a 64-item instrument which the present investigators reduced to 32 items because of previously reported overlap in various scales of the original instrument. Unfortunately, they failed to report reliability coefficients for the full or shortened version used in previous studies. Therefore, even though they reported reliabilities for the shortened version used in this study, the reader has no information to make comparisons. The investigators also made another adaptation in the working of the items to reflect a health care setting and provided examples. However, because they did not provide examples of the original items, again the reader is left to make the assumption that the changes made did not substantively alter the intent of the instrument.

The second instrument used was the Minnesota Satisfaction Questionnaire (MSQ). The MSQ is a 20-item instrument which provides a global measure of job satisfaction. The investigators provided very little information about the instrument. To allow the reader to ascertain if the predicted relationship between satisfaction and climate was reasonable, the investigators needed to describe the underlying conceptualization of the MSQ. However, the only rationale given for using the MSQ was that it was "an individual's evaluative perceptions of an outcome variable thought to be important as it related to organizational climate." Later, the investigators state that job satisfaction, as measured by the MSQ, is presumed to be relatively stable. Even if one could accept that job satisfaction is a stable attribute, the question would be for how long. The MSQ was given several months after the NOCDQ-A. It is difficult to accept that an individual attribute, such as job satisfaction, could remain stable over such a long period of time. An additional problem in interpreting the results is that those who responded to the MSQ may or may not have been the same people who responded to the NOCDQ-A.

After the investigators found low reliabilities on the NOCDQ-A instrument, they did a factor analysis to determine if a new set of more homogeneous items would emerge. The result was a reformulation of items under a six-factor scale with a shifting of two items to Scale 1 Humanistic/Thrust. Then they did an analysis of variance on the new climate scale (NOCDQ-B) using the individual scores of respondents across all NICUs. Results indicate that indeed the scores varied significantly across the 18 units. The eta-square values ranged from .08 to .24 with a median value of .12, meaning that there are considerable variables among the individuals within each unit with regard to their ratings of organizational climate. Although the units could be differentiated, because of the variation within each unit, it may be concluded that this instrument is an imperfect measure of climate. If it were a good measure, a higher level of consensus among individuals would be present.

Part III: Believability of Results

In general, the sampling and statistical methods employed by the investigators were appropriate, so results can be accepted with certain caveats. The instrument (NOCDQ-B) needs further work before being used to plan management strategies. Essential information is omitted, the first having to do with subjects' participation in the study. The investigators state that subjects were registered nurses employed in 18 NICUs, a subset of a larger randomly selected sample of NICUs throughout the United States, and that from the total of 901 nurses who were employed in these 18 NICUs, 682 of them participated in "part or all" of the study. The investigators do not explain the meaning of "part or all" and we have no way of knowing how the nonparticipants compare with participants.

Second, the investigators provide little information on how the 18 NICUs were selected from the larger sample of NICUs except that the sample was purposive and represented a broad range of turnover rates (09–72 percent crude turnover). They state that there is a "disproportionate number of low turnover units" and go on to say that this "means that this sample is atypical of the general NICU population." Confusion arises when the investigators further state that "In fact, the over-representation of low turnover rates is not extensive" and "it ensures that the obtained findings are generalizable to units with a broad range of turnover rates." Additional information about the rationale for this sampling strategy and the turnover rate of each of the 18 NICUs would have been helpful. Certainly, the desire to assess NICUs with high as well as low turnover rates is acceptable. However, the investigators do not provide the reader with sufficient information on the number of units in each category.

A third problem is that the lack of relationship between the MSQ and the NOCDQ-B makes construct validity questionable.

In conclusion, results of this study do not support use of the NOCDQ-B instrument at this time.

Part IV: Generalizability of Results

This study was an initial effort to test the applicability of an instrument used frequently in business and industry for health care organizations. Results using the adopted instrument were less than encouraging. Therefore, further work should be done before general use in practice can be accepted. The sample was limited to NICU nurses so generalization beyond this group is inappropriate.

In conclusion, this research is appropriate to the practice of nursing administration and provides useful information. However, it should only be considered a first step.

Part V: Other Factors to Consider in Utilization

It is important that research that helps us describe the practice environment of our institutions continues. Organizational climate assessment is one way to do this. There is greater risk in being ignorant about the climate in our institutions than there is in identifying and changing those elements of climate that lead to low morale and productivity. It is incumbent on nurse administrators to create the optimal climate for professional practice. Unlike many of the financially driven changes the nurse administrator faces, changes in climate can be a low cost and highly effective way to reduce turnover in nursing. Continued research in organizational climate is important to changing practice.

Correlations of Two Quality of Nursing Care Measures

Marlene R. Ventura
Associate Chief of Nursing Service (Research)
Veterans Administration Medical Center
Buffalo, NY

Paul T. Hageman
Former Research Associate
Veterans Administration Medical Center
Buffalo, NY

Malcolm J. Slakter
Professor
State University of New York
Buffalo, NY

Richard N. Fox
Doctoral Student
State University of New York
Buffalo, NY

A correlational design was used to examine two process instruments designed to measure the quality of nursing care: the Quality Patient Care Scale (Qual-Pacs) and the Methodology for Monitoring Quality of Nursing Care (Rush-Medicus). Pearson product-moment correlations indicated that the Physical and Psychosocial subscales of the instruments were unrelated; in a replication, the subscales were weakly correlated. The results indicate that these two process instruments measure different dimensions and underscore the idea that quality of nursing care is complex and multidimensional.

Measuring the quality of nursing care is essential for nursing practice. However, because of the complexity of this aspect of nursing, quality of care is difficult to define and measure appropriately.

As we learn more about quality nursing care, and as the concept becomes more complex, the criteria by which it is evaluated will become more stringent and demanding. Therefore, we need a comprehensive definition of quality and a valid and reliable method of measurement.

There have been many attempts to define quality nursing care. In the early 1930's, Eldredge (1932) attempted to define "quality nursing." Lindeman (1975) considered the determination of valid and reliable indicators of quality of nursing care the first priority for investigating nursing impact on patient welfare. On this basis, the measurement of quality of care was established as the priority for targeted research efforts of the Western Interstate Commission of Higher Education (WICHE) Regional Program for Nursing Research Development (Krueger, Nelson, & Wolanin, 1978).

Donabedian (Note 1) reviewed literature on quality assessment and assurance and made recommendations for further research in assessing and monitoring the quality of medical care. Although his work almost exclusively dealt with the services of physicians, nurses have attempted to identify and define quality of nursing care. The results include a multiplicity of approaches to quality assessment, i.e., structure, process, outcome, and concurrent or retrospective process-outcome-type approaches. Various methodologies measuring the quality of nursing care

(Haussmann, Hegyvary, & Newman, 1976; Horn & Swain, 1977; Phaneuf, 1976; Wandelt & Ager, 1974) are currently available. These methodologies differ in conceptual frameworks, implied definitions of quality, and methods of data collection. The existence of such variation among methodologies poses problems for the investigator involved in conducting evaluation research where quality is a criterion measure.

Wandelt and Ager (1974) identified the need for a validation study between the Quality Patient Care Scale (QualPacs) and the Phaneuf Nursing Audit (Phaneuf, 1976). They stated: "It seems that such a test for validity is most likely one with the tools currently available for measuring the quality of care received by patients" (Wandelt & Ager, 1974, p. 68). The need for such a study preceded the availability of the Rush-Medicus Methodology for Monitoring Quality of Nursing Care (Haussmann, et al., 1976).

Although we do not know of any validational studies between the QualPacs and the Rush-Medicus tool, a review of the literature revealed one study in which the QualPacs scores were correlated with the scores obtained from another quality of nursing care instrument. Dyer, Monson, and Cope (1975), in a study examining the interrelation among written goal-setting approaches, performance counseling, and the quality of patient care, correlated the scores obtained from the QualPacs and from the Veterans Administration Nursing Care Quality Evaluation Form (Veterans Administration, Note 2). On three occasions, using the Pearson r statistic, the correlations between the total scale scores for these two instruments were reported as .25, .42, and .54, respectively; these were significant at the .05 level. In an earlier study, Linn, Linn, Greenwald, and Gurel (1974) found a low correlation between the ratings of patient status derived from chart review and those made by direct care providers.

The present study was part of a larger research effort (Ventura & Hageman, Note 3), which included examination of the linkages of nursing process measures to outcome measures. In this study, the investigators examined the relationship between two existing instruments designed to measure the quality of the nursing care, the QualPacs and the Rush-Medicus tool. These instruments were selected because of their widespread use in nursing evaluation and research, and because both instruments used a concurrent process approach to evaluate the quality of nursing care.

METHOD

Sample

The setting for the study was an 872-bed hospital. Two hundred and seventy-three patients, admitted to either of two 36-bed surgical care units, were included in the data collection. In the larger study (Ventura & Hageman, Note 3) examined patient outcomes pertaining to selected surgery and to medications. Approximately 25% of the subjects in the present data analysis were selected because they participated in a preoperative teaching program and 22% participated in a medication teaching program. The remaining 53% were selected because of their availability.

Instruments

The QualPacs is an instrument consisting of 68 items designed to measure the quality of nursing care received by a patient or a family on behalf of the patient. These items are arranged according to the following six subsections: (a) Psychosocial individual (15 items), (b) Psychosocial Group (8 items), (c) Physical (15 items), (d) General (15 items), (e) Communication (8 items), and (f) Professional Implications (7 items). A set of cues are available which present concrete illustrations of the items. According to Wandelt and Ager (1974), the QualPacs measures the quality of nursing care received by a patient in any setting where nurse-patient interactions occur. Measurements are made on all nursing care a patient receives, regardless of the qualifications of the personnel providing the care. The standard of measurement is "care expected of a first-level staff nurse," i.e., safe, adequate, and therapeutic care. The standard of measurement is held constant for all ratings made with the scale. Care is rated on a five-point scale with 5 = best care, 3 = average care, 1 = poorest care, and 4 and 2 are unspecified.

The Rush-Medicus instrument consists of 257 items applicable to medical, surgical, and pediatric units, as well as to normal newborn nurseries and recovery rooms. There are 205 patient specific items; the remaining 52 items are unit specific. For this study, the items for Nursery/Recovery Room Patient and Nursery/Recovery Room Unit were removed and 207 items remained.

The items are grouped into homogenous clusters to define these six nursing objectives: (a) Plan of Care Is Formulated (30 items), (b) Physical Needs Are Attended (69 items), (c) Nonphysical Needs Are Attended (46 items), (d) Achievement of Objectives Is Evaluated (11 items), (e) Unit Procedures Are Followed for the Protection of All Patients (8 items), and (f) Delivery of Nursing Care Is Facilitated by Administrative and Managerial Services (43 items). These six objectives are further delineated into 28 subobjectives. Each individual subobjective can be considered an independent characteristic for which a performance measure can be obtained. Patients are classified as types I, II, III, or IV, according to their level of self-sufficiency. Each item used in the methodology is coded according to the type of patient to which it is most applicable.

To keep the actual quality-monitoring process manageable, not all items were used in evaluating the nursing process with regard to a single patient and unit setting. Instead, the master item list was placed in a computer file by the developers of the instrument. From this file, subsets of 30 to 50 items, depending on patient type, had been selected systematically and grouped into observation worksheets (Hegyvary & Haussmann, 1975).

The instrument package includes a computer program which produces scores for the objectives and subobjectives. According to the orientation manual prepared by the Medicus Corporation (Note 4), the score for each subobjective is the average of the scores within the subobjective. The scores for the major objectives are the average values of the subobjective scores within a given objective. The computer program was designed by the test developers to produce scores on a unit basis and was adapted by Veterans Administration project personnel to produce scores on a patient basis.

Procedure

Eight registered nurses were recruited from outside the agency to serve as nonparticipant observers. They were selected because of their level of educational preparation and the amount and recency of their nursing experience. The nurses were assigned randomly for training as observers for either the QualPacs or the Rush-Medicus instrument. The training program and method of determining interrater reliability are reported elsewhere (Ventura, Hageman, Slakter, & Fox, 1980).

Data were collected in two time periods. Period 1 lasted 3 months; period 2 lasted 6 months. Using the QualPacs, two patients were observed simultaneously. Approximately 4 hours were allotted for the observation. This included 1 hour for chart review and development of care plan, 2 hours for direct observation of care, and 1 hour for retrospective rating. For the Rush-Medicus instrument, two patients were interviewed within the same specific 2-hour time frame. This included time for direct observation, patient and staff interview, as well as review of the chart. Both procedures were carried out as outlined by the respective developers of the instruments.

Interrater reliability was determined before Period 1 and Period 2. The average intraclass correlation coefficients (ICC) across the two pairs of raters for the Rush-Medicus Physical and Nonphysical subscales were .84 and .88 in Period 1 and .93 and .94 in Period 2. For the QualPacs in Period 1, the ICC value for the Physical subscale was .38; for the Psychosocial Individual subscale, .54; and for the Psychosocial Group subscale, .24. The second period values were .33, .69, and .68, respectively.

The nature of the two instruments did not allow us to obtain data simultaneously on the same patient. It was also felt that the simultaneous use of both instruments would interfere with normal nursing care delivery. The next option considered was to collect patient data using one of the instruments in the morning and the other in the evening. However, other investigators, using the QualPacs, reported differences in total scores between the day and evening shifts (Taylor & Serafin, Note 5). Therefore, in this study, the care received by each patient was observed by different nurse observers at the same time of day on successive days. Data on each patient were collected by alternating the use of the instruments. In 58% of the observations, the QualPacs was completed first; the Rush-Medicus instrument preceded in the remaining observations (42%).

To perform correlational analysis, two subscales of the QualPacs, (Psychosocial: Individual and Psychosocial: Group) were averaged together to yield a single score considered equivalent to the Rush-Medicus subscale titled Nonphysical Needs Are Attended. Both instruments had subscales measuring the category of Physical Needs.

RESULTS

The Pearson product-moment correlations between the Physical and Nonphysical subscales for the two instruments for the 3- and 6-month periods are presented in Table 1. The correlations for data collected in the 3-month period ($n = 96$) are not significantly different from zero at the .05 level. In the 6-month period ($n = 177$), the correlations are significantly different from zero, but are nearly negligible in magnitude.

To provide an explanation for the low correlations, a content analysis of the instruments was conducted to identify differences in the definition of quality of nursing care. For example, the QualPacs was developed in an educational setting and is designed to measure nursing staff-patient interactions. The Rush-Medicus instrument was developed by operations researchers and is designed to examine the overall delivery of nursing care as a system, i.e., examination of the structure of the system including equipment availability, as well as examination of process and staff-patient interactions. The time frames for data collection are also different. The QualPacs measures primarily, but not exclusively, interactions that occur during the two-hour direct observation period; the Rush-Medicus instrument measures the care process over a more extended time, i.e., at the time of admission, in the past 24 to 48 hours, in the last 5 or 7 days, or at the time of the observation.

Both the Rush-Medicus instrument and the QualPacs use specific questions or statements to measure the quality of nursing care. With the Rush-Medicus instrument, observers interview nurses and patients separately. Nurses are asked procedural questions, i.e., "If the patient depends on prosthetic devices for activities or daily living, is this recorded within the first 24 hours of admission to this unit?" and "Is bowel function recorded daily?" Patients respond to questions about the nursing care they received, i.e., "In the past two days, did you usually receive pain medication promptly after you asked for it?" and "For the past two nights, have you been able to sleep or rest without interruptions for at least several hours?" The observer reviews the patient's care for the previous 5 days or for the length of time the patient remained on the unit, if it was less than 5 days.

These staff and patient interviews are not required for the QualPacs. With this instrument, the indicators of quality are observed directly. Observers record their impressions of the nursing care to times listed on the QualPacs. These items include: "Action is taken to meet the patient's needs for adequate hydration and elimination;" "Environment is maintained that gives the patient a feeling of being safe and secure;" and "Expectations of patient's behavior are adjusted and acted

Table 1
Correlations Between Physical and Psychosocial Subscales of the QualPacs and the Rush-Medicus Instruments

Subscales	3-month period ($n = 96$)	6-month period ($n = 177$)
Physical	−.02	−.15*
Psychosocial°	.07	.19*

°For the QualPacs, includes average of Psychosocial: Group and Psychosocial: Individual.
*$p < .05$.

Table 2
Percentage Distribution of Items by Method of Data Collection for QualPacs

Subscales	No. of items	Direct observation	Direct/indirect observation	Indirect observation
Psychosocial (group & individual)	23	78.3	21.7	0.0
Physical	15	60.0	40.0	0.0
General	15	73.3	26.7	0.0
Communication	8	25.0	50.0	25.0
Professional implications	7	14.3	85.7	0.0

upon according to the effect the medication has on the patient."

The lack of correlation between the instruments could also be accounted for by variations in the methods used to collect data. The QualPacs relies heavily on direct observation of staff and patient interactions while the Rush-Medicus instrument relies more on document review and patient or staff interview. Analysis of the distribution of items by method of data collection illustrates the differences between the two instruments. In Table 2, the percentage distribution of items by data collection method for the QualPacs instrument is shown. For the Psychosocial area (Individual and Group categories) approximately three-fourths (78%) of the items are rated by direct observation and those remaining (22%) by direct/indirect observation. For the Physical domain, a little less than two-thirds (60%) of the items are by direct observation.

The percentage distribution of items by method of data collection for the Rush-Medicus instrument is listed in Table 3. For the Psychosocial area (Nonphysical Needs category), slightly less than three-fourths (72%) of the items are rated by patient interview. This is followed by interview of nursing personnel, review of record, observation of nursing personnel, and observer inference. For the Physical Needs area, data can be collected by all seven methods. One-fourth of the items (25%) can be rated by patient interview and approximately another one-fourth (22%) by patient observation. The remaining items are rated by review of patient record, observation of patient environment, interview of nursing personnel, observation of nursing personnel, and observer inference.

Other basic differences exist in the measurement techniques used for the two instruments. For instance, the Rush-Medicus items are not held constant for use with all patients. Since patients are separated by identified nursing needs into one of four different classifications with five worksheets for each, an individual patient could be evaluated on any one of twenty different worksheets, each containing a distinct set of items. In contrast, the QualPacs instrument contains 68 items which remain constant, regardless of the patient's classification, even though selected items may be rated as Not Observed or Not Applicable.

All these factors, as well as the achievement of only moderately acceptable levels of interrater reliability (Ventura et al., 1980), undoubtedly contributed to the lack of correlation found between these two instruments. Immediately preceding the 6-month period of data collection, the interrater reliabilities were somewhat higher than for the period immediately before the 3-month period (Ventura et al., 1980). Increased observer standardization possibly contributed to the statistical significance of the correlations for the 6-month period. However, since both nonchance correlations are small, and the one between the Physical

Table 3
Percentage Distribution of Items by Method of Data Collection for the Rush-Medicus Instrument

		\multicolumn{3}{c}{Patient}	\multicolumn{2}{c}{Nursing personnel}		
Objectives	No. of items	Record	Observation	Interview	Interview	Observation	Environment Observation	Observer inference
Planning	30	90.0	0.0	0.0	6.7	0.0	0.0	3.3
Physical needs	69	18.8	21.7	24.6	11.6	2.9	18.8	1.5
Nonphysical needs	46	8.7	0.0	71.7	10.9	6.5	0.0	2.2
Evaluation	11	100.0	0.0	0.0	0.0	0.0	0.0	0.0
Unit procedures	8	12.5	0.0	0.0	37.5	37.5	12.5	0.0
Management services	43	18.6	0.0	2.3	51.2	0.0	20.9	7.0

subscales is negative, the low agreement of the scales cannot be caused totally by rater error.

DISCUSSION

The results of this research indicate that there is no relationship between these two instruments. The construct of quality is multidimensional and measures of the same underlying dimension would be expected to show substantial correlations. The negligible correlations between the QualPacs and Rush-Medicus instruments reported here strongly suggest that they may not be measuring the same dimensions of nursing care pertaining to quality. In addition, each uses different methods of data collection. Individuals conducting research using these instruments as measures of quality of care should be aware that they could obtain different findings depending on which instrument is selected. Investigations should evaluate the conceptual and operational definitions of the instruments currently available to assess nursing care quality. Since there are similarities and differences among the approaches of the various instruments, a choice should be made that most closely matches the measures with the specific objectives of the investigative effort.

The correlational design used in the study controlled for variables, such as patient and time of day. However, the provider of nursing care and exact time of measurement were not controlled and may constitute study limitations. These uncontrolled variables would tend to lower the correlations. Replication of this correlational design using tandem observations is needed. Such an approach should control for the variation of care providers and time difference between measurements.

Observers were trained to use one instrument or the other, but not both. Replication using a design with individual observers trained to use both instruments should be considered. Replication using a crossed design should be considered also. Future replications might develop estimates of the relative amounts of variance in nursing care quality measures attributable to the patient, provider of nursing care, nonparticipant observers, and method of data collection.

REFERENCE NOTES

1. Donabedian, A. (1978, February 28). Proposals for research in assessment and monitoring of the quality and utilization of medical care. In Information Letter 15-78-2 *Solicitation of proposals dealing with research issues in evaluation of quality or utilization of care.* Washington, DC: Veterans Administration, Department of Medicine and Surgery, Research and Development.

2. Veterans Administration. (1969). *Nursing care quality evaluation* (VA form 10-204663 NR). Washington, DC: Author.
3. Ventura, M., & Hageman, P. (1978). *Testing for the reliability, validity, and sensitivity of quality of nursing care measures* (Final Report, HSR&D 264). Washington, DC: Health Services Research and Development Service, Veterans Administration.
4. Medicus Corporation. (1977). *Orientation manual for observers: Nursing quality monitoring methodology.* Unpublished manual. (Available from Medicus Corporation, 500 S. Racine Avenue, Chicago, Ill. 60680.)
5. Taylor, D., & Serafin, B. (1977). Systematized patient-family data: An educational approach (Final Report: Special Projects Training Grant 5D10-NU-01028). Bethesda, MD: U.S. Department of Health, Education and Welfare.

REFERENCES

Dyer, E., Monson, M., & Cope, M. (1975). Increasing the quality of patient care through performance counseling and written goal setting. *Nursing Research, 24,* 138–144.

Eldredge, A. (1932). What is quality nursing? *American Journal of Nursing, 32,* 1189–1196.

Haussmann, R., Hegyvary, S., & Newman, J. (1976). *Monitoring quality of nursing care: Part II, Assessment and study of correlates* (DHEW publication HRA 76-7). Washington, DC: U.S. Government Printing Office.

Hegyvary, S. T., & Haussmann, R. K. (1975). Monitoring nursing care quality. *Journal of Nursing Administration, 5(5),* 17–26.

Horn, B., & Swain, M. (1977, February). *Development of criterion measures of nursing care* (2 vols.). Ann Arbor: University of Michigan Department of Hospital Administration, School of Public Health. (NTIS No. PB 267 004 and 267 005.)

Krueger, J., Nelson, A., & Wolanin, M. (1978). *Nursing research: Development, collaboration and utilization.* Germantown, MA: Aspen System.

Lindeman, C. (1975). Delphi survey of priorities in clinical nursing research. *Nursing Research, 24,* 434–441.

Linn, B., Linn, M., Greenwald, S., & Gurel, P. (1974). Validity of impaired ratings made from medical records and from personal knowledge. *Medical Care, 12,* 363–368.

Phaneuf, M. (1976). *The nursing audit: Self-regulation in nursing practice* (2nd ed.). New York: Appleton-Century-Crofts.

Ventura, M., Hageman, P., Slakter, M., & Fox, R. (1980). Interrater reliabilities for two measures of nursing care quality. *Research in Nursing and Health, 3,* 25–32.

Wandelt, M., & Ager, J. (1974). *Quality patient care scale.* New York: Appleton-Century-Crofts.

This article is printed with permission of *Research in Nusing and Health.*
Copyright © 1982 John Wiley & Sons.